Trounce's Clinical Pharmacology for Nurses and Allied Health Professionals

Trounce's Clinical Pharmacology for Nurses and Allied Health Professionals

Nineteenth Edition

RUMA ANAND, MBBS, BSC(HONS), MRCGP, DRCOG

General Practitioner, Maidenhead, UK
GP appraiser, NHS England

STEPHEN DEWILDE, MBBS, BSC(HONS), DRCOG, MD, FRCGP

General Practitioner, London, UK
Senior Lecturer, Public Health Research Institute, St George's, University of London, UK

CLIVE P. PAGE, OBE, BSC, PHD

Director, Sackler Institute of Pulmonary Pharmacology and Professor of Pharmacology, Institute of Pharmaceutical Science, King's College London, London, UK

Nursing Advisors

RUTH PATERSON, PHD, MPHIL, FHEA, RN, V300 Prescriber

Associate Professor
School of Health and Social Care, Edinburgh Napier University, Edinburgh, Scotland, UK

MICHELE GARDNER, DIP AP SCI, BA Nursing

Registered Nurse RGN
Flinders University of South Australia, Adelaide, Australia

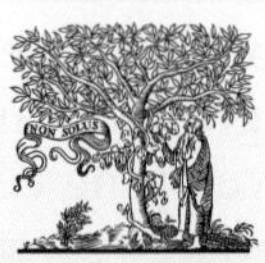

ELSEVIER London New York Oxford Philadelphia St Louis Sydney Toronto 2022

Notice

Practitioners and researchers must always rely on their own experience and knowledge in evaluating and using any information, methods, compounds or experiments described herein. Because of rapid advances in the medical sciences, in particular, independent verification of diagnoses and drug dosages should be made. To the fullest extent of the law, no responsibility is assumed by Elsevier, authors, editors or contributors for any injury and/or damage to persons or property as a matter of products liability, negligence or otherwise, or from any use or operation of any methods, products, instructions, or ideas contained in the material herein.

ISBN: 978-0-7020-6705-1
International ISBN: 978-0-7020-6704-4
e-ISBN: 978-0-7020-6722-8

Printed in Poland

Last digit is the print number: 9 8 7 6 5 4 3 2 1

Content Strategist: Poppy Garraway
Content Development Specialist: Veronika Watkins
Project Manager: Joanna Souch
Designer: Patrick Ferguson
Illustration Manager: Teresa McBryan

CONTENTS

CONTRIBUTORS

DHEERAJ THAPAR, VRACH, MRCPSYCH

CCT in Forensic and Learning Disability Psychiatry,
Bank doctor, London, UK

Chapter 20 Nervous system 2: opioid analgesics
Chapter 22 Drugs used in psychiatric disorders: antipsychotics, antidepressants, anxiolytics, hypnotics and anti-dementia drugs
Chapter 23 Drug dependence and drug abuse

1 THE USE OF PHARMACEUTICALS

CHAPTER OUTLINE

LEARNING OBJECTIVES

At the end of this chapter, the reader should be able to:

- describe the factors that dictate the choice of dose
- list the various routes of drug administration
- list the factors that affect absorption and distribution of drugs in the body
- discuss the consequences of metabolism and excretion on drug efficacy and duration
- define the terms agonist, antagonist, partial agonist and ligand
- describe the cellular sites of drug action
- explain the basic properties of the dose–response curve

DRUG DEVELOPMENT

The science of pharmacology is the discovery and characterization of chemicals to the point where they can be used to treat or prevent illness (e.g. aspirin to treat pain or inhibit platelet aggregation). Drugs are also designed to intervene in the normal functions of the body (e.g. contraceptives).

Medicinally useful drugs can be discovered quite by accident, as was the case with penicillin and the oral sulphonylureas for the treatment of adult-onset (type 2) diabetes (see Chapter 16). More usually, however, a deliberate attempt is made to introduce a new drug by modifying an existing natural or synthetic substance to increase its performance, i.e. increase its potency, modify the duration of action, improve its absorption, change the route of administration or to minimize unwanted effects. For example, modifying the chemical structure of the hormone adrenaline (epinephrine) has led to the discovery of beta blockers (for the treatment of a variety of conditions, see Chapters 5 and 6) and β_2 agonists (for the treatment of asthma, see Chapter 9).

Advances in the understanding of physiological processes can also result in new drugs. The discovery that Parkinson's disease results from the selective destruction of certain dopaminergic nerve pathways in the brain led to the invention of the drug levodopa to try to counteract some of the symptoms of the disease, such as tremor, slowness of movement and rigidity (see Chapter 21). The discovery of the physiological role of the peptide tumour necrosis factor-alpha (TNF-α) in the human immune system led to the use of the very potent and effective anti-TNF-α drugs for the treatment of rheumatoid arthritis (see Chapter 13).

In some cases, pharmaceutical researchers will search for novel natural molecules and then examine large numbers of these to identify their pharmaceutical properties in an effort to find uses for them. This approach has been much used in the search for new antibiotics. The antifungal agent nystatin was first discovered by this method in 1950, in bacteria growing in a soil sample in **N**ew **Y**ork **Stat**e – from which comes the name.

Drug discovery is time consuming and expensive. Most promising drugs never make it to the market, failing at some point in the testing stage. In 2018, it was estimated that only 13.8% of promising new drugs make it from Phase I trials to approval and marketing. This is an improvement on past performance, but many compounds are tested and never even make it to Phase I trials (see later). Given this, it is not surprising that new drugs are often very expensive when first introduced. Pharmaceutical companies only have a limited time to recoup their costs before the patent on a new drug expires and generic manufacturers can produce it at much lower cost. In the UK, a drug patent lasts for 20 years, but often it will take 10 years or more for a patented drug to make it to market. In 2019, the average cost of bringing a new drug to market was estimated at US$2.6 billion. Although 'Big Pharma' is often criticized for the cost of new drugs, this criticism is not always justified.

BASIC PHARMACOKINETICS

Pharmacokinetics is about how the body deals with drugs: What are the factors that determine the maintenance of a therapeutically useful level of the drug in the body? For any new drug, the following pharmacokinetic principles must be investigated:

- **The dose:** How much of the drug should be used to get the desired effect while minimizing unwanted effects?
- **Route of administration:** By what route should the drug be administered?
- **Absorption and distribution:** How is the drug absorbed and compartmentalized in the body, e.g. does most of it dissolve in the aqueous (water) or in the lipid (fatty) components? How is it carried in the blood? Is it concentrated in any particular organ? For example, when iodine is administered, most of it is concentrated in the thyroid gland.
- **Metabolism and excretion:** How long does the drug stay in the body? The body's way of dealing with drugs is to try and remove them as soon as possible through metabolism and excretion. The effects of altered physiology, as in pregnancy, childhood or old age should also be considered, as should possible excretion in breast milk.

CLINICAL NOTE

By investigating the principles of pharmacokinetics (absorption, distribution, metabolism and excretion) the dose, frequency and route will be determined. The aim is to achieve maximum therapeutic effect while minimizing side-effects. The route of administration will be determined by the pharmacokinetic properties of the drug. For example, glyceryl trinitrate is given sublingually because when given orally, the drug is 100% metabolized by the liver rendering it inactive. The sublingual route avoids metabolism by the liver allowing the drug to be distributed directly into the systemic circulation.

The Dose

Pharmacology and therapeutics are how we optimize dosing of a drug to achieve a desired beneficial effect

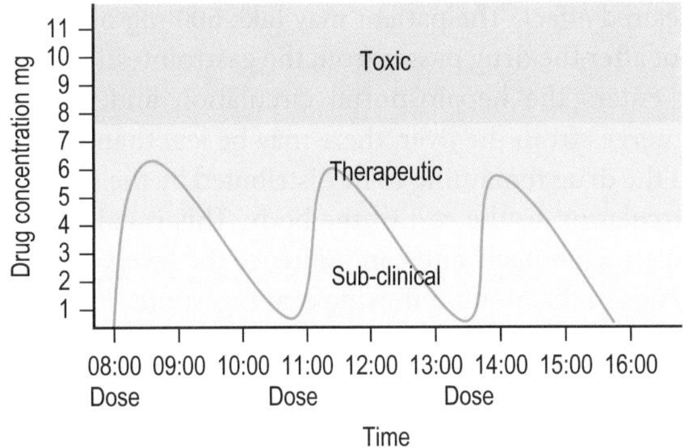

Fig. 1.1 ■ The relationship between dose frequency and therapeutic effect of a drug. (This drug has a short half-life and a moderate Therapeutic Index.)

while minimizing side-effects. This is called the 'therapeutic window'. Ideally, we want to obtain a therapeutic effect with no side-effects, but this is rare, as all drugs have the potential to cause unwanted adverse effects.

The Therapeutic Index

The Therapeutic Index (Fig. 1.1) is a measure of the difference between the dose of the drug producing a desirable effect and the dose producing unwanted effects. There is no absolute value for the Therapeutic Index, but the greater it is, the safer the drug is. However, sometimes a low Therapeutic Index is accepted if the drug is used to treat a dangerous or life-limiting condition. Important drugs such as gentamicin, aminophylline, lithium, digoxin and warfarin have a low Therapeutic Index.

Choosing and Adjusting the Dose

In a perfect world, all adults would respond equally to a given dose. In practice, however, there may be considerable interpersonal variation in plasma concentrations of a given dose of a drug. When the Therapeutic Index is low, this often demands regular plasma monitoring of the drug and dose adjustment as needed. Some commonly used drugs that usually require close monitoring include:

- ciclosporin, used for suppressing transplant rejection and for rheumatoid arthritis
- digoxin for treatment of cardiac disease

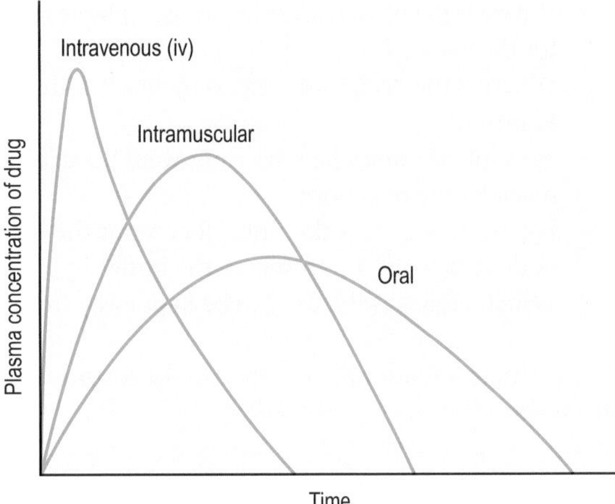

Fig. 1.2 ■ Effects of the route of administration of a single dose of a drug on its plasma levels with time.

- warfarin for anticoagulation therapy
- gentamicin and other aminoglycoside antibiotics
- lithium for treatment of bipolar disorder
- methotrexate for treatment of rheumatoid arthritis and cancer
- phenytoin for treatment of epilepsy.

CLINICAL NOTE

There will be local guidelines and protocols in place to guide the frequency and type of therapeutic drug monitoring. Careful planning with patients about timing and frequency of monitoring is vital. Dosing will be determined by the plasma concentration in the blood and the dose will vary from patient to patient. While drug levels may be low due to the patient not taking the medicines as prescribed, how an individual absorbs, distributes, metabolizes and excretes a drug will vary. Practitioners should familiarize themselves with populations and drug–drug interactions that may affect therapeutic index. Any unexpected low or high levels should be highlighted and clinical notes and drug history reviewed and discussed with the patient and interprofessional team to establish possible reasons. Possible reasons will be discussed later in the chapter.

Route of Administration

When considering the route of administration, several questions need to be addressed (Fig. 1.2):

- Which is the most convenient or acceptable route for the patient?
- Where is the drug to act, e.g. skin, heart, kidneys, brain, etc?
- How quickly does the prescriber want the drug to reach its site of action?
- For how long does the prescriber want the dose of drug to work, i.e. to stay in the body?
- Which organs is the drug to be kept away from?

The route of administration can have profound effects on:

- the onset of the action of the drug
- the plasma concentrations achieved
- the length of time that the drug will remain in the body.

Terminology

Before describing routes of administration, it is important to understand the related terminology:

- Internal and external environments
- Bioavailability
- Specific routes of drug administration.

Internal and External Environments. Physiologists talk about the internal and external environments of the body. When a drug is swallowed, it remains in the specialized external environment of the gastrointestinal tract until it, or one of its breakdown products, passes across the wall of the gastrointestinal tract to enter the bloodstream where it can the circulate within the body. A cherry pip, if swallowed, may be inside the gastrointestinal tract for a while, but normally will never get into the internal environment of the body and is excreted unchanged in faeces. This is also true of some drugs, such as osmotic laxatives like macrogols (see Chapter 10), which act only in the external environment of the gastrointestinal tract.

Bioavailability. Another important concept is that of bioavailability. The term 'bioavailability' generally means that the drug has reached the circulation and is therefore available to all the tissues to exert the desired effect. The patient may take 600 mg of a drug, but after the drug passes from the gastrointestinal tract it enters the hepato-portal circulation and, once it emerges from the liver, there may be less than 600 mg of the drug remaining to be distributed by the systemic circulation to the rest of the body. This is called 'first pass metabolism' and can influence the levels of many drugs in the blood following oral ingestion.

CLINICAL NOTE

Bioavailability is expressed as a proportion of 1 or as a percentage (%). Drugs given by the intravenous, sublingual or rectal route have a bioavailability of 1 or 100% because the drug enters the systemic circulation direct, avoiding first pass metabolism, and all the drug is available for distribution. A drug with low bioavailability will have a low percentage of the drug available following first pass metabolism. This helps us to understand differences in oral and intravenous drug dosing. For example: when giving 10 mg intravenous atenolol, an equivalent oral dose is 100 mg. This is because when the drug is given orally, 90% is metabolized by the liver rendering only 10% available for distribution. Thus, bioavailability of the drug is 0.1 or 10%.

Specific Routes of Drug Administration

The various routes of administration are as follows:

- oral
- topical
  - transdermal
  - rectal and vaginal
  - inhalation and intranasal
- injection (parenteral)
  - intravenous
  - intramuscular
  - intradermal
  - subcutaneous
  - intrathecal.

Oral Drugs

The medication is taken by mouth and preparations comprise:

- tablet
- capsule
- powder
- mixture
- emulsion
- linctus.

Tablets and Capsules. Tablets are prepared by mixing a drug with a base that binds the two together so that the tablets will not disintegrate in the body before they are meant to. They are usually coated and may be coloured. Capsules are made of gelatine or a similar substance and contain a drug that is liberated when the wall of the capsule is digested in the stomach or intestine. Be aware of cultural and religious issues: gelatine is often made of pork and is not kosher or halal and may not be acceptable to vegetarians. The actual formulation of tablets and capsules is very important and determines how satisfactorily the drug is released, which governs their absorption and bioavailability. A great deal of care is taken in the manufacture of tablets to ensure the maximum bioavailability. It is also possible, by coating the tablets, modifying the capsule or by binding the drug to some inert substance, to slow down the release of the active ingredient and thus prolong its absorption and effect. These may be called sustained-release, modified release or retard preparations.

Liquids. Mixtures are liquids that contain several ingredients dissolved or diffused in water or some other solvent. An example is kaolin mixture for diarrhoea, when insoluble kaolin powder is suspended in the aqueous liquid. An emulsion is a mixture of two immiscible liquids (e.g. oil and water) in which one is dispersed through the other in a finely divided state, e.g. milk of magnesia. A linctus is a liquid that contains a sweet syrupy substance used for its soothing effect on coughs. It may also contain a cough suppressant such as dextromethorphan.

When liquid drugs are prescribed, manufacturer's information and correct measuring syringes or spoons should be used. Liquid medications are often prescribed for children, and it is important that the parents/carers are involved in the prescribing process and understand the mechanism of actions and potential side-effects.

Advantages of Oral Administration.

- *Oral administration of drugs is extremely convenient for the patient.* The drug can be taken at home and does not need the attendance of a carer or health professional unless the patient is physically or mentally incapable of self-medication.
- Oral administration avoids the fear of needles.
- The gastrointestinal tract provides a huge surface area for absorption and drugs are pumped from the gastrointestinal tract lumen into the gastric mucosa against concentration gradients (see later).

Disadvantages of Oral Administration.

- *Absorption can be variable* and depends on the chemical nature of the drug, e.g. its ionization, solubility and stability.
- *Absorption can also depend on the stomach contents.* For example, the absorption of some tetracycline antibiotics from the gastrointestinal tract is inhibited in the presence of milk. If a drug is taken with or after a meal, it is absorbed more slowly. This is due to delayed emptying of the stomach, where little absorption occurs, and because certain drugs become temporarily bound to food. When a rapid effect is required, the drug should be given on an empty stomach. Some medications may irritate the stomach, and should be given with food.
- *Rate of gastric emptying and drug interactions.* Drugs may affect gastric emptying (emptying of the stomach) and this may modify absorption. For instance, atropine-like drugs delay gastric emptying, whereas metoclopramide, which is often used for nausea, increases the speed of gastric emptying and thus the rate of absorption. Although patients are often concerned that drugs may not work if taken together, this is very rarely a problem in practice.
- *All drugs that are taken by mouth will undergo first pass metabolism*, which will reduce the final bioavailability, i.e. plasma level. This means that the dose of drug must be increased to take first pass metabolism in the liver into account. Some

drugs that are completely inactivated during first pass metabolism, e.g. glyceryl trinitrate, which is used to treat anginal pain, are nevertheless put in the mouth and placed under the tongue (sublingual) or in the buccal cavity, where they are rapidly absorbed from the oral mucosa, thus bypassing the liver. This route of administration also has the advantage or producing a rapid onset of action.

NURSING NOTE

If your patient self-administers glyceryl trinitrate (GTN) tablets, it is important that the drug is not swallowed, rather the spray is directed under the tongue and the tablet is placed in the buccal cavity.

- The patient has to remember to take the drug, and this could be extremely important, for example when oral anticoagulant drug or antibiotics are prescribed. Confused patients may not remember to take the drugs or may mix up the doses of the different drugs they take. Optimizing adherence will be discussed more fully in Chapter 2 and physical aids such as dosette boxes may be used

Topical

Dermal. The skin is the most accessible part of the body for the administration of drugs. Most of the preparations for topical administration to the skin are used for treating skin disorders. There is a huge range of non-pharmaceutical topical products for cosmetic or recreational use and these will not be described in any detail here, except when their use results in the need for treatment. Skin preparations are formulated mainly into lotions, creams, ointments, foams and powders and are used for a wide variety of purposes, e.g. for the symptomatic relief of an itch or to treat fungal infections such as athlete's foot. They are convenient for the patient, who can use them at home, and, because the drug is generally poorly absorbed, this makes them relatively safe. The one tissue most at risk from the use of these preparations is the skin itself, and caution should be taken to ensure there are no side-effects and long-term use should be monitored.

Transdermal. Transdermal administration involves putting an adhesive patch against the skin, similar to an adhesive plaster. The patch has a pad impregnated with the drug. The drug is absorbed through the skin into the bloodstream. This avoids first pass metabolism. Absorption is slow and so patches are not used if rapid onset of drug action is required. Patches are used, for example to administer nicotine, to help wean smokers off cigarettes. They are useful for long-term administration of hormones for contraceptive use, as well as hormone replacement therapy (HRT) in peri-menopausal and menopausal women. Opiates such as fentanyl and buprenorphine are available as self-adhesive patches for the treatment of chronic pain and some formulations may only need to be replaced once a week.

CLINICAL NOTE

Skin irritation is one of the most common side-effects reported when using transdermal patches. To reduce this side-effect, patches are applied to clean, unbroken skin on the trunk or arms, or on the postauricular area (behind the ears). The patch should labelled with the date and time it was applied and checked daily. Some report the use of low dose topical corticosteroids may also reduce irritation (Paudel et al., 2010).

Advantages.

- Long-acting, therefore replacement can be infrequent.
- Consistent symptom relief over long periods.
- Eliminates the need to remember to take a dose.

Disadvantages.

- Absorption may be variable.
- Possible adverse skin reactions.

Rectal and Vaginal. Drugs can be administered rectally in suppositories and are absorbed into the bloodstream. This, too, bypasses the liver and may be helpful when vomiting prevents oral absorption. Patient acceptability may be a limiting factor, and there are marked cultural differences in the acceptability of rectal administration of drugs. Suppositories are useful when a local action is wanted. Haemorrhoids ('piles') can be treated with suppositories that contain a local anaesthetic. Constipation can be treated with glycerine suppositories. Bacterial or fungal infections of the vagina can be treated with pessaries.

Inhalation. Inhalation is used to apply drugs directly to the lungs to treat, for example, asthma and chronic obstructive pulmonary disease (COPD). The medication may be in gaseous, aerosol or dry powder form. Antiinflammatory steroids such as beclomethasone diproprionate are inhaled, as are the β_2-adrenoceptor agonist bronchodilator drugs such as salbutamol (albuterol) (see Chapter 9). The β_2-receptor agonists work through receptors on the surface of airway smooth muscle cells to relax the muscle surrounding the airways to cause bronchodilation and thus symptomatic relief of airway obstruction. As β_2-receptors are found on other tissues in the body (such as skeletal muscle where stimulation can cause muscle tremor), by inhaling this drug a rapid clinical benefit is achieved while keeping the majority of the drug out of the blood, reducing unwanted side-effects and thus improving the therapeutic window. In contrast, some drugs are given by inhalation in order to benefit from the large surface area of the lung to achieve rapid blood levels, e.g. gaseous general anaesthetics are administered by inhalation during surgical procedures (see Chapter 19). Drugs that would be destroyed by enzymes in the gastrointestinal tract, such as insulin, can sometimes be given by inhalation as an alternative to injection, or topically to the nasal mucosa in the case of calcitonin. Intranasal drugs can also bypass the blood–brain barrier (see later) and this may become an important route of administration for new treatments for neurological diseases.

Advantages.

- High local concentrations of the drug can be achieved in the relevant tissues.
- It can produce rapid relief of symptoms.

Disadvantages.

- Requires specialist delivery devices for the drug, such as nebulisers or metered dose inhalers, which can provide difficulties for some patients, particularly those with poor hand/eye coordination such as the elderly and young children. Careful education on the use of these devices is very important to ensure successful treatment.
- Some powder formulations can be irritant and cause coughing, and advice about oral hygiene is important for inhaled corticosteroids.

CLINICAL NOTE

Effective inhaler technique is important to maximize drug effect. This is of particular importance when patients are prescribed inhalers for respiratory conditions. Time should be taken, on a regular basis, to verify effective patient inhaler technique. Asthma UK (2019) have excellent instructional videos, which can assist patients to improve their technique between asthma or respiratory reviews.

Intravenous (IV) Injection

- The drug is injected directly into a vein, usually in the arm or hand.

Advantages.

- A rapid onset of action is achieved.
- The entire injected dose is almost instantly bioavailable, since it bypasses the gastrointestinal tract and first pass metabolism.
- A lower dose is administered than if the drug was given orally.
- Administration is useful for drugs that are irritant when administered intramuscularly (see later).

Disadvantages.

- The drug must be administered by a trained person.
- Any puncture of the skin carries the risk of bruising, bleeding and infection.
- Inadvertent injection into an artery can cause arterial spasm with resulting tissue damage.
- Correct dosage may require more complex calculation than with oral medication and is therefore more open to accidental overdose. Accidental overdose by this administration route may be more dangerous than by other routes.

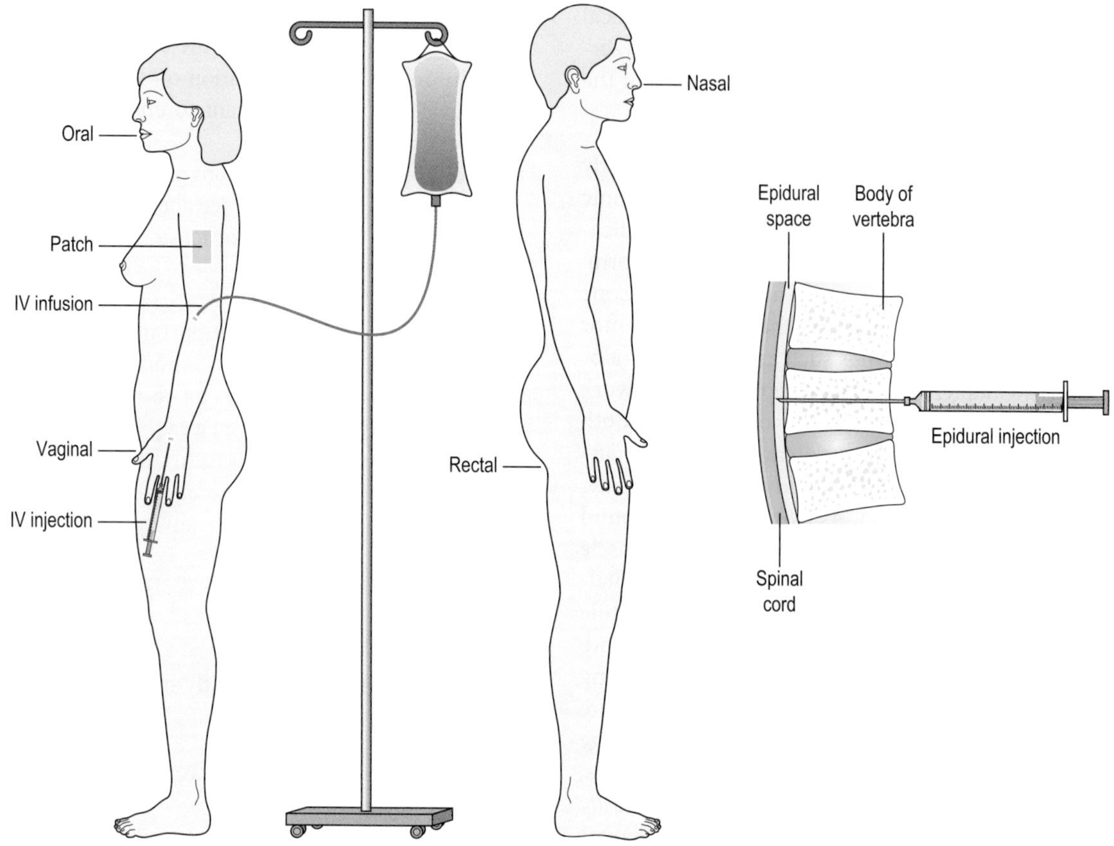

Fig. 1.3 Routes of drug administration.

Examples of drugs given IV are: thiopental for induction of general anaesthesia, some antibiotics (see Chapter 26) and adrenaline (epinephrine) for the treatment of cardiac arrest (see Chapter 8). Some drugs are administered continuously or intermittently by IV infusion using a motorized syringe-driver. This is an important part of patient-controlled analgesia (PCA). Drugs are sometimes injected directly into arteries – for example, the use of radio-opaque chemicals for X-ray purposes – but this is a rare route for the parenteral administration of drugs.

Intramuscular (IM) Injection

The drug is injected into a muscle. Absorption is variable, depending on which muscle is used, being most efficient from the deltoids of the arms, and least from the buttocks (Fig. 1.3). Absorption depends on the blood flow through the muscle and is increased by exercising the muscle or rubbing the site of injection. The rate of absorption will be reduced in shock. Drugs used for premedication before surgery are sometimes given via the IM route (see Chapter 19). Certain drugs, for example some steroids used for HRT (see Chapter 18), are implanted IM and released slowly from the implant.

Advantages.

- This injection is technically easier than IV.
- The gastrointestinal tract and first pass metabolism are avoided.
- A long-term effect from a single dose can be achieved if the drug is formulated as a 'depot', e.g. some formulations of insulin.

Disadvantages.

- Injections can be painful.
- Self-administration is difficult.
- Rarely, abscesses can form at the site of injection.
- The needle may puncture a small blood vessel and cause bruising of the skin.

Intradermal Injection

The needle is inserted into the skin without penetrating into the subcutaneous space. This is an important route for local anaesthetics, especially in dental surgery. It is an unusual route for drug administration outside dentistry. The aim is to localize the injection as much as possible in order to minimize more general effects and maximize the local effect.

Subcutaneous (SC) Injection

The subcutaneous route of injection is widely used. Common sites for injection include the thigh or upper arm. The skin is pinched, and the needle inserted so that the drug is administered under the layer of skin. Insulin is often injected SC by the patient. Some local anaesthetics are administered SC and a vasoconstrictor, such as adrenaline (epinephrine), may be added to the drug to minimize absorption away from the site of injection and thus maximize the local effect.

Advantages.

- Absorption is slower than after IM injection.
- The patient can self-administer the drug.

Disadvantages.

- Care has to be taken not to inject IV.
- Absorption is, as with IM injection, dependent on local blood flow, being increased with exercise and decreased in shock.
- The needle may puncture a small blood vessel and cause bruising of the skin.

NURSING NOTE

Refer to local patient self-administration policy. All patients who are able to administer their drugs via SC injection should be educated to do so.

Intrathecal Injection

Intrathecal injection is the administration of drugs directly into the central nervous system (CNS), thus bypassing the blood–brain barrier. The needle is passed through the dura (sometimes called the theca), the connective tissue sheath that surrounds the brain and spinal column, and the drug is injected into the subarachnoid space, through which the cerebrospinal fluid circulates, bathing the surfaces of the brain and spinal cord. This is a potentially hazardous procedure, which should only be attempted by trained, experienced personnel, since the spinal cord can be inadvertently damaged. Intrathecal injection is a route for direct application into the CNS of drugs such as local anaesthetics and antiviral agents. A 'spinal' anaesthetic involves this procedure and can provide total abolition of pain for major operations while the patient remains awake.

An epidural injection is the injection of a local anaesthetic into the epidural space in the lumbar region of the spinal cord, and can be used to alleviate the pain of labour. It is an uncomfortable procedure and is not always effective. In some cases, the dura is accidentally punctured as an epidural is being administered. The resulting leak of cerebrospinal fluid can, occasionally, lead to a very severe headache, requiring treatment with an epidural blood patch.

ABSORPTION, DISTRIBUTION AND ELIMINATION

The concentration of an administered medication in a body tissue depends on the absorption, distribution and elimination of that medication.

Absorption

Absorption of a drug means the transfer of the drug from the external to the internal environment of the body. Drug formulations (tablets, liquids) and route of administration have an immediate effect on absorption but then, in order to get into the body, the drug needs to get across cell membranes. These membranes are designed to very strictly control the movement of chemicals across them. Only dissolved substances can cross a membrane but even then, chemicals that ionize in solution can only cross these membranes with difficulty. This means that if taken orally, a drug that is a weak acid will be absorbed primarily in the acidic environment of the stomach, whereas a drug that is a weak base will be absorbed in the alkaline environment of the small intestines. Cell membranes regulate the ionic composition of the cell very tightly, or else they would be unable to function properly. Uncharged molecules, such as the steroids and ethyl alcohol, move freely across cell membranes. Aspirin, however, will ionize in the small intestine, which hinders absorption.

Absorption can occur through:

- passive diffusion
- facilitated transport
- active transport
- pinocytosis.

Passive diffusion is the movement of substances down a concentration gradient and the process does not require energy. Most drugs are absorbed by passive diffusion. Drugs that are more lipid soluble, are largely un-ionized in solution, and are composed of smaller molecules, are most likely to be absorbed by passive diffusion. The statins are examples of drugs absorbed by passive diffusion.

Facilitated transport (also called 'facilitated diffusion') is the transport of chemicals across the cell membrane by carrier proteins in the cell membrane that do not require energy to function. The carrier proteins can be thought of as pores in the membrane that can carry specific molecules across the membrane. The carrier proteins will not work against a concentration gradient and can also be a target for drugs. For example, glucose is carried across the cell membrane by facilitated transfer, and the numbers of glucose carriers in the membrane are increased by insulin. Vitamin B12 is absorbed from the gut by this mechanism, and failure of this mechanism causes B12 deficiency and pernicious anaemia.

Active transport is the pumping of chemicals across the membrane against a concentration gradient, requiring energy to do so. Ions such as sodium and potassium are actively transported across cell membranes. Drugs can modify the function of these active mechanisms, and some drugs, such as iron salts or levodopa, are themselves transported into cells by these mechanisms.

Pinocytosis is a process by which cells envelop an external liquid with a layer of cell membrane and draw the liquid (and any dissolved chemicals) into the interior of the cell. The process is energy intensive and is probably only of importance in the absorption of protein-based drugs.

CLINICAL NOTE

Some drugs are deactivated by gastric enzymes, e.g. insulin, which is always given by injection.

Distribution of the Drug in the Body

It is important to understand what happens to a drug when it enters the body and how long it stays there. It needs to get to and stay in the tissue where it acts if it is to do its job effectively. Ideally, a diuretic such as furosemide would target the kidney selectively; or, if it were intended to act on the heart to regulate the heart rate – such as bisoprolol – then ideally such a drug would target cardiac muscle selectively. Again, ideally, such drugs would not enter certain tissues or organs. However, in reality, once a drug gets into the bloodstream it is carried to all parts of the body and therefore will come into proximity with virtually all tissues and organs, and that fact explains many of the side-effects associated with orally ingested and systemically administered drugs. Blood flow is a key determinant of drug distribution and tissues with a high blood flow will tend to have higher concentrations of a drug than those with a lower blood flow. Fatty tissue has a much smaller blood flow than glandular tissue, for example. Some organs preferentially absorb certain substances, e.g. the thyroid gland absorbs iodine.

Some organs block the distribution of many drugs. The placenta and the blood–brain barrier are the most important examples.

Drugs and the Placenta

Many drugs cannot pass the placenta. Those that can tend to be highly lipid soluble.

It is particularly important to determine whether a drug will cross the placenta and thus potentially affect the fetus, if it is to be made available for women of child-bearing age.

Drugs and the Blood–Brain Barrier

There is a highly specialized physiological barrier called the blood–brain barrier, which actively prohibits many substances from getting across from the

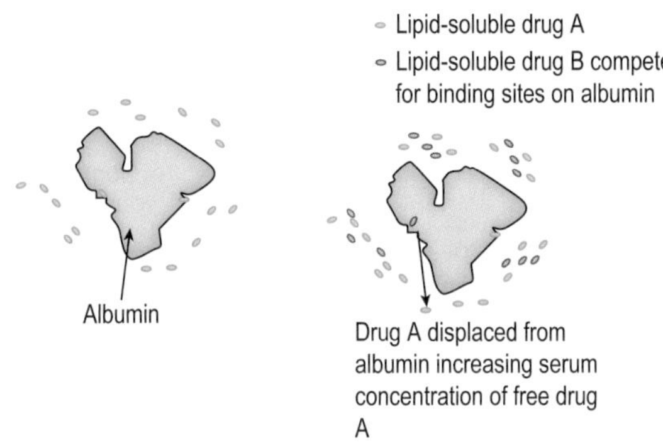
Lipid-soluble drug A
Lipid-soluble drug B competes for binding sites on albumin
Albumin
Drug A displaced from albumin increasing serum concentration of free drug A

Fig. 1.4 ■ Plasma protein binding of drugs.

bloodstream into the CNS and protects the brain from many chemicals. Thus, if a drug is to be designed to work in the brain, it must be able to cross the blood–brain barrier. In general, drugs that are lipid soluble are able to cross the blood–brain barrier by passive diffusion, although other mechanisms also exist. Parkinson's disease is treated by replacing lost dopamine in the brain. As dopamine itself will not cross the blood–brain barrier, a drug called levodopa is used, which can cross the blood–brain barrier and is then converted to dopamine. Such a drug is referred to as a 'pro-drug'.

Plasma Protein Binding of Drugs

The blood contains several proteins that can bind some hormones and drugs (Fig. 1.4). When these are bound to plasma proteins they can be protected from first pass metabolism (see later), which may be beneficial. However, plasma protein binding renders substances pharmacologically inert because they cannot get into the cell to interact at their site of action. Drugs or hormones that bind to plasma proteins usually bind reversibly to the protein such that an equilibrium is set up between bound and free hormone or drug. Only the free drug can be metabolized or interact with target tissues. The more tightly bound the chemical is to the plasma protein, the longer its circulation time, or *half life* (see later), will be. The sex steroids, for example, are so tightly bound to a plasma protein (called sex hormone-binding globulin, SHBG), that less than 5% of the plasma hormone is available to the tissues at any given moment. Similarly, most of the circulating thyroid hormone thyroxine is tightly bound to a plasma protein that recognizes the hormone specifically.

CLINICAL NOTE

Plasma protein binding of drugs can have serious clinical implications. Some drugs will displace others from plasma proteins and this can cause unacceptably high free – i.e. pharmacologically active – plasma levels of the drug. The anticoagulant warfarin, for example, displaces many drugs from plasma proteins and must be monitored carefully when used alongside certain other drugs. A potentially serious drug interaction is caused when warfarin is prescribed alongside a non-steroidal antiinflammatory drug (NSAID). NSAIDS are more tightly bound to plasma proteins resulting in more warfarin 'free' to exert its effect. Plasma levels of warfarin will rise and INR will increase, resulting in greater risk of bleeding.

First Pass Metabolism

First pass metabolism occurs when some drugs are metabolized in the liver as soon as they are absorbed from the gut. This may have an important effect on how much of a dose of an oral drug is actually available to work in the body. All substances that are absorbed from the gastrointestinal tract are carried in the portal blood system to the liver, where one of several things can happen:

- The drug escapes from the liver unchanged, e.g. certain oral contraceptive steroids.
- All or some of the drug is converted to an inactive metabolite that is excreted, e.g. 67% of an oral dose of morphine is inactivated in the liver. All of an oral dose of glyceryl trinitrate will be inactivated if it is swallowed, hence the reason this drug is administered sublingually to treat angina.
- The drug is metabolized to an active metabolite that exerts its therapeutic effect, e.g. the analgesic codeine is converted to the active metabolite morphine, which is around 10 times more powerful a painkiller than codeine itself.

The process of altering a drug in the liver during first pass metabolism is referred to as biotransformation, and as noted earlier, may lead to increased, decreased or unchanged pharmacological activity of the metabolite, compared to the original drug. Most drugs that undergo first pass metabolism do this in two phases:

Phase I metabolism chemically alters the drug through *oxidation*, *reduction* or *hydrolysis*. Commonly, the liver enzyme systems known as cytochrome P450 oxidases (CYP450) are involved in this process. There is a great deal of genetically mediated variation in the activity of these enzyme systems, discussed further later. Some drugs have the effect of increasing (*inducing*) the activity of the Phase I enzyme systems that metabolize them (and other drugs – leading to drug interactions – see later). These drugs *induce their own metabolism*, which means they become less effective with continued use. Many anticonvulsants, such as phenytoin, have this effect.

Phase II metabolism involves *conjugation* in which the metabolite is joined to an electrically charged molecule such as glutathione, generally as a precursor to elimination from the body. Drugs that have undergone Phase II metabolism tend to be less pharmacologically active than their precursors.

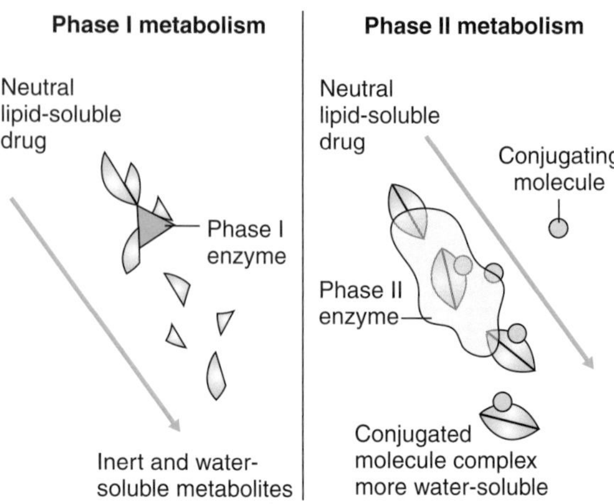

Fig. 1.5 First pass metabolism: Phase I and Phase II metabolism. (Note: Most drugs undergo Phase I and then Phase II metabolism. A few drugs undergo only one Phase or the other.)

Drug interaction with other drugs often occurs as a consequence of altering the effects of first pass metabolism. An example is the herbal preparation St John's Wort (*Hypericum perforatum*). This is available without prescription and is an effective antidepressant. However, it strongly increases the activity of CYP450 and this can lead to increased first pass metabolism of many important drugs, thus reducing their effectiveness. Such drugs include warfarin, ciclosporin, many epilepsy drugs and many anti-HIV drugs.

If a drug is given by any other route apart from the gastrointestinal tract, it escapes first pass metabolism (Fig. 1.5). Sometimes first pass metabolism can be used to improve the therapeutic window. For example, a high percentage of inhaled drugs are swallowed during the process of inhalation (hence the importance of teaching inhaler technique), so by designing an inhaled corticosteroid that undergoes extensive first pass metabolism, the systemic exposure to the swallowed portion can be very significantly reduced, thus reducing unwanted systemic side-effects.

Elimination of Drugs

The rate at which the body eliminates drugs is a major determinant of their duration of action. Generally, drugs are metabolized, mostly by Phase I and Phase II metabolism in the liver, although other tissues may also metabolize them. This process of metabolism occurs so that the drug can be eliminated more easily via the lungs, kidneys or the gut. Of these routes of elimination, the kidney is by far the most important. Reduced kidney function affects the elimination of many drugs. It is often necessary to reduce the dose of a drug in patients with reduced renal function, in order to prevent drug toxicity or unwanted effects. An example would be the anticoagulant drug apixaban, which needs dose reduction when renal function is very reduced, in order to prevent uncontrolled bleeding.

It is important to know how and where drugs are metabolized. Take, for example, a diabetic patient whose kidneys have been damaged by the disease. It is necessary to avoid giving this patient drugs such as certain oral sulphonylureas that are excreted via the kidneys. The liver itself can become damaged, e.g. after paracetamol overdose or in alcohol-induced cirrhosis or cardiac failure. Here, the action of a drug may be prolonged beyond its desired duration.

Drug Efflux

Drug efflux is a mechanism by which cells actively transport specific molecules that have entered them

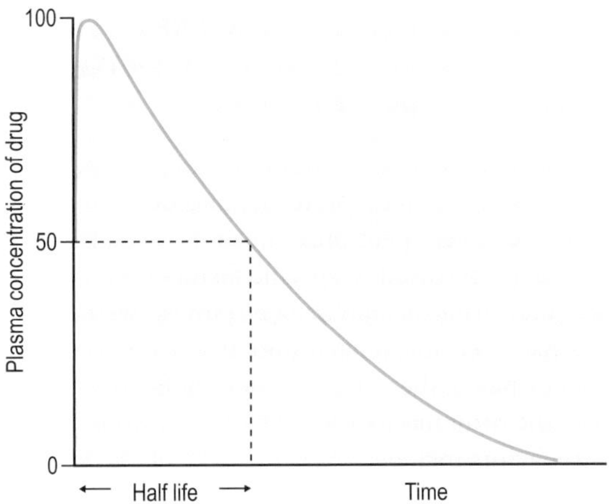

Fig. 1.6 ■ Plasma levels and half-life of a drug after a single intravenous injection.

back across the cell membrane into the outside environment where they can be eliminated. This mechanism is an important way in which bacteria eliminate antibiotics from themselves – leading to *antibiotic resistance*. In human cells, a similar mechanism is the common way in which cancer cells can become resistant to anti-cancer drugs.

Plasma Half-Life of a Drug (t½)

The blood is the only liquid compartment in the internal environment that is easily accessible to the clinician, and in which levels of a drug in the body can be conveniently monitored. The plasma half-life is an important and easily measured parameter of a drug's pharmacokinetics.

The plasma half-life of a drug is defined as the time taken for the plasma concentration of the drug to decline to one-half of its value after administration. It can be measured by giving a dose of the drug, sampling blood at intervals and plotting the results on a graph. A typical result is shown in Fig. 1.6.

The shape of the graph tells us a great deal about how the body eliminates the drug. Ideally, one would like to give a single dose of a drug that maintains steady levels at a therapeutically effective concentration – the so-called **steady state**. In reality, this is seldom achieved, and it is often required to keep giving doses at intervals to maintain the effective concentrations in plasma. After the first dose, blood levels of the drugs start rising, and further doses may be needed to

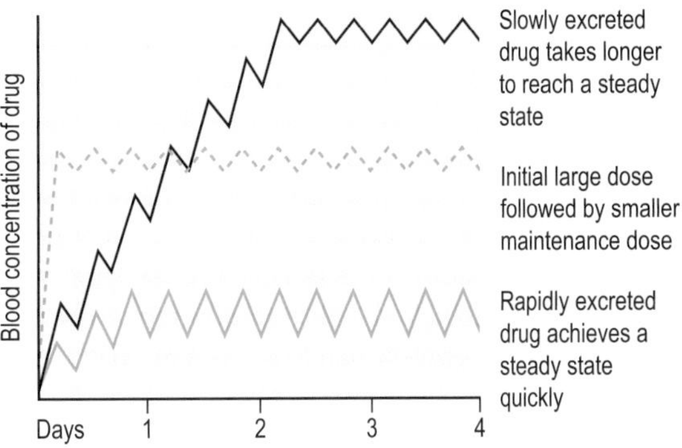

Fig. 1.7 ■ Steady-state concentrations of drugs.

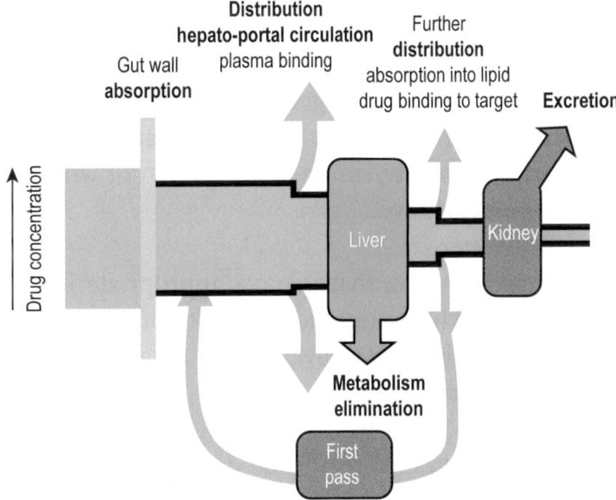

Fig. 1.8 ■ Absorption, distribution and elimination of an oral drug.

achieve and then maintain the desired level. Clearly, from Fig. 1.6, levels are falling. From working out the half-life of a drug it has been found that the time taken to reach the steady state is approximately five times the half-life of the drug. For example, the antidysrhythmic drug digoxin has a half-life of 36 h; therefore the patient must be given 5 doses regularly every 36 h, i.e. 180 h, to attain the steady state. The process can be observed graphically by monitoring drug levels with time (Fig. 1.7).

In practical terms, to speed up the process of getting to steady-state levels with a drug that has a longer half-life, it may be necessary to give an initial high 'loading dose' of the drug, followed by smaller maintenance doses. The fate of the administered drug is summarized in Fig. 1.8.

CLINICAL NOTE

We can work out half-life based on the dosing regimen of particular drugs, e.g. drugs such as digoxin or amiodarone have a long half-life and are prescribed as a daily dose. This also means that the drug will take a long time to reach 'steady state' and in the acute phase of an illness, a loading dose may be given. Drugs with a short half-life have to be given more frequently, e.g. aciclovir which is prescribed five times per day.

SUMMARY

In summary, some of the important factors that dictate how much of a drug we need to give, how often and by which route are listed below. Clearly these are generalities and the choice of drug, dose and route of administration will vary with the individual patient's needs. The points below are simply a distillation of what has been discussed above.

- Choose a drug that is most appropriate for the patient's condition and the route of administration that is most convenient to take, e.g. oral or topical or perhaps parenterally if the patient is unable to swallow.
- For a very rapid effect, the drug may be administered IV if it can be given safely through this route or sublingually.
- For a delayed onset, but a longer-lasting effect, the drug can be administered SC, IM or as a patch.
- Avoid administering drugs to patients with poor or damaged kidney or liver function if it is eliminated via these organs. Doses may need to be adjusted in such patients.
- For a longer effect, choose a drug that is metabolized more slowly.
- Drugs with shorter half-lives will need more frequent administration, perhaps even continuously by IV infusion.
- To speed up attainment of steady-state levels of a drug, give a high loading dose, followed by smaller maintenance doses.
- In patients receiving multiple drugs be aware of drug-to-drug interactions, e.g. drugs that induce liver enzymes will clear other drugs from the body more rapidly.

FACTORS THAT MAY MODIFY THE EFFICACY AND CHOICE OF DOSE OF A DRUG IN PATIENTS

The fact of inter-person variation in drug response that may require plasma monitoring and dose adjustment has already been mentioned. In some cases, this variation has been traced to specific factors such as lack of particular drug metabolizing enzymes. Even after the drug has been formulated into an injection, mixture, tablet or patch, there are a number of factors that may make the drug more or less effective in some patients. These factors include:

- patient age and size
- genetic factors, including single nucleotide polymorphisms (SNPs)
- ethnicity
- nutritional factors
- intercurrent illness
- drug–drug interactions
- psychological factors.

Patient Age and Size

There are considerable variations in response related to patient age and size and these are considered in more detail in Chapter 32. However, it is important to note that children are not to be considered as small adults for the purposes of drug dosing.

CLINICAL NOTE

Drug dosing in adults is calculated according to the standard adult weight of around 70 kg and those who are obese or extremely underweight will require their weight to be taken into account. In addition, people who are very underweight may also have low albumin levels, which is a plasma protein that some drugs bind to. If albumin levels are low it will result in higher concentrations of free drug, which may result in toxic drug levels. In children, drug dose is generally calculated by dose/kg and children are defined as ranging from 1–17 years. In most cases of prescribing for children, the adult dose should not be exceeded. In overweight children the dose of drug should be based on ideal rather than actual body weight.

Genetic Factors

There are a large number of inherited variations in medication response that are mostly related to differences in medication elimination. Most drugs are broken down by enzymes (usually in the liver) and this terminates their actions and makes them easy to eliminate. There are considerable inter-person differences in the activity of these enzymes. Many of these differences are caused by genetic variations (polymorphisms) known as single nucleotide polymorphisms (SNPs – pronounced 'snips'). A SNP is a change in one of the building blocks of a person's DNA – a nucleotide. Each person will have 4–5 million SNPs, most of which have no functional effect. However, if the SNP is in a gene, then it may affect the function of the protein that gene codes for. If the protein is an enzyme that metabolizes a drug (such as CYP450, discussed earlier), then the enzyme may have more, less or no activity, compared to the general population. With many drugs it is possible to distinguish between populations of people: some with a highly active enzyme system that can break the drug down rapidly and others with a less active system and relatively slower breakdown of the drug. SNPs are of increasing importance and testing of patients for specific SNPs will soon become routine in higher income countries, enabling the development of **personalized medicine**, where a drug is prescribed with a clear knowledge of how a patient will respond to it, and what side-effects they might expect. A new field of pharmacology has developed recently, studying the effect of SNPs and how this knowledge informs the development of personalized medicine. This is known as **pharmacogenomics**.

Examples

The TB drug, isoniazid is inactivated by acetylation, a process involving enzyme action. In the UK, 40% of the population are so-called 'fast acetylators' (with highly active acetylator enzymes) and 60% are considered 'slow acetylators'. This is an inherited characteristic and the ratio of fast/slow acetylators varies in different parts of the world. The Inuit of North America are without exception, rapid acetylators, whereas 80% of Egyptians are slow acetylators.

Differences in acetylator status do not usually matter in the UK, except when a high dose of the drug is used when there is a slightly increased risk of toxic effects in subjects who are slow acetylators. In low-income countries, where, for reasons of expense, very minimal doses may be necessary, those who are rapid acetylators may have less effective treatment of their TB.

Another example of genetic polymorphism is deficiency in the enzyme glucose-6-phosphate dehydrogenase (G6PD). This involves largely Africans and Indians, affecting about 100 million people. This polymorphism is due to an abnormal G6PD enzyme in red blood cells that results in the breakdown of these cells when exposed to the antimalarial drug, chloroquine, for example.

While differences in acetylator status and G6PD activity have been recognized for many years, SNPs affecting the metabolism of many other drugs have now been identified. Examples include:

- Codeine – some patients get very little pain relief from this drug.
- Clopidogrel – some patients show 'clopidogrel resistance' to this important antiplatelet drug.
- Warfarin – different SNPs lead to either resistance to the effects of this anticoagulant, or undue sensitivity to its effect.
- Salbutamol (albuterol) – some people have little response to this commonly used inhaled asthma drug.
- Simvastatin – people with one of two SNPs are at higher risk of myopathy with this cholesterol lowering drug, but conversely, people with another SNP benefit from a greater reduction in cardiovascular mortality than the average population, when given this drug.

This is a developing field of study and there are new discoveries all the time (https://www.SNPedia.com). It is important to realize that in most cases, genetic factors do not have a binary response/no response effect. Instead, they have degrees of effect, from little or no effect of the drug, through moderate effect to unusually high effect. Understanding how an individual's genetic make-up affects their response to drug treatment will be of increasing importance in the coming decades.

Ethnicity

The increasingly multicultural nature of many societies means that the health worker may be looking after patients from diverse ethnic groups. Genetic polymorphisms, as described previously, occur in different patterns in human populations who have developed in geographically separate areas, and so different ethnic groups may show different responses to drugs. Some of this variation may also be due to different lifestyles, particularly different diets. It has, for instance, long been known that ACE inhibitor drugs such as ramipril lower blood pressure less effectively in many people with African genes, and so these are not first-line choices as antihypertensives in Africans, Afro-Caribbeans or African-Americans. Similarly, some people with African genes respond relatively poorly to the β-blockers given for heart failure. This is known to be related to a number of genetic polymorphisms in the β_1 receptor that are more common in these populations. The development of pharmacogenomics will inform our understanding of ethnic differences in drug response but will probably also make such crude distinctions obsolete in due course, with the development of personalized medicine.

Nutritional Factors

Severe malnutrition can modify responses to drugs. Loss of body mass leads to reduction of body proteins, some of which are the enzymes that metabolize and thus inactivate drugs. Therefore, malnutrition can result in prolonged action of drugs, which could be deleterious to the patient.

Malnutrition as such is not common in high and medium income countries, except in certain populations such as individuals who practice extreme forms of dieting, or patients with alcoholism or suffering from cachexia due to diseases such as cancer.

Intercurrent Illness

Intercurrent illness is the occurrence of an illness that may modify the course and treatment of another illness (comorbidity) that is present at the same time. This may modify drug elimination and is an important cause of altered response to a drug. Most drugs are either broken down by the **liver** or excreted by the **kidneys**, so disease of these organs with diminished function can lead to accumulation of the drug with a more intense and prolonged action, which can sometimes be dangerous.

CLINICAL NOTE

A patient with a long-term history of alcohol abuse may develop cirrhosis of the liver. This disease results in a loss of enzyme-containing liver cells and distortion of liver anatomy, such that blood may bypass the liver. These cells play a role in drug metabolism and, if a drug is not metabolized into a substance that can easily be eliminated, it will remain in the systemic circulation for longer and may result in an increase in side-effects. For example, if the patient was prescribed morphine for pain, a drug that is normally inactivated in the liver, side-effects could occur. Morphine causes slight depression of respiration, even in therapeutic doses, but if its breakdown is impaired, the patient may get an overdose of morphine due to accumulation of the drug with repeated dosing, and therefore may suffer severe respiratory depression. **This the reason why drug formularies may recommend that dose is reduced in people with liver disease.**

Medication metabolism may be altered even if the liver is not damaged. For example, in heart failure the blood flow through the liver is reduced, and thus heart failure may indirectly cause a reduction in the rate of drug metabolism by the liver.

The Kidney

Kidney function may also modify the response to drugs. Many drugs are excreted by the kidney via urine and when considering the dosage of a drug, creatinine clearance (renal function) needs to be taken into account. Gentamicin (see Chapter 26) is excreted via the kidneys and, when renal function is reduced, serious accumulation occurs with normal dosage. Gentamicin is toxic, particularly to the ear, even with slightly raised blood levels. Therefore, careful monitoring of blood levels, with subsequent modification of doses, is required when gentamicin is given, particularly in patients with renal disease.

CLINICAL NOTE

In renal and liver disease, drugs are often prescribed at 50% of the usual dose, or avoided to prevent toxic side-effects. Referral to drug formularies, for example the *British National Formulary* (BNF) are of great importance when prescribing, administering or monitoring drug treatment in these groups.

Drug Interactions

One drug can modify the response to another drug in several different ways. This is a very important topic and is discussed more fully in Chapter 33. Drug–drug interactions are a major cause of illness and are often preventable.

Psychological Factors

Psychological factors may also be important in the patient's response to a drug. Expectation of a successful outcome may appear to improve the results of treatment. For example, analgesics are more effective if the patient believes they are effective. It has been shown that the colour and shape of pills and the branding on their packaging also has an effect on the response to the drug (MacKrill et al., 2019). This is known as the **placebo effect**, and it is very powerful. This is also the reason that a placebo arm is necessary (where it is ethical) in clinical trials of new drugs to check for the true efficacy of the drug.

In summary, most drugs are given in doses that have been found to be satisfactory from clinical trials and clinical practice, although the dose may need to be modified because of the factors discussed earlier. As a result, formularies usually give a range of doses. In the light of the clinical response, some alterations may be needed (e.g. the dose of hypotensive drugs is adjusted until a satisfactory fall in blood pressure is achieved).

CLINICAL NOTE

In addition to the placebo effect, there is also evidence that patients may decide to refuse drug treatment because they believe the treatment has harmful, negative side-effects. This may be caused by negative expectations or previous experience of treatment (Faasse, 2019). This is known as the 'nocebo' effect and as a practitioner, it is important to explore those concerns with the patient and come to a shared understanding about the benefit of the proposed or prescribed treatment.

BASIC PHARMACODYNAMICS

Pharmacodynamics is the study of how drugs exert their effects on the body to bring about clinical benefit. Understanding how drugs work also aids in the development of new and better ones to treat disease. Most drugs bring about their effects by interacting with protein structures on the cell surface called **receptors**, or by interacting with **ion channels** or **enzymes** in cells.

Receptors as Targets for Drug Actions

There are now known to be a wide range of families of receptors, but they all broadly share the same important functions:

- to recognize and bind the body's own chemical messengers, such as hormones and neurotransmitters
- to convert the binding event into a signal that the cell can recognize and respond to in some way, such as: divide, secrete, relax or contract.

Drugs have several important properties that need to be understood to explain how they work and how they can produce side-effects:

- selectivity
- affinity
- efficacy
- potency.

Selectivity

Specific substances, whether natural or artificial (drugs), are recognized by receptors and bind to them selectively. For example, the receptors for adrenaline (epinephrine), known as α and β adrenoceptors, will bind to both adrenaline and noradrenaline (norepinephrine), but they will not bind to, e.g. acetylcholine or progesterone. By chemically modifying the natural structure that recognizes a particular receptor type, pharmacologists can exploit this specificity to develop drugs that recognize the same receptor to either activate it (an **agonist**) or block the ability of the natural substance to recognize the receptor (an **antagonist**). Agonists and antagonists are discussed later. Drugs will vary in how selective they are for a particular receptor. Some are highly selective and others may activate more than one type of receptor. A substance that binds to a receptor or enzyme protein target is also called a **ligand**.

Affinity

Substances – again whether natural, such as hormones, or artificial, such as drugs – need to bind to receptors for long enough (*tightly* enough) in order to initiate the biochemical processes in the cell and bring about a cellular response. Substances that bind to their receptors very tightly are described as having a high affinity. This property of affinity is very important and again can be exploited by pharmacologists. Drugs that have very high affinity and are poorly reversible following binding to the receptor, often behave as antagonists, preventing the ability of the naturally occurring signalling molecule from activating the receptor.

Efficacy

Efficacy, or intrinsic activity, refers to the ability of a drug to trigger a response when it is bound to a receptor on a cell. Some drug types will produce a bigger effect than others when they bind to a receptor. A drug with higher efficacy will produce more of an effect on a cell than a drug with lower efficacy, even if both drugs have bound to the same number of receptors on the cell.

Potency

Potency is a function of both affinity and efficacy and so depends on both properties of a drug. A highly potent drug will bind tightly to receptors and when bound, will exert a bigger effect than a low potency drug. In terms of dose, a highly potent drug will require a lower dose than a less potent drug. Alprazolam is a more potent drug than diazepam, although both are of the same class of benzodiazepine drugs used in the short-term treatment of anxiety.

Agonists and Antagonists

Agonists

Adrenaline is a naturally occurring hormone that can activate different cell types depending on the adrenergic receptors present on the cell. There are different adrenergic receptor types, which are distinct proteins found on the surface of different cell types that when activated by adrenaline lead to different physiological responses:

- $\alpha 1$ – found on blood vessels (lead to vasoconstriction and cause an increase in blood pressure).
- β_1 – found in cardiac tissue (stimulates the heart).
- β_2 – found on airway smooth muscle (relaxes the bronchioles).

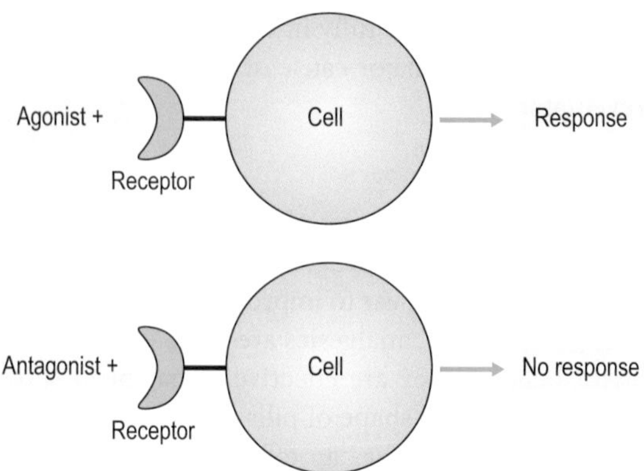

Fig. 1.9 ■ Action of agonist and antagonist on the cell.

We refer to adrenaline as an adrenergic agonist and it can activate a range of tissues that express adrenergic receptors. However, the drug salbutamol (albuterol) is known as a β_2 selective agonist as it only binds to β_2 receptors and therefore only mimics the action of adrenaline on airway smooth muscle and not on the heart or blood pressure.

Antagonists

If a patient has too high a level of adrenaline in the blood, this can lead to an increase in blood pressure. One class of antihypertensive drugs are called 'alpha blockers' or '$\alpha 1$ receptor antagonists', as these are drugs that bind to the α receptors in blood vessels, but produce no effect themselves. However, they prevent adrenaline from binding to $\alpha 1$ receptors and thus reduce the ability of adrenaline to initiate a contractile response in the blood vessel and thus reduce blood pressure. Doxazocin is an example of an $\alpha 1$ antagonist (Fig. 1.9).

Partial Agonists

Partial agonists are drugs that bind to a receptor but do not have full efficacy at that receptor, compared to a full agonist. They therefore provoke a less than maximal response when they bind. By binding at the receptor, they also block it from being bound by a full agonist and can therefore act as a partial (competitive) antagonist to that receptor, if the dose given is sufficient clinically. Important examples include the opioid analgesics, buprenorphine and tramadol. In the case of tramadol, its partial agonist activity may account for the reduced risk of respiratory depression associated with its use. Other examples include aripiprazole and buspirone.

Functional Consequences of Agonist–Receptor Interaction

The functional consequences of agonist ligand–receptor interactions depend very much on the cell type. For example:

- When adrenaline binds to β_2 receptors on airway smooth muscle, it leads to bronchodilation, which can be exploited therapeutically in the treatment of patients with asthma.
- When adrenaline binds to β_1 receptors on heart muscle cells, this will generate contraction of the muscle and will increase heart rate.
- When adrenaline binds to its liver cell receptor, it will cause glycogen stored inside the cell to be broken down to glucose.
- When hydrocortisone binds to its receptor inside a skin cell, it will stimulate changes in protein synthesis inside the cell that result in an antiinflammatory response.

Ion Channels and Enzymes as Targets for Drug Actions

While receptor interactions are very important and should be thoroughly understood, drugs can also exert their action by other means, of which interactions with ion channels and enzymes are the most important. Ion channels can be thought of as pores through cell membranes that can be opened and closed to specific stimuli. When open, they allow the passage of charged atoms or molecules (ions) in and out of the cell. Ion channels are involved in nerve and muscle function, blood pressure control and electrolyte balance. Drugs have been developed which act on ion channels to open or close them, with consequent effects on cell function. Important examples of ion channel modulating drugs include amlodipine, zolpidem, alprazolam, the sulfonylureas, repaglinide and nateglinide.

Enzyme systems within cells are the biochemical machinery of life, and some drugs will bind to certain enzymes and alter their function, often by inhibiting them. Aspirin is an example of a drug that works by inhibiting the enzyme cyclooxygenase and so reduces the formation of inflammatory substances called 'prostaglandins'. Antibiotics such as penicillin block the action of enzymes in bacteria that are used to make bacterial cell walls, thus leading to their destruction.

Both ion channel blocking drugs and enzyme inhibitors exhibit properties analogous to the selectivity, affinity, potency and efficacy of drugs that act on receptors, and they are often discussed using these terms.

Other Targets for Drug Action

Drugs may also work at sites on or in the cell that are not receptors, ion channels or enzyme systems. An important class of drugs work on **transporter** molecules that carry large molecules into cells. The selective serotonin reuptake inhibitors (SSRI) antidepressants work by inhibiting uptake of serotonin at nerve synapses.

Another important group of drugs affect the structure of cells by altering the production of microtubules within them. Colchicine, which is used to treat gout, works in this manner. The taxane group of cancer chemotherapy drugs (e.g. paclitaxel) also affect microtubule function.

Other types of cancer chemotherapy work by chemically altering cell DNA and so lead to cell death. The nitrogen mustard group of drugs (e.g. cyclophosphamide) work in this manner.

CLINICAL NOTE

In some cases, antagonists are given to reverse the effect of an agonist. For example, when a patient takes an overdose of morphine (an agonist at μ receptors), the patient can be treated by injecting another drug called naloxone (which is an antagonist). This drug also binds to the same receptors and has a greater affinity to μ receptors and can be used as an antidote to morphine. Note that if naloxone is given, it will not only reverse the side-effects of morphine (e.g. respiratory depression) but will also reverse the analgesic effect of morphine. It will therefore be important to consider an alternative form of pain management for the patient or to give morphine at a reduced dose.

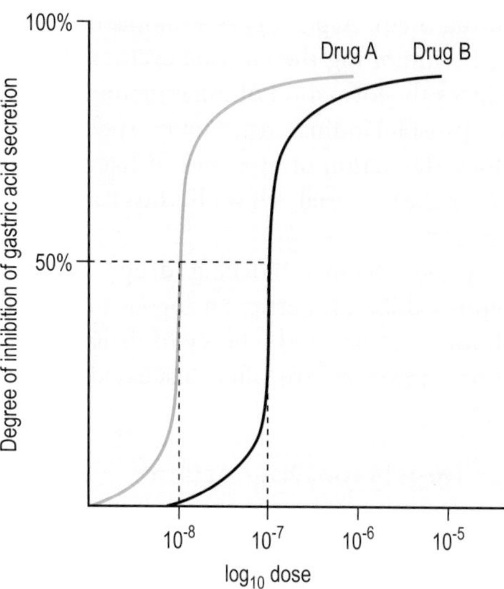

Fig. 1.10 ■ Inhibition of gastric acid secretion by two drugs, A and B. The dose–response curves are for two drugs acting on the same histamine H_2 receptors, but drug A is more potent than drug B.

The Dose–Response Curve

An important tool in understanding and quantifying drug actions is the dose–response curve. This simple graph can yield much information about the effectiveness of a drug. For example, we can use the dose–response curve to determine a drug's potency.

Consider, in Fig. 1.10, the dose–response curves showing the degree of inhibition of gastric acid secretion by two different histamine H_2 receptor antagonists. We learn some important information from the graph:

- The curves have identical shapes, especially over the linear rising parts. This suggests that both drugs are acting on the same receptor system in order to lower gastric acid secretion.
- Both drugs are capable of the same maximum effect, i.e. have similar **efficacies.**
- At 50% inhibition of acid secretion, drug B has only one-tenth the **potency** of drug A.

All else being equal, it would be preferable to give drug A to the patient, since 10 times less of a foreign chemical would be introduced into the body, even if drug B at a high enough dose will suppress acid secretion to the same extent. Drug A is more potent, but both drugs have the same efficacy. This is because both produce the same maximum response. The term 'efficacy' used here, is a reflection of how effective the drug is at activating its receptor to produce an effect and is not to be confused with effectiveness of a drug in a patient in clinical practice. This depends on many factors, such as how well it is absorbed from the gastrointestinal tract and the degree of metabolism of the drug through first pass metabolism before it can get to its site of action.

CLINICAL NOTE

In day-to-day practice, it may be necessary to explain to patients that a change of drug from one to another, which has a greater number of milligrams in the daily dose, does not necessarily mean that they are being given a 'stronger' drug than the first one – just different.

SUMMARY

- Receptors, enzymes and ion channels are important protein targets for drugs.
- Antagonists are drugs that block the normal cellular function that a receptor triggers.
- Agonists have the opposite effect and trigger a cellular function when they bind to a receptor.
- The dose–response curve is an important tool for quantifying the action of a drug.
- High potency means that relatively little of the drug is required in order to achieve a powerful effect, and usually means it has a high affinity for the receptor it acts upon.

REFERENCES AND FURTHER READING

Asthma, U.K., 2019. How to Use Your Inhaler. https://www.asthma.org.uk/advice/inhaler-videos.

Corrie, K., Hardman, J.G., 2011. Mechanisms of drug interactions: pharmacodynamics and pharmacokinetics. Anaesth Intens Care Med. 12 (4), 156–159.

Faasse, K., 2019. Nocebo effects in health psychology. Aust. Psychol. 54 (6), 453–465.

Gallimore, D., 2006. An overview of how drugs are designed and developed. Nurs. Times 102 (47), 30–31.

Goldacre, B., 2012. Bad Pharma. Fourth Estate, London.

MacKrill, K., Kleinstäuber, M., Petrie, K.J., 2019. The effect of rebranding generic medicines on drug efficacy and side effects. Psychol. Health 34 (12), 1470–1485.

McGavock, H., 2016. How Drugs Work: Basic Pharmacology for Healthcare Professionals, fourth ed. Taylor & Francis, Boca Raton.

Muñoz, C., Hilgenberg, C., 2005. Ethnopharmacology: understanding how ethnicity can affect drug response is essential to providing culturally competent care. Am. J. Nurs. 105 (8), 40–49.

National Institute of Healthcare Research (NIHR), 2019. The Role of a Clinical Research Nurse. https://www.nihr.ac.uk/documents/the-role-of-the-clinical-research-nurse/11505.

Paudel, K.S., Milewski, M., Swadley, C.L., et al., 2010. Challenges and opportunities in dermal/transdermal delivery. Ther. Deliv. 1 (1), 109–131.

Wallin, M., Tagami, T., Chen, L., et al., 2018. Pulmonary drug delivery to older people. Adv. Drug Deliv. Rev. 135, 50–61.

USEFUL WEBSITE

SNPedia. https://www.snpedia.com.

2 THE ROLE OF NURSES IN DRUG ADMINISTRATION

CHAPTER OUTLINE

LEARNING OBJECTIVES

At the end of this chapter, the reader should be able to:

- understand the types of non-medical prescribers
- have an awareness of the prescribing competency framework
- promote patients' understanding of the purpose of their treatment and improve adherence to drugs
- list the regulations governing drug administration
- obtain a reliable drug history from patients
- list the essential details that need to be included on a drug prescription
- state the responsibilities of the nurse in ensuring that the prescription is interpreted accurately and in understanding and knowing the reason for action and dose of the drug
- describe the procedure for drug dispensing to patients when two nurses are involved
- list the safety factors for drug supervision in the clinical area
- describe the procedures for administration to the patient of drugs by oral, rectal and vaginal routes and by injection
- explain how to gain the cooperation of children and older patients when administering drugs to them
- explain the reasons for drug errors
- state the legal and professional responsibilities of the nurse concerning drugs

NON-MEDICAL PRESCRIBERS

Medication therapy plays a major part in the treatment of patients. Traditionally, medicines have been prescribed by physicians, and the nurse's responsibility has been to ensure safe, reliable administration and to monitor side-effects. Globally, many countries have introduced prescribing for healthcare professionals other than doctors, with Australia, the USA, Scandinavia, and some European countries widely adopting the practice (Kroezen et al, 2011). The UK has the most liberal prescribing legislation in the world and this section outlines the evolution of practice in the UK and its benefits to patients.

In 1998, it became possible for all appropriately qualified community nurses in the UK to prescribe from a limited nursing formulary. From 2003, any registered nurse could undertake training to enable them to become a nurse prescriber and prescribe from a broader *Nurse Prescribers' Extended Formulary*. Since then, legislation has evolved and nurses can prescribe any medicines within their sphere of competence including controlled drugs, unlicensed and off-label medicines. Prescribing practice has also extended to other professions, resulting in the UK having the most liberal prescribing legislation in the world. Nurses, midwives, pharmacists and allied health professionals (AHPs; physiotherapists, podiatrists, radiographers, dieticians) are all eligible to prescribe following completion of a prescribing programme. This growth reflects the effectiveness of the role and growing need for prescribers in response to changes in workforce and service user demographics. This has resulted in five categories of prescribers in the UK. These are:

I. V300 independent and supplementary nurse or midwife prescriber
II. V100 or V150 nurse or midwife prescribers (community nurse formulary)
III. Physiotherapist, podiatrist, therapeutic radiographer and paramedic independent and supplementary prescriber
IV. Dietetic, diagnostic radiographer, supplementary prescriber
V. Pharmacist independent and supplementary prescriber.

CLINICAL NOTE

Nurse prescribing programmes are regulated by the Nursing and Midwifery Council and upon completion, registrants will gain entry onto that part of the register. Nurses can now undertake a V150 prescribing qualification immediately after qualifying and enrol on the V300 prescribing course 1 year after qualifying. As part of revalidation, once qualified as a prescriber, registrants must provide evidence of their prescribing practice and have this verified by their confirmer. In 2018, the NMC standards of proficiency for nurse and midwife prescribers was replaced by the RPS competency framework, an interprofessional competency framework adopted by the Health and Care Professions Council and Pharmacy Prescribers, which has standardized prescribing practice across professions.

Independent Prescribers must Ensure that they have Professional Indemnity

All prescribers must maintain competency and follow the recent competency requirements from The Royal Pharmaceutical Society. The standards of proficiency for nurse and midwife prescribers (2006) were replaced by the Royal Pharmaceutical Society's Competency Framework for all Prescribers, on 28 January 2019. All prescribers must also maintain their registered status with the Nursing and Midwifery council (NMC) of the UK.

The Prescribing Competency Framework

The Prescribing Competency Framework developed by the Royal Pharmaceutical Society helps to instil competencies required for prescribing, regardless of whether you are an independent or a supplementary prescriber. It helps to streamline and update the competencies relevant to doctors as well as non-medical prescribers. This allows the setting of good prescribing standards. An outline of the main competences follows (please refer to the framework through the Royal Pharmaceutical Society for a detailed review).

The framework lists a total of 10 competencies, divided within the areas of The Consultation (which comprises competencies 1–6) and Prescribing Governance (competencies 7–10).

The Consultation

1. Assess the patient
2. Consider the options
3. Reach a shared decision
4. Prescribe

5. Provide information
6. Monitor and review

Prescribing Governance

7. Prescribe safely
8. Prescribe professionally
9. Improve prescribing practice
10. Prescribe as part of a team.

CLINICAL NOTE

Nurse prescribers should ensure that as part of revalidation they include a reflective account on prescribing, maintain their competency document and discuss prescribing with their revalidator. Nurses who have the annotation of prescriber on their registration must complete an appropriately recognized training course, the new prescribing framework and keep up-to-date with the latest prescribing trends.

A number of studies have demonstrated the positive effect that nurse prescribing has on cost, patient satisfaction and patient outcomes (Gielen et al., 2014). The positive effect of nurse prescribing has resulted in over 73,000 (11%) registered as practicing prescribers in the UK (Dowden, 2016). The need for nurse prescribers is in response to the increasing ageing population and people living with more complex health needs and medication regimens. This has resulted in a need for greater emphasis on prescribing in pre-registration programmes and from 2020, prescribing and pharmacology theory will be an integral theme throughout the UK.

High rates of polypharmacy and complex drug regimens may increase the risk of drug errors, the cost of which is estimated at US$42 billion per annum. The World Health Organization (WHO) has a global programme of work on Medicines Safety, which includes management of polypharmacy, medicines adherence and reduction of harm due to adverse drug events (WHO, 2017). The risk of adverse drug events can, in part, be mitigated by care provided by well-informed clinicians working collaboratively and service users and carers treated as partners.

In legal terms, 'prescribing' is taken to mean the ability to make a personal, professional and independent assessment of the patient. Based on this, a free choice is made from the drug formularies and evidence-based guidelines of the most appropriate medication or treatment (Box 2.1). A doctor's opinion is not required. The nurse signs the prescription form and remains professionally and legally accountable for his or her actions. In primary care, each individual NHS prescription issued and dispensed is identified and monitored by the Prescription Pricing Agency (PPA).

BOX 2.1

CONTROLLED DRUGS WHICH MAY BE PRESCRIBED BY INDEPENDENT NURSE PRESCRIBERS

- Diamorphine, morphine, diazepam, lorazepam, midazolam or oxycodone for use in palliative care
- Buprenorphine or fentanyl for transdermal use in palliative care
- Diamorphine or morphine for pain relief in suspected myocardial infarction or to relieve acute or severe pain after trauma, including postoperative pain
- Chlordiazepoxide hydrochloride or diazepam to treat initial or acute withdrawal symptoms from people habituated to alcohol
- Codeine phosphate or dihydrocodeine tartrate or co-phenotrope

One area to be aware of is that a breakdown of communication is possible after the patient is discharged from hospital, and when there is the potential for drugs to be prescribed by more than one person. However, the new prescribing–dispensing process means greater contact between the nurse and pharmacist, especially when problems arise.

The prescribing record should contain details of previous and current drugs along with any drug allergies. When prescribing or altering the drug prescriptions, it is good practice to be aware of over-the-counter drugs as well as other herbal or homeopathic therapies. These could have potential interactions but the information regarding these may not always be volunteered by the patient without specific enquiry. When prescribing, the prescriber will need to consider psychosocial as well as physical factors and the need for patient education must be recognized. The record should monitor the response to drugs and reasons for discontinuing their use. This is particularly important as information about adverse effects about the drug can be collated and future prescribing cautions regarding the drug class can be carefully considered by the prescriber.

Irrespective of whether or not they are permitted to prescribe and the setting in which they are employed, all nurses need to help patients understand the purpose of their treatment and to promote compliance with taking the prescribed drugs. The nurse must be aware of his or her responsibilities in giving drugs. Drugs are governed by the Misuse of Drugs Act 1971 and the Misuse of Drugs (Amendment) Regulations 2005, for controlled drugs; and the Medicines Act 1968, for prescription-only drugs, together with additional regulations formulated locally. All trusts have their own procedures and policies. The NMC code of conduct, in laying down the general responsibilities of the nurse, stipulates that his or her actions should put the patient's safety and well-being first at all times.

The National Institute of Health and Care Excellence (NICE) in the UK provided guidance on the safe use and management of controlled drugs in 2016. The guidelines provide recommendations for record-keeping, prescribing, obtaining, handling and supplying controlled drugs (NICE, 2016). They are designed to improve good practice in hospital and community settings. Where controlled drugs are prescribed by non-medical prescribers in community settings, the patient's general practitioner (GP) should be informed, and full details of the treatment plan should be provided with arrangements for monitoring and reviewing treatment. When opioid analgesics are prescribed, particular care must be given to possible side-effects, dosage, tolerance and possible interactions with other drugs

In hospital, the custody and administration of drugs is the responsibility of the ward sister/charge nurse, who may delegate this responsibility as instructed by the employing authority's policy. Although it is usual for a qualified nurse to give drugs, with a second nurse checking to prevent error, the NMC takes the view that registered nurses should be seen as competent to administer drugs on their own and be responsible for their actions. Student nurses will take part in drug administration and senior student nurses who have shown competence may be allowed to act as the senior person giving drugs with supervision. The actions of nurses in relation to drug administration will be legally covered by the employing authority when the rules are followed.

CLINICAL NOTE

NMC standards for medicines management were withdrawn in 2018 and replaced by Professional Guidance on the Administration of Medicines in Healthcare Settings, published by the Royal Pharmaceutical Society and Royal College of Nursing (2019). This outlines safe practice for drug administration, covert drug administration and transcribing. Local policy will also apply to student and registered healthcare professionals and this should be considered prior to administering any medicines in a healthcare setting and patient's homes. The person administering the drug must be appropriately trained and must meet professional regulatory standards (e.g. The Code). This means the person administering the medicine must have an overall understanding of the medicine being administered, including (but not limited to):

- the drug name, class and normal dose
- how the drug acts on the body
- why it is being given
- any potential side-effects or interactions with other drugs or foodstuffs and how long it will be given for.

DRUG HISTORY

A reliable drug history should be obtained from the patient and, if necessary, from relatives or friends, a doctor's letter, the patient's drug list, an electronic record or verification from a relative or significant other. This is known as drug reconciliation. The history should also include previous exposure to drugs, current drugs, over-the-counter, herbal or complimentary drugs and use of any recreational drugs. Nurses have a responsibility to record all drugs being taken, all drug allergies or past allergies and any other drug-related information that could prove necessary to the patient's history. If the illness is of a recurrent nature, the efficacy of any drugs used in previous episodes should be noted.

CLINICAL NOTE

For more detailed information on taking an accurate medication history, please refer to, *Alexander's Nursing Practice* (Peate, 2020) or review some of the further reading at the end of this chapter.

THE PRESCRIPTION

In hospital it is normal practice for all drugs to be prescribed. This enables the pharmacist to supply the appropriate drugs and provide advice concerning their safe administration. The prescription, which can be documented in many different forms – paper-based prescription or drug chart, electronic prescription, electronic drug record – is the primary document for the prescription of drug for a patient. The prescription must be headed with the patient's full name, age, hospital number, ward and allergies. The prescription must be clearly and indelibly written or typed and must contain the date, the approved name of the drug (preferably in block letters), the dose (using metric dosage), the route and frequency of administration with the validity period and signature of the prescriber. If any of these details are omitted, the drug should not be given until the prescription has been amended. Frequency of dosage can be ordered by filling in allocated time spaces rather than using Latin abbreviations. Administration is recorded by initialling the relevant box on the prescription sheet. The exact format of this sheet will vary and nurses must familiarize themselves with documents in use when moving to a new health authority.

Electronic prescribing is now standard practice within primary care, and there is a drive for its implementation in secondary care. It provides useful data for audit purposes as well as calculating cost implications. Electronic prescribing helps in improving safety as it can highlight interactions with other prescribed medication, which in turn can help reduce adverse drug events. However, it remains important to enquire with patients regarding over-the-counter medication as well as adherence to drugs prescribed, to gain a complete understanding of possible interactions.

CLINICAL NOTE

Many hospitals have now moved to an electronic prescribing system. All parts of the electronic prescription should be assessed when giving drugs to ensure that all drugs are administered. They should also ensure they are aware of all local policies that govern drug administration in the environment within which they are working.

Generic Prescribing

All the drugs in this book are referred to by their **generic** names (with a few exceptions where branded drug names are also shown, in italics, next to the generic name). The generic name of a drug is also known as the International Non-proprietary Name (INN) and is an internationally recognized name for the drug. However, many drugs are marketed by their manufacturers under trade or brand names, which are usually snappy and easy to remember. In many countries, if a drug is prescribed by its trade name, then that brand of drug must be dispensed. However, when a drug patent has expired, it may be manufactured by any licensed and regulated manufacturer as a generic drug, using the INN. Such generic drugs are often much less expensive than branded drugs and yet are chemically identical and so have the same effect. It is good practice to prescribe by INN rather than brand in most cases. This is because the generic drug is likely to be much less expensive for the patient or health system, but also because it avoids confusion, as brand names often differ between countries. This can make it difficult to identify just what drugs an international traveller may be taking if they present to a clinician in a different country. Some drugs, mainly modified release preparations, some anticonvulsants and all biologics and biosimilars, should be prescribed by brand, as generic versions of these agents may not have identical bioavailability.

Controlled Drugs

In hospital, controlled drugs must always be given by two people and it is common practice for one to be a qualified nurse. Both nurses must sign the book following each administration at the bedside or in the presence of the patient. The prescription requires the number of doses in words and figures. An additional record is kept in a specially designed book so that every tablet or ampoule is accounted for when used, both nurses signing the book following each administration. The controlled drug record book is retained on the ward for 2 years after the date of the last entry. These are legal requirements for controlled drugs, but some health authorities apply similar rules to other medicines liable to misuse or if there has been a local incident that needs additional processes to be put in place.

Drug Protocols

Protocols, often known as clinical guidelines or standards, have long been used in hospital and community settings to provide written documentation for an agreed method of performing a particular procedure, to achieve continuity and to standardize care. Some clinics and departments standardize administration of drugs according to protocols in both hospital and the community; for example, nurses may administer immunizations or oral contraception under a patient group direction (PGD), or patient specific direction. The use of protocols or PGDs are distinct from prescribing, as the nurse does not have to be a prescriber and is unable to make an independent choice of drug or treatment – this will already have been specified within the PDG. The PGD or protocol is operating as a substitute prescription authorized and signed by a doctor, or authorized by a drug and therapeutics committee who remains legally and professionally accountable for the treatment of the patient. Nevertheless, the nurse remains professionally and legally accountable for his or her decisions within the use of the protocol.

CLINICAL NOTE

If an area has drug protocols or patient group directions for the nurse to follow, it is the nurse's responsibility to ensure they have an adequate understanding of the drug and drug administration policy and have received a reasonable level of instruction to safely work within the protocol. Documentation of the drug protocol and the decisions made within the protocol boundaries is essential and must be completed in a timely manner following administration.

NURSING ASPECTS OF ADMINISTRATION

The nurse is responsible for interpreting the prescription accurately, recording that the drug has been given and observing the patient's response. Prior to administration the nurse must know the reason for the prescription and the usual dosage of the drug; this should enable the nurse to recognize and question mistakes in prescribing. When in doubt about a prescription, advice should be sought and, if necessary, the doctor or pharmacist should be consulted. If a prescription cannot be clearly viewed, it should not be given and clarification should be sought. Observations should be made for therapeutic and adverse effects. The nurse should realize that the patient's condition may alter the effect of a drug and that there may be interactions with concurrent treatment. The nurse is greatly assisted in these circumstances by the pharmacist, with whom a good working relationship will enhance the safety of patient care.

In the community, most patients, or a family member, are responsible for drug administration, although the nurse may also have a role to play. Many people are now discharged within a few days or hours of surgery and the average length of stay for medical patients has been reduced. People returning home are often still taking drugs, which in the past may have been administered in a hospital setting, so monitoring for adverse effects is an increasingly important aspect of the community nurse's role. The nurse must also be aware that some drugs, even if stopped before discharge, may still exert an action or cause side-effects. Careful counselling of patients on common adverse effects on discharge is crucial, with clear instructions on course of action should adverse effects develop.

The Committee on Safety of Drugs requests that adverse reactions are reported (yellow cards or online reaction reporting) and, in addition, may require that a special watch is kept on certain drugs.

CLINICAL NOTE

If a nurse suspects a prescribed dose is unusually high (or low), the dosage should be checked in the *British National Formulary* and hospital formulary, and discussed with the prescriber. If, after discussion, the dose is confirmed, a rationale for dosing outwith the normal dose range should be entered into the patients record by the prescriber. When in doubt, the dose should be withheld until clarification of dose is sought. The Committee on Safety of Medicines requests that adverse reactions are reported (yellow cards or online reaction reporting) and, in addition, drugs new to the market require close monitoring. Any suspected adverse drug reaction should be recorded through the yellow card system. Healthcare professionals, patients and carers can report suspected reactions. The information is stored on a national database and will detect any safety issues associated with drugs that may result in modifications to guidance or in some cases, withdrawal of the drug. There are a number of education modules that may help develop your understanding of this role, which can be accessed through their website (MHRA, 2018).

Administration of Drugs on the Ward

Drugs may be given to the whole ward by the same nurses or to a smaller group of patients by those directly involved in their care. The second method is preferable, as timing is more accurate and the nurse will know the patients well and can cater for individual needs; this may include a patient self-administering, education around administration, discharge preparation, swallowing the drug or assessment of the action of the drug. Time can be spent teaching patients about their drugs and student nurses can take part to gain experience in relating drugs to the patient's condition.

Patient education and enabling self-administration of drugs by patients, for example by arranging Nomad dispensing trays – sealed medication trays for patients who need support in ensuring they take all their daily drugs as prescribed, e.g. patients with mild cognitive impairment or those with complex drug regimens, allows patients to continue their drug routine independently or with appropriate carer support upon discharge from the hospital. The nurse remains responsible for the drug therapy in these cases and should assure themselves that the patient can properly administer their drugs in a different setting. If there are concerns regarding this, then this should, with consent, be communicated to carers for safe discharge to the destination organized for the patient.

Drug flexibility may not always be possible, e.g. antibiotics are more effective if doses are spread evenly throughout the day, and insulin must be given before meals. Other drugs such as non-steroidal antiinflammatories (NSAIDs) are best given with or after food, to help minimize adverse effects of gastritis. Clear discussion with patients and explanation of the drugs and routine that is being followed is important for drug compliance.

CLINICAL NOTE

With some potent medicines, variations in times of dosing may lead to a loss of efficacy. Taking medication before, during or after food can also significantly alter its clinical effect. For example, for maximum efficacy, bisphosphonates should be taken 30 min before breakfast to promote maximum absorption.

Rules of Drug Administration

Specific rules of drug administration must be followed to prevent errors. The principles behind the rules which require the nurse's undivided attention are: that the right patient must receive the right dose of the right drug in the right form by the right route at the right time, and that the fact is duly recorded. This is often described as the 5 rights.

When two nurses are involved, instructions should be read aloud:

1. Read the patient's full name from the drug chart.
2. Read the prescription, checking the validity and time of last administration.
3. Read the name of the drug from the label when removing the container from storage.
4. Check the label of the container for the name, strength and dose of the drug, the route of administration where relevant and the expiry date against the prescription.
5. Measure or count the correct dose. Avoid contact with the drug, as allergies can develop. When measuring liquids, shake the bottle, hold the measure at eye level, placing the thumbnail on the meniscus, and pour from the back of the bottle to keep the label clean. A calibrated measure should be used. When a fractional dose is required, calculations should be made independently before checking the dose.

CLINICAL NOTE

For liquid drugs, a bottle stopper should be used to help ensure correct dosage, a syringe for oral use (usually a different colour than an IV syringe) can be used if a bottle stopper is in place to aid in administration.

6. Recheck the label before returning the container to storage.
7. Both nurses must verify the patient's identity by checking the details on the drug chart with the

patient's identity bracelet. If this is absent, ask the patient to state his or her full name. If this is not possible (e.g. if the patient is comatose, has severe dementia or is a paediatric patient), identification must be confirmed by a member of the family or permanent staff.

8. Ensure the patient is in a fit state to receive the drug.
9. Give the dose and see that it has been swallowed.
10. Record the administration. Also record when a drug is not given and the reason.

CLINICAL NOTE

Reasons, including a patient's ideas, concerns and expectations, should be explored in those refusing to take a drug. The drugs should not be disguised, hidden in food or crushed for patients with intact mental health capacity.

SAFETY POINTS

- Do not leave drugs unlocked, on the side table or on the patient locker. They may be placed on a drug trolley or another dispensing apparatus, or in a cupboard.
- Do not give drugs from memory; a drug chart must always be used.
- Do not give a drug from a container that is not correctly labelled.
- Do not give a drug prepared by someone else.
- Do not return an unused dose to a stock bottle.
- Unused drugs may be returned to the pharmacy, where they will be checked and used for another patient. Drugs returned by outpatients should be destroyed.

Correct disposal of drugs should always be adhered to and disposed of in a timely manner.

DOSAGE CALCULATIONS

Patients may be prescribed doses of a drug not precisely equivalent to a single tablet, ampoule or a 5 mL spoonful. In this case, it is necessary to calculate the quantity of drug preparation that contains the dose prescribed, and this is a common source of error in drug administration. The ward pharmacist should always be asked to annotate the prescription with the precise quantity of drug preparation, which will contain the prescribed dose. If the dose must be given before the ward pharmacist has seen the prescription, then any calculation made must be checked by a second person, and if there remains any doubt, advice must be sought before the drug is administered. Remember that the most common error when calculating drug dosage is a misplaced decimal point, i.e. the patient receives 10 times too much or only one-tenth of the dose, either of which could cause problems for the patient.

The ability to calculate drug dosages accurately and safely is an important responsibility and a useful resource in this regard is Lapham's (2015) *Drug calculations for nurses: a step-by-step approach.* Many universities which provide nurse training provide their own in-house learning resources.

AIDS TO TAKING ORAL DRUGS

- Ensure the patient is sitting up whenever possible, to facilitate swallowing.
- Prepare a drink before giving the drug and see that an adequate amount of fluid is taken with the drug, to prevent oesophageal irritation/ulceration.
- Liquid preparations are given via an oral syringe. Soluble tablets should be dissolved completely before giving them. If a patient has difficulty holding a tablet, it can be administered by a tablet dispenser.
- If a patient has difficulty swallowing a tablet, remove it, give a drink and try again. Many drugs can be prepared and given in liquid form if necessary. Do not crush or dissolve a drug that does not have instructions to do so, as it will damage the integrity of the drug.
- If a drug tastes unpleasant, it may be followed by a flavoured drink or mouthwash.

Although many drugs will be given orally, the nurse will also be required to administer some medicines by other routes including by injection, rectal or vaginal routes. In all cases the above rules must be followed.

Rectal Medicines

These are given in suppository form using protective gloves and a small amount of lubricant to ease insertion. It is important that the method is explained to the patient beforehand and that correct positioning is used with the patient lying on his or her left side with hips and knees flexed. It has been shown that insertion of the blunt end of the suppository aids comfort and retention. Long-term treatment may be given by this route, in which case patients can be taught self-administration most effectively.

Vaginal Medicines

Vaginal pessaries and creams are inserted with the patient lying on her side or back. Clean (rather than sterile) gloves are satisfactory, except during labour or after delivery, when sterile gloves are preferred to prevent ascending infection. A lubricant is used and the drug inserted into the posterior fornix of the vagina. In some circumstances, a pad may be worn after insertion as leakage can occur. Again, patients can be instructed on self-medication by this method. Pessaries are best inserted last thing at night as they tend to become dislodged. Many women are able and prefer to administer pessaries themselves.

Injections

The nurse will be responsible for giving drugs by intradermal, subcutaneous and intramuscular routes. Qualified nurses may give drugs intravenously through an established route. Fractional dosage may be required in these circumstances and careful calculation is vital as errors in dose measurement can occur, the danger of this being compounded by the more rapid action of drugs by injection. When giving injections, sterile equipment must be used and strict aseptic techniques observed. Local guidelines for skin cleansing before an injection should be followed – there is varying research showing little benefit to this when giving a subcutaneous or intramuscular injection. However, where the skin is contaminated or the balance of flora changed, as in debilitated patients, cleansing of the skin may be necessary. If used, the alcohol should be allowed to dry before inserting the needle.

Intradermal Injection. The two most common reasons for giving intradermal injections are testing for sensitivity to allergens and immunization. In the former case, there is risk of an anaphylactic reaction, so adrenaline (epinephrine) should be readily available. A very small amount of fluid (≤0.1 mL) is given using a 1 mL syringe, graduated in 0.1 mL divisions, through a short, fine needle (26 gauge × ⅜-inch, Fig. 2.1). This is introduced just under the skin at an angle of 10 to 15 degrees, which will raise a small weal. The area should not be massaged after removing the needle. The usual site of injection is the lightly pigmented area of the forearm, where the reaction can be easily observed.

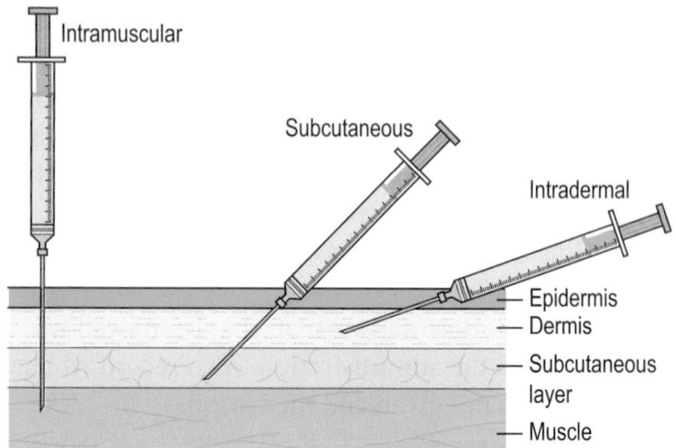

Fig. 2.1 The position of the needle for intramuscular, subcutaneous and intradermal injections.

CLINICAL NOTE

This form of injection is usually performed by a specialist nurse in a controlled environment.

Subcutaneous Injection. A subcutaneous injection is given into the fatty layer just under the skin (see Fig. 2.1). Small amounts of fluid are injected (0.5–2 mL) using a 25 gauge × {15/16}-inch needle. A fold of skin is raised between the thumb and forefinger and the needle is inserted at an angle of 45 degrees (see Fig. 2.1). After insertion, the plunger is withdrawn slightly to ensure a blood vessel has not been entered. If this occurs, the needle should be removed, pressure applied to the area and a new injection prepared. For injections of heparin or insulin, shorter needles are used. These may be the very short, fine needles integral with insulin syringes or 25 gauge × ⅝-inch needles. In these instances, the needle enters the skin at 90 degrees. The area is not massaged after withdrawing the needle, but firm pressure is used to prevent haematoma formation when heparin is given and to ensure uniform absorption rates in patients

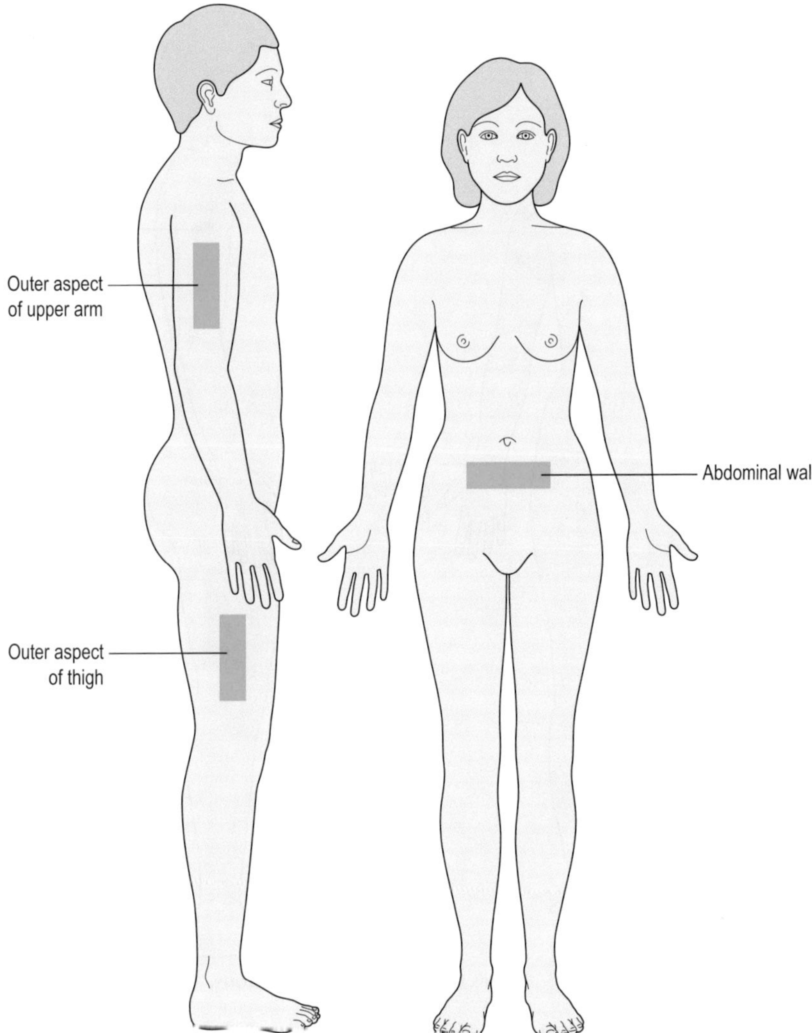

Fig. 2.2 ■ Sites for subcutaneous injections.

with diabetes. Other modifications which may be made when giving insulin are discussed on Chapter 16.

The usual sites for subcutaneous injections are the outer aspect of the upper arm, the outer aspect of the upper thigh and the skin of the abdominal wall (Fig. 2.2). Patients injecting subcutaneous insulin should rotate their injection sites to prevent complication of lipodystrophy (abnormal fat distribution), which can subsequently interfere with insulin absorption.

Intramuscular Injection. This is given into muscle, so larger amounts can be injected, e.g. 1–5 mL (Fig. 2.3). The best site is the outer aspect of the thigh, locating the area in the middle third of the space between the knee and greater trochanter of the femur. The upper outer quadrant of the buttock is also used (see Fig. 2.3). It is vital to determine the sites carefully, to avoid damage to the sciatic nerve and major blood vessels. Alternatively, the upper outer aspect of the arm may be used if the muscle is big enough. To aid relaxation, the patient should be positioned comfortably; for buttock injections, either lying on the abdomen with the toes turned in or lying on the side with the lower leg extended and the upper leg flexed. For thigh injections, the limb

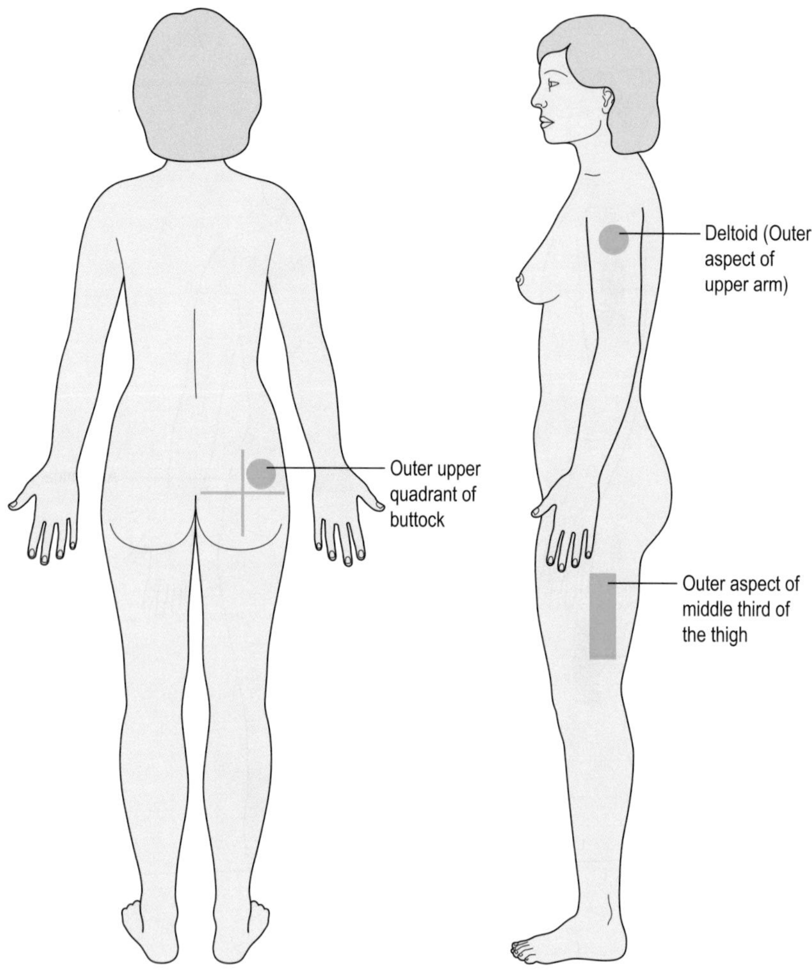

Fig. 2.3 Sites for intramuscular injections.

should be slightly flexed and supported. When giving an intramuscular injection, the skin is held taut and a 21 gauge × 1½-inch needle introduced at 90 degrees (see Fig. 2.1). As in the subcutaneous technique, the plunger is withdrawn to check for inadvertent puncturing of a blood vessel. The fluid is then injected slowly, the needle withdrawn quickly, pressure applied initially and then the area massaged gently.

CLINICAL NOTE

When preparing injections, care should be taken to prevent skin contamination, as contact dermatitis can occur. Hands must be cleansed thoroughly before and after the procedure. Drugs may be absorbed by the skin and so care in preparation should be observed. Special precautions are taken when using cytotoxic drugs.

When injecting substances that cause skin discolouration, such as iron, the Z-track method can be used. In this technique, the skin is pulled to one side before inserting the needle, and a few seconds are allowed to elapse before it is withdrawn, at which point the skin is released, thus achieving the Z-track.

Intravenous Injections and Additives. From 2020, responsibility for drug administration by the intravenous route is the responsibility of all registered nurses and will be part of pre-registration nurse education in the UK. It has been estimated that 12% of patients have an intravenous infusion at some time during their stay in hospital, usually for one or more of the following reasons: fluid replacement treatment, drug treatment, monitoring central venous pressure, hyperalimentation or to provide emergency access to a vein. Responsibility for drug administration by the intravenous route is part of the nurse's extended role. The intravenous route is most often used for heparin, cytotoxic medicines and antibiotics. Individual drugs may be given as a bolus or added to the infusion fluid, in which case careful mixing and labelling are vital, and it is important to check that drugs do not interact with each other in the infusion bottle. Intravenous drugs need very careful monitoring and the nurse requires an adequate knowledge of potential side-effects. It is therefore essential that student nurses involved in checking and observing the effects of drugs given by this route are closely supervised. When the flow rate is mechanically controlled, it is still necessary to check independently that the correct dose is being delivered. Any adjustment to dosage must be undertaken only by trained nurses.

Infection is a known hazard of intravenous cannulation and is increased when drugs or additives are given, because the apparatus is handled more often. Patients must therefore be observed for signs of local infection at the site of the cannula and their temperature monitored carefully. Continuous infusion of drugs by a gravity feed infusion apparatus is not very accurate, although the use of a paediatric volume control administration device will render the flow rate more easily controllable.

For accurate dosage, an infusion pump should be used; accurate set up of this pump is essential and regular checking of the pump should be maintained to ensure infusion of drugs is continuous without interruption or interference. Two staff should set up the pump and independently check the infusion rate prior to commencing administration. Many drugs are given by an infusion pump for safety and accuracy.

CLINICAL NOTE

Needle-stick injuries pose an occupational hazard to nurses and may result in the transmission of blood-borne infection – hepatitis B, hepatitis C or, more rarely, HIV. A recent systematic review of 11 articles noted needle-stick injuries were mostly in nurses and noted factors associated with needle-stick injury were age, level of education, number of shifts per month and history of related training (Motaarefi et al., 2016). Risks can be reduced by ensuring that you have received appropriate education and by disposing of the needle and the syringe immediately after use, without attempting to recap the needle, as research studies indicate that recapping is particularly likely to result in injury. All sharps should be placed in a designated container, which should be disposed of when more than two-thirds full. Sharps should never be transported in the hands or in pockets, and hands should never, under any circumstances, be inserted into the sharps container. Injuries, when they occur, should be recorded with local policy and medical opinion should be sought.

Administration of Drugs to Children

Obtaining cooperation from children is very important and a simple, honest explanation helps to achieve this. Children are more likely to take the prescribed drugs from a familiar person and, where appropriate, parents and relatives can actually give them and be observed by the nurses who have prepared them. As paediatric doses are so different from those of adults, it is important for nurses familiar with children's care to be involved in checking medicines, adhering to local policies. Fractional dosage is used and needs careful calculation. Most drugs are given in liquid form, and should be accurately withdrawn from bottles and ampoules. For very young children, a drug dispenser is useful. This is a special 1 mL syringe into which the required dosage is drawn via a special bottle adaptor. With the child sitting up, the dispenser is inserted into his or her mouth with the tip pointing to the inside of the cheek and the plunger is depressed slowly, allowing the drug to be swallowed naturally. For older children, a special graduated syringe is used.

Administration of Drugs to Elderly Patients

Many patients dislike taking oral drugs and it is important to elicit the patient's expectations and beliefs about drugs. A simple explanation should be provided in the first instance. If swallowing tablets proves difficult, it may be possible to prescribe the drug in liquid form; concurrently it may also be important to investigate any new structural problems that may be causing the issue. Support of speech and language therapists should be sought if an issue is detected, as they can help provide assessment and management of safe swallow for individuals (which in turn can reduce harm to patients, e.g. reducing risks of aspiration through use of thickeners if swallowing is impaired). If there is doubt as to whether drugs have been swallowed, inspection of the mouth of the patient may be needed.

DRUGS ADHERENCE

Drugs adherence is the extent to which a patient's actions match the recommendations from the healthcare professional. Previous terminology used was 'medicines concordance' or 'compliance'; however, 'concordance' was a term not clearly understood and 'compliance' was associated too closely with blame. Therefore, 'adherence' is currently the term defining how effectively patients take their drugs. Prescribing recommendations from healthcare professionals maximizes therapeutic effects, alleviates clinical symptoms, minimizes adverse drug events and ensures safe and timeous drugs consumption.

However it is estimated that only 30%–50% of medicines are taken as prescribed, and non-adherence is a major public health issue due to the negative impact on health, and the financial consequences of wasted medicines. The WHO purports that drug non-adherence is one of the biggest threats to health (WHO, 2017). In response to this, a major Europe-wide project is underway to assess in greater depth the prevalence and factors associated with adherence. This assessment will assist clinicians to identify why a patient is not taking drugs and allow strategies to be developed to optimize treatment.

Drug adherence is a complex behaviour which, outside of the hospital environment, is regulated by service users and/or carers. There are a number of factors reported to influence drug adherence (or non-adherence), which include practical, cognitive and socioeconomic factors (WHO, 2003). Practical factors influencing adherence include dexterity to open packs or bottles; cognitive factors include remembering or being able to follow instructions related to taking the medicines; socioeconomic factors are cited as the ability to pay for treatment regimens.

Psychological factors imply that a person's actions will be influenced by how they think, feel and behave. In the context of drug adherence, this suggests that beliefs and attitude about illness and proposed treatment will influence how well a patient will adhere to their drug regimen. Therefore, as a healthcare professional, when prescribing or administering drugs, it is important to understand the patient's perspective and come to a shared understanding about how prescribed treatment can be optimized.

In hospital, the nurse is in an expedient position to fulfil this role by being the person primarily involved in medicine administration and having continued contact with the patient. The aim of developing a shared understanding is to help the patient to gain insight into the way drugs can be used to treat his or her disorder. Implicit in this is the nurse's knowledge of the disease process and drug action. Answering patients' questions will impart a certain amount of information, but this must be accompanied by a more structured approach.

In 2015, NICE published guidance on how to develop a shared understanding of drugs. This involves establishing effective communication and encouraging patients to ask questions about their condition and treatment. Consideration of any factor that may impede understanding is also important. For example, cognitive impairment, intellectual disability, sight/hearing problems or language barriers may hinder the patient's ability to consider the risks, benefits and alternatives to drug treatment. Translators, easy-read materials and written or recorded information may assist communication. Discussing treatment options, adopting a non-judgemental approach and using open-ended questions promote a shared understanding and contributes to optimizing drug adherence.

Illness or drug beliefs may impede a patient's desire to take medicines. Anxiety about the harmful effects of chemicals and addiction to drugs may concern some patients and will hinder learning if not overcome. It is also important to ascertain whether any dietary or bought over-the-counter medicines will interact with prescribed drugs; for example the interaction between grapefruit juice and statins or the concomitant use of antacids with tetracycline reduces absorption rates. At this time, drugs brought in by the patient are seen by the doctor and permission gained, if possible, to dispose of them, explaining the dangers of error if a different regimen is prescribed on discharge.

Drugs advice during transitions of care are often hurried and impeded by the patient's anxiety due to moving from one area of care to another. At this time, it is vital that the healthcare professional ensures that the patient is fully cognizant of the drugs prescribed. Having a family member or carer present, providing written and oral instructions and giving the patient contacts or resources should they wish to clarify any instructions are all important strategies that may reduce adverse drug events due to suboptimal adherence.

CLINICAL NOTE

Around 7%–10% of hospital admissions are related to adverse drug events and a proportion of those are related to medicines' non-adherence (Pirmohamed et al., 2004). Nurses have an important role in drug advice and treatment advice should be given in verbal and written formats, allowing time for the patient to ask questions. Patients should also be advised about what to do when they are unwell and advice may be given according to Sick Day Rules, a Scottish Patient Safety Programme adopted across the UK to minimize adverse drug events during short periods of illness (SPSP, 2019).

PATIENT EDUCATION

CLINICAL NOTE

Self-administration of medicines by patients and or carers during a hospital stay is now encouraged as best practice and the patient/carer should have appropriate training and assessment prior to carrying this out. Training should involve both the nurse and the pharmacist to ensure that the patient and family member are aware of any specific instructions. Drugs information should be given in written and verbal format. Patient information leaflets and websites can assist in educating the patient about their treatment and are useful resources to refer back to, both for the patient as well as for carers who may be involved in administration of the drugs.

Patients vary as to the amount of information they need, so this must be tailored to individual requirements, but should include the following:

1. The name and purpose of the drug, emphasizing its positive effects
2. Frequency and timing of administration according to home routine, including advice about 'as required' drugs
3. Method of administration with explanation where special equipment will be required for routes other than oral
4. Proposed length of treatment – short or long term
5. The importance of not stopping or starting drugs without advice and where to obtain that advice
6. How and where to obtain further supplies and safely dispose of unwanted drugs
7. Adverse effects to be reported and how to carry out special tests and observations to show if they are developing

The aim is to give adequate information without causing unnecessary alarm. Most drugs produce side-effects, some of which are minor, but others are potentially serious. In some cases, it may be possible to advise on the relief of side-effects. If sufficient information is not given, patients may just stop taking the drugs rather than report the adverse effects, or they may stop treatment when symptoms subside, as in the case of, e.g. antibiotic treatment. A well-informed patient able to participate in his or her own care will feel more in control and thus more responsible, contributing to optimum adherence.

CLINICAL NOTES

Adherence to drugs is a particular problem in people living with long-term conditions, e.g. asthma, diabetes, high blood pressure and cardiovascular disease. Living with a long-term condition can affect mood and depressive symptoms can develop, which is known to be a major factor associated with adherence. For others, drug adherence is a far more practical issue: swallowing, poor vision or poor manual dexterity, dislike of inconvenient or embarrassing side-effects (e.g. the need to frequently empty the bladder when treated with diuretics) or apathy resulting from depression. It is important to explore the reasons for non-adherence and try to find solutions that will optimize how drugs are managed.

Missed Doses

The preceding discussion has emphasized the importance of taking drugs in the correct dose, via the correct route and following particular instructions. It has highlighted the problem of non-adherence, which continues to be a major stumbling block in therapeutics. In hospital, the nurse is in a strong position to influence patients' adherence and to provide explanations and allay anxieties as they occur. Time spent listening to patients' ideas and exploring their concerns is helpful to both nurses and patients.

In the community, drug non-adherence is less closely monitored through direct daily observation (unless the drugs are being administered by carers in specific groups of patients) and is likely to occur due to patient's beliefs, miscommunication or perhaps adverse effects of the drug. There are a few exceptions such as opiate dependent patients who take substitute medication, e.g. methadone under observation at the pharmacy or specialized clinic to help improve safety and compliance. Directly observed therapy is also a strategy that has been endorsed by the WHO to improve compliance in patients requiring treatment for tuberculosis. Furthermore, regular blood tests for certain drugs such as anticoagulants, e.g. warfarin or disease modifying drugs, help to closely monitor adherence and if issues are detected, they can be rectified more promptly, which is of importance in helping to ensure drug safety.

Prescribers must remember:

1. It is sensible to choose drugs whose efficacy is unlikely to be affected by the occasional missed dose.
2. Drugs should not be used at the limits of their duration of action – a drug with an intermediate duration of action is more efficacious if taken twice daily rather than stretched to once daily by taking a higher dose.
3. Drugs that are eliminated slowly and accumulate in the body are the least impaired by poor adherence.

Useful Points

1. Drugs prescribed for others should not be taken, even if the problems appear similar.
2. Drugs may deteriorate from moisture if kept in bathroom cabinets.
3. Different drugs should not be put in the same container as errors may occur. The drugs may also interact chemically.
4. All drugs should be kept out of the reach of children, preferably in a locked cupboard. They should never be referred to as 'sweets'.

In all situations, it is useful to have verbal information reinforced by written instructions, as it is well known that anxiety limits retention of information. It is especially important that this is done where there is memory impairment. Instruction should be kept simple; memory aids such as tear-off calendars and recording cards can be of value. Special dose boxes, e.g. the dosette pill dispenser or Nomad trays, which hold up to 1 week's supply of medicines, can be used, but may be too complicated for some patients who still require another person/carer to help.

Containers must be labelled with adequate-sized lettering and/or colour coding. Information on the label as to the purpose of the drug, e.g. 'heart tablets' or 'water tablets', may be helpful for older patients. Braille labels can be used for blind patients.

Drug manufacturers can also contribute to drug adherence by appropriate packaging and presentation of drugs. The container should be easy to open; child-resistant containers are used increasingly, but are very difficult for older patients and those with arthritis to handle. Many people are unaware that ordinary screw-top bottles are available. Caps with wings can be supplied where necessary; the occupational therapist will be able to assess the patient's need and offer other helpful suggestions.

Despite these aids, there will still be some patients who are unable to cope with drug administration independently. In these cases, education of other family members or those involved with the patient's care may need to be counselled. A number of trials of self-administration of drugs in older patients have been carried out in some parts of the country in preparation for discharge from hospital and to improve compliance. These programmes aim to identify individual patient problems well before discharge, but require the total commitment of all staff involved and continued counselling and follow-up in the community. It appears that these programmes have proved useful in training older patients and it may be that special self-administration programmes could have a wider application.

Drug Errors

Occasionally, drug errors are made by nursing staff. Such episodes not only have the potential to cause harm to patients, but also have a serious effect on the self-esteem and confidence of the prescribers and need to be investigated fully and objectively so that any lessons learnt can be used to reduce the risk of future errors. There is increasing evidence that drug errors, like other adverse medical incidents, are often accidents waiting to happen and are more likely to occur in chaotic, disorganized settings.

Reasons for drug errors can be multifold and include:

1. *The patient*: failure to understand self-administration systems; failure to recognize adverse effects when they occur; poor adherence; interactions with self-administered alternative treatment.
2. *The nurse*: failure to take an adequate medication history with particular reference to previous adverse effects; failure to identify the patient correctly; failure to educate the patient adequately; lack of knowledge of the properties and actions of the drug involved; confusion over the names of drugs; errors in calculation or measurement of the dose or in the mode and site of administration.
3. *Organizational*: inadequate control of ordering and storing of drugs; errors in labelling and inaccurate prescriptions; failure to guard constantly against errors; failure to investigate the cause if errors occur or to take steps to prevent their recurrence.

CLINICAL NOTE

The most common reasons for drug error when drugs are given by health professionals are: giving the wrong dose, omitting the drug altogether or giving the wrong drug. Nursing staff should ensure they are competent in drug calculations and if they are unsure of a dose, ask a colleague to independently check the calculation. This should never be done together.

NON-PRESCRIPTION DRUGS

For years, social scientists have been interested in the 'sick role' phenomenon and the factors that cause people to decide they are ill and behave accordingly by taking drugs or going to bed. It has also become apparent that some people visit their doctors more frequently than others, whereas some diagnose themselves as not ill enough to 'trouble' a doctor or nurse but, nevertheless, take some form of drug. Indeed, few households are without some mild form of analgesic or antiseptic. Most people who travel abroad wisely purchase anti-diarrhoeal drugs and every year large numbers of people dose themselves for coughs, motion sickness and constipation.

Healthcare professionals need to know what the patient is taking and this extends to over-the-counter as well as prescribed drugs. Aspirin is widely available, but many people do not realize the full range and potency of its therapeutic effects. Paracetamol, another mild analgesic, can cause severe and fatal liver damage in overdose. Both these drugs are incorporated into numerous proprietary drugs. For example, several branded drugs, e.g. *Anadin* are marketed containing different amounts of aspirin and in some cases paracetamol, with its implications in overdose or if prescribed drugs are also needed. When the nurse assesses the patient on hospital admission or the initial community visit, they should enquire not only about prescribed drugs, but *any* drug and, if possible, see it. The commercial preparation *Lomotil* for diarrhoea contains atropine, which in overdose may cause atropine toxicity or interact with other drugs. Some expectorants induce drowsiness and a few contain appreciable amounts of alcohol. Patients need to be aware of the likely side-effects and actions of these drugs as much as with those which are prescribed.

REFERENCES AND FURTHER READING

Cloete, L., 2015. Reducing medication errors in nursing practice. Nurs Stan. 29, 50–57.

Dowden, A., 2016. The expanding role of the nurse prescriber. Prescriber 27, 24–27.

Edwards, S., Axe, S., 2015. The 10 'R's of safe multidisciplinary drug administration. NursePrescribing 13, 398–406.

Felzmann, H., 2012. Adherence, compliance and concordance: an ethical perspective. NursePrescribing 10, 446–450.

Gielen, S.C., Dekker, J., Francke, A.L., et al., 2014. The effects of nurse prescribing: a systematic review. Int. J. Nurs. Stud. 51 (7), 1048–1061.

Kroezen, M., van Dijk, L., Groenewegen, P.P., Francke, A.L., 2011. Nurse prescribing of medicines in Western European and Anglo-Saxon countries: a systematic review of the literature. BMC Health Serv. Res. 11, 127.

Lapham, R., 2015. In: Drug Calculations for Nurses: A Step-by-step Approach, fourth ed. CRC Press, Boca Raton.

Lowry, M., 2016. Rectal drug administration in adults: how, when, why. Nurs. Times 112, 12–14.

MHRA, 2018. Committee for Safety of Medicines. The Yellow Card System. Medicines and Healthcare Products Regulatory Agency. https://yellowcard.mhra.gov.uk.

Motaarefi, H., Mahmoudi, H., Mohammadi, E., Hasanpour-Dehkordi, A., 2016. Factors associated with needlestick injuries in health care occupations: a systematic review. J. Clin. Diagn. Res. 10 (8), IE01–IE04.

NICE, 2015. Medicines Optimisation: The Safe Use of Medicines to Enable to Best Possible Outcome [NG5]. https://www.nice.org.uk/guidance/ng5/chapter/introduction.

NICE, 2015. Medicines Management in Care Homes [QS85]. http://www.nice.org.uk/guidance/qs85/chapter/quality-statement-6-covert-medicines-administration.

NICE, 2016. Controlled Medicines: Safe Use and Management. https://www.nice.org.uk/guidance/ng46/chapter/recommendations.

Nute, C., 2014. Reducing medication errors. Nurs. Stand. 28, 45–51.

O'Grady, I., 2015. Minimising harm from missed drug doses. Nurs. Times 111, 12–15.

Ogston-Tuck, S., 2014. Subcutaneous injection technique: an evidence-based approach. Nurs. Stand. 28, 53–58.

Peate, I., 2020. Alexander's Nursing Practice. Elsevier, London.

Pirmohamed, M., James, S., Meakin, S., et al., 2004. Adverse drug reactions as cause of admission to hospital: prospective analysis of 18 820 patients. BMJ 329 (7456), 15.

RPS, 2011. Pharmaceutical Issues when Crushing, Opening or Splitting Oral Dosage Forms. Royal Pharmaceutical Society, Edinburgh.

RPS/RCN, 2019. Professional Guidance on the Administration of Medicines in Healthcare Settings. Royal Pharmaceutical Society and Royal College of Nursing. https://www.rpharms.com/Portals/0/RPS%20document%20library/Open%20access/Professional%20standards/SSHM%20and%20Admin/Admin%20of%20Meds%20prof%20guidance.pdf.

SPSP, 2019. Medicines Sick Day Rules Cards. Scottish Patient Safety Programme. https://ihub.scot/improvement-programmes/scottish-patient-safety-programme-spsp/spsp-medicines-collaborative/high-risk-situations-involving-medicines/medicines-sick-day-rules-card.

Stone, M., 2014. Prescribing in patients with dysphagia. NursePrescribing 12 (10), 504–507.

WHO, 2003. Adherence to long term therapies: evidence for action. https://www.who.int/chp/knowledge/publications/adherence_introduction.pdf.

WHO, 2017. The Third WHO Global Patient Safety Challenge. Medication without harm https://www.who.int/initiatives/medication-without-harm.

USEFUL WEBSITES

NHS Professionals. Guidelines for the administration of medicines. https://www.nhsprofessionals.nhs.uk/e-library/useful-information/cg3-guidelines-for-the-administration-of-medicines.

NMC. Standards for prescribing. Nursing and Midwifery Council. https://www.nmc.org.uk/standards/standards-for-post-registration/standards-for-prescribers/standards-for-prescribing-programmes.

NMC. The Code. Nursing and Midwifery Council. https://www.nmc.org.uk/standards/code/read-the-code-online.

3 ADVERSE REACTIONS TO DRUGS, TESTING OF DRUGS AND PHARMACOVIGILANCE

CHAPTER OUTLINE

LEARNING OBJECTIVES

At the end of this chapter, the reader should be able to:

- explain what is meant by type A and type B adverse reactions to drugs, and list the four causes of type B reactions
- explain what is meant by an acute anaphylactic reaction and appreciate the possibility of drug interactions in patients on large numbers of drugs
- list the five main sites in the body where drug interactions can occur
- explain how certain types of drugs such as monamine oxidase inhibitors (MAOIs) are strongly associated with drug and food interactions
- list commonly occuring drug interactions
- give an account of the processes involved in the introduction and testing of new drugs and explain what is meant by Phases I, II and III in clinical trials and what is meant by a double-blind trial
- describe the pivotal role of the nurse in the running of these trials
- explain what is meant by pharmacovigilance and pharmacoeconomics, and how they affect the patient

TYPES OF ADVERSE REACTIONS

During recent years, adverse reactions to drugs have become increasingly common. They are responsible for about 5% of admissions to hospital and occur in 10%–20% of hospital inpatients (Zhang et al., 2009; Davies et al., 2010). This is probably due to the enormous increase in the range and number of drugs now in use. It is particularly important for healthcare practitioners to be aware of the possibility of drug reactions as they may be the first to realize that something is wrong, and so the drug can be stopped promptly following detection of an adverse reaction.

Drugs most commonly causing adverse reactions are:

- Warfarin
- Diuretics
- Digoxin
- Sedatives
- Antibacterials
- Steroids
- Potassium

- Antihypertensives
- Drugs for treatment of Parkinson's disease
- Antineoplastic drugs.

The classification of adverse reactions to drugs can be divided into type A reactions and type B reactions.

- **Type A reactions** are more common and are due to the normal pharmacological actions of the drug, which for various reasons are greater than would normally be expected. They are therefore predictable.
- **Type B reactions** (idiosyncratic) are considerably less common and are unrelated to the drug's normal pharmacological action. They are therefore unpredictable and may not be related to the dose of the drug.

NOMENCLATURE NOTE

In some texts, the terms 'types *C*, *D* and *E*' may be found with reference to adverse effects. These refer not to actual reaction types, but to the characteristic of the reaction. Thus, *C* refers to Continuous chronic occurrences of the reaction, *D* refers to *D*elayed adverse reactions and *E* refers to *E*nd-of-use reactions.

Type A Reactions

They can be due to **incorrect dose** or excessive absorption, which is uncommon; **decreased elimination** of drugs or **undue sensitivity** of organs.

Decreased Elimination

This is due to slower breakdown or poor excretion by the kidneys. This in turn leads to accumulation of the drug in the body and then adverse effects. Examples are the slow breaking down of morphine by the liver in patients with liver damage, causing excess sedation and even coma, and poor elimination of gentamicin by the kidneys in renal failure, causing accumulation of the antibiotic and ototoxicity.

Undue Sensitivity

Undue sensitivity to the action of a drug can produce symptoms of overdose or abnormal responses. Examples include the increased sensitivity of the heart to digoxin, leading to toxicity, in patients with potassium deficiency, and the undue sensitivity of the respiratory centre of the patient with chronic lung disease to opioids, so that normal therapeutic doses cause symptoms of overdose.

This type of reaction is usually related to the dose of the drug and can be relieved if a lower dose is given or the drug is stopped for a time.

Type B Reactions

These are bizarre and unexpected reactions, and are not dose-related. In many cases, the reason for and mechanism of this type of adverse reaction is not known, e.g. chloramphenicol causes severe depression of the bone marrow in about 1:30,000 treatment courses. It is very difficult to relate the adverse effect to the drug when it occurs in such a small proportion of patients.

Among the known causes of type B reactions are:

- Genetic factors
- Host factors
- Environmental factors
- Allergic reactions.

Genetic Factors

A tendency to certain reactions of this type is related to the genetic make-up of the individual. For example, subjects of tissue type HLA-DR3 are more likely to suffer from gold toxicity.

Genetic factors may make the drug act in a completely abnormal way. For example, primaquine, an antimalarial agent, causes breakdown of red blood cells in a number of people of African and Indian descent. This has been shown to be due to a deficiency in the red blood cells of the enzyme glucose-6-phosphate dehydrogenase (G6PD). The same enzyme deficiency is responsible for favism, in which red blood cells break down as a result of eating beans.

Host Factors

Host disease may predispose to a certain adverse reaction. For example, patients with infectious mononucleosis (glandular fever) are liable to get a rash if given ampicillin.

Environmental Factors

These have been little studied, but it is possible in certain individuals that diet, tobacco or alcohol consumption and other, as yet unknown, factors may influence the response to a drug. There are a few examples of drug interactions, which can occur due to ingestion of certain foods. Statin absorption can be altered by grapefruit consumption. Vitamin K-rich foods (e.g. spinach and kale) can antagonize the anticoagulation effects of warfarin, which normally works by inhibiting vitamin K.

Allergic Reactions

Allergy plays an important part in unexpected drug reactions, although here the mechanism is only partially understood.

This type of reaction implies that the patient has been exposed to the drug on some previous occasion. This exposure has resulted in the production of an antibody against the drug. Antibodies are proteins formed in the body as the result of the introduction of a foreign substance (antigen). They often serve a useful purpose, e.g. antibodies formed against bacteria combine with and destroy the bacteria. Several different types of antibodies are produced in response to drugs. Sometimes these antibodies combine with a drug in such a way as to cause damage to tissue and so produce the symptoms of an allergic reaction. Four types are described here:

- **Type I** The antibody (produced in response to a drug) may become attached to the surface of certain cells called 'mast cells', which are scattered throughout the body. If the drug is given on a second occasion, the drug (antigen) and antibody combine on the surface of the mast cells, which are destroyed, liberating substances such as histamine, which causes an acute anaphylactic reaction (see later).
- **Type II** The antibody may become attached to the surface of red blood cells. On second exposure to the drug, the combination occurs on the surface of the red blood cells, which are destroyed, producing a haemolytic anaemia.
- **Type III** Antigens and antibodies may combine in the bloodstream to form immune complexes. They may penetrate various organs, where they are deposited, together with a further substance called 'complement', which is present in the blood. The antigen/antibody/complement combination stimulates inflammation, which may affect the skin, kidneys and other organs.
- **Type IV** Drugs acting as antigens may sensitize lymphocytes, which, on further contact with the antigen, will cause tissue damage. This type of reaction usually causes rashes.

Although the exact mechanism of all allergic reactions is not understood, some form of drug/antibody combination is always involved.

Clinical Disorders Caused by Allergic Reactions

Allergic reactions cause a number of clinical disorders:

- Acute anaphylaxis
- Serum sickness
- Rashes
- Renal disorders
- Other allergies.

Acute Anaphylaxis

This may be caused by certain foods (especially nuts, eggs and fish), by drugs (notably penicillin), by wasp and bee stings, by injection of foreign serum and by contact with latex rubber. The onset is usually rapid.

Mild cases present with urticaria, nausea and coughing. More severe attacks include bronchospasm, facial oedema, hypotension, substernal pain and collapse. Severe anaphylaxis can be fatal.

Treatment. Acute anaphylaxis should be avoided whenever possible. Patients must always be questioned about previous reactions before they are given a drug or a vaccine, especially one such as a flu vaccine, which has been prepared in eggs. Particular care is required with sufferers from certain allergic disorders, notably asthma, hay fever and infantile eczema, as they are more prone to anaphylactic reactions.

The treatment depends on the severity of the reaction, if severe, utilize the following guidelines:

1. The patient should be recumbent.
2. Ensure a clear airway and give 100% oxygen.
3. Give adrenaline (epinephrine) 1:1000 solution 500 micrograms intramuscularly and repeat as required at 5-min intervals.

4. Give hydrocortisone 200 mg intravenously or intramuscularly, although its effect may be delayed.
5. Give chlorphenamine 10 mg intravenously or intramuscularly.
6. Give an intravenous infusion of 500–1000 mL of colloid if circulatory collapse occurs.
7. Use a nebulised bronchodilator (e.g. 5 mg salbutamol) if bronchospasm is marked.
8. Nurses should never leave the patient alone and escalate changes to observations.
9. Follow-up to determine the cause of the reaction and to prevent a recurrence (e.g. specialist referral should be sought and consideration for an adrenaline autoinjector prescribed).

Serum Sickness

This develops about a week after the serum or drug has been administered. There is usually an urticarial rash with stiffness and swelling of joints, sometimes a mild nephritis and lymph node enlargement. Spontaneous recovery is usual, but calamine lotion applied to the rash and oral chlorphenamine, together with prednisolone for a few days in more severe cases, will relieve the symptoms and speed recovery.

Rashes

Rashes may occur as a result of drugs allergy, but not all rashes which occur when drugs are given are due to allergy. An example of a non-allergic drug rash is the typical erythematosus rash, which often occurs when ampicillin is taken for glandular fever.

Renal Disorders

Damage to the glomerulus by several drugs, including penicillamine and gold, can cause gross proteinuria. Non-steroidal antiinflammatory drugs (NSAIDs) and angiotensin-converting enzyme (ACE) inhibitors can cause renal failure and there are a number of other types of drug-induced renal disease.

Other Allergies

Other allergies have been implicated as the cause of various other disorders, including depression of the bone marrow leading to leukopenia, thrombocytopenia and anaemia, haemolysis (breakdown) of red blood cells, jaundice and renal damage. These drug reactions are not always caused by allergic mechanisms and in many cases, the exact way in which a drug damages the tissues and organs is not known.

CLINICAL NOTE

Adverse reactions cannot be eliminated entirely, but they can be minimized by the following:

1. Take a drug history to discover whether patients are already taking drugs and whether they have had adverse effects from drugs in the past.
2. Reduce prescribing to a reasonable minimum number of necessary medicines.
3. Remember that certain patients (i.e. the elderly, those with liver or renal disease) may not handle drugs in the usual way and dose modifications may be required.
4. Monitoring and following up the effect of a drug on a patient is important, this may include therapeutic drug monitoring with some drugs, e.g. digoxin, some antiepileptic drugs and some antibiotics, e.g. gentamicin.
5. Always remember that some unexpected change in a patient's condition may be due to an adverse reaction to a drug.

NURSING NOTE

Safety note: Drugs safety updates are available in the UK. The medicines and Healthcare products Regulatory Agency (MHRA) publish drug safety updates and similar agencies are located in Europe in the form of the European Medicines Agency (EMA) and Federal Drug Agency (FDA) in the USA. These agencies provide up-to-date reports of adverse reactions to drugs and updates on drug–drug interactions.

Looking at a drug chart of an inpatient can often show patients receiving up to half a dozen separate drugs. Polypharmacy, which has become a feature of medical practice, has brought with it the danger that certain drugs may interact, occasionally with disastrous consequences. Dangerous interactions are particularly liable to occur:

- in seriously ill patients because they will probably be taking several drugs at the same time;

- in elderly patients because they may be very sensitive to relatively small changes in the blood concentration of certain drugs;
- when there is only a small difference between the toxic and therapeutic dose of the drug.

Interactions may occur before the drugs enter the body. Intravenous infusions are commonly used, particularly in very ill patients, and two or more drugs may be mixed prior to administration. This commonly occurs in palliative or critical care environments. Some of these drugs may be incompatible in solution, and precipitation or modification may occur. It is therefore very important that when drugs are given via an infusion, they should, wherever possible, be given as a bolus injected into the plastic tubing and flushed into the patient. If drugs have to be mixed in the infusion devices prior to administration, the advice of the pharmacist should be sought.

Sites of Drug Interactions

After administration of drugs, interactions can occur at numerous sites (Fig. 3.1):

- In the gastrointestinal tract
- In the blood
- At the site of action of the drugs
- At the sites of elimination of the drugs:
  - liver
  - kidney

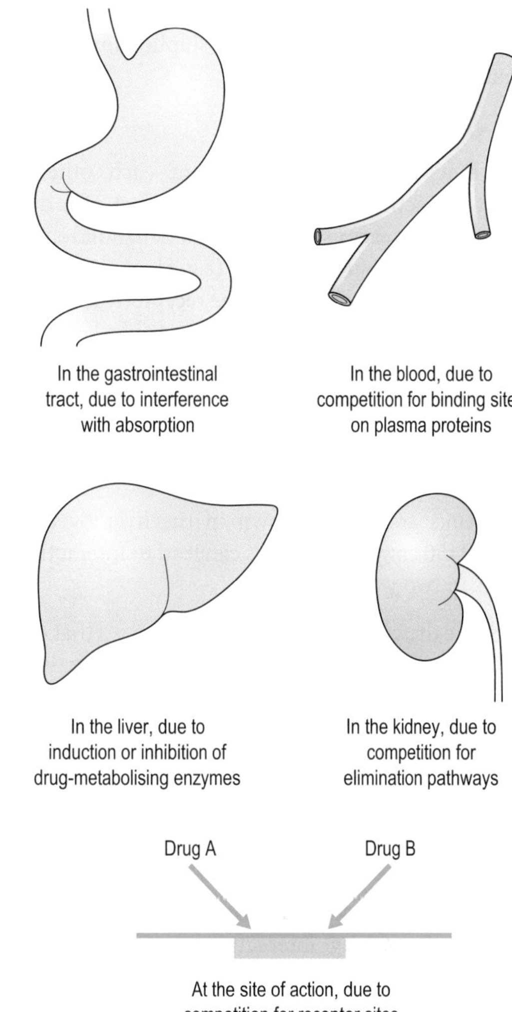
In the gastrointestinal tract, due to interference with absorption
In the blood, due to competition for binding sites on plasma proteins
In the liver, due to induction or inhibition of drug-metabolising enzymes
In the kidney, due to competition for elimination pathways
Drug A
Drug B
At the site of action, due to competition for receptor sites

Fig. 3.1 ■ Main sites at which drug interactions can occur.

The Gastrointestinal Tract

Most drugs are absorbed by diffusion through the gut wall. If a drug which is well absorbed becomes attached to a drug which is poorly absorbed, the well-absorbed drug will be held in the gastrointestinal tract and absorption will be decreased. For example, if tetracycline and iron are given together, the tetracycline is held in the gastrointestinal tract by the iron, which is poorly absorbed.

The Blood

Many drugs are transported partially attached to the plasma proteins and partially free in the blood. Only the free drug can have any pharmacological action. If two drugs A and B that can bind plasma proteins are given together, they may compete for sites of attachment to the carrier plasma protein. Drug A may then be displaced from the carrier sites on the protein by drug B so that there is more drug A available to produce an increased pharmacological action. For example, the anticoagulant warfarin is largely carried by the plasma proteins. If chloral hydrate is given to a patient taking warfarin, the warfarin is displaced from the carrier protein and more of the free warfarin becomes available, resulting in increased pharmacological action (anticoagulation) and bleeding.

Drugs which will displace others from the plasma protein include NSAIDs, sulphonamides and tolbutamide.

At the Site of Action

Drugs may antagonize or augment each other at their site of action: for example, the effect of a drug depressing the nervous system (e.g. a benzodiazepine) enhanced by another depressant (e.g. alcohol).

There may be antagonism at the receptors: for example, β-agonists (e.g. salbutamol) and β-blockers (e.g. propranolol) compete for receptors in the walls of the bronchi and thus produce bronchodilatation or bronchoconstriction, depending on their relative concentrations.

At Sites of Elimination

Many drugs are broken down in the liver by cytochrome P450 enzymes and this can lead to interactions of drugs in two ways:

- Some drugs cause enzyme induction, so that other drugs are broken down by the same enzymes more rapidly and their effect is consequently decreased. Phenytoin, rifampicin and erythromycin are powerful enzyme inducers.
- Some drugs can suppress enzyme activity. The antibiotic chloramphenicol is an enzyme suppressor.

Monoamine Oxidase Inhibitors. One of the most important drug–drug interactions involves another class of enzymes called 'monoamine oxidases' that break down some naturally occurring substances such as adrenaline and noradrenaline (referred to as catecholamines). There are a group of drugs that inhibit these enzymes, called 'monoamine oxidase inhibitors' (MAOIs), which are used to treat depression. If patients receiving MAOIs are given certain drugs or even foods containing amines, these substances will accumulate in the body and cause an abrupt and serious rise in blood pressure.

Drug examples:	**Food examples:**
Adrenaline (epinephrine)	Cheese
Noradrenaline (norepinephrine)	Broad beans
Amphetamine	Marmite and Bovril

In addition, the effects of some drugs are potentiated, particularly those of:

- pethidine (meperidine)
- barbiturates
- anaesthetics.

Drugs may also be excreted via the kidney and in many cases they are passed through the renal tubule cell into the urine. At this site, competition can occur. Perhaps the best-known examples are probenecid and penicillin, both of which are excreted via the renal tubule cells. Probenecid blocks the excretion of penicillin and this fact is used when very high levels of penicillin are required. Similarly, thiazide diuretics block the renal excretion of lithium and small increases in blood levels of lithium lead to severe and dangerous toxicity.

Important Interactions

The number of drug reactions which have been described is now very large and many of them are of little or no clinical importance. In general, those interactions which are important will occur when the dose of a drug is critical and a small change in the blood concentration or the patient's sensitivity to the drug results in toxicity or, conversely, a lack of therapeutic effect. It is impossible for the nurse or doctor to remember them all, but most of the important ones of concern are:

ACE inhibitors	Rifampicin
Lithium	Digoxin
Anticoagulants/ warfarin	Theophylline
Oral contraceptives	Erythromycin
β-Blockers	Hypoglycaemic agents
Phenytoin	Cimetidine

When these drugs are being given to a patient, the possibility of interactions must be considered if further drugs are added to the treatment regimen.

CLINICAL NOTE

Patients in the community may be taking over-the-counter drugs, including items such as dietary supplements and herbal remedies, which they do not think of as drugs. Emerging evidence suggests there are serious and often unpredictable drug–herbal interactions that may affect patients choosing to take herbal remedies in addition to, or instead of, licensed medicines (Parvez and Rishi, 2019) For example, patients would not consider alcohol as a drug, but nevertheless it can cause serious interactions and should therefore be avoided when certain drugs are taken (Chan and Anderson, 2014).

- **Disulfiram**, **griseofulvin**, **procarbazine**, **metronidazole** and **chlorpropamide** interfere with the metabolism of alcohol, causing flushing, headaches, sweating and nausea.
- **Hypnotics** and **sedatives** are potentiated by alcohol.
- **Warfarin's** anticoagulant action is enhanced with an acute overdose of alcohol.
- **MAOIs** can precipitate a hypertensive crisis, particularly with Chianti.
- **Metformin** carries a risk of lactic acidosis with alcohol.
- **Aspirin and other NSAIDs** carry an increased risk of gastric bleeding, although this risk is small and many people take alcohol and aspirin without disaster.

CLINICAL NOTE

Charts are available which show the most important interactions and it is good practice to display these in every ward and outpatient department. If you are accessing online prescribing or administration charts, then you will be alerted electronically to interactions. Research suggests that these alerts can be overridden and quickly bypassed when prescribing and administering drugs (Bell et al., 2019). Do not ignore these alerts; act on them and ensure you assess the patient when administering the drug.

Beneficial Interactions

Not all interactions are harmful and some are used deliberately to enhance a therapeutic effect. For example, antibiotics may be combined to increase their efficacy and/or prevent the emergence of bacterial resistance, as in the combination of drugs used to treat tuberculosis. In hypertension, two agents acting in different ways (e.g. ACE inhibitors and diuretics) help to reduce blood pressure.

THE INTRODUCTION AND TESTING OF NEW DRUGS

There are two ways in which newly introduced drugs can be licensed for use in the UK.

The European Agency for the Evaluation of Medicinal Products (EMEA), which is based in London, covers all member states in the European Union, and is the only agency that can approve biotechnical products as well as other drugs.

Most countries also have their own licensing bodies. In the UK, this is the Medicines and Healthcare Regulatory Authority (MHRA) and in the USA it is the Food and Drug Administration (FDA). There are increasing attempts to share data on drugs between regulatory authorities and to harmonize the development of drugs.

The introduction of a new drug is a costly and protracted affair. It takes about 10–12 years from the time a chemical entity is discovered until its marketing approval to be used as a therapeutic agent. Most recent estimates are that it costs up to one billion US dollars to develop a new drug.

In the past, many substances were screened for an action which could be useful in treating disease. With greater understanding of the nature of drug action, it is now possible to design drugs which might be expected to have the desired effect. These are then synthesized in the laboratory. Certain proteins are very complex and difficult to synthesize, but this can be achieved by biotechnology. Genes responsible in human or animal cells for the manufacture of specific substances, such as hormones, can be introduced into bacteria or yeasts, which then produce these substances in large quantities. When harvested, they can be used therapeutically. Human insulin and growth hormone are produced in this way. The drugs are then tested in animals to ensure that they have the required pharmacological action at dose levels that do not have toxicity.

All drugs have to be thoroughly tested for toxic effects, which is done in two stages for acute and chronic toxicity. In the latter stage the drug has to be administered for up to 28 days to two species of animal (a rodent and a non-rodent) and the toxicity determined, including examining whether there are any histological changes in the various tissues and organs

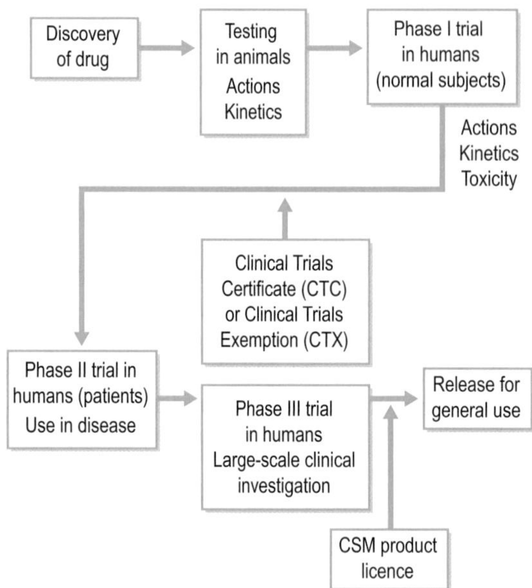

Fig. 3.2 ■ Stages in introducing a new drug, indicating when licences are required. A clinical trials certificate (CTC) requires full information about a drug. CSM, the Committee on Safety of Medicines.

of the body at postmortem. Only if this testing shows satisfactory results is the drug given to humans (Fig. 3.2). If the early clinical trials show promise with a new drug, further animal toxicity studies may be required to establish whether the drug produces any fetal abnormalities in pregnant animals or an increased risk of developing cancer after long-term use. There are three phases of drug testing in humans:

- **Phase I** The first time a new drug is used in humans typically involves administering ascending doses of the drug to young and healthy volunteers, starting with very small doses which are then increased until some adverse effect is observed. The subjects are kept under close observation either in hospital or in a special unit. Safety is evaluated and measurements are made of the various actions of the drug, and estimation of blood levels determine the rate and degree of absorption and elimination. The Phase I trial determines the highest safe dose that can be subsequently used in further clinical trials.
- **Phase II** If the preliminary studies are satisfactory, permission must be obtained from the licensing authority for limited clinical trials of the new drug in relevant patients groups to find out whether the drug is useful in treating disease. About 250 patients are involved in Phase II studies. Often studies undertaken during Phase II are 'blinded' to help reduce bias.
- **Phase III** If these Phase II trials are successful, then two larger clinical trials involving several thousands of patients are undertaken to confirm the safety and efficacy of the drug using pre-approved clinical end-points.

Only after this process will a product licence be given, which allows the use of the drug in patients, although the licensing authority may require a so-called **Phase IV** post-marketing surveillance study to gain further evidence on the effectiveness and possible adverse effects.

It is important to note, however, that at the point of approval of the new drug, only a few thousand patients will have been exposed to the drug, which may not have been sufficient to pick up rarer or idiosyncratic adverse reactions and therefore it is important to have ongoing surveillance of new drugs, and some drugs are actually withdrawn even after approval as more is understood about the safety of the drug used in wider populations.

Post-marketing Surveillance and Pharmacovigilance

Voluntary Adverse Reaction Reporting

Practising healthcare professionals and dentists are asked to fill in a yellow card or an online reporting advice form to regulatory authorities if they suspect an adverse reaction to a drug. For older drugs, only severe or unusual reactions should be reported, but for recently introduced drugs, designated by a black triangle in the *British National Formulary,* doctors should report any unusual effect. This method is limited by under-reporting and probably only 5%–10% of these untoward reactions are recorded on the yellow cards.

CLINICAL NOTE

Suspected adverse drug reactions can be reported by healthcare professionals, service users and carers. Therefore, healthcare professionals should be aware of types of adverse reactions and when to report. Member states of the World Health Organization created a central reporting system and, to date, have over 3 million reports of adverse drug reactions (WHO, 2020) All verbalized drug and food sensitivities should be recorded in the patients clinical notes. It is every member of staff's responsibility to document allergies reported by the patient.

A Study of the National Statistics

Statistics such as causes of death may, rarely, give a clue to some adverse reactions, an example being the rise in sudden deaths in young people suffering from asthma, which was probably due to overuse of pressurized inhalers containing isoprenaline, in the 1960s. Another is the withdrawal of COX-2 inhibitors used for the treatment of the pain associated with arthritis that caused unwanted cardiovascular side-effects and sometimes death.

Monitored Release and Prescription Event Monitoring

When a new drug is released for the first time for general use it may be limited to certain doctors, who are asked to report any untoward reactions. Alternatively, the names of doctors who are using a certain drug can be obtained from prescription returns and they may be asked specifically whether they have noticed any untoward event in a patient. This method may become popular as a means of following up a newly introduced drug when it is released. It depends, however, on the collaboration of the doctors concerned, who must be willing to fill in the appropriate reports.

Cohort Studies

This method involves a large number of patients, who are divided (randomly, if possible) into a group taking the drug and a control group. They are then monitored for a long period and the frequency of adverse effects compared between the two groups. Although the results can be useful, it is very expensive and laborious.

Case–Control Studies

This method captures a cluster of patients with similar symptoms, which have occurred for no obvious reason; the possible causes are then investigated. One problem with this technique is that even if taking a certain drug is a common factor, it does not prove that it is the cause of the symptoms.

Record Linkage

This method involves studying the medical records of groups of patients over very long periods to ascertain whether delayed adverse effects emerge.

None of these methods is by any means perfect and, in spite of much effort, adverse effects still pose a difficult problem. One of the most important factors in early detection is from effective history taking by healthcare professionals. History taking is key in relating an adverse effect to a drug reaction, rather than a presenting symptom of a distinct disease.

Therapeutic Trials

In the past, opinion as to the usefulness of a drug depended on impression and anecdote. As a result, many drugs in common use were worthless, some of them having no therapeutic effect at all. One important advance has been the introduction of the randomized controlled clinical trial as a means of assessing the true value of a drug.

Defining the Question

First of all, the question to be answered by the trial should be defined. For example, it may be a simple one such as the prolongation of life or the cure of a disease; or it may be a more difficult question such as the relief of anxiety or improved quality of life. The challenge is then to determine what constitutes quality of life and how to measure it, or to determine what is an acceptable level of anxiety and how to measure it. In these cases, psychometric scales are commonly used.

Trial Design

It is not always easy to assess the efficacy of a drug in practice and its trial requires careful planning. Patients in the population to be studied are randomly allocated to one of two groups. One group receives the drug under trial and the other group, namely the control group, receives a placebo (a placebo being an inert substance similar in appearance to the drug that is being tested) or possibly another active drug against which the trial drug is being compared. This is necessary because suggestion plays a considerable part in the relief of certain symptoms and may be responsible for some apparent therapeutic action of a drug.

The usefulness of the active drug is then compared with the placebo by noting the beneficial effect in both groups. It is also important that the nurses and doctors who are looking after the patients during the trial do not know who is receiving the active drug and who the placebo, as even they may bias the result by unconsciously communicating their hopes and fears to the patients. This is known as a 'double-blind trial'.

The trial is designed so that the number of subjects involved is sufficient to give a clear answer as to the drug's efficacy. When completed, the results are subjected to statistical analysis, which will allow an estimation of the drug's therapeutic value.

CLINICAL NOTE

Nurses play a key role in research and should be aware of any drug trial that their patients may be undergoing. Documentation of the trial drug and continued compliance to the trial parameters is essential.

The Placebo Response

A placebo drug may be defined as a substance which has no pharmacological action but which, when used, produces a therapeutic effect.

There is now good evidence that with a wide variety of symptoms, including pain, cough, headache, etc., the administration of an inert substance (the placebo) will produce marked improvement in about 30% of subjects. It is important to realize that this does not mean that the patient's symptoms were imaginary. The mechanism whereby this improvement is produced is not known, but is obviously connected with the powers of suggestion.

The placebo effect has a number of important implications:

- It is possible in some patients to control symptoms without using active drugs.
- In assessing the effectiveness of new drugs, the placebo response must be remembered and, as far as possible, excluded.
- Further study of the placebo response might be useful in opening up new methods of treatment of symptoms by suggestion, thus making it possible to relieve symptoms without resorting to pharmacologically active drugs.

Meta-Analysis

Even with a well-designed controlled trial it is not always certain whether a particular new drug is more effective than those in current use. This is usually because the differences between the treated and control groups are small and the number of patients involved is not large enough to give a clear result.

To further assess the effectiveness of any drug, the technique of meta-analysis has been introduced. This takes an overview of all properly controlled randomized trials of a particular drug or treatment. This technique has become very sophisticated and gives useful information and guidance as to the best treatment in certain clinical circumstances. For example, meta-analysis of the trials in the use of streptokinase in coronary thrombosis has firmly established that it reduces mortality.

Risk–Benefit Analysis

When a drug is licensed for use to treat a patient, it is important to consider the benefits which will result from its use and the possible risks involved.

When granting a product licence, regulatory authorities need to be convinced not only that the new drug is effective but also that the risks entailed in its use are acceptable in the context of the disease being treated (e.g. greater risks are reasonable for an anti-cancer drug than for a hypnotic or yet another H1 receptor antagonist). It is essential that prescribers explain clearly to the patient the benefits and possible adverse effects of any drug they prescribe.

It may not be easy for nurses to obtain up-to-date information about drugs, but prescribers should have a current edition of the *British National Formulary* available and should use (if possible) drugs which are frequently administered in the prescriber's clinical setting.

Ethics Committees

Trials of new drugs, like all research studies involving people, must be approved by an independent ethics committee before commencement. Committee membership involves a wide medical representation and, in addition, nursing and lay members, who often include experts in law. Their main task is to protect participants from unnecessary risk, to ensure every safeguard is provided and that individuals are fully informed about the purpose of the research, and of their rights to refuse or withdraw permission to take part in research. Committees also see that participants in research receive proper compensation if something goes wrong. Increasingly, ethics committees assume the responsibility of criticizing, if necessary, the design of the research and ascertaining that the work is worth doing.

Generic Prescribing

When a new drug is introduced it is given two names: a generic (approved) name and a brand name applied by the pharmaceutical manufacturer. If a drug is prescribed by its brand name, the pharmacist must dispense that brand.

On introduction, there is usually only a single brand of a drug, so the generic and brand names apply to the same product. However, when the patent expires (after 20 years), several manufacturers may produce a particular drug, each giving it a different brand name.

For many years there has been a move to use generic names only and to abolish brand names. This would eliminate the confusion due to a drug having several different names and would reduce the cost, particularly after the patent has expired. Against this it is argued that different brands may differ in quality and the doctor should know which brand is being dispensed. Also, it would reduce the profitability of the drug to the company which had introduced it and had spent millions of pounds on its development.

FORMULARIES

Formularies and pharmacopoeias were originally introduced as reference books and were mainly concerned with the preparation and composition of drugs in an attempt to achieve some uniformity of composition. The first formulary in England was published by the Royal College of Physicians in 1618. Since then, formularies have become more concerned with which drugs are available or approved and their actions and uses.

The *British National Formulary* (BNF)

The BNF lists the drugs and pharmacological preparations available in the UK together with indications for their use, dosage, adverse effects and cost. It also includes notes on the treatment of many conditions and useful guidance on a variety of problems encountered when using drugs. A copy should be available in every ward, outpatient department and doctor's surgery. It is also available online and may be accessed by members of the public. There is no charge.

The BNF is updated twice a year. The BNF, however, is not selective: for example, the current edition lists at least 10 β-blockers, and it is obviously wasteful and extravagant for a hospital pharmacy to stock all of these. A number of hospital trusts and clinical commissioning groups (CCGs) have constructed their own formularies, which list the drugs available in the pharmacy, chosen on the basis of efficacy and cost; these may also contain background information. Local formularies have reduced prescribing costs and have had some educational benefits by stimulating interest in rational and sensible prescribing.

PHARMACOECONOMICS

In recent years there has been concern over the rising cost of health care. This has to some extent been caused by an increase in the number of elderly people, the introduction of new and more costly methods of treatment, and the increased expectations from medical care.

In the UK, the drug bill, at approximately 10% of the NHS budget, is the third largest area of NHS expenditure. The available resources are insufficient to meet all needs and so various attempts are being made to control this expenditure. Methods used include increasing the patient's contribution to the drug costs (i.e. raising prescription charges); introducing restrictive formularies, which evaluate drugs and indicate which are considered most useful in patient care, i.e. 'best value for money'; limiting the drugs prescribable on the NHS; appointing pharmaceutical advisers who help general practitioners to prescribe in a cost-effective manner; and through the work of the National Institute for Clinical Excellence (NICE).

Pharmacoeconomics has emerged as a branch of health economics relating specifically to the area of drug usage. It is a tool that allows the comparative assessment of the costs and consequences of various uses for the available resources. Choices have to

TABLE 3.1

Four Types of Pharmacoeconomic Evaluation

Type of Analysis	Definition
Cost-minimization	Determines the least costly of two interventions that produce clinically identical outcomes
Cost-effectiveness	Costs[a] are compared with outcomes measured in natural units; for example, per life saved, per symptom-free day
Cost-utility	Costs[a] are compared with outcomes measured in 'utility-based' units - that is, quality adjusted life years
Cost-benefit	Places monetary values on both costs and outcomes

[a]All relevant costs are measured in monetary terms.

be made, as resources used for one treatment cannot be used for another; pharmacoeconomics provides a framework to aid the decision-making process. Resource allocation does not only limit costs, but should maximize the benefit received from the use of these resources.

All healthcare workers, administrators and the pharmaceutical industry will increasingly need to participate in the practical application of pharmacoeconomics. This will be important as audit and the development of treatment protocols begin to define what should be used, how it should be used and who should receive it. This will move the emphasis of drug decision-making away from acquisition costs and therapeutic efficacy towards the total effect of drug treatment on the life of the patient.

The four main types of pharmacoeconomic evaluation, differing in how the consequences (outcomes) are measured, are (Table 3.1):

- cost-minimization
- cost-effectiveness
- cost–utility
- cost–benefit analysis.

Each of these methods involves the systematic identification, measurement and, where appropriate, valuation of all relevant costs and consequences of the treatment options under review. The costs and benefits will vary according to the viewpoint used in the analysis, for example, the patient or the hospital. The broadest viewpoint is that of 'society in general'.

CASE HISTORY 3.1

Mr. H had suffered from rheumatoid arthritis for over 20 years. He had previously had operations on both his hands and both feet to insert artificial knuckles. His doctor had recommended knee replacements for both knees, but Mr. H declined. He was on methotrexate injections (15 mg subcutaneously per week), folic acid and low-dose prednisolone (5 mg three times a week) and Celebrex (celecoxib) when needed. The arthritis was clearly not controlled and he had frequent flares. His consultant rheumatologist decided to apply to the local health authority to use infliximab and, after reviewing his history, it was agreed that he should be given a course of infliximab. He was admitted as a day-case patient for infusion, and, after routine urine tests and blood pressure, was given a bed and cleared for intravenous infusion of infliximab, which took 2 hours. He was kept in hospital for a further 2 hours and then allowed to go home. After the first infusion of infliximab Mr. H reported a remarkable effect and said he had not felt so free from stiffness and pain for years. He has infliximab infusions every 2 months and to-date has suffered no ill effects.

Pharmacoeconomics may seem at first to readers to be an interesting, if somewhat academic, concept until the implications for the patient are experienced in the clinical situation, and this is best exemplified by an actual case history (see Case History 3.1).

This case history is an example of pharmacoeconomics in action. Clearly the dramatic effects of drugs such as infliximab will produce an intense demand for the drug and decisions will be made on the basis both of need and of economic realities until the price of newer 'biologic' drugs such as infliximab comes down. The long-term effects of these drugs still need to be discovered, and that will also be factorized into the decision once these effects are known. The needs of the patient should come first, and this principle should be put before all other considerations. Unfortunately, the practice of 'postcode' prescribing has dictated that the drugs the patient gets depends on where that patient happens to live. Decisions about whether to provide expensive treatments have been taken locally by regional or district health authorities, and patients in one part of the country might get a particular drug that patients in another might not. This, understandably, has generated a great deal of anguish and anger.

Given the increasing cost of modern drugs, it is not surprising that disciplines such as pharmacoeconomics have come into being.

The decision to approve infliximab involved not only the patient's history but also the cost of the treatment, which is probably in excess of £8000 per annum. This excludes the costs to the hospital for providing the bed, labour and resources made available. The doctor's decision was in-line with the NICE guidance for the use of infliximab (see the BNF).

REFERENCES AND FURTHER READING

Ainsworth, S., 2006. Medicines on trial: TGN 1412 and the implications for future drug testing. NursePrescribing 4 (3), 121–123.

Bell, H., Garfield, S., Khosla, S., et al., 2019. Mixed methods study of medication-related decision support alerts experienced during electronic prescribing for inpatients at an English hospital. Eur. J. Hosp. Pharm. 26 (6), 318–322.

Cadogan, C.A., Ryan, C., Hughes, C.M., 2016. Appropriate polypharmacy and medicine safety: when many is not too many. Drug Saf. 39 (2), 109–116.

Chan, L.N., Anderson, G.D., 2014. Pharmacokinetic and pharmacodynamic drug interactions with ethanol (alcohol). Clin. Pharmacokinet. 53 (12), 1115–1136.

Davies, E.C., Green, C.F., Mottram, D.R., et al., 2010. Emergency readmissions to hospital due to adverse drug reactions within 1 year of the index admission. Br. J. Clin. Pharmacol. 70 (5), 749–755.

Farre, A., Heath, G., Shaw, K., et al., 2019. How do stakeholders experience the adoption of electronic prescribing systems in hospitals? A systematic review and thematic synthesis of qualitative studies. BMJ Qual. Saf. 28 (12), 1021–1031.

Green, L., 2011. Explaining the role of the nurses in clinical trials. Nurs. Stand. 25 (22), 35–39.

Hughes, D.A., 2012. Pharmacoeconomics. Br. J. Clin. Pharmacol. 73 (6), 968–972.

Kaufman, G., 2016. Polypharmacy: the challenge for nurses. Nurs. Stand. 30 (39), 52–60.

Keers, R.N., Williams, S.D., Cooke, J., Ashcroft, D.M., 2013. Causes of medication administration errors in hospitals: a systematic review of quantitative and qualitative evidence. Drug Saf. 36 (11), 1045–1067.

Parvez, M.K., Rishi, V., 2019. Herb–drug interactions and hepatotoxicity. Curr. Drug Metab. 20 (4), 275–282.

Patton, K., Borshoff, D.C., 2018. Adverse drug reactions. Anaesthesia 73 (Suppl. 1), 76–84.

Powrie, K., 2018. Identification and management of drug allergy. Nurs. Stand. 33 (1), 45–50.

WHO, 2020. World Health Organization, Upsala Monitoring Centre. https://www.who-umc.org.

Zhang, M., Holman, C.D., Price, S.D., et al., 2009. Comorbidity and repeat admission to hospital for adverse drug reactions in older adults: retrospective cohort study. BMJ 338, a2752.

USEFUL WEBSITES

Adverse Drug Reactions. https://www.blackwellpublishing.com/content/BPL_Images/Content_store/Sample_chapter/9780632045860/cobertsample.pdf.

BMA. https://www.bma.org.uk/ap.nsf/Content/AdverseDrugReactions.

European Medicines Agency. https://www.ema.europa.eu/en/human-regulatory/post-authorisation/pharmacovigilance/periodic-safety-update-reports-psurs.

MHRA. https://www.gov.uk/drug-safety-update.

National Institute of Clinical Research (NIHR). 2020. The role of the clinical research nurse. https://www.nihr.ac.uk/documents/the-role-of-the-clinical-research-nurse/11505.

NICE. https://pathways.nice.org.uk/pathways/drug-allergy.

WHO. Upsala Monitoring Centre. https://www.who-umc.org.

4 THE AUTONOMIC SYSTEM

CHAPTER OUTLINE

LEARNING OBJECTIVES

At the end of this chapter, the reader should be able to:

- describe the anatomy of the autonomic nervous system
- name the neurotransmitters and receptors of the autonomic nervous system
- give examples of sympathomimetic and parasympathomimetic drugs
- give examples of selective α and β agonists and antagonists
- describe the effects of sympathetic and parasympathetic stimulation on visceral organs
- explain the action and uses of drugs that block the action of acetylcholine

INTRODUCTION TO THE AUTONOMIC NERVOUS SYSTEM

The autonomic nervous system is the part of the nervous system that supplies the viscera as distinct from the voluntary muscles.

The **viscera** include:

- the gastrointestinal tract
- the respiratory and urogenital systems
- the heart and blood vessels
- the intrinsic muscles of the eyes
- various secretory glands.

The autonomic nervous system consists of two divisions, called the **sympathetic** and **parasympathetic** systems. Nerves from both these divisions supply most of the viscera. In general they have opposite effects on the various viscera they supply, and they also differ in both their anatomical arrangement and mechanism of function. They are responsible for controlling and regulating the internal organs and involuntary functions of the body, including the heart rate, respiratory rate, blood pressure, body temperature, digestion and sexual arousal.

COMPONENTS OF THE AUTONOMIC NERVOUS SYSTEM

Sympathetic Nervous System

The sympathetic nervous system is thought to cause the body's 'fight or flight' response, which may be triggered by fear-inducing situations or exercise. It consists of a chain of ganglia lying on either side of the vertebral column and extending from the thoracic to the lumbar vertebrae. Sympathetic nerve fibres, after passing out from the spinal cord, leave the anterior nerve root and pass to one of these ganglia. Here they form a synapse or junction with further nerve cells whose fibres are distributed to the viscera.

Some sympathetic fibres, after leaving the spinal cord, pass through the ganglia and form their synapses in ganglia situated peripherally; the group of ganglia surrounding the coeliac artery is a good example of this arrangement.

Parasympathetic Nervous System

The parasympathetic nervous system stimulates the body to cause a 'rest and digest' response. The parasympathetic fibres leave the central nervous system (CNS) and are distributed with certain cranial nerves (III, VII, IX and X) and with the sacral nerves. Cranial nerve X, called the 'vagus nerve', has a number of different functions but is crucial in the contribution towards the parasympathetic system. The relay ganglia of the parasympathetic system are situated peripherally, near the organs supplied (Fig. 4.1).

Non-adrenergic Non-cholinergic Nerves

There are also nerves within branches of the autonomic nervous system that are neither sympathetic nor parasympathetic. These non-adrenergic non-cholinergic nerve pathways (NANC) utilize nitric oxide as their neurotransmitter and stimulation of these nerves leads to relaxation of a number of peripheral tissues such as the blood vessels in the corpus cavernosum of the penis leading to an erection and airway smooth muscle in the bronchial tree eliciting bronchodilation.

Sensory Fibres

The autonomic system also carries a large number of sensory nerves, which carry information from the organ to the CNS. They enter the spinal cord, where they may form a spinal reflex arc with the autonomic nerves leaving the cord or they may ascend to the brain where more complex reflexes are built up, which may be influenced by impulses arising from the higher levels of the brain. Some visceral sensation may enter consciousness and events in consciousness may themselves stimulate various visceral effects. The rapid beating of the heart after a fright is a typical example.

CHEMICAL TRANSMISSION OF NERVE IMPULSES

Stimulation of a nerve liberates a substance called a **neurotransmitter** at the nerve ending, which activates a **receptor** in the organ supplied or in another nerve cell. This is known as the chemical transmission of nerve impulses and is an important concept because many drugs act by interfering with this process. In the autonomic nervous system, transmission occurs in this way in the sympathetic, parasympathetic and NANC divisions, but the neurotransmitter released onto the target organ differs, being acetylcholine in the parasympathetic division, noradrenaline in the sympathetic division and nitric oxide in the NANC nerves.

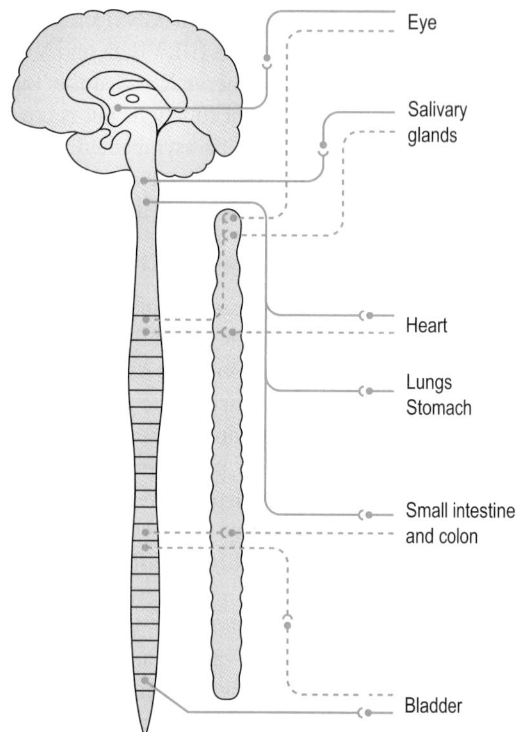

Fig. 4.1 ■ The anatomy of the autonomic nervous system. Dashed line, sympathetic; solid line, parasympathetic.

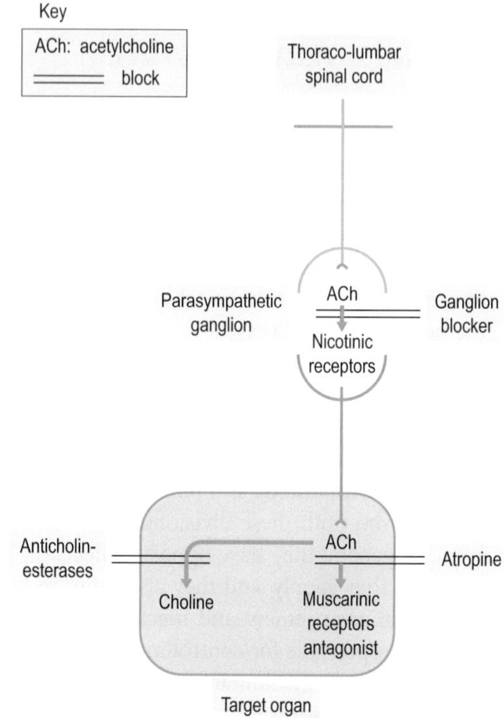

Fig. 4.2 ■ Principal neurotransmitter and its receptors in the parasympathetic division of the autonomic nervous system and sites of receptor blocking drugs.

The Parasympathetic System (Fig. 4.2)

Following stimulation of a parasympathetic nerve, **acetylcholine** (ACh) is liberated at the nerve ending; ACh acts on so-called 'muscarinic receptors' on the organ supplied by the nerve. There are five types of muscarinic receptor, called M1, M2, M3, M4 and M5. M1 receptors for example are found on a number of smooth muscle types and, when activated by ACh, these cause contraction of the muscle. M2 receptors are found in cardiac tissue, but also have another very important function being found on the presynaptic nerve terminals of the parasympathetic nerves where activation of these receptors causes a reduction of further ACh release in response to electrical stimulation of the nerves. These are so-called 'autoreceptors' and play a vital role in the maintenance of homeostasis to ensure just the correct amount of ACh is released. A further important control mechanism exists to prevent the effect of ACh being too prolonged and powerful, which is the presence in the synapse of an enzyme called **acetylcholinesterase**, which rapidly breaks down the ACh and terminates its effect. There are a number of drugs that interfere with the parasympathetic nerves, which are discussed later.

The Sympathetic System (Fig. 4.3)

The sympathetic nerves release the neurotransmitter **noradrenaline** from stores at the nerve endings in the peripheral tissues. In addition, the sympathetic system releases **adrenaline** (90%) and noradrenaline (10%) from the medulla of the adrenal gland; these substances enter the bloodstream and produce widespread effects. Noradrenaline and adrenaline produce these effects by combining with specific sympathetic adrenoceptors on the target organs. There are several types of sympathetic receptors:

Adrenoreceptors

Types of adrenoreceptors:

- α_1
- α_2

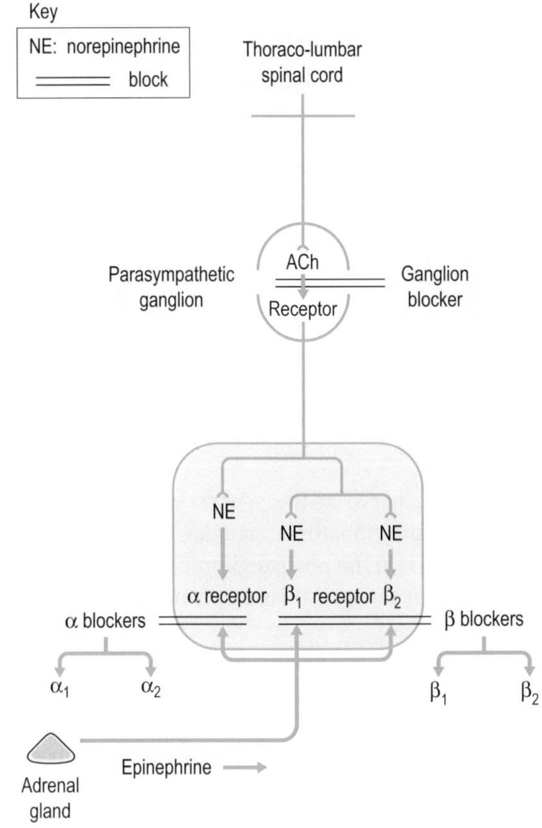

Fig. 4.3 ■ Neurotransmitters and receptors of the sympathetic division of the autonomic nervous system and sites of receptor blocking drugs.

- β_1
- β_2
- β_3.

α_1 *Receptors*

These receptors occur on target tissues opposite the nerve terminal and are stimulated by noradrenaline released from sympathetic nerve endings and by circulating adrenaline released during stressful situations. Stimulation of this receptor type produces constriction of blood vessels, causing a rise in blood pressure and reflex slowing of the heart, and dilatation of the pupil. Stimulation of α_1 receptors is blocked by several drugs which are commonly used to treat symptoms of benign prostatic hyperplasia in men, e.g. tamsulosin.

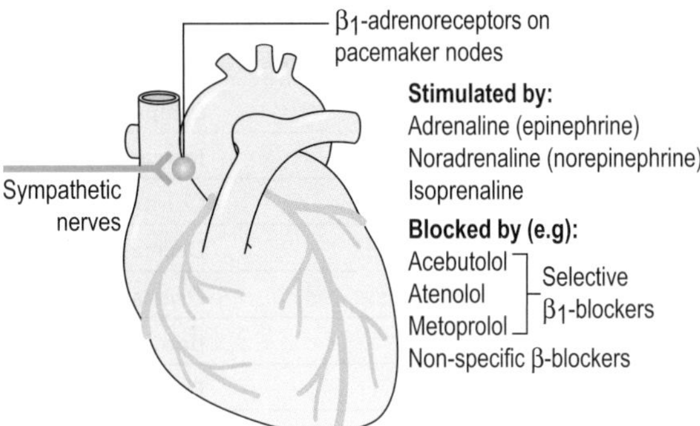

Fig. 4.4 ■ Examples of β_1-adrenoreceptor agonists and antagonists.

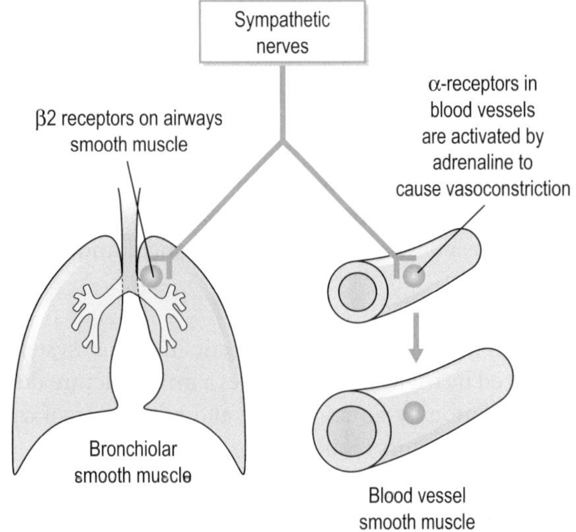

Fig. 4.5 ■ β_2 Receptors are stimulated by β agonists, e.g. noradrenaline (norepinephrine), adrenaline (epinephrine) and selective β_2 agonists, e.g. salbutamol, causing dilatation.

α_2 *Receptors*

These receptors occur on the nerve terminal from which noradrenaline is released, and when noradrenaline binds them, they limit further release of noradrenaline, thus forming a release control mechanism. The α_2 receptors are targets for drugs such as clonidine, which stimulate them selectively to inhibit further noradrenaline release, and were useful to treat hypertension for decades but are now less commonly used.

β_1 *and* β_2 *Receptors*

These receptors (Figs 4.4 and 4.5) are both stimulated by isoprenaline and adrenaline (epinephrine). In

TABLE 4.1

The Main Effects of Sympathetic and Parasympathetic Activity

	Sympathetic Activity	Parasympathetic Activity
Heart rate	Increased	Slowed
Blood vessels	Constricted	Dilated
Stomach and intestine	Decreased activity and secretion	Increased activity and secretion
Salivary and bronchial glands	Decreased secretion	Increased secretion
Urinary bladder	Body relaxed, sphincter contracted	Body contracted, sphincter relaxed
Bronchial muscle	Relaxed	Contracted
Blood sugar	Raised	–
Eye	Pupils dilated	Pupils constricted, accommodates for near vision

addition, the neurotransmitter noradrenaline (norepinephrine) acts as a β_1 stimulator on the heart, and the drug salbutamol produces a β_2 response largely on the bronchi. The effects are:

- β_1 responses – increase in rate and excitability of the heart with increased cardiac output
- β_2 responses – dilatation of bronchi and blood vessels.

Overactivity of the sympathetic nervous system produced by fright or anger causes a mixed picture due to stimulation by noradrenaline and adrenaline of α_1, β_1 and β_2 receptors (Table 4.1).

β_3 Receptors

These receptors have been reported in cardiac muscle and in fat tissue. They are negatively inotropic, i.e. they depress the rate and force of contraction, and can influence fat deposition. β_3 receptors can also be found on the bladder. Mirabegron is a drug which is a β_3 adrenergic agonist and is used for the treatment of overactive bladder with symptoms of urge incontinence, urgency and urinary frequency. This drug is contraindicated in patients with uncontrolled high blood pressure and in new patients in whom the medication is initiated, it is recommended the blood pressure is closely monitored.

Transmission at Autonomic Ganglia

The nerve that arrives at an autonomic ganglion from the CNS is termed a **preganglionic nerve**. The nerve with which it synapses in the ganglion, and which carries the impulse away to the target organ, is called the **postganglionic nerve**. ACh is liberated by the preganglionic nerve at the synapses in both sympathetic and parasympathetic ganglia, binds to muscarinic receptors on the postganglionic nerve and is thus responsible for the transmission of the nerve impulse.

SYMPATHOMIMETIC DRUGS

Sympathomimetic drugs have effects similar to those produced by activity of the sympathetic nervous system and comprise:

- adrenaline (epinephrine)
- noradrenaline (norepinephrine)
- isoprenaline
- selective β_2 agonists.

Adrenaline (Epinephrine)

Adrenaline is released from the medulla of the adrenal gland when the sympathetic system is activated. For clinical use, however, it is prepared synthetically. It acts on the sympathetic receptors located on the visceral organs. Adrenaline (epinephrine) is destroyed by gastric acid and is therefore not effective if taken orally. It is usually given by subcutaneous or intramuscular injection, its effects being produced more rapidly from the latter site. Following injection, its various actions become apparent within a minute. They are:

- An increase in the force and rate of contraction of the heart (β_1 effect), so that the patient may report palpitations.

- A rise in systolic blood pressure due to the increased cardiac output (β_1 effect). The diastolic pressure shows little change as adrenaline (epinephrine) produces vasoconstriction only in the skin and in the splanchnic area (mixed α_1 and β_2 effects), but vasodilatation in arteries in muscle (β_2 effect).
- Adrenaline (epinephrine) relaxes non-vascular smooth muscle, including that of the bronchial tree (β_2 effect).
- Adrenaline (epinephrine) raises blood sugar by mobilizing glucose from tissues.

Following injection, adrenaline (epinephrine) is rapidly broken down in the body by the enzymes monoamine oxidase and methyl-O-transferase, and therefore its effects last for only a few minutes.

Adrenaline (epinephrine) is used less now than in former times, but it still remains the best immediate treatment for serious anaphylactic reactions (see Chapter 8). In anaphylactic reactions, adrenaline (epinephrine) causes constriction of blood vessels and thus relieves oedema and swelling, as well as stimulating the heart in cardiac arrest.

CLINICAL NOTE

Adrenaline (epinephrine) stimulates adrenergic receptors and is predominantly used in critical care to control hypotension. In these cases, the drug is given intravenously and the patient should be constantly monitored and frequently with an arterial line in situ. Most commonly it will be given in a cardiac arrest as an intravenous bolus or intramuscularly to treat anaphylactic shock. It is also used in combination with lidocaine when administering local anaesthetic for minor surgery causing vasoconstriction and reducing the risk of bleeding.

Noradrenaline (Norepinephrine)

Noradrenaline (norepinephrine) is chemically closely related to adrenaline (epinephrine) and is the neurotransmitter released from sympathetic nerves at the target organs and tissues. Its most important action is to produce widespread vasoconstriction and thus a rise in both systolic and diastolic blood pressure (α_1 effect). The body rapidly inactivates noradrenaline (norepinephrine); to produce a continuous effect on the blood pressure, it is given by intravenous (IV) infusion.

Noradrenaline (norepinephrine) has been used in the treatment of various forms of shock, which is usually associated with a very low blood pressure.

CLINICAL NOTE

The surviving sepsis campaign recommend noradrenaline as the first-line treatment for a patient in septic shock with a mean arterial blood pressure of <65 mmHg alongside fluid resuscitation. Widespread vasoconstriction puts the patient at risk of tissue ischaemia due to extravasation (Kim et al., 2012) when the drug is given via peripheral vein, therefore it is recommended that the drug is administered via a central line.

Opinion has moved against using noradrenaline (norepinephrine) to raise blood pressure except in extreme circumstances, for although a satisfying rise in blood pressure can be obtained due to vasoconstriction, this also reduces the blood flow in essential organs, particularly the kidney, with troublesome results.

Isoprenaline

Isoprenaline is a synthetic drug related to adrenaline (epinephrine); however, unlike adrenaline, which stimulates all sympathetic receptors, isoprenaline stimulates only β_1 and β_2 receptors and not α receptors. It is well absorbed from the oral mucosa and following inhalation. It relaxes smooth muscle, including that of the bronchial tree, and also stimulates the heart, but has little or no effect on the blood pressure. It is important to avoid overdosage as it can cause dangerous cardiac arrhythmias. It is rapidly inactivated after absorption and its effects are short-lived.

Adverse effects include palpitations, nausea, headaches and tremors.

CLINICAL NOTE

Isoprenaline is now usually only used for emergency situations by IV injection/infusion in high dependency units for stimulating heart rate in patients with bradycardia or heart block.

Selective β_2 Agonists

These drugs stimulate predominantly β_2 receptors, so that although they are effective bronchodilators, they have minimal effects on the heart. This is an important improvement over drugs such as isoprenaline, as the risk of cardiac arrhythmias is reduced. This drug class is generally inhaled for the treatment of asthma and chronic obstructive pulmonary disease (COPD) to relieve symptoms of bronchoconstriction.

Salbutamol

Salbutamol is the most widely used β_2 agonist. It is a powerful bronchodilator (Fig. 4.6). Salbutamol is used to treat bronchospasm due to asthma or COPD. It may be taken to relieve an attack, but is no longer recommended for regular treatment, unless being used in conjunction with an antiinflammatory glucocorticosteroid (see Chapter 9). It can be given via various routes:

- Inhalation is the most commonly used route of administration (Fig. 4.7), and given in this way in the treatment of bronchospasm it is possible to get the maximum effect on the bronchi with minimal effects elsewhere. Even so, only 10% of the dose reaches the bronchial tree if the patient inhales directly from the aerosol puffer, the rest being swallowed during self-dosage (Fig. 4.8).
- The nebulised form is commonly used in acute management of exacerbation of both asthma and COPD. Potentially serious hypokalaemia can result from nebulised administration, therefore 'back-to-back' nebuliser administration should prompt close monitoring of electrolytes so that hypokalaemia can be detected and managed appropriately.
- By IV bolus and if subsequently required, then by IV infusion to treat an acute severe or life-threatening asthmatic attack. This is rarely necessary, as a nebuliser is usually very effective. Salbutamol through the IV route requires careful monitoring for cardiac arrhythmias, and the nurse has an important role to play in monitoring the patient for cardiac arrhythmias when salbutamol is administered IV. This would normally require monitoring in a high dependency unit or an intensive care unit.
- It can be given orally but this is not commonly used as relatively larger doses are required because of the large first pass metabolism by the liver (see Chapter 1) as well as side-effects (tremors and palpitations).

In addition to its use in asthma, salbutamol is used to inhibit premature labour (see Chapter 18), and for treatment of hyperkalaemia. There are other selective β_2 agonists, which are very similar to salbutamol, e.g.

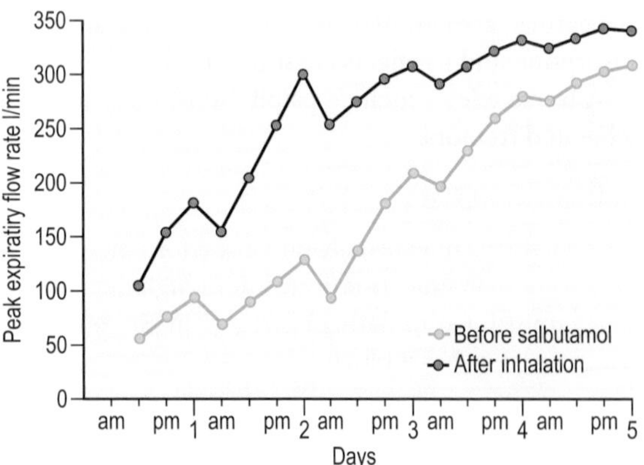

Fig. 4.6 The effect of inhalations of salbutamol on a patient with severe asthma. Note the progressive improvement in respiratory function and the morning dips, which are characteristic of asthma.

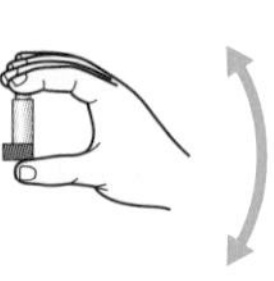

1. Remove the mouthpiece cover and shake the inhaler well

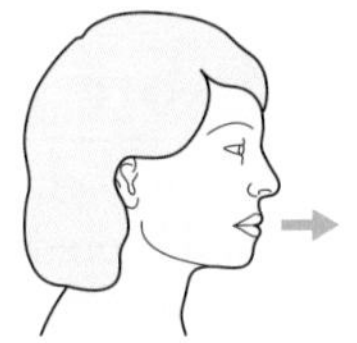

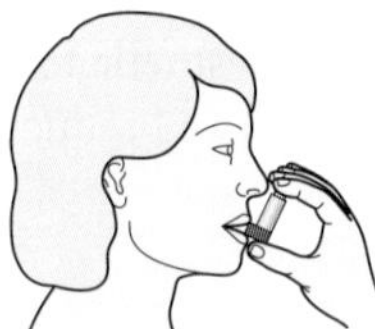

2. Breathe out gently, but not completely

3. Put the inhaler mouthpiece into the mouth and close your lips around it.
Start breathing in deeply through your mouth and press the inhaler plunger firmly.
Continue to breathe in.

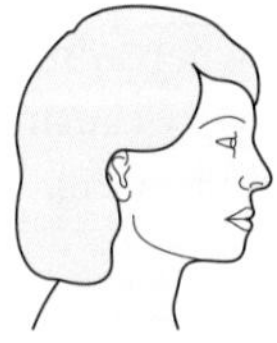

4. Hold your breath for as long as is comfortable (usually about 10 seconds) and then breathe out slowly.
If you intend to take another dose, wait 30 seconds to one minute before taking it

Fig. 4.7 How to use a pressurized metered dose inhaler (pMDI) properly.

terbutaline, fenoterol, reproterol and bambuterol (an orally active prodrug that liberates two molecules of terbutaline).

CLINICAL NOTE

Due to the immediate effect of salbutamol, it is often described as a reliever inhaler. It has a quick onset of action (5–15 min) and is intended to produce an immediate relief of bronchospasm (see Fig. 4.6). People with asthma are encouraged to carry a salbutamol inhaler with them at all times. During acute and prolonged asthma attacks salbutamol is given via a nebuliser. Side-effects such as tremor and palpitations are as a result of stimulation of B2 cells, which are located throughout the body, including the heart.

Long Acting β_2 Receptor Agonists (LABAs) – Salmeterol and Formoterol

These drugs are long-acting β_2 agonists. They are effective after about 30 min and their action lasts for about 12 h; therefore they should not be used for rapid effect in treating an acute attack, but given twice daily, by inhalation, as a preventative. They must not be used alone and should be combined with an inhaled steroid (see later). Ultra-LABAs have been approved for the

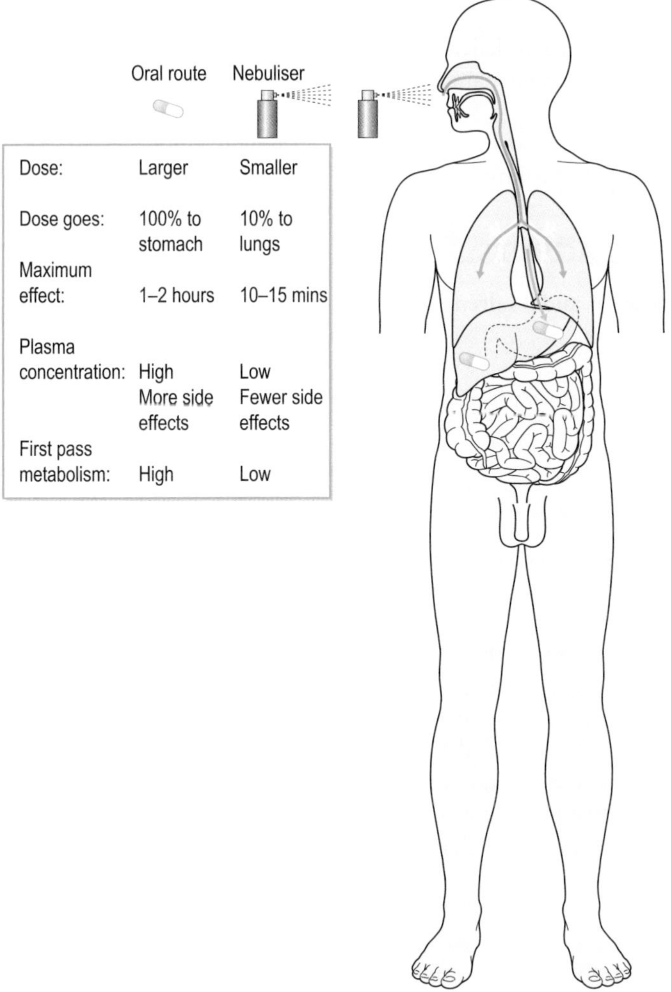

Fig. 4.8 ■ Comparison of inhalation and oral dose of, e.g. salbutamol for asthma.

treatment of COPD that provide bronchodilation for up to 24 h following a single inhalation; this in theory helps to improve compliance in patients; an example is vilanterol (e.g. Relvar Ellipta).

OTHER SYMPATHOMIMETIC DRUGS

Amphetamine and **dexamphetamine** are similar drugs whose main effect is on the CNS. They produce some euphoria, abolish fatigue, increase activity and reduce appetite. They are taken orally and act primarily on α_1 receptors. They carry a considerable risk of dependence and their therapeutic use is now confined to:

- patients with narcolepsy (recurrent, uncontrollable episodes of sleep)
- patients with a diagnosis of attention deficit hyperactive disorder (ADHD), on whom, paradoxically, they have a sedative effect.

They should not be used for appetite control.

ADRENERGIC BLOCKING AGENTS

It is possible to block (antagonize) α- and β-adrenergic receptors selectively.

α_1-Adrenergic Blockers

Examples of use:

- hypertension
- bladder neck obstruction.

Hypertension

α_1-Adrenergic blocking drugs are used in the treatment of hypertension but are often third- or fourth-line. By removing the vasoconstrictor action of noradrenaline, these drugs dilate arterioles and thus lower blood pressure. They are also used in the diagnosis of phaeochromocytoma – a rare adrenaline- and noradrenaline-releasing tumour of the adrenal gland – when phentolamine is used.

Bladder Neck Obstruction

α_1-Adrenergic receptors control the smooth muscle round the neck of the bladder. By blocking these receptors it is possible to relax this muscle and partially relieve bladder neck obstruction due to an enlarged prostate. Several α-blockers, including tamsulosin, can be used first-line or when surgical treatment is contraindicated.

β-Adrenergic Blockers

This group of drugs, which block the effects of adrenaline and noradrenaline on β-adrenergic receptors, are widely used and are a more important group of drugs than are the α-blocking drugs. In general, the therapeutic effects and uses of the various β-blockers are very similar, but individual members of the group show some differences:

- Some β-blocking drugs block predominantly β_1 adrenoceptors (i.e. cardiac β receptors) and are called **selective β-blockers**; others block both β_1 and β_2 receptors (i.e. cardiac + bronchial + peripheral blood vessel receptors) and are called **non-selective β-blockers.**
- Members of the group differ in their speed and site of elimination and in their duration of action.

CLINICAL NOTE

The first β-blocker introduced was **propranolol**, which is still in use, and historically used for the treatment of hypertension. It is, however, non-selective, and will block both β_1 and β_2 receptors, which makes it dangerous in patients with asthma since it can cause life-threatening bronchospasm by blocking the beneficial effects of endogenous adrenaline in the airways. There are some drugs (e.g. bisoprolol and atenolol) which are more cardioselective and may need to be given in patients with coexisting well-controlled respiratory conditions (e.g. asthma/COPD), for example following a myocardial infarction or in stable heart failure. These drugs are not, however, cardiospecific and although they may have a reduced effect on the airways resistance, they may not be completely free of this side-effect.

General Actions of β-Blockers

- **Cardiovascular actions.** When β_1 receptors in the heart are blocked, the heart rate is slowed, the cardiac output is reduced and the work done by the heart is thus decreased. This is particularly marked when there is increased activity of the sympathetic nervous system such as occurs with excitement or exercise. In addition, the excitability of heart muscle is reduced as β-blockers lower blood pressure.

- **Respiratory actions.** Blocking β_2 receptors with β-blockers cause bronchospasm, particularly in patients with asthma. This is particularly marked with non-selective β-blockers such as propranolol. This is usually of little consequence in healthy people, but in patients with asthma, it may make bronchospasm worse and increase dyspnoea. Selective β_1-blockers (sometimes referred to as cardioselective β-blockers) have less effect on β_2 receptors.
- **Metabolic actions.** Some β-blockers prevent the rise in blood glucose, which normally follows increased sympathetic activity.
- **CNS actions.** It is believed that at least some β-adrenergic blockers penetrate the CNS. Some sedation is fairly common in patients receiving β-blockers and occasionally this may be severe. In addition, vivid dreams and, more rarely, hallucinations may occur.

Many of the symptoms of anxiety such as palpitations, sweating and tremor are mediated via the sympathetic nervous system. These symptoms can often be relieved by β-blockers. Whether this is only a peripheral action or whether in addition there is some other effect on the brain is not known (Table 4.2).

Examples of Uses of β-Blockers

- Angina pectoris (see Chapter 7), because they reduce the work of the heart, especially on effort or excitement
- Cardiac arrhythmias, because they reduce the excitability of the heart
- Thyrotoxicosis and anxiety, because they reduce the increased sympathetic activity which occurs in these disorders
- Essential tremor, a rare familial condition characterized by severe skeletal muscle tremor
- Prevention of migraine attacks.

Labetalol and **carvedilol** are combined α- and β-blockers, which are used to treat hypertension.

TABLE 4.2

Features of Some β-Blockers in Common Use

		ELIMINATION		
Drug	**Selectivity**	**Hepatic**	**Renal**	**Half-life (h)**
Propranolol	$\beta_1 + \beta_2$	+	–	3
Oxprenolol	$\beta_1 + \beta_2$	+	–	2
Sotalol	$\beta_1 + \beta_2$	(+)	+	12
Timolol	$\beta_1 + \beta_2$	(+)	(+)	5
Nadolol	$\beta_1 + \beta_2$	–	+	16
Metoprolol	$\beta_1 > \beta_2$	+	–	4
Acebutolol	$\beta_1 > \beta_2$	(+)	(+)	6
Atenolol	$\beta_1 > \beta_2$	–	+	12
Bisoprolol	$\beta_1 > \beta_2$	(+)	(+)	10
Betaxolol	$\beta_1 > \beta_2$	?	(+)	16
Esmolol	$\beta_1 > \beta_2$	?	?	Very short

Blocking α receptors dilates the arterioles, thus reducing blood pressure; blocking the β receptors prevents the reflex speeding up of the heart ('palpitations') that occurs when cardiac β_1 receptors are activated in response to the fall in blood pressure. Although β-blockers are effective at reducing the blood pressure, there are other drugs more effective at reducing complications of hypertension such as strokes and myocardial infarctions. To reflect this, hypertension guidelines emphasize the use of other antihypertensives (see Chapter 6) for preferential treatment for hypertension. However, for the treatment of hypertension in pregnancy, β-blockers, e.g. labetalol, remain useful.

Adverse Effects

Adverse effects, other than exacerbation of unstable heart failure and of bronchospasm, can be troublesome, but are not usually serious. Occasionally, this drug class causes vivid dreams and hallucinations, and by decreasing cardiac output they reduce the blood flow to the extremities, causing the patient to feel cold, and are best avoided in patients having peripheral vascular disease. β-Blockers also mask the usual warning symptoms of hypoglycaemia and can be dangerous in patients with diabetes who are taking insulin (see Chapter 16). Active people may feel less energetic while taking these drugs.

PARASYMPATHOMIMETIC DRUGS

Parasympathomimetic drugs have effects similar to those produced by activity of the parasympathetic nervous system. Examples of parasympathomimetic drugs are:

- acetylcholine
- carbachol
- bethanechol
- pilocarpine.

Acetylcholine

Acetylcholine (ACh) is released from the parasympathetic nerve endings throughout the body and also from motor nerve endings in skeletal muscle. ACh is also the neurotransmitter at the neuromuscular junction and the release of ACh here causes contraction of skeletal muscle that is essential for initiating all voluntary movements. At the neuromuscular junction ACh acts on nicotinic receptors on skeletal muscle. The organs are innervated by the parasympathetic nervous system, where ACh acts on muscarinic receptors. The effects as a result of ACh released from parasympathetic nerves are shown in Table 4.1. The action of ACh is very short-lived, as it is quickly broken down by the enzyme cholinesterase to choline and acetate, so it is not used therapeutically. However, a prolonged effect can be produced either by giving an acetylcholine-like drug, which is not broken down or by using a drug that inhibits the action of cholinesterase, thus prolonging and intensifying the actions of naturally occurring acetylcholine. This latter type of drug is called an **anticholinesterase** and such drugs can be used to prolong the action of ACh at the skeletal neuromuscular junction in the treatment of patients with myasthenia gravis.

Carbachol and Methacholine

Carbachol is a synthetic substance chemically related to acetylcholine. Its actions resemble those of parasympathetic stimulation. It is not broken down by cholinesterases and its actions are therefore much more prolonged than those of acetylcholine. Carbachol may be given by subcutaneous injection or by mouth.

Methacholine is another stable analogue of ACh. This also mimics the actions of ACh, but has a more prolonged action and can be inhaled as a diagnostic aid, called a bronchoprovocation test, in patients with asthma.

Uses of Carbachol. The most important therapeutic use of carbachol is in the treatment of urinary retention following a surgical operation or childbirth when there is no mechanical obstruction. It causes contraction of the bladder muscle, resulting in the passage of urine. Carbachol is not licensed for UK use.

Administration and Effects of Carbachol after Injection. Carbachol may be given by subcutaneous injection or by mouth. After subcutaneous injection, flushing and sweating appear in about 20 min, followed by increased intestinal peristalsis, sometimes with colic and contraction of the bladder muscle. *Other adverse effects* include colic, diarrhoea and a marked fall in blood pressure. These actions last up to an hour and are a reflection of the drug mimicking stimulation of the parasympathetic nervous system. These adverse effects can be controlled by muscarinic receptor antagonists such as atropine (see later).

Bethanechol

Bethanechol is another acetylcholine-like drug, which, like carbachol, is not broken down by cholinesterase.

Pilocarpine

Pilocarpine is used only as eye drops, where it causes constriction of the pupil.

THE ANTICHOLINESTERASES

These drugs prevent the breakdown by cholinesterase of ACh produced at nerve endings throughout the body. The actions of ACh are thus intensified at their two sites of action:

- on tissues innervated by the parasympathetic nerve endings
- on skeletal muscle.

As ACh is the neurotransmitter at ganglia (both sympathetic and parasympathetic), at the neuroeffector junction of the parasympathetic nervous system and at the skeletal neuromuscular junction, potentiating its effects with an anticholinesterase drug can produce mixed actions. The actions on tissues innervated by the parasympathetic nerve endings usually predominate, and the action on voluntary muscle is only seen under special circumstances such as in patients with deficient innervation of skeletal muscle, e.g. patients with myasthenia gravis.

Important Effects of Anticholinesterases

- **The eye**: some anticholinesterases are absorbed through the conjunctiva and following application to the eye cause constriction of the pupil and spasm of accommodation.
- **Gastrointestinal tract**: anticholinesterases cause increased tone and motility.
- **Urinary tract**: anticholinesterases cause contraction of the bladder.

Clinically Used Anticholinesterases

Several anticholinesterases are used to treat a variety of disorders, depending on where their actions are most pronounced:

- neostigmine
- physostigmine
- pyridostigmine
- edrophonium
- distigmine
- donepezil
- galantamine
- rivastigmine.

Neostigmine is a synthetic anticholinesterase with actions very similar to those of physostigmine, but with an effect on the neuromuscular junction of voluntary muscle and less on the eye and cardiovascular system. It is rapidly effective following subcutaneous or intramuscular injection and is also absorbed after oral administration, although this route requires larger doses.

Uses of Neostigmine. Neostigmine is used widely in the treatment of disorders of the skeletal neuromuscular junction (e.g. myasthenia gravis – a form of muscular paralysis through ACh receptor failure), and has been used in cases of paralytic ileus and atony of the bladder.

Physostigmine is a naturally occurring anticholinesterase that is relatively short-acting.

Pyridostigmine and **edrophonium** are anticholinesterases used in the treatment of myasthenia gravis. Edrophonium has a very short-lived action and is used more in the diagnosis of myasthenia gravis.

Distigmine has widespread actions and may be used for urinary retention and myasthenia gravis. It can be given orally or by injection.

CLINICAL NOTE

Myasthenia gravis is a long-term incurable condition affecting around 20,000 people a year. It causes weakness in skeletal muscles and can, in extreme cases, affect breathing requiring invasive or non-invasive ventilation. Neostigmine assists in stimulating the skeletal muscle, thus reducing skeletal weakness (Sanders et al., 2016). Drugs should be taken early in the day when muscle weakness and fatigue are most severe. Other uses of acetylcholinesterase inhibitors are in people with dementia (excluding vascular dementia, frontotemporal dementia or cognitive impairment by multiple sclerosis). Alzheimer's disease is the most common type of dementia. These drugs all prevent acetylcholinesterase from breaking down acetylcholine in the brain. First-line treatment for mild to moderate Alzheimer's disease is monotherapy with **donepezil**, **galantamine** or **rivastigmine**. For severe Alzheimer's disease, **memantine** (NMDA receptor antagonist) is the drug of choice.

Adverse Effects of the Anticholinesterases

All the anticholinesterases produce broadly similar adverse effects due to the prolonged action of ACh. The symptoms include:

- abdominal cramps and diarrhoea
- sweating and salivation
- constricted pupils
- slow pulse
- low blood pressure.

Treatment. The immediate treatment is to use a muscarinic receptor antagonist such as atropine given intravenously.

Non-clinical Uses of Anticholinesterases

There are a number of other anticholinesterase preparations not used therapeutically, but which are extensively employed as insecticides and are also potential lethal weapons for use in war. As some are absorbed through the intact skin and produce powerful anticholinesterase effects, they have been termed 'nerve agents'. These are the organophosphate anticholinesterases. Examples are malathion and parathion insecticides, and the nerve agents sarin and Novichok that was recently used in anger against a former Russian spy on UK soil. These agents are dangerous because they combine irreversibly with the cholinesterase enzyme and new enzyme has to be produced. If organophosphate poisoning is suspected, the drug pralidoxime must be administered fast before the poison forms an irreversible bond with the enzyme.

DRUGS INHIBITING THE ACTION OF ACETYLCHOLINE

The drugs that inhibit the action of ACh after it has been released from parasympathetic nerve endings are called 'muscarinic receptor antagonists'. **Atropine** was the first muscarinic receptor antagonist to be described and was originally extracted from the belladonna plant. This plant was originally used by Italian women to cause pupil dilation, seen at the time as a way to make themselves more beautiful and hence the name of the plant being called 'bella donna'. We now know that this effect is due to atropine in the plant antagonizing muscarinic receptors in the eye. Another natural example of a muscarinic receptor is **hyoscine**. These drugs produce their effect by blocking the action of ACh on the cholinergic muscarinic receptors in the various organs innervated by the parasympathetic nervous system.

Effects of Blockade of the Parasympathetic Division of the Autonomic Nervous System

The blockade of the parasympathetic division of the autonomic nervous system produces the following symptoms:

- Gastrointestinal tract: diminished motility of the stomach, and both small and large intestines, with relief of spasm.
- Secretions: decrease in salivary secretion and reduction of gastric acid secretion.
- Heart: diminished cardiac vagal tone, leading to an increase in pulse rate.
- Lungs: blockade of vagal (parasympathetic) action, leading to some relaxation of the bronchial muscle; diminished secretion from the bronchial glands.
- Involuntary muscle: relaxation of other involuntary muscles, notably those of the biliary and renal tracts.
- Eye: blockade of the parasympathetic nerve supply to the eye, leading to dilatation of the pupil and paralysis of accommodation with an inability to see near objects clearly.

CLINICAL NOTE

Patients receiving drugs that block the parasympathetic response (e.g. hyoscine, some antihistamines, antidepressants) frequently report a dry mouth. To avoid this, patients can be advised to drink water frequently. In some instances, these drugs can be given for hypersalivation, e.g. in people with cerebral palsy. Anticholinergic drugs should also be used with caution in older people due the risk of cognitive and functional impairment (Nishtala et al., 2016).

Atropine

Uses of Atropine

Atropine has several therapeutic uses, the most important of which are:

- *Relief of involuntary muscle spasm*: most forms of smooth muscle spasm are relieved by atropine, given subcutaneously or intravenously. It is useful in the relief of intestinal, biliary or renal colic.
- *Eye conditions*: atropine may be applied locally to the eye as an eye drop to dilate the pupil. Homatropine or tropicamide are often used for this purpose because their effects are not as prolonged as are those of atropine. Ophthalmologists may use a short-acting atropine-like drug such as **tropi-**

camide to dilate the pupil to facilitate examination of the eye.
- *Preoperative medication (pre-med)*: pre-med is not used as much as in the past. Short-acting muscarinic receptor antagonists were given preoperatively by subcutaneous injection to dry up the salivary and bronchial secretions, and to protect the heart from undue vagal depression.
- *Bronchospasm*: an atropine derivative (**ipratropium bromide**) is given by inhalation to relieve acute bronchospasm in patients with asthma or COPD (see Chapter 9).

CLINICAL NOTE

Ipratropium bromide promotes bronchodilatation by blocking muscarinic receptors, it has the same effect as salbutamol but achieves this in a different way, by blocking receptors in the parasympathetic nervous system rather than stimulating β_2 receptors. In acute exacerbations of COPD or asthma, it is given in conjunction with salbutamol as it has an additive effect and reduces bronchospasm more effectively (see Case History 9.1).

Administration, Absorption and Elimination of Atropine

Atropine is well absorbed from the intestine after oral administration; it can also be given subcutaneously, intramuscularly or intravenously. Atropine is largely broken down by the liver. Its effects last 2 h or longer.

Adverse effects are dose-related. Dry mouth, constipation, difficulty with micturition (in the elderly) and paralysis of ocular accommodation are common. After toxic doses, restlessness, hallucination and delirium can occur. The patient appears flushed and the skin is hot to the touch.

CLINICAL NOTE

It is important that atropine or similar medicines should not be given to those with a history of glaucoma. In this disorder, the drainage of fluid from the eye is reduced and the pressure rises within the eyeball. Atropine further reduces the flow of fluid from the eye and may precipitate an acute attack of glaucoma (see Chapter 31).

Hyoscine

Hyoscine (scopolamine) is the drug traditionally beloved of mystery fiction writers, who call it the 'truth drug'. The peripheral actions of hyoscine are the same as those of atropine. Its action on the CNS differs, however, in that hyoscine, even in small doses, is a CNS depressant, leading to drowsiness and sleep. Hyoscine is particularly used for its central as well as peripheral effects. It is used preoperatively by injection and can be taken orally as an antiemetic. Several proprietary travel sickness preparations contain hyoscine.

Synthetic Atropine-like Drugs

These drugs were originally developed to have shorter acting drugs, e.g. tropicamide for use in the eye, or to target certain specific subtypes of the muscarinic receptor. For example, trihexyphenidyl is used clinically to treat Parkinson's disease since it is claimed selectively to target M1 muscarinic receptors in the brain. Longer acting muscarinic receptor antagonists (LAMAs) have been developed for inhalation for the maintenance treatment of COPD (see Chapter 9).

Among those available are:

- dicycloverine
- mebeverine
- propantheline
- oxybutynin
- flavoxate
- tolterodine
- tiotropium (inhalation).

DRUGS AFFECTING THE NON-ADRENERGIC NON-CHOLINERGIC SYSTEM

Nitric oxide (NO) is now recognized at the neurotransmitter in the third branch of the autonomic nervous system, the non-adrenergic non-cholinergic (NANC) system. Once released from these nitrergic nerves, NO activates an enzyme called 'guanylate cyclase' in the vascular smooth muscle to bring about relaxation. This discovery has allowed us to explain how a number of widely used drugs work. For example the use of the vasodilator glyceryl trinitrate (GTN) to treat the symptoms of anginas can be explained by the GTN being able to mimic the actions of NO on vascular smooth muscle to bring about vasodilation. Inhaled NO is now used for the treatment of pulmonary hypertension because of its ability to relax vascular smooth muscle in the pulmonary vascular bed. Very recently a new drug has been introduced called 'riociguat', the first synthetic guanylate cyclase agonist, which is approved for the treatment of adults with pulmonary hypertension. An intriguing story related to NO arises from the discovery that NO was the neurotransmitter at the corpus cavernosum of the penis and that the effect of NO in this tissue could be potentiated by the phosphodiesterase-5 inhibitor sildenafil citrate, which led to this drug being approved for the treatment of erectile dysfunction (Viagra). Subsequent studies have shown that sildenafil also potentiates the effect of NO in the pulmonary vasculature, which has led to the approval of this drug also for the treatment of pulmonary hypertension.

SUMMARY

- Adrenaline (epinephrine) is used as an intramuscular (IM) injection in the treatment of anaphylactic shock, but be careful not to inject into a vein.
- Adrenaline (epinephrine) is used for cardiac arrest, but do not use the same IV line used for sodium bicarbonate.
- Noradrenaline (norepinephrine) can be used to treat shock associated with large drops in blood pressure, but is not commonly used to raise blood pressure because it reduces blood flow through the kidneys.
- Isoprenaline is no longer used to treat asthma because it stimulates both β_1 (heart) and β_2 (lung) receptors, and can cause fatal arrhythmias. Selective β_2 agonists such as salbutamol are used for asthma and to inhibit premature labour.
- β-Blockers lower blood pressure but are primarily now used to reduce the pulse rate.
- Drugs influencing NO can be used for the treatment of pulmonary hypertension and erectile dysfunction.
- Muscarinic receptor antagonists are used to treat urinary incontinence and, when given by inhalation, for the treatment of COPD.
- Nicotinic receptor antagonists are used as relaxants of the skeletal muscle.
- Acetylcholinesterase inhibitors are used to diagnose and treat myasthenia gravis. They are also used in the treatment of dementia.

REFERENCES AND FURTHER READING

Barnes, H., Brown, Z., Burns, A., Williams, T., 2019. Phosphodiesterase 5 inhibitors for pulmonary hypertension. Cochrane Database Syst. Rev. 1, CD012621.

BNF, 2013. Mirabegron for overactive bladder syndrome. Drug Ther. Bull. 51, 90–92.

BTS/SIGN, 2019. BTS/SIGN British Guideline on the Management of Asthma. British Thoracic Society/Scottish Intercollegiate Guidelines Network. https://www.brit-thoracic.org.uk/quality-improvement/guidelines/asthma.

Davis, G., 2007. The central, peripheral and nervous system: an overview. NursePrescribing 5 (1), 16–21.

Howell, M.D., Davis, A.M., 2017. Management of sepsis and septic shock. J. Am. Med. Assoc. 317 (8), 847–848.

Kim, S.M., Aikat, S., Bailey, A., 2012. Well recognised but still overlooked: norepinephrine extravasation. BMJ Case Rep. https://doi.org/10.1136/bcr-2012-006836. https://casereports.bmj.com/content/casereports/2012/bcr-2012-006836.full.pdf.

Morice, A.H., Wrench, C., 2001. The role of the asthma nurse in treatment compliance and self-management following hospital admission. Respir. Med. 95 (11), 851–856.

Nishtala, P.S., Salahudeen, M.S., Hilmer, S.N., 2016. Anticholinergics: theoretical and clinical overview. Exp. Opin. Drug Saf. 15 (6), 753–768.

Sanders, D.B., Wolfe, G.I., Benatar, M., et al., 2016. International consensus guidance for management of myasthenia gravis: executive summary. Neurology 87 (4), 419–425.

UKGOV, 2018. Novichok nerve agent use in Salisbury: UK government response. March–April 2018. https://www.gov.uk/government/news/novichok-nerve-agent-use-in-salisbury-uk-government-response.

USEFUL WEBSITES

Guidelines for Nurses. http://guidelinesfornurses.co.uk/respiratory/nice-chronic-asthma-management-guideline.

Living with pulmonary hypertension. https://www.phauk.org/living-with-pulmonary-hypertension.

Myasthenia gravis. https://www.musculardystrophyuk.org/about-muscle-wasting-conditions/myasthenia-gravis/myasthenia-gravis-factsheet.

5 CARDIOVASCULAR SYSTEM 1

Drugs Acting on the Heart

CHAPTER OUTLINE

LEARNING OBJECTIVES

At the end of this chapter, the reader should be able to:

- list the factors that determine cardiac output
- describe the causes and consequences of heart failure
- describe the main approaches to the treatment of heart failure and the major types of drug used
- describe the overall strategies for care as well as drug treatment of patients with heart failure
- give an account of the normal cardiac cycle of the spread of electrical excitability and muscle contraction
- discuss the nature of arrhythmias due to cardiac overexcitability and conduction defects in the bundle of His
- list the names of drugs used to treat different types of arrhythmias, how they are classified and their basic mechanism of action

DRUG TREATMENT IN TWO MAJOR DISORDERS OF HEART FUNCTION

These disorders are:

- cardiac failure
- cardiac arrhythmias.

CARDIAC FAILURE

The Cardiac Output

The heart is a muscular pump receiving blood from the systemic and pulmonary veins and driving it, under pressure, into the pulmonary arteries and the aorta. The volume of blood passing through the heart each minute is known as the cardiac output. This is largely determined by four factors:

- **The preload:** the pressure in the venous system filling the heart and stretching the cardiac muscle. In health, a rise in venous pressure causes a rise in cardiac output.
- **The afterload:** the arterial pressure, that is, the resistance against which the heart must pump.
- **The heart rate:** an increase in rate leads to an increased output until the heart rate becomes too fast for the heart to fill adequately in diastole.
- **The contractile efficiency of the cardiac muscle:** measured as the 'ejection fraction' (EF), which is the proportion of the volume of blood in the filled ventricle in diastole which is ejected in systole. An important distinction that guides treatment of heart failure is whether the EF is preserved or reduced. About 50% of cases of heart failure have a reduced EF.

In good health, the cardiac output varies considerably depending on the needs of the body, being low at rest and rising with exercise. The healthy heart has a great functional reserve and can cope with demands for increased output that sometimes occur.

Causes of Cardiac Failure

If the pumping efficiency of cardiac muscle is reduced through disease, this may lead to the symptoms associated with cardiac failure. Cardiac failure is essentially 'pump failure', and is not the same as cardiac arrest, although to many patients 'cardiac failure' means that the heart has stopped or will soon do so. It is important to realize this when discussing the diagnosis, which may seem very frightening to patients.

Cardiac failure may be acute or chronic. Acute cardiac failure often occurs as a sudden worsening of preexisting chronic cardiac failure.

Cardiac failure is conceptually complex, and its symptoms will vary according to its causes, which may include:

- Heart muscle damage by ischaemic heart disease or by cardiomyopathy weakens the power of the heart muscle. In these cases, the EF is often reduced.
- High blood pressure or heart valve leakage or narrowing may cause an increased workload over a long period, which ultimately causes the heart to fail.
- The heart muscle may become thicker and/or stiffer for various reasons. In diastole it therefore fails to relax completely. Filling of the ventricles in diastole is diminished and therefore the total amount of blood that the ventricles expel in systole is reduced. In these cases, the EF is often preserved.
- Diseases that cause the heart to beat faster, such as arrythmias or thyrotoxicosis, or that cause increased demand on the heart, such as liver failure or anaemia, can lead to cardiac failure. Fluid overload from chronic kidney disease or mismanaged intravenous fluids may also precipitate cardiac failure. Alcohol and cocaine use may lead to cardiac failure, and some prescribed drugs, such as β-blockers (but see later), some calcium channel blockers and non-steroidal antiinflammatory drugs (NSAIDs) may worsen it.

CLINICAL NOTE

It is estimated that 23 million people worldwide have heart failure (Roger, 2013). In developed countries, the prevalence of heart failure is around 1%–2%, rising to more than 10% in people over the age of 70. Reduced cardiac output is characterized by increasing shortness of breath, often at night, ankle swelling and fatigue, which may be accompanied by clinical signs such as bibasilar crackles, elevated jugular venous pressure and peripheral oedema. It is commonly caused by ischaemic heart disease, valve disorders, immune or metabolic conditions. It can also be caused by exposure to toxins, e.g. alcohol and some drugs.

Consequences of Cardiac Failure

- If the ventricles fail to empty properly, the heart may become enlarged.
- The veins leading to the heart (including those in the neck) become distended with blood and the heart cannot respond to the increased filling pressure (preload) by raising output. At first this is only apparent on exercise, but later occurs at rest.
- The increased venous congestion can lead to oedema (fluid retention and swelling) in peripheral

tissues and in the lungs, the latter being responsible for marked dyspnoea (shortness of breath), which is a common feature of patients with cardiac failure. In acute cardiac failure, the dyspnoea may be very marked and of sudden onset.

- The pump output becomes insufficient for the needs of the body, and various organs receive an inadequate blood and oxygen supply. This is particularly important in the kidney, where it activates the renin-angiotensin system (see later), causing the kidney to retain salt and water, which may worsen oedema. Angiotensin is also responsible for constriction of arterial smooth muscle, which increases the work (afterload) of an already labouring heart. This is further aggravated by an increase in sympathetic activity, causing additional vasoconstriction and tachycardia.
- The low cardiac output carries less oxygen to the tissues. The oxygen supply to the heart and brain is kept up at the expense of other organs, which are starved of oxygen, and this accounts for the fatigue, which may be a prominent symptom of patients with chronic cardiac failure (Fig. 5.1).
- Cardiac failure is a serious life-limiting condition with a high morbidity and mortality. About 50% of people with heart failure die within 5 years.

In the past, the terms 'right heart failure' and 'left heart failure' were used depending on whether the predominant symptoms were due to congestion in the systemic (right) or pulmonary (left) veins. 'Congestive heart failure' was a term used when there was evidence of sodium and water retention. However, these distinctions are not especially helpful in guiding treatment and are falling out of general use.

The severity of heart failure in a patient can be assessed and documented using the New York Heart Association Classification, which assigns a functional score between 1 and 4, depending on the effect of the heart failure on the patient's life.

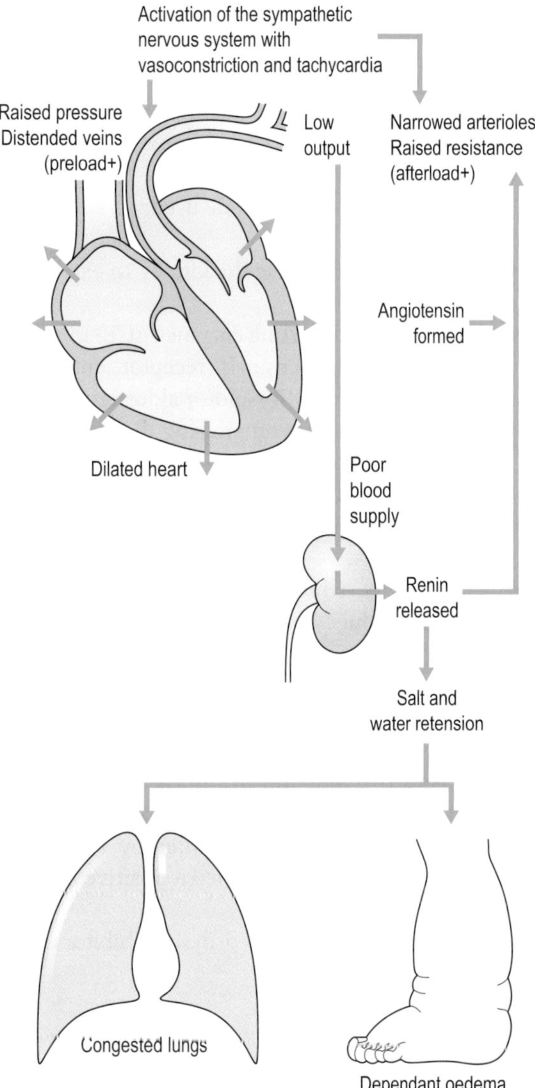

Fig. 5.1 ■ Processes in cardiac failure.

CLINICAL NOTE

Care of people with heart failure is often in the community, and is frequently delivered by nurse specialists or advanced practitioners with prescribing knowledge and skills. In addition to medication reviews and, where necessary, adjustment to treatment, they provide patients and families with psychological support akin to palliative care nursing. A systematic review (Bryant et al., 2015) of 13 samples concluded that heart failure nurse specialists reduced hospital readmission, reduced cost and improved patient satisfaction and treatment adherence. This is similar to findings from a Cochrane review (Takeda et al., 2012) concluding that an interprofessional team including clinical nurse specialists is vital when caring for this group of patients.

DRUGS USED IN THE TREATMENT OF CARDIAC FAILURE

Pharmacological approaches mainly aim to reduce the workload on a failing heart and relieve the associated symptoms.

Four main groups of drugs are used:

- Diuretics, which cause the kidney to excrete excess salt and water.
- Angiotensin-converting enzyme (ACE) inhibitors (ACEI) or angiotensin-II receptor antagonists (AIIRA or often 'ARB') and/or aldosterone antagonists, which act by suppressing the angiotensin-renin-aldosterone mechanism, which is overactive in cardiac failure.
- β-Blockers, which reduce inappropriate sympathetic activity.
- Vasodilators, which lower peripheral resistance and thus reduce cardiac work.

In addition, there is a limited role for:

- Positive inotropic drugs, which are drugs that improve the function of the cardiac muscle so that the heart contracts more powerfully and empties more completely, thereby raising the cardiac output. This is called a positive inotropic effect.
- New treatments – the neprilysin inhibitors.

Diuretics

Diuretics increase urine production. They are considered in detail in Chapter 12. Both thiazide-like (metolazone) and loop diuretics (furosemide, bumetanide) are used in the treatment of patients with cardiac failure.

Mechanism of Action

- Diuretics reduce oedema and pulmonary congestion by increasing the excretion of salt and water.
- Diuretics also relieve distension of the heart by reducing blood volume.

Disadvantages

- Renin production by the kidney is activated by reduced blood volume, and this may partially reverse the diuretic's beneficial effects by stimulating fluid retention and increased blood pressure.
- Vasoconstriction will occur in response to reduced blood volume, and this will increase blood pressure and the work of the heart.
- Both thiazide-like and loop diuretics increase potassium loss via the kidney. If small doses are used, this is unlikely to require correction. If large doses of diuretic are used, if dietary potassium is deficient (e.g. in those whose diet is poor, or in the elderly), or if concurrent digoxin is given, this loss of potassium ions needs to be corrected.

Nevertheless, the benefits of diuretics usually outweigh the disadvantages and this class of drug is widely used for the relief of acute and chronic cardiac failure. For mild heart failure, thiazide-like diuretics may be adequate, but more severe heart failure will require a loop diuretic such as furosemide. NSAIDs such as ibuprofen will reduce the efficacy of diuretics.

CLINICAL NOTE

When administering diuretics, timing of the dose should be considered. This is particularly important when a twice daily dose is prescribed. Advice should be that the second dose should be taken early afternoon, thus avoiding having to pass urine during the night. In addition, furosemide is a common cause of adverse drug events resulting in hospital admission (Pirmohamed et al., 2004) and to reduce the risk of dehydration and acute kidney injury, it may be appropriate that the diuretic is withheld for 24 h if the patient is acutely unwell, especially if they have diarrhoea or vomiting. In these circumstances, the patient should be advised to contact a prescriber. Angiotensin-converting enzyme inhibitors (ACEI) (such as ramipril) and angiotensin II receptor antagonists (AIIRA) (such as losartan) were originally developed to treat hypertension, but have become key drugs in the management of chronic heart failure. Use of ACEI substantially reduces mortality in cardiac failure. Aldosterone antagonists (such as spironolactone) may be used as an additional treatment in more severe cardiac failure.

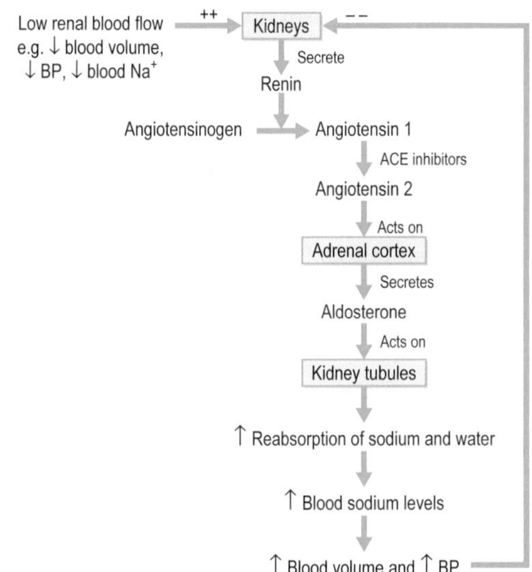

Fig. 5.2 ■ Action of angiotensin-converting enzyme inhibitors.

Mechanism of Action

Both ACEI and AIIRA block the overactive renin-angiotensin mechanism (Fig. 5.2). This results in a reduction of salt and water retention by the kidneys; in addition, by dilating arterioles, they lower the resistance to blood flow from the heart (afterload), reduce cardiac work and raise cardiac output. High levels of angiotensin also trigger the production of the hormone aldosterone from the adrenal glands. Aldosterone leads to sodium and water retention from the kidneys. Aldosterone antagonists block the action of this hormone.

Disadvantages

The initiation of treatment with ACEI and AIIRA requires some care. The main danger is a profound fall in blood pressure after the first dose, which is especially liable to occur in patients already taking diuretics and in patients whose cardiac failure is related to heart valve disease. In most cases, this danger can be avoided by starting on a low dose and gradually titrating the dose upwards, sometimes over a period of weeks. A sudden decline in renal function may be seen in patients with previously undetected renal artery stenosis. Renal function should be assessed before and shortly after starting treatment with these drugs. Around 20% of patients develop a chronic dry cough on ACEI. Rashes, particularly urticaria (hives), are also relatively common. Patients with these side-effects should be changed to an AIIRA.

Renal function and electrolytes need to be carefully monitored during treatment with aldosterone antagonists. Spironolactone also blocks the action of male hormones and can lead to breast development (gynaecomastia) in male patients.

NURSING NOTE

The initial dose of ACEI should be low and the blood pressure should be closely monitored. For unwell patients in hospital, this should be at least 4-hourly for 24 h. ACEIs can be nephrotoxic and regular monitoring of urea and electrolytes should be scheduled when treating the elderly and frail who are prescribed an ACEI.

β-Blockers

The use of β-blockers to treat cardiac failure is a relatively recent, but very important, development. Historically, they were avoided as their negative inotropic action may lead to worsening of cardiac failure. However, sympathetic nervous system overactivity with tachycardia and peripheral vasoconstriction is a prominent feature of cardiac failure and small doses of β-blockers reduce this overactivity. The β-blockers carvedilol, metoprolol and bisoprolol have been shown to reduce mortality in cardiac failure with reduced EF. They should not be used as initial treatment of acute or severe cardiac failure or if there is severe hypotension or ECG evidence of sino-atrial (SA) or second- or third-degree A-V block. They should not be prescribed in patients with severe asthma or severe chronic obstructive pulmonary disease, although **nebivolol** may be safe in less severe asthma.

Vasodilators

Vasodilators reduce the work of the heart by lowering peripheral resistance and, by dilating the veins, lower the venous pressure and allow the heart to beat more effectively. Nitrate vasodilators (glyceryl trinitrate, isosorbide mononitrate, isosorbide dinitrate and sodium nitroprusside), are used as intravenous infusions to treat acute cardiac failure but have not been shown to reduce mortality when given in their oral forms for chronic cardiac failure. There is research interest in the possible role of non-nitrate vasodilators in cardiac failure, but none are currently in routine clinical use.

Positive Inotropic Drugs

Positive inotropic drugs increase the strength of the heart muscle. They have a role in intensive and coronary care units for short-term intravenous use in acute cardiac failure with reduced EF. Phosphodiesterase (PDE)-3 inhibitors (e.g. milrinone) and β-adrenergic receptor agonists (e.g. dobutamine) are relatively widely used for this purpose. Calcium-sensitizing agents (e.g. levosimendan) are also used in some countries, but are not currently approved for use in the UK or USA. Digoxin (see later) has been used intravenously to treat heart failure but is rarely used intravenously in current medical practice.

Digoxin

Digoxin has been used by physicians for hundreds of years, but its use has declined markedly. It was originally extracted from Foxglove and in 1785 William Withering described the use of this plant in the treatment of 'dropsy' (oedema) and noted that it appeared to act on the heart. It is now produced synthetically and is available for oral use. It has a positive inotropic effect and also slows the heart rate, particularly in atrial fibrillation. In most countries it is no longer used to treat cardiac failure, except when associated with atrial fibrillation. Treatment with digoxin does not reduce mortality from cardiac failure and appears to increase all-cause mortality, possibly because of its small therapeutic window and consequent high risk of toxicity. If it is used, then plasma levels of the drug should be monitored, as should plasma electrolytes. Drugs such as diuretics, which reduce potassium levels, may precipitate digoxin toxicity and several other drugs also interact with digoxin. The most dangerous toxic effects are a marked slowing of the pulse to <60 beats/min or coupled beats, where ventricular extrasystoles follow normal beats and can be a warning of fatal arrhythmias. Confusion is also common in elderly people suffering digoxin toxicity. Digoxin still has a role in clinical practice but needs to be used cautiously and monitored carefully.

The Neprilysin Inhibitors

Neprilysin is an enzyme found in many tissues, particularly the kidney. Inhibiting its action in the kidney leads to vasodilatation and sodium and water excretion. The neprilysin inhibitor **sacubitril**, used in combination with the ACEI **valsartan**, has shown benefit in symptom control (Jhund and McMurray, 2016) and reduced risk of death in patients with cardiac failure with reduced EF. **This is an emerging area of treatment that may become important**.

There is new evidence that in diabetic patients, the use of GLP2 inhibitors (the gliflozins; see Chapter 16) may reduce the likelihood of cardiac failure in this vulnerable group.

CARE AND TREATMENT OF PATIENTS WITH CARDIAC FAILURE

The main objectives in treating cardiac failure are:

- to relieve the acute and chronic symptoms associated with cardiac failure, particularly shortness of breath and oedema.
- to increase the efficiency and output of the heart, so that there is sufficient blood and oxygen supply to the various organs.
- to try where possible to remove or diminish the factor(s) that caused the heart to fail.

Non-drug Management of Cardiac Failure

Drugs are only part of the treatment of patients with cardiac failure. In acute cardiac failure, patients should be nursed in a sitting position so that the accumulated fluid from oedema drains away from the lungs and abdominal viscera to the legs, to improve breathing. Although the legs may be slightly elevated on a stool when the patient is sitting out of bed, they should not be raised above the horizontal, as this may shift fluid to the abdomen and lungs. Controlled oxygen with monitoring is usually required for acute cardiac failure.

Constipation may be a problem requiring modification of diet and, sometimes, laxative treatment. Dyspnoea, oedema, fatigue and malaise impair appetite, and patients with chronic cardiac failure may be malnourished. Low volume, high energy, protein-rich foods or supplements may be helpful. Retention of salt is as important as retention of water by the kidneys in producing oedema. Diuretics will usually enable the kidneys to excrete salt and a low-salt diet is rarely required. It is not usually necessary to restrict fluid intake. However, in severe heart failure or when sodium deficiency has developed as a result of prolonged and intensive diuretic treatment, fluid intake may need to be restricted, with careful monitoring of input and output, weight and electrolytes. Patients in hospital with cardiac failure are at high risk of venous thromboembolism (VTE) and local guidelines on VTE prevention should be followed. All patients with chronic cardiac failure should be considered for antiplatelet treatment.

Some patients with acute cardiac failure may require ventilatory support. Diuretic resistant acute cardiac failure occasionally requires ultrafiltration therapy. Severe low output cardiac failure can be improved with mechanical support devices such as intra-aortic balloon pumps, where suitable facilities exist. A small proportion of patients may be suitable for cardiac transplantation.

There is good evidence to support supervised graduated exercise therapy in improving outcomes in chronic stable cardiac failure, and patients should be offered this if appropriate. Annual influenza vaccinations and a single pneumococcal vaccination should be offered. It is important to understand and address the patient's knowledge, concerns and fears about their disease and to consider their wishes about treatment. Education about the condition is important, as is psychological support. Depression is common in patients with cardiac failure and formal or informal screening for this should be undertaken. Advance care planning and advance decisions should be discussed early in the progress of the disease and not left to the end stages.

It is important to consider treating modifiable causes of cardiac failure, both drug and non-drug, and the patient's comorbidities should not be forgotten.

CLINICAL NOTE

A review conducted in 2010 suggested that depression and anxiety was underreported and can result in poor treatment adherence, worsening anxiety and psychological symptoms being masked by physical symptoms, e.g. dyspnoea (Yohannes et al., 2010). There is limited evidence on the effect of psychological interventions such as cognitive behaviour therapy; however, healthcare professionals should be aware of the high prevalence of depression and anxiety in this population, and provide support, advice and professional interventions as required.

Drug Management of Cardiac Failure

In acute heart failure presenting in hospital, initial treatment will be with oxygen and intravenous loop diuretics. Very distressed patients may benefit from small doses of opiates, such as diamorphine, to help dyspnoea. Patients not responding to diuretics alone may require intravenous vasodilators and some will require intravenous positive inotropes in a coronary care or high dependency unit.

Drug treatment of chronic heart failure is guided by knowledge of the EF, usually estimated by echocardiography. Measurement of the level of brain natriuretic peptide (BNP) in the patient's blood may aid diagnosis and help in assessing severity, and also response to treatment.

Patients with a normal EF are treated with diuretics, usually furosemide, in low to medium doses (up to 80 mg) to relieve symptoms of fluid overload. There is insufficient evidence to support the routine use of other cardiac failure drugs. Antiplatelet drugs and statins may also be prescribed.

Patients with reduced EF are initially treated with loop diuretics, usually furosemide. The dose is titrated according to symptoms and physical signs, including blood pressure and weight. Very high doses (up to 1.5 g/day by IV infusion) may be needed. Occasionally, the thiazide-like diuretic metolazone may be used in low doses in conjunction with furosemide, every few days. This combination can provoke very substantial diuresis, but with an increased risk of dehydration and electrolyte imbalances. An ACEI and a β-blocker licensed for cardiac failure should also be started, but not simultaneously. If the patient has significant fluid overload or diabetes, it is most appropriate to start the ACEI first. If the patient has angina, then it may be more appropriate to start the β-blocker first. When stabilized, the other drug should be introduced. The β-blocker dose should be gradually increased to the maximum dose tolerated. This may require a temporary increase in the diuretic dose. If the ACEI is not tolerated – usually due to provoking a chronic cough – then an AIIRA may be used instead. These drugs should be started at low doses and the dose gradually increased according to response, blood pressure and electrolytes. Moderate to severe cardiac failure usually requires the addition of an aldosterone antagonist as an adjunct (such as 25–50 mg of spironolactone). It is important to monitor serum potassium when these drugs are added.

NURSING NOTE

Patients with marked oedema and unstable cardiac failure often benefit from daily weighing to help guide their diuretic dose, which may vary from day-to-day. If it is remembered that 1 litre of water (i.e. oedema) weighs 1 kg, it will be appreciated how important and useful this simple measurement can be.

CLINICAL NOTE

Unless the underlying cause can be removed, most patients with chronic heart failure will require some medication for the rest of their lives. It should be explained to them that the main objectives of treatment are to give them a reasonable exercise tolerance and to keep them free of oedema. The importance of taking their drugs regularly should be stressed. Patients should be told of the main adverse effects, particularly those producing symptoms. All patients with chronic heart failure should be seen regularly, either as outpatients, by their family doctor and/or community nurses (see Case History 5.1). The psychosocial factors associated with life with a chronic condition should always be considered.

CASE HISTORY 5.1

Mr. CS is 68 years old and has a past history of two ST elevation myocardial infarctions, the most recent one being 7 months ago. Following the last episode, he stopped smoking and was put on a combination of low-dose aspirin, 2.5 mg β-blocker bisoprolol and 40 mg atorvastatin. He has not had any further coronary episodes and does not have angina, but he has noticed gradually increasing shortness of breath on exertion, with a decreased ability to exercise and occasions when he has woken up short of breath and had to get up out of bed and breathe at the open window. He finds it more comfortable to sleep with two pillows. He has noticed that his ankles are a little swollen.

His GP noted that his blood pressure was normal but he had pitting oedema of the ankles. A brain natriuretic peptide blood test was raised, suggesting cardiac failure, and in consequence, an echocardiograph was organized. This showed a reduced EF. The diagnosis was: cardiac failure with reduced ejection fraction. He was initially treated with furosemide, 80 mg/day, to relieve the oedema. His renal function was checked before and after starting this treatment and again after an ACE inhibitor – ramipril – was started. He was already on a good dose of an appropriate β-blocker, so the dose of ramipril was gradually increased with monitoring of his blood pressure and renal function, while the furosemide dose was reduced and eventually stopped. His GP was guided by his symptoms until an effective dose of the ramipril was reached.

CARDIAC ARRHYTHMIAS

The Normal Cardiac Cycle

In the normal, healthy heart, the initial electrical stimulus for contraction starts in the SA node (the pacemaker of the heart), situated at the junction of the superior vena cava and the right atrium (Fig. 5.3). The rate of discharge from the node is under the control of parasympathetic (vagus) and sympathetic nerves. Vagal activity slows the heart rate and sympathetic activity increases it. The wave of electrical stimulation spreads over both atria, causing them to contract and forcing blood into the ventricles. The stimulus then pauses for a fraction of a second at the atrio-ventricular (AV) node before passing down the bundle of His and spreading through the muscles of both ventricles, which contract and drive blood into the pulmonary artery and the aorta. Immediately after this, the heart muscle enters a brief recovery (or refractory) phase, in which it cannot respond to electrical stimulation. During this phase, the heart relaxes, refills with venous blood and awaits the next stimulus for contraction.

The ECG is used to diagnose arrhythmias and a knowledge of the normal ECG and the way it correlates with heart action is important in aiding understanding (Fig. 5.4).

Some Useful Definitions

- **Arrhythmia:** variation from the normal rhythm of the heartbeat, encompassing abnormalities

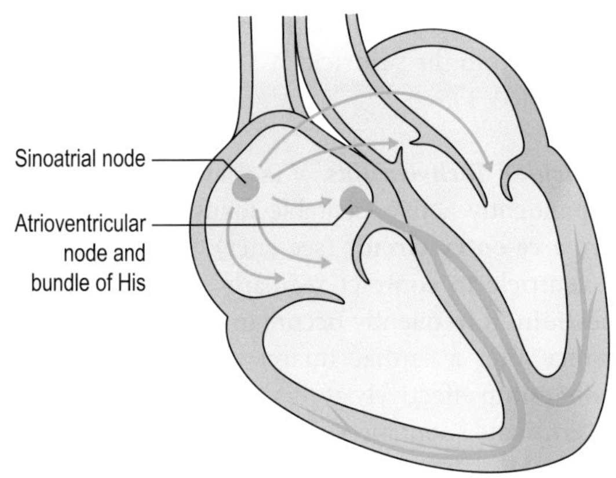

Fig. 5.3 ■ The heart, showing the sino-atrial node and conducting system (atrio-ventricular node and bundle of His).

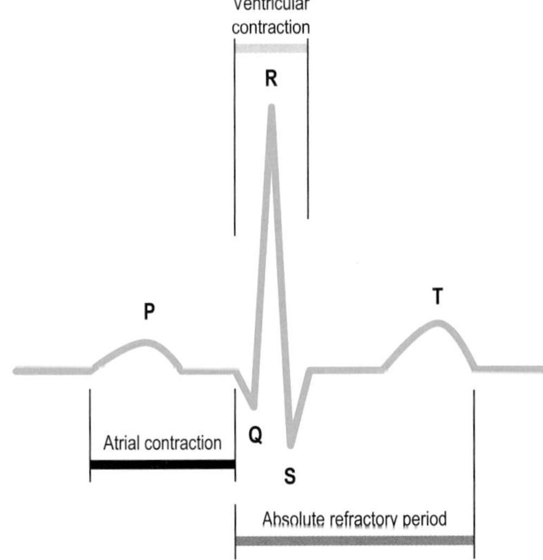

Fig. 5.4 ■ The ECG and cardiac activity. A typical ECG tracing of the cardiac cycle (heartbeat) consists of a P wave (atrial depolarization), a QRS complex (ventricular depolarization) and a T wave (ventricular repolarization).

of rate, regularity, site of impulse origin and sequence of activation.

- **Atrial fibrillation:** atrial arrhythmia marked by rapid, randomized contraction of small areas of the atrial myocardium, causing an irregular and often rapid ventricular rate.
- **Bradycardia:** slowing of the heart rate; pulse rate falls below 60.
- **Cardioversion:** restoration of the normal rhythm of the heart by the application of a controlled direct current shock to the heart of an anaesthetized patient using electrodes placed on the chest wall.
- **Coupled rhythm:** heartbeats occurring in pairs, the second beat usually being a premature ventricular beat.
- **Defibrillation:** the use of a direct current shock to terminate ventricular fibrillation.
- **Ectopic rhythm:** a heart rhythm originating outside of the SA node.
- **Extrasystole:** a premature cardiac contraction independent of the normal rhythm, which arises in response to an impulse outside of the SA node.
- **Sinus rhythm:** the normal heart rhythm that originates in the SA node.
- **Supraventricular rhythm:** any cardiac rhythm originating above the ventricles but not originating from the SA node.
- **Tachycardia:** very rapid heart rate.
- **Ventricular fibrillation:** cardiac arrhythmia marked by fibrillary contractions of the ventricular muscle due to rapid, repetitive excitation of myocardial fibres without coordinated ventricular contraction and by absence of atrial activity. There is no cardiac output and so it is fatal, unless treated rapidly by defibrillation.

Disorders of Cardiac Rhythm

Disorders of cardiac rhythm can be divided into:

- those due to **overexcitability of the heart**, which are by far the most common
- those due to **conduction defects** in the bundle of His.

Arrhythmias Due to Overexcitability

These can be divided into:

- extrasystoles (ectopic beats)
- paroxysmal tachycardia – types include supraventricular tachycardia (SVT) and ventricular tachycardia (VT)
- atrial flutter
- atrial fibrillation.

Extrasystoles (Ectopic Beats). Extrasystoles are caused by an electrical focus, either in the atria or in the ventricles, which stimulate the heart to contract while relaxed and awaiting the next normal stimulus. A normal stimulus which immediately follows it does not stimulate a normal contraction as the heart muscle is in its refractory phase, and there is a pause before normal rhythm is resumed. Extrasystoles are very common in healthy people and although they are sometimes associated with heart disease, they are usually of little significance. They are sometimes related to smoking or to excessive tea, coffee or alcohol consumption. They rarely require treatment, other than reassurance.

Paroxysmal Tachycardias. Paroxysmal tachycardias may arise from the ventricle (VT) or from the atria or AV node (SVT).

Ventricular Tachycardias. VTs may be caused by an independently active excitable focus in the ventricle or by a **re-entry circuit** (see later), which stimulates the ventricle to contract regularly at about 160–180 times/min. It frequently occurs in diseased hearts, for instance after a cardiac infarct (Fig. 5.5). The heart cannot pump effectively at this rate and if the VT does not terminate spontaneously, it needs to be ended, by

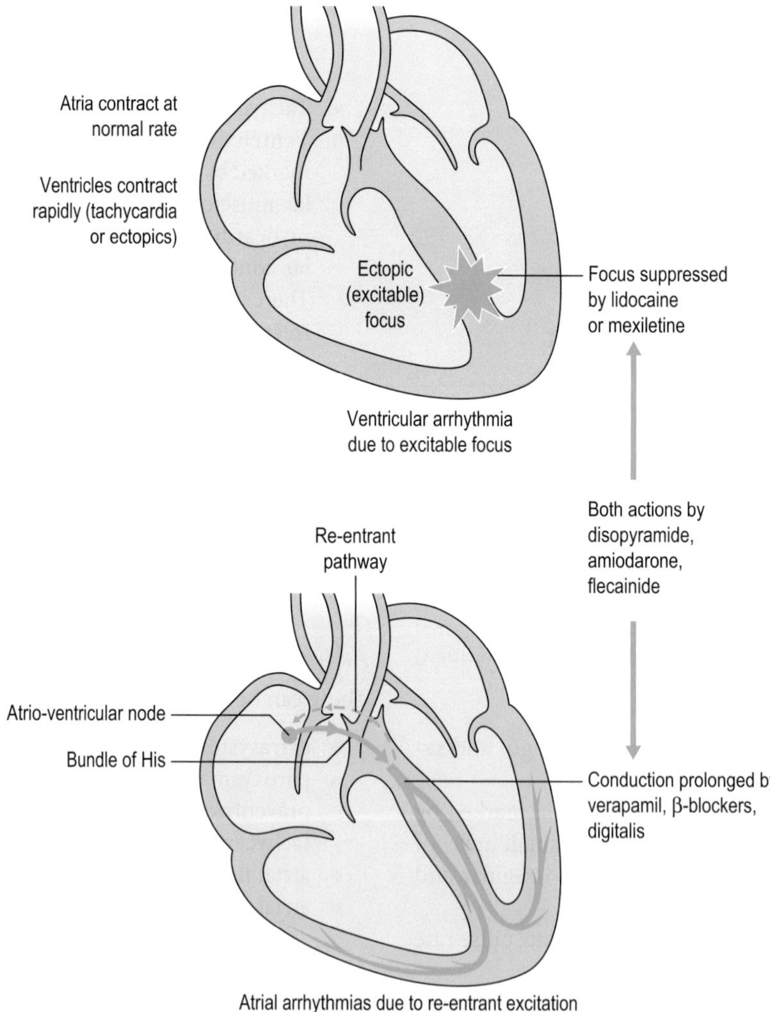

Fig. 5.5 The mechanisms of paroxysmal tachycardias.

cardioversion or medication. VT can also be provoked in people who have a congenitally long QT interval on their ECG. Certain drugs can further prolong the QT interval and can provoke a particularly dangerous VT (known as torsades des pointes) in susceptible people, particularly if given in combination. The antibiotic erythromycin and the antidepressant citalopram are examples of common drugs that should not be given together to people with a prolonged QT interval. Abnormal blood levels of potassium, calcium or magnesium may also provoke this condition.

Reentry circuits (sometimes called 'circus rhythms') underlie many VTs and also SVTs (see later). When an area of heart muscle is abnormal – either congenitally or through damage (commonly ischaemia or infarction) – the area cannot conduct the electrical impulses that course through the heart muscle. This can result in a local circular movement of impulses around the damaged area (hence '*circus*'). These electrical impulses can *re-enter* a previously stimulated area and stimulate it again in a kind of positive feedback loop, setting up a local focus that produces arrhythmias. Interestingly, and usefully, these foci are more easily suppressed by antiarrhythmic drugs than are the normal flows of current through the heart muscle.

Supraventricular Tachycardias. SVTs tachycardias (SVTs) are quite common and are generally less serious than VTs. Attacks of paroxysmal tachycardia may last for anything from a few seconds to hours or even days. They may occur in quite healthy people or they may complicate heart disease.

They are often due to a 'reentry circuit' within the AV node, which fires off ventricular contractions via the bundle of His at about 160/min. They may sometimes be due to abnormal excitability of the AV node without reentry and sometimes may be due to a rapid ventricular response to abnormal atrial activity. Drugs may be effective treatment, but increasingly, ablation (see later) is used to treat the problem. Less commonly, there is an abnormal *accessory* (extra) conducting pathway between the atria and the ventricles, which is involved in the reentrant phenomenon (see Wolff–Parkinson–White syndrome, later).

Atrial Flutter. Sometimes, the atria may contract regularly, but at high speed, usually about 240–300/min. This is called 'atrial flutter'. Under these circumstances, the ventricles are unable to 'keep up' with the atria and therefore respond to every other, or perhaps every third, atrial contraction, a condition known as 2:1 or 3:1 heart block.

Atrial Fibrillation. In atrial fibrillation (AF), each individual bundle of muscle fibres in the atria contracts individually at a rate of about 450 contractions/min. This results in irregular and ineffective atrial contraction, while the ventricles are bombarded, via the bundle of His, with rapid and irregular electrical stimuli and beat irregularly and less efficiently than when in normal sinus rhythm. The cardinal sign of AF is an *irregularly irregular* pulse. AF, which may be persistent or paroxysmal, is usually associated with heart disease (coronary disease, hypertension, cardiomyopathy or valvular disease). It can also be a complication of thyrotoxicosis, various acute illnesses and alcoholism. Sometimes, however, there is no apparent cause. AF may be continuous or paroxysmal.

Arrhythmia Due to Conduction Defects

Sometimes, the bundle of His may fail to transmit the impulse from the atria to the ventricles. This condition is known as **heart block**. If there is no association between atria and ventricles, the block is said to be complete; if only a proportion of impulses get down the bundle, the block is said to be partial. This may, as mentioned earlier, also lead to 2:1 or 3:1 heart block. Complete block leads to a dangerously slow heartbeat; partial blocks will lead to some degree of bradycardia. More commonly, it is only noted on the ECG as a prolonging of the PR interval.

NURSING NOTE

Much of the treatment of cardiac arrhythmias takes place in hospital with continuous monitoring of the heart by ECG, often in an intensive care unit. Careful observations are required and changes in rhythm must be noted as they may indicate the need to stop a drug or change treatment. When there is a change in rhythm, and the patient is cardiovascularly stable, a 12-lead ECG is performed. Any loss of consciousness will require immediate intervention by a medical emergency or cardiac arrest team. This is discussed further in Chapter 8.

Drugs Used to Treat Arrhythmias

Cardiac arrhythmias can be terminated and normal rhythm restored by certain classes of drug. If, however, the heart is functioning poorly, it is safer to stop the arrhythmia by direct-current (DC) cardioversion, or, if it is a conduction defect, to use electrical pacing.

Vaughan Williams Classification of Antiarrhythmic Drugs

Vaughan Williams and Singh introduced a classification of antiarrhythmic drugs in 1970 which is still used today, although it has been modified with time and is not perfect. It does organize the drugs into a form that facilitates remembering them and is included here with examples. The drugs are broadly classified according to their mechanism of action (Table 5.1). Other classifications have been proposed more recently and may be preferred, in due course. The following is a simple approach to understanding the effects of individual drugs.

TABLE 5.1

Vaughan Williams Classification of Antiarrhythmic Drugs

Class		Mechanism	Drugs
I		Na^+ channel blockers	
	Ia		Procainamide Disopyramide
	Ib		Lidocaine Mexiletine
	Ic		Flecainide Propafenone
II		β-Blockers	Propranolol Labetalol Carvedilol
III		Mainly K^+ channel blockers	Amiodarone Sotalol (also has β-blocking activity)
IV		Ca^{2+} channel blockers	Diltiazem Verapamil
V		Miscellaneous action	Adenosine Digoxin

Functional Classification of Antiarrhythmic Drugs

When the arrhythmia is due to an **excitable focus** in the heart muscle (usually in the ventricle), drugs that reduce excitability are appropriate and include:

- lidocaine.

When the arrhythmia is due to a **re-entry circuit**, as in SVTs, drugs that slow conduction in the AV node are used. They include:

- adenosine
- verapamil
- β-blockers
- digoxin.

In addition, three drugs that have **both actions** and can therefore be used in both types of arrhythmia are:

- disopyramide
- amiodarone
- flecainide.

Lidocaine

Lidocaine is a local anaesthetic that suppresses the excitability of the ventricular muscle with only moderate depression of the heart's action. Lidocaine is sometimes used to treat arrhythmias due to ventricular excitability that are liable to occur in the first few days after a myocardial infarction (MI), particularly if amiodarone (see later) is not available or not tolerated. It must be given intravenously because, if it is given orally, it is very rapidly broken down by the liver after absorption from the intestine (first pass effect).

NURSING NOTE

In patients with cardiac failure or shock, the breakdown of lidocaine by the liver is much slower, and dangerous accumulation can occur with continuous infusion. In these circumstances the infusion rate should be slower.

Contraindications and Adverse Effects. Lidocaine should be avoided in shocked patients, when it may further depress cardiac function. It should not be given if the conducting system of the heart is damaged. It is no longer routinely administered as a prophylactic drug after an MI. The most common adverse effects are caused by stimulation of the central nervous system, with restlessness, tremor and possibly convulsions. It can also cause a fall in blood pressure and bradycardia, particularly if heart function is already compromised.

Verapamil (and Diltiazem)

These are calcium antagonists that act selectively on the heart. They block the flow of calcium ions into the muscle cells of the heart. This reduces the force of contraction of the heart muscle and slows conduction in the AV node, and is thus useful in the treatment of SVT as it breaks the circus wave of stimulation.

Because of their depressant effect on cardiac muscle contraction, they should not be used if a β-blocker has been given in the preceding 24 h, as the combination can seriously reduce cardiac efficiency and may cause cardiac arrest. They may be given to control ventricular rate in AF if β-blockers are not tolerated. Verapamil is the more commonly used drug for these purposes.

Drug Interactions. β-Blockers (see earlier). Verapamil reduces the excretion of digoxin; so, if the two are combined, the dose of digoxin should be reduced.

β-Blockers

Mechanism of Action. The general pharmacology of this group of drugs is considered in Chapter 6. By preventing the stimulation of β-adrenergic receptors by adrenaline, β-blockers decrease the excitability of the heart and thus stop arrhythmias due to a supraventricular circus movement. **Bisoprolol** is the most commonly used oral preparation for this purpose, while esmolol is used as in infusion for short-term use.

β-Blockers can be used to prevent ectopic beats or SVTs and for rate control in AF. They are frequently prescribed after MI, where they improve the prognosis. **Sotalol** is a β-blocker with additional Class III effects and may be useful in the treatment of ventricular arrhythmias.

Drug Interactions. β-Blockers may seriously exacerbate the depressant effect on heart muscle of drugs such as verapamil.

Safety point: β-blockers may exacerbate or precipitate heart failure in patients whose hearts are under stress from some disease. Despite this, small doses of β-blockers are used to treat heart failure with reduced EF (see earlier).

Adenosine

Mechanism of Action and Use. Adenosine suppresses conduction through the AV node and is used to terminate supraventricular arrhythmias. Adenosine is given intravenously and its action begins very rapidly and only lasts a very short time, but this is usually sufficient to restore sinus rhythm.

Adverse Effects. Adverse effects are flushing, chest pain and dyspnoea, coming on immediately after injection and lasting up to 30 s.

CLINICAL NOTE

Adenosine is only administered in the presence of a resuscitation team while a patient is being constantly monitored. Immediately following administration, it is not uncommon to have period of asystole, resulting in the patient experiencing flushing, chest pain and dyspnoea. It is important that the patient is warned that this is to be expected and that it will resolve soon after administration.

Digoxin

Digoxin is sometimes used in the treatment of certain cardiac arrhythmias, although its use has declined:

- Supraventricular arrhythmias: by slowing conduction, digoxin may abolish the arrhythmia or control the ventricular rate.
- Atrial fibrillation: by suppressing conduction between the atria and ventricles, digoxin controls the ventricular rate in AF whether there is associated cardiac failure or not. It does not, however, abolish the fibrillation.
- Atrial flutter: digoxin may change the arrhythmia into AF. If the drug is then stopped, normal sinus rhythm may be restored.
- See also Wolff–Parkinson–White syndrome (later).

Disopyramide

Mechanism of Action. Disopyramide decreases excitability and slows conduction, so it can be used for both SVTs and VTs. Disopyramide can be given either orally or intravenously. Disopyramide is excreted via the kidneys and reduced dosage is necessary if renal function is impaired.

Adverse Effects. These include dry mouth, worsening of glaucoma and difficulty with micturition, all due to an anticholinergic action. Disopyramide may also cause nausea, vomiting and diarrhoea.

Amiodarone

Amiodarone is effective in both ventricular and supraventricular arrhythmias, but because of its adverse effects it is mainly used to treat the more serious and difficult to treat ventricular arrhythmias.

Mechanism of Action. Amiodarone acts by prolonging the refractory period of heart muscle. This is the short period after each contraction of the heart when the muscle will not respond to any stimulus. Its other important property is that, unlike most antiarrhythmic drugs, it has little depressant effect on cardiac function.

Adverse Effects. Adverse effects of amiodarone are common and limit its use. They include:

- Photosensitivity - high factor sun protection should be used. Also a bluish-grey pigmentation of exposed areas.
- Amiodarone contains a high concentration of iodine and thus may cause both hypothyroidism and thyrotoxicosis. Thyroid function tests (TSH, T3 and T4) should be performed every 6 months in those patients receiving long-term treatment with amiodarone.
- Pulmonary fibrosis can occur and should be suspected if a patient develops progressive cough or shortness of breath.
- Deposits in the cornea of the eye occasionally cause visual haloes. Regular eye checks are important.
- Rarely, liver damage and neuropathy. Liver function should be checked 6-monthly.
- Rapid IV injection causes marked hypotension.

Drug Interactions. Amiodarone potentiates the actions of warfarin and digoxin. When used with various combinations of drugs used in the treatment of Hepatitis C, there is a risk of severe bradycardia and heart block.

Flecainide

Mechanism of Action. Flecainide reduces excitability and slows conduction in the AV node and bundle of His, so it can be used for both ventricular and supraventricular arrhythmias, including those complicating the Wolff–Parkinson–White syndrome. Flecainide can be given by slow IV injection (over 10 min) to terminate arrhythmias. Given orally, it is also useful in preventing ventricular arrhythmias.

Adverse Effects. Dizziness is quite common. It should not be used in patients with conduction defects as it may provoke complete heart block. Rarely, it actually provokes, rather than diminishes, ventricular arrhythmias. Although flecainide is an effective drug, it can induce dangerous arrhythmias in patients who have poorly functioning or damaged ventricular muscle, particularly following MI, and should be avoided in this group.

CLINICAL NOTE

As noted earlier, flecainide should be avoided in heart failure or post-myocardial infarction. It is generally used in the younger population following exclusion of any cardiomegaly or ischaemic heart disease.

Propafenone

Propafenone is effective in suppressing ventricular and some supraventricular arrhythmias and those complicating the Wolff–Parkinson–White syndrome. It can be given orally in divided doses and has also been used intravenously. Its efficacy is similar to that of lidocaine and flecainide. The dose may need to be individualized, as there may be considerable difference in the blood levels for a given dose due to variations in drug metabolism. It has a weak β-blocking action and should be avoided in patients who are susceptible to bronchospasm. It should also be avoided in ischaemic heart disease.

Direct Current Cardioversion

A DC shock is applied to the heart via electrodes placed on the chest. The patient is briefly anaesthetized or heavily sedated for the procedure. The shock obliterates the ectopic focus or circus movement that causes the arrhythmia and allows normal rhythm to be resumed. This form of treatment is often used in treating AF and about 70% of these patients can be converted to sinus rhythm. Unfortunately, many patients relapse within a few months, although maintenance drug treatment (discussed later) reduces relapse rates.

ABLATION

Ablation, also known as catheter ablation, is increasingly used to treat arrythmias.

It uses either heat (radiofrequency ablation) or freezing (cryoablation) via a cardiac catheter to the abnormal area of the heart. This treatment creates scar tissue, which may break abnormal circuits in the heart or destroy areas of the heart muscle that are triggering arrhythmias.

An ablation is started using the same technique as an electrophysiology (EP) study and is often carried out at the same time. The EP study can discover the abnormal electrical pathways in the heart. Ablation is only available in centres specializing in heart problems, as it is highly technical and expensive. It may remove the need for drug treatment, and has been used to treat many types of arrhythmia, including SVTs and AF, particularly paroxysmal AF.

Electrolytes and Arrhythmias

A low plasma potassium concentration (hypokalaemia) increases the risk of developing an arrhythmia and makes the arrhythmia more difficult to terminate. This is particularly liable to occur after an infarct or in patients taking diuretics. It can also be a problem in patients administered large doses of β_2 agonists.

Magnesium deficiency also predisposes to arrhythmias and an infusion of magnesium sulfate may be used as part of the treatment of serious arrhythmias, such as torsades des pointes.

Treatment of Individual Arrhythmias

Atrial Fibrillation

Treatment of persistent AF aims to improve symptoms and reduce the risk of stroke. Strategies for this include control of the ventricular rate, or restoration of normal sinus rhythm. If AF is of proven recent onset (within 48 h), then rhythm control is preferable, and may be by DC cardioversion or by pharmaceutical means, using flecainide or amiodarone (the relatively new drugs, **ibutilide** or **vernakalant**, may also be used for this purpose in some countries). If the AF onset is more than 48 h previously, DC cardioversion is preferable to pharmaceutical cardioversion in most cases. The patient should be anticoagulated for 3 weeks before and 4 weeks after conversion, to reduce the risk of thrombi forming in the atria and becoming emboli. Relapse is common, but maintenance treatment with a standard β-blocker may reduce this risk. If this is ineffective or cannot be used, then sotalol, flecainide, propafenone or amiodarone (or possibly the relatively new drug **dronedarone**) may be used. These drugs may also be used to prevent paroxysmal AF.

If the patient is unfit for DC cardioversion, or does not wish to have this treatment (which is often the case), or relapse occurs, the ventricular rate should be controlled. A β-blocker, verapamil or diltiazem, may be used for this. If this is ineffective, then combinations may be used, including adding digoxin. Digoxin is no longer used for rate control on its own as it only slows heart rate at rest. It is useful when AF accompanies cardiac failure, particularly in elderly patients who may be sedentary.

AF greatly increases stroke risk. All patients with persistent AF should have their stroke risk assessed using a clinically validated algorithm such as the CHA2DS2-VASc tool. Most will be advised to have lifelong anticoagulation therapy (see Chapter 7).

Atrial Flutter

Atrial flutter is managed with similar principles to the management of AF. However, drug treatment tends to be less effective than in AF, and DC cardioversion or ablation is the preferred treatment, if available. Stroke prevention follows the same principles as in AF.

Ventricular Tachycardia

Pulseless VT or ventricular fibrillation should be treated with immediate defibrillation.

Patients with VT who deteriorate with signs of hypotension or reduced cardiac output, should receive DC cardioversion to restore sinus rhythm.

Haemodynamically stable patients can be treated with intravenous antiarrhythmic drugs. Amiodarone is the most appropriate. Flecainide, propafenone and lidocaine have all been used.

Following restoration of sinus rhythm, many patients require treatment to prevent further episodes. β-Blockers, sotalol and amiodarone can be used. Increasingly, patients are treated with an implantable cardioverter defibrillator where such devices are available.

Supraventricular Tachycardia

Depressing conduction through the AV node and thus breaking the circuit terminates acute attacks. This may be achieved if the patient performs the Valsalva manoeuvre (expiring against the closed glottis), which causes reflex vagal stimulation and slows AV conduction. A similar effect can be produced by pressure over **one** carotid sinus. Drinking very cold water may also be effective.

NURSING NOTE

The Valsalva manoeuvre or carotid massage should be carried out with the patient lying flat, where it is more effective and the patient is less liable to faint.

Drug Treatment. Adenosine, given as a rapid IV injection under ECG monitoring, is the treatment of choice for stopping a sustained SVT. The alternative drug is verapamil, but not if the patient is on β-blockers. If drug treatment fails, DC cardioversion may be used.

Recurrent episodes of SVT can be treated by catheter ablation, or prevented with drugs. Diltiazem, verapamil, β-blockers, sotalol, flecainide or propafenone have all been used.

The Wolff–Parkinson–White Syndrome

The Wolff–Parkinson–White (WPW) syndrome is a congenital abnormality that occurs in about 1.5/1000 of the population. It is due to an extra (accessory) conducting system between the atria and the ventricles. In itself it causes no trouble but is associated with supraventricular arrhythmias due to re-entry (i.e. down one bundle and up the other) and AF, which are occasionally dangerous. There are characteristic changes on the resting ECG which may help make this diagnosis.

The accessory bundle may not respond to drugs in the same way as the normal conducting system. In particular, digoxin and verapamil enhance rather than depress conduction through the accessory bundle. This is important if these drugs are used to treat AF in a patient with previously undiagnosed WPW.

Ablation is increasingly used to treat patients who are found to have this condition.

Arrhythmias Due to Conduction Defects

Atropine is the first-line drug for emergency treatment of acute symptomatic bradycardia in hospital. Otherwise drugs have little role in the treatment of bradycardia due to conduction defects, which normally require the implantation of a cardiac pacemaker.

CLINICAL NOTE

NICE have published a treatment summary of management of patients with arrhythmias to further support learning (NICE, 2019). This guidance is updated frequently and provides an evidence-based approach to treating and supporting people with arrythmias.

REFERENCES AND FURTHER READING

Bryant, L.D., Carter, N., Reid, K., et al., 2015. The clinical effectiveness and cost—effectiveness of clinical nurse specialist—led hospital to home transitional care: a systematic review. J. Eval. Clin. Pract. 21 (5), 763–781.

Correale, M., Monaco, I., Tricarico, L., et al., 2019. Advanced heart failure: non-pharmacological approach. Heart Fail. Rev. 24 (5), 779–791.

Jhund, P.S., McMurray, J.J. V., 2016. The neprilysin pathway in heart failure: a review and guide on the use of sacubitril/valsartan. Heart 102 (17), 1342–1347.

NICE, 2019. Treatment Summary Arrhythmias. https://bnf.nice.org.uk/treatment-summary/arrhythmias.html.

Pirmohamed, M., James, S., Meakin, S., et al., 2004. Adverse drug reactions as cause of admission to hospital: prospective analysis of 18 820 patients. BMJ 329 (7456), 15.

Ponikowski, P., Voors, A.A., Anker, S.D., et al., 2016. ESC guidelines for the diagnosis and treatment of acute and chronic heart failure: the Task Force for the diagnosis and treatment of acute and chronic heart failure of the European Society of Cardiology (ESC). Developed with the special contribution of the Heart Failure Association (HFA) of the ESC. Eur. Heart J. 37 (27), 2129–2200.

Roger, V.L., 2013. Epidemiology of heart failure. Circ. Res. 113 (6), 646–659.

Takeda, A., Taylor, S.J.C., Taylor, R.S., et al., 2012. Clinical service organisation for heart failure. Cochrane Database Syst. Rev. 9, CD002752.

Yohannes, A., Willgoss, T., Baldwin, R., Connolly, M., 2010. Depression and anxiety in chronic heart failure and chronic obstructive pulmonary disease: prevalence, relevance, clinical implications and management principles. Int. J. Geriatr. Psychiatry 25 (12), 1209–1221.

6 CARDIOVASCULAR SYSTEM 2
Drugs Used for Blood Pressure

CHAPTER OUTLINE

LEARNING OBJECTIVES

At the end of this chapter, the reader should be able to:

- describe blood pressure control
- list the causes of hypertension
- give examples of drugs that:
  - lower total peripheral resistance
  - lower cardiac output
  - decrease blood volume
  - act centrally
- describe the treatment of resistant hypertension, hypertensive emergencies and hypertension in pregnancy
- discuss the principles and practical aspects of taking blood pressure
- describe the treatment of hypotensive shock and the problems treating peripheral vascular disease

THE NORMAL CONTROL OF BLOOD PRESSURE

The physiological control of blood pressure depends on:

- the peripheral vascular resistance
- the output of blood from the heart
- the volume and viscosity of the blood.

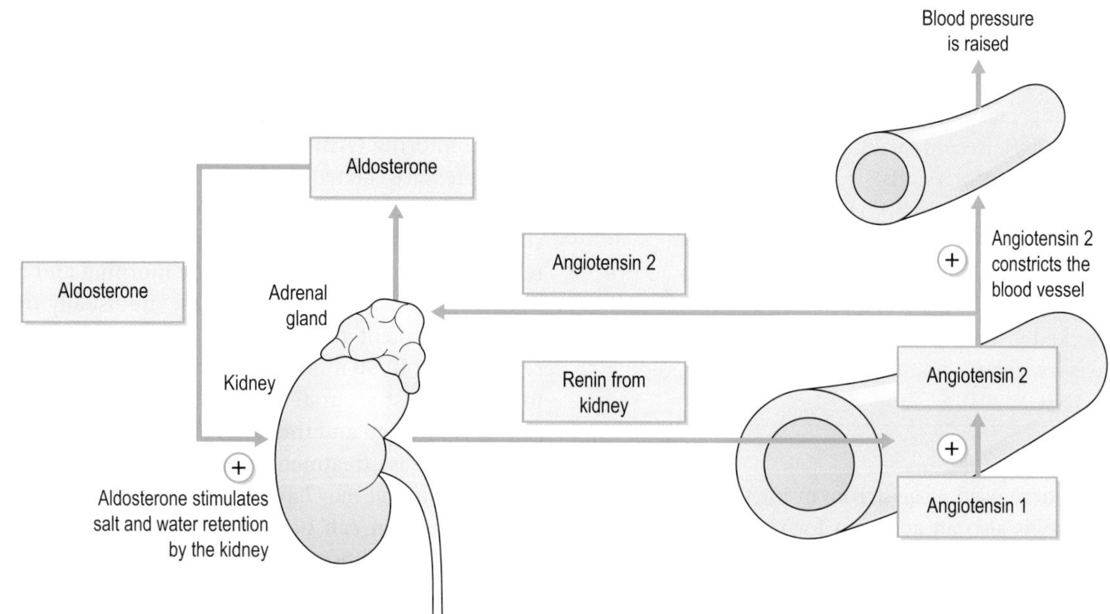

Fig. 6.1 ■ Diagram showing how blood pressure is raised and water and salt are converted by the kidneys when blood pressure falls due to the actions of renin, angiotensin and aldosterone.

By changing one or more of these factors it is possible to change the blood pressure.

The peripheral vascular resistance depends on the cross-section of the smaller arteries (arterioles). The walls of these arteries contain circular muscle fibers, which are controlled by the sympathetic nervous system (see Chapter 4). Stimulation of this system releases noradrenaline, which causes these muscles to contract and leads to narrowing of the arterioles and a rise in blood pressure. As a counterbalance, the endothelial cells lining the blood vessels are continually producing nitric oxide and prostacyclin, which are vasodilator substances that tend to lower blood pressure. *Angiotensin* (see later) is another endogenous factor that causes constriction of blood vessels and therefore a rise in blood pressure.

The output of blood from the heart, or the cardiac output, depends on several factors, but one important control is again the sympathetic nervous system, which, by releasing noradrenaline, causes a rise in pulse rate and cardiac output.

The volume and viscosity of the blood is ultimately controlled by the kidneys. There are receptors that 'sense' changes in the blood volume; if it falls, the kidney secretes a substance called renin, which, via a complex series of changes, leads to retention of salt and water by the kidneys (Fig. 6.1) and the formation of angiotensin II, which causes vasoconstriction, both of which raise the blood pressure.

In addition to reducing volume, drugs such as the diuretics are used to reduce the body's stores of sodium, which is believed to contribute to hypertension by increasing blood vessel stiffness, possibly through a sodium–calcium exchange that increases intracellular calcium levels in vascular smooth muscle.

Measurement of Blood Pressure

When blood pressure is measured using a sphygmomanometer, two values are noted, namely, the systolic and diastolic pressures. The **systolic pressure** is the blood pressure at systole, when the ventricles contract and pump blood into the arterial circulation. Here, the pressure of the pumping heart is a major component of the value recorded. The **diastolic pressure** is the pressure recorded at diastole, when the heart is filling, and the value obtained reflects predominantly the total peripheral resistance (TPR) in peripheral vascular beds.

CLINICAL NOTE

Accurate measurement of blood pressure is dependent on a number of factors including patient positioning, cuff size and how relaxed a patient is (Alexis, 2009). Recent qualitative research explored the healthcare professionals perspective on barriers to measurement accurate BP (Hwang et al., 2018). This included staff training, time factors and patient position. Accuracy of automated blood pressure measurement is affected by an irregular pulse and this should be checked prior to measuring blood pressure. If the pulse is irregular, a manual blood pressure should be taken (NICE, 2019).

TPR, here used as an acronym for total peripheral resistance, is also an acronym for temperature, pulse and respiration.

A typical reading, e.g. 120/75 mmHg (millimetres of mercury), where 120 is the systolic pressure and 75 is the diastolic pressure. Diastolic values of 90 or more indicate an abnormally high peripheral resistance. The aim for clinic blood pressure is below 140/90 in people aged under 80 years old and below 150/90 in people aged over 80 years old. It is important to look at individualized care for patients and special consideration should be made, particularly in patients who are frail, to balance the tolerability of blood pressure lowering drugs (antihypertensives) against the likely benefit from them. The new NICE guidelines (NICE, 2019) suggest that patients who are having postural symptoms (e.g. feeling light-headed on standing) or those who are over 80 years of age should have standing blood pressures measured and it is this reading that should be used to compare against the target values. Blood pressures measured during periods of stress or pain will often give spuriously high systolic values and the clinician should be aware of this when taking readings, including a fear of healthcare professionals or 'white coat syndrome'.

HYPERTENSION

Hypertension is the term used to describe blood pressure that is **chronically** raised above acceptable levels and contributes to detrimental health. If the blood pressure is consistently raised above normal limits, this can be due to a raised peripheral resistance secondary to vasoconstriction, although the kidneys also play a part.

According to NICE guidelines, diagnosis of hypertension is confirmed following ambulatory blood pressure monitoring (ABPM, which is a measurement of blood pressure carried out over a 24-h period during a patient's typical day) or alternatively home blood pressure monitoring (HBPM, which is usually a twice daily recording of blood pressure, in the morning and evening for 7 consecutive days). These are usually organized subsequent to increased clinic blood pressure readings of 140/90 mmHg or higher. ABPM is thought to be the most accurate method by which hypertension is confirmed and the rationale for its use is that it should decrease treatment in people who do not have hypertension but may have 'white coat syndrome'.

Hypertension can be classified into stages, which can help the healthcare professional manage urgency of treatment.

The stages of hypertension can be divided as:

- **Stage 1:** clinic BP readings of 140/90 mmHg (ABPM daytime average blood pressure average/ HBPM 135/85 mmHg or higher).
- **Stage 2:** clinic BP readings 160/100 mmHg (ABMP daytime average/ HBPM 150/95 mmHg or higher)
- **Stage 3/severe hypertension:** clinic BP readings 180 mmHg systolic or diastolic 120 mmHg or higher
- **Malignant/accelerated hypertension:** is a medical emergency, needing prompt management to improve prognosis. It is defined as diastolic above 130 mmHg accompanied by end organ damage (e.g. hypertensive retinopathy).

Causes of Hypertension

In the majority of patients the cause of hypertension is not known; however, genetic and environmental factors can contribute to its development. This is known as *essential hypertension*.

Other rarer causes of a raised blood pressure are secondary to kidney or endocrine disorders. In patients aged under 40 years, a thorough clinical work-up is usually required to exclude secondary causes of hypertension, usually via a specialist. Examples of secondary causes of hypertension include:

- phaeochromocytoma, a catecholamine-secreting tumour of the adrenal medulla, which is usually treated surgically by removal of the tumour
- renal artery stenosis (constriction)
- Cushing's disease (see Chapter 17)
- primary aldosteronism/Conn's syndrome (see Chapter 17).

The actual elevation of blood pressure, unless severe, rarely produces symptoms, but over a period of time, hypertension can lead to damage to the brain, heart, blood vessels, retina and kidneys, which can lead eventually to coronary thrombosis, heart failure, blindness, strokes and less often, to renal failure. It is therefore logical to prevent these complications by lowering the blood pressure with lifestyle measures as well as antihypertensive drugs.

HOW DRUGS CAN LOWER BLOOD PRESSURE

Drugs can lower the blood pressure in a number of ways. They can:

- lower the total peripheral resistance
- lower cardiac output
- reduce blood volume and body sodium stores
- act centrally in the CNS.

MEDICINES TO LOWER TOTAL PERIPHERAL RESISTANCE

- **Angiotensin-converting enzyme (ACE) inhibitors**
- **Vasodilators**
- **Sympathetic blocking drugs.**

Angiotensin-converting Enzyme Inhibitors

Mechanism of Action

Angiotensin-converting enzyme inhibitors (ACE) inhibit the conversion of angiotensin I to angiotensin II in the circulation. This reduces the vasoconstricting effect of angiotensin II and, by inhibiting the release of aldosterone, causes less sodium retention (Fig. 6.2). The overall effect is a fall in blood pressure. ACE inhibitors are used to treat hypertension and cardiac failure. They may actually improve the structure of thickened arteries and help preserve cardiac function by preventing remodelling of the heart. This drug class also reduces proteinuria in diabetic patients with kidney disease and slows the decline in renal function.

Therapeutic Use and Preparations Available

An ACE inhibitor may be used as a single drug to lower blood pressure and is often first-line treatment for stage 1 hypertension in patients aged under 55 and they may also be preferred option for diabetic patients due to their protective effects on the renal system. They can also be combined with other hypotensive drugs such as diuretics. ACE inhibitors are particularly useful if hypertension is complicated by heart failure (see Chapter 5). Several of these drugs are now available, with similar actions and uses.

Preparations and Uses

Ramipril is one of the most commonly used long-acting ACE inhibitors. Ramipril is a prodrug converted to its active metabolite ramiprilat in the liver. The peak effect is reached within 3–6 h after oral intake and the antihypertensive effect of a single dose normally lasts for 24 h. However, the maximum effect of continued treatment with ramipril is usually evident after 3–4 weeks.

Other examples include **lisinopril** and **enalapril**.

CLINICAL NOTE

High blood pressure is more difficult to control in some populations. As outlined in Chapter 1, ethnicity may affect how a population responds to a drug, and one such group is the Afro-Caribbean population. A 25-year longitudinal study has reported suboptimal blood pressure control in this group and that ACE inhibitor therapy is not as effective as in the general population. Therefore, although NICE recommends ACE inhibitors as first-line treatment for most populations, in the Afro-Caribbean population without diabetes, calcium antagonists are the recommended drugs of choice. Second-line treatment in this group is an ARB rather than an ACE inhibitor.

Effects of ACE Inhibitors

A marked fall in blood pressure occurs occasionally with the first dose of an ACE inhibitor, especially if the patient is already taking a diuretic. For

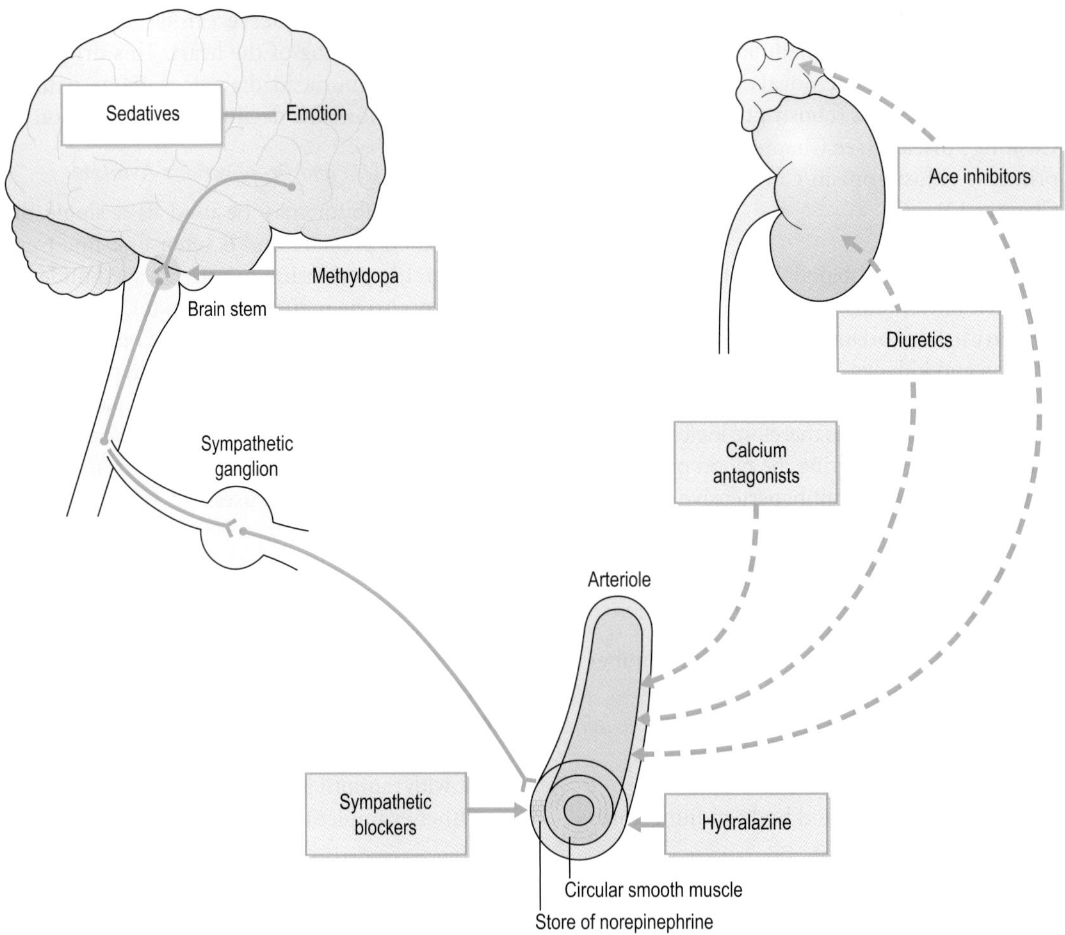

Fig. 6.2 ■ Site of action of some hypotensive drugs.

this reason, the initial dose should be low and taken before going to bed; patients should be warned of the possibility of a sharp fall in blood pressure if they get up during the night. Before starting treatment, electrolytes and renal function should be measured, which should then be repeated within a couple of weeks following initiation and any change of dose. It is recommended that discussion with a specialist should be sought if there is a rise in creatinine by 30% or a decrease of 20% in the estimated glomerular filtration rate (eGFR).

Contraindications for ACE Inhibitors

ACE inhibitors are contraindicated in pregnancy, as they may damage the fetus. They are also contraindicated in renal artery stenosis and severe aortic stenosis. Patients with a history of angioedema of any cause should not be prescribed this class of drugs or if the baseline potassium on checking the kidney function is over 5.5 mmol/L.

Adverse Effects and Interactions

- Dry cough (10%) and/or bronchospasm (5%) particularly in patients with underlying airway diseases such as asthma. Cough is one of the most common reasons to discontinue ACE inhibitors and substitute them with angiotensin II receptor blockers (see later).
- A few patients develop renal failure with ACE inhibitors. This is particularly liable to happen in elderly patients and those with stenosis of the renal arteries. Plasma creatinine should

therefore be measured in the first few weeks of treatment and thereafter at least anually (if the patient does not have chronic kidney disease).
- Rashes (particularly urticaria are common).
- Fatigue, headaches, diarrhoea.
- Hyperkalaemia (raised potassium) in patients with renal disease or those who are taking potassium-sparing diuretics or supplementary potassium. Declining renal function if combined with non-steroidal antiinflammatory drugs (NSAIDs). ACE inhibitors should be discontinued if potassium concentration increases to 6 mmol/L and other drugs responsible for hyperkalaemia have been stopped (e.g. NSAIDs, potassium sparing diuretics such as spironolactone).

CLINICAL NOTE

To optimize blood pressure control and medicines adherence patients should be informed of the risks, benefits and alternatives to drug treatment. The British Heart Foundation (BHF, 2019) has excellent resources that may assist in informing patients on how ACE inhibitors work to control blood pressure.

Angiotensin II Receptor Blockers (ARB)

Angiotensin II is an extremely powerful vasoconstrictor that acts on specific angiotensin II receptors on the blood vessel wall. Drugs have been developed that bind to the angiotensin II receptor and block the vasoconstrictor action of angiotensin II. These angiotensin receptor antagonist medicines will therefore have similar effects to those of medicines such as the ACE inhibitors. Examples of drugs in use:

- **losartan**
- **valsartan.**

Their hypotensive action is thus very similar to that of the ACE inhibitors and trials suggest that they have much the same efficacy. Some clinical trials of losartan have produced results suggesting that the medicine not only reduces blood pressure, but also improves left ventricular mass and improves ventricular contractility. An update of the 2019 NICE guidelines suggest that an ARB is to be considered instead of an ACE inhibitor in patients of black African/Caribbean origin.

Adverse Effects

The adverse effects are broadly similar to those of the ACE inhibitors, although ARBs are much less liable to cause a cough. Therefore they are usually used second-line in patients who do not tolerate an ACE inhibitor, e.g. if they develop a cough.

CLINICAL NOTE

Dry cough with ACE inhibitors is thought to be linked to the accumulation of bradykinin and its accumulation in the lungs, stimulating cough. The cough is often worse at night, when the patient lies down and is more common in women and in the East Asian population (Sato and Fukuda, 2015; Nishio et al., 2011). Patients should be informed of this side-effect and be advised to consult with their prescriber if it is affecting sleep and how they take medicines.

Vasodilators

Vasodilators comprise the following:

- **calcium channel antagonists (blockers)**
- **hydralazine**
- **minoxidil**
- **nitrovasodilators (e.g. sodium nitroprusside).**

Calcium Channel Antagonists (Blockers)

Mechanism of Action. The entry of calcium ions into the muscle cell is necessary for vascular smooth muscle fibres to contract. This group of medicines block the entry of calcium ions into the vascular muscle cells in the arterial walls, resulting in relaxation of the muscle and dilatation of the arteries.

Uses.

- Calcium channel antagonists are used to lower blood pressure in hypertension, to dilate coronary arteries in angina (see Chapter 7) and one calcium antagonist (verapamil; see later) slows conduction in the atrioventricular (AV) node and is also used to treat cardiac arrhythmias.

- At present, there is no clearly preferred drug for hypertension, although the longer-acting preparations are more convenient for patients (see later).
- Calcium channel antagonists may be used alone or combined with other hypotensive medicines to manage hypertension.
- Although their actions and uses are similar, calcium channel antagonists differ in their duration of action. They are all given orally and are broken down by the liver.

Short-Acting Calcium Antagonists Used for Hypertension or Angina.

- **Diltiazem**
- **Nifedipine**
- **Nicardipine.**

These need to be administered twice or three times daily.

Nifedipine is also the most common agent used in the treatment of autonomic dysreflexia, which can result following spinal cord injury at or above the sixth thoracic vertebrae. Typically it causes acute hypertension and bradycardia. It is often precipitated by painful stimuli (commonly bladder distention or constipation) below the level of injury, which results in widespread vasoconstriction through sympathetic drive. As well as the use of nifedipine for acute management of the raised blood pressure, it is important to identify the noxious stimulus and treat it (e.g. through catheterization for the management of urine retention to resolve bladder distention).

Long-Acting Calcium Antagonists Used for Hypertension or Angina.

- **Amlodipine**
- **Felodipine.**

These drugs are usually administered once daily.

Calcium Antagonists Used for Hypertension Only.

- **Lacidipine**

Calcium Antagonists Used for Hypertension, Angina and Cardiac Arrhythmias.

- **Verapamil**

Adverse Effects of Calcium Antagonists.

- Headache, flushing and ankle oedema due to vasodilatation can occur with all these medicines, but are more common with nifedipine and nicardipine. Verapamil can also cause constipation, which can be particularly problematic for the elderly.
- Depression of cardiac function is bound to be a feature of calcium antagonists since they also antagonize the entry of calcium ions into cardiac muscle cells. This effect is particularly marked with verapamil and to a lesser extent with other medicines in this class.
- Great care is necessary if calcium channel blockers are given to patients with heart failure, as this may be made worse.
- There is some evidence of increased mortality in patients taking large doses of the short-acting preparation of nifedipine, particularly in patients with coronary artery disease. The longer-acting preparations appear safe, but ACE inhibitors (see later) are to be preferred in hypertensive patients with diabetes.

Drug Interactions. The actions of nifedipine and nicardipine are increased by cimetidine, a drug used to treat gastric ulcers (see Chapter 10).

CLINICAL NOTE

For patients with suboptimal blood pressure control on an ACE inhibitor or ARB, a calcium antagonist may be added. However, prior to prescribing any additional therapy medicines, adherence should be explored. As outlined in Chapter 2, factors such as forgetting to take medicines, fear of side-effects, illness perceptions or regimen complexity will all affect whether a patient is adherent to medicines and establishing reasons for non-adherence allows for person-centred strategies to be put in place. There are a number of ways to explore medicines adherence with a patient, including monitoring prescription refills, monitoring effects of prescribed treatment through biological parameters, e.g. blood pressure, or self-report adherence tools. One self-report tool, validated for use in people with hypertension, is the Morisky Medication Adherence Scale (MMAS-8), an 8-item scale that is simple to administer to establish how adherent a patient is and reasons for non-adherence (Moon et al., 2017).

Hydralazine

Hydralazine is chemically a hydrazine derivative, which has been clinically available for many years.

Mechanism of Action and Pharmacokinetics.

- Hydralazine directly dilates arterioles but not veins to produce its antihypertensive effects.
- The hypotensive action of a given dose becomes successively less effective, a phenomenon known as tachyphylaxis. This limits the use of hydralazine for the treatment of hypotension to only be prescribed together with other antihypertensive drugs.
- Hydralazine is administered orally and is well absorbed, but rapidly metabolized during first pass metabolism. This reduces its bioavailability considerably.
- The metabolism of hydralazine is partly by acetylation. The general population consists of those who are either fast or slow acetylators of drugs. Fast acetylators will derive less benefit from a single dose than people who are slow acetylators.
- The half-life of hydralazine is 2–4 h, although the hypotensive effect may persist after plasma levels have declined. This is because the drug binds tightly to arteriolar tissue.

Use of Hydralazine.

- Hydralazine is generally not used alone, but in combination with other drugs, to help counteract tachycardia and fluid retention adverse effects.
- Hydralazine has now been largely replaced by newer antihypertensive medicines and is rarely used except in exceptional circumstances for the treatment of resistant hypertension, under specialist guidance.

Adverse Effects of Hydralazine.

- Nausea, headaches, palpitations (due to reflex tachycardia) and anorexia are the most common side-effects.
- Hydralazine may precipitate angina or ischaemic arrhythmias in patients with ischaemic heart disease, due to the reflex tachycardia.
- Rarely, hydralazine may cause peripheral neuropathy (functional or pathological changes in the nervous system).
- At high doses, especially in slow acetylators, hydralazine may cause arthralgia (joint pain), myalgia (muscle pain), fever and skin rashes – a set of symptoms very reminiscent of the disease systemic lupus erythematosus (lupus; SLE). This medicine-induced syndrome is reversible, and symptoms should disappear on ceasing treatment with hydralazine.

Minoxidil

Minoxidil is another direct vasodilator of arterioles that is very effective, but it has some potentially serious adverse effects. Its indication is for severe hypertension.

Mechanism of Action and Pharmacokinetics.

- Minoxidil, like hydralazine, dilates arteriolar, but not venous smooth muscle, by opening potassium channels.
- Minoxidil is taken orally and is well absorbed from the gastrointestinal tract.
- After absorption, minoxidil is converted to minoxidil sulphate, the active metabolite.
- The half-life of minoxidil in the circulation is about 4 h. It is not protein-bound in the blood.
- Despite the relatively short plasma half-life, the antihypertensive effects of minoxidil may last up to 24 h or more, possibly because of a longer half-life of minoxidil sulphate and its ability to bind to arteriolar tissue.

Use of Minoxidil.

The use of minoxidil is confined to patients who are resistant to more usual treatments. It causes salt and water retention and reflex sympathetic stimulation of the heart, which results in an increased heart rate. Therefore, minoxidil must be prescribed together with a diuretic and a β-blocker.

Adverse Effects of Minoxidil.

If diuretics and β-blockers are not used, or if inadequate doses of these other medicine classes are given, minoxidil causes:

- oedema
- tachycardia

- palpitations
- angina.

Patients may also complain of sweating, headache and hirsutism. This last-mentioned adverse effect has resulted in the use of topical preparations of minoxidil to stimulate scalp hair growth in baldness.

Sympathetic Blocking Drugs

- **Prazosin**
- **Doxazosin**
- **Terazosin.**

Mechanism of Action and Uses

- Prazosin, doxazosin and terazosin block the vasoconstrictor sympathetic nerve supply to the small arteries and arterioles by blocking α_1 receptors on the blood vessels, and the resulting vasodilatation causes a fall in blood pressure. With these medicines there is little compensatory rise in pulse rate or cardiac output.
- The fall in blood pressure is inclined to be postural (greater on lying than standing).
- Prazosin is short-acting and dosage is required two or three times daily, which makes control of blood pressure difficult. Doxazosin and terazosin have a longer action, so once-a-day dosage is adequate.
- α-Blockers also improve the flow of urine in patients with bladder neck obstruction and are used in mild cases of prostatic enlargement. These medicines may be combined with other hypotensive agents. Adverse effects are unusual except for postural hypotension. Occasionally, these medicines cause urinary incontinence, particularly in women.

CLINICAL NOTE

When a patient complains of palpitations, this could be because of a vasodilator drug. When blood pressure falls due to a decrease in the total peripheral resistance, this fall is detected by the central nervous system, which immediately activates the sympathetic drive to the heart to speed it up (tachycardia). The patient experiences the tachycardia and complains of 'palpitations.' The initial dose of an α_1-blocker can sometimes cause a profound fall in blood pressure with fainting, so it is advisable that this dose is given before going to bed and that it should be low. Subsequent doses rarely provoke this problem, but the blood pressure should be taken standing and lying down to assess any postural fall. The dose is increased at weekly intervals until satisfactory control is achieved.

Nitrovasodilators Exemplified by Sodium Nitroprusside

Sodium nitroprusside is a very powerful vasodilator used to treat hypertensive emergencies and severe cardiac failure. It dilates both arterial and venous blood vessels, which results in reduced peripheral resistance and venous return. Nitrovasodilators act by mimicking the effects of nitric oxide released by the vascular endothelial cells lining blood vessels.

Use of Sodium Nitroprusside

Sodium nitroprusside must be given intravenously and is therefore only suitable for treating a hypertensive crisis and some patients with acute heart failure. It is given by infusion and it is usual to start at the lower end of the dose range and increase the dose of the drug until the blood pressure is satisfactorily controlled. This will require close observation and is usually carried out in an intensive care unit.

CLINICAL NOTE

There are five important practical points in the use of sodium nitroprusside:

1. The contents of the ampoule should be dissolved in 2 mL of 5% dextrose solution and then diluted in dextrose or saline.
2. The infusion must be protected from the light and discarded after 24 h.
3. It should also be discarded if the colour changes from pale orange to dark brown or blue.
4. Infusion should not be continued for more than 72 h.
5. If infusion is prolonged, blood cyanide and thiocyanate levels should be measured to guard against the development of cyanide poisoning.

Adverse Effects of Sodium Nitroprusside

- Headaches
- Dizziness
- Palpitations
- Chest pain.

Other nitrovasodilators such as glyceryl trinitrate can be administered sublingually to treat the coronary vasoconstriction that causes angina pectoris.

DRUGS TO LOWER CARDIAC OUTPUT

β-Blockers for Treating Comorbidities

β-Blockers are useful for treatment in angina, cardiac arrhythmias, post-myocardial infarction and heart failure. They are no longer used as first-line treatment in hypertension (except in pregnancy where, e.g. labetalol is used), as studies have found that treatment of hypertension with β-blockers had little or no effect on mortality. They will however, lower the blood pressure to a satisfactory level in about 40% of patients with hypertension, but the hypotensive effect may be delayed for several weeks after starting treatment. It is not known exactly how these drugs produce this effect. By interfering with the sympathetic nervous system, they certainly prevent the rise in cardiac output and blood pressure, which occur with excitement or effort. It may be that this damping down of the cardiac output ultimately causes a permanent fall in blood pressure. β-Blockers may also decrease renin release by the kidney, which would tend to lower the blood pressure (see Fig. 6.1), and some of them (particularly propranolol) have some central sedative action. β-Blockers are reserved as fourth-line treatment for hypertension.

The effect of some β-blockers is predominantly on the heart by acting on β_1 receptors and they are called 'selective' β-blockers; others also affect the bronchi and possibly the peripheral circulation by acting on β_2 receptors and are known as 'non-selective' β-blockers, although this selectivity is not absolute (see Chapter 4). Therefore, particularly non-selective β-blockers should not be used in patients with asthma or chronic obstructive pulmonary disease as they can cause life-threatening adverse effects.

DRUGS TO DECREASE BLOOD VOLUME

Diuretics

Diuretics are considered step 2 of antihypertensive treatment, provided they are not contraindicated, e.g. in pregnancy. The fall in blood pressure is due to a reduction in blood volume (by increased urination) and to a vasodilating effect on the walls of the arterioles. They are relatively inexpensive, relatively easy to use and serious side-effects are rare.

Therapeutic Use of Diuretics

Thiazide diuretics are the most suitable. The dose should be relatively low; raising the dose causes little further fall in blood pressure, but increases the incidence of adverse effects.

Examples include:

- Indapamide
- Bendroflumethiazide
- Xipamide.

Contraindications and Adverse Effects

- Diuretics cause uric acid retention and can subsequently increase the risk of developing gout.
- In diabetes, diuretics decrease glucose tolerance and thus make control of the disease more difficult.
- In pregnancy, diuretics may damage the fetus.
- Diuretics can cause impotence in about 20% of males.
- High dosage can lead to hypokalaemia, due to increased urinary loss of potassium. This is rare with low dosage, but the blood potassium should be checked within 1 month after starting treatment as hypokalaemia can precipitate arrhythmias.

Drug Interactions

- NSAIDs reduce the efficacy of diuretics.
- Diuretics raise blood levels of lithium and the dose of lithium may require adjustment if these drugs are co-prescribed.

CLINICAL NOTE

NSAIDs are available as an over-the-counter medication and are safe in low dose for short periods of time; however, long-term use and prescription strength non-steroidals should be used with caution in the elderly and those prescribed antihypertensive medication (Moore et al., 2015).

DRUGS THAT ACT CENTRALLY

Methyldopa

Methyldopa lowers blood pressure by an action on the brain that results in decreased activity of the sympathetic system. The antihypertensive effect of methyldopa is not really fully understood, but is probably due to its metabolism to alpha-methylnoradrenaline, which then lowers arterial pressure by stimulation of central inhibitory alpha-adrenergic receptors, false neurotransmission (as this metabolite is not as active at affecting blood pressure as noradrenaline itself), and/or reduction of plasma renin activity. Methyldopa has been shown to cause a net reduction in the tissue concentration of serotonin, dopamine, norepinephrine, and epinephrine.

Therapeutic Use

Methyldopa was formerly used widely in the treatment of hypertension. It is effective and easy to use because the fall in blood pressure is not precipitous. However, it has a number of common adverse effects that patients sometimes find unacceptable and its use has declined considerably. It is still, however, widely used in treating pregnancy-related hypertension.

Adverse Effects

- Drowsiness and depression often occur early in treatment, but may pass off after a few weeks.
- More rarely, fluid retention producing oedema can be troublesome, but this can be controlled by a diuretic.
- Haemolytic anaemia and drug induced fever have also been reported.

Moxonidine

Moxonidine acts centrally to reduce activity of the sympathetic nervous system. At present, it is indicated if other hypotensive agents are not satisfactory and is given orally, once or twice daily.

Adverse Effects

These include tiredness, headache and nausea.

The sites of action of the various antihypertensive agents are shown in Fig. 6.2.

THE TREATMENT OF HYPERTENSION

When raised blood pressure is detected, it is important to exclude underlying renal or endocrine causes, although essential hypertension is responsible in more than 90% of cases. Hypertension by itself rarely causes any symptoms and the object of treatment is to prevent the development of complications, e.g. stroke, coronary thrombosis, cardiac and renal failure. Many hypertensive patients live for years without these complications and this means that the drugs used in treatment should be safe and as free as possible from adverse effects. Unfortunately, no antihypertensive drug entirely fulfils these criteria.

It is generally accepted that severe hypertension carries a poor prognosis and adequate treatment considerably reduces morbidity and mortality. It is in patients with milder degrees of hypertension that a decision to embark on these treatments is more difficult.

In healthy subjects with no evidence of cardiac, vascular or renal complications, it is justifiable to observe the patient with regular measurement of blood pressure for 3–6 months because, in some people, it may return to normal levels, particularly if they have instigated lifestyle measures (see later). If, however, the blood pressure remains persistently above 140/90 in clinic, and particularly if there are special risk factors (hyperlipidaemias, diabetes, smoking or a family history of cardiovascular disease), it is usual to start treatment with a single drug, and, if this fails, a combination of different classes of antihypertensive drug should be given, as highlighted earlier. However, commonly treatment is a combination of different drug classes in lower doses, which are generally more effective than a single drug up to its maximum dose. As mentioned previously, the aim is to maintain the blood pressure around 140/90 in patients under 80 years old or below 150/90 in patients above 80 years old. However, tighter control of 130/80 is required in diabetics, due to added cardiovascular risk posed by the disease.

Ideal blood pressure readings are not easy to achieve and a substantial proportion of treated subjects will still have blood pressures well above the target of 140/90. There have been many trials of antihypertensive medicines in this group of patients and the results can be roughly summarized as follows:

- There was some reduction in overall mortality, probably about 20%.
- The incidence of stroke was halved, but there was less reduction of coronary thrombosis.
- In elderly patients, the incidence of stroke was reduced by about 35% and there was some reduction in the occurrence of coronary thrombosis (20%).

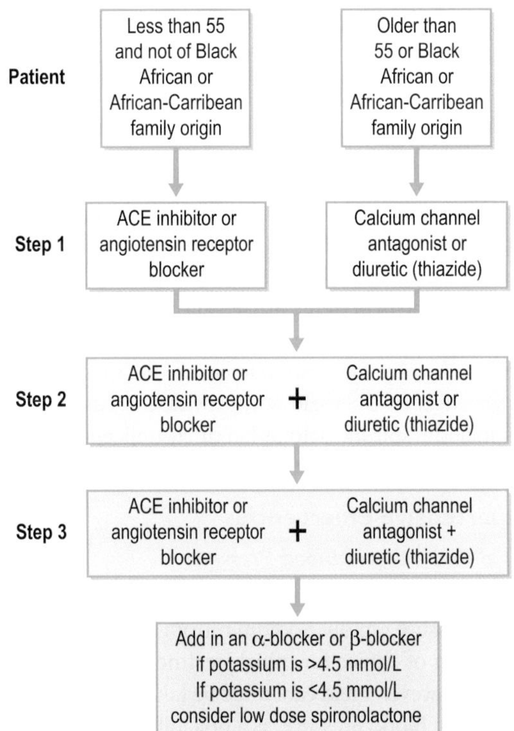

Fig. 6.3 ■ The British A/CD algorithm for treatment of hypertension. *ACE,* Angiotensin-converting enzyme. (Reproduced with kind permission of the British Hypertension Society – now called the British and Irish Hypertension Society.)

As a wider variety of antihypertensive drug classes are now available, the optimal drug class or combination of drugs for treatment of hypertension continues to be investigated. The usual approach is to start with ACE inhibitors in younger patients or those with diabetes. In older patients over the age of 55 years or those who are Black African or African-Carribean family origin, preference to calcium channel blockers is given (Fig. 6.3).

There is, however, increasing concern about the quality of life of many patients receiving treatment for hypertension, as these regimens may be associated with various adverse effects, which, although usually minor, can be troublesome. ACE inhibitors, though not entirely trouble-free, have a place in initial treatment, especially for diabetics, in whom they help to preserve renal function. α-Blockers and calcium channel blockers may also be used and there are numerous possible combinations where the effects are at least additive. It is usually possible to plan a regimen that is therapeutically effective without interfering with the patient's lifestyle.

Elderly patients are a little more prone to side-effects, but usually tolerate treatment well. Low-dose thiazides, ACE inhibitors and calcium channel blockers are all satisfactory.

ACE inhibitors are indicated if there is any evidence of heart failure or diabetes, and α-blockers may be helpful if there is prostatic obstruction.

Hypertension is primarily managed in primary care. Very few patients require admission to hospital, e.g. those with suspected malignant hypertension. Young patients, under 40 years of age or those with resistant hypertension need specialist review to exclude secondary causes of hypertension.

British and Irish Hypertension Society Guidelines for Hypertension Management

The British and Irish Hypertension Society has published guidelines for the treatment of hypertension with drugs and some of their recommendations for the use of antihypertensives are summarized in Fig. 6.3.

1. Some patients do not realize that once treatment is initiated it is likely to continue lifelong, although it may be altered or attenuated over time.
2. There are several lifestyle factors that can be implemented. Avoiding addition of salt in food or cooking will help reduce blood pressure and enhance the effect of drugs. However, some patients find this spoils the joy of eating. Various forms of relaxation, meditation and stress reduction produce a small but useful fall in blood pressure in many patients.
3. Exercise, currently recommended at 30 minutes five times/week should be encouraged, e.g. going for brisk walks, swimming, social dancing, cycling or even walking up and down stairs. Modern technology, through the use of apps, can help encourage patients to increase and track their activity.
4. It is crucial to address the risk factors alongside hypertension management, which can otherwise increase their liability to the complications of hypertension. The following advice should be given:
   a. Smoking cessation
   b. Reduce weight if overweight or obese
   c. Treat hyperlipidaemia

   d. Reduce alcohol consumption if excessive of 14 units/week
   e. The place of diet and exercise in lowering blood pressure is more controversial, but a 'Mediterranean diet', which contains plenty of fruit and vegetables, combined with an exercise programme within the competence of the patient, should be encouraged.
5. Patients should be warned of the main adverse effects of the drugs prescribed for them.
6. It is impossible for patients to know and understand all the possible interactions, but if given a new drug, they should remind the prescriber that they are already receiving medication.
7. Some patients can be taught to take their own blood pressure and thus obtain a more accurate assessment of day-to-day levels. It is also now gold standard to use ambulatory blood pressure for diagnosis of hypertension. This helps to prevent overdiagnosis of hypertension and is particularly useful for patients suffering with 'white coat hypertension'.

CLINICAL NOTE

It is important to take an holistic, person-centred approach to supporting people with hypertension. A systematic review of 20 studies concluded that adherence to pharmacological and non-pharmacological treatment had a positive impact on quality of life. Healthcare professionals should consider how they can support patients to focus on making small lifestyle changes, in addition to optimizing medication adherence. As outlined in Chapter 2, adherence is a complex interaction between cognitive, psychological and physical factors and a Cochrane Review in 2014 (Nieuwlaat et al., 2014) concluded complex interventions may be the most effective, but there was insufficient evidence to recommend anything more specific. Interventions that may help are cognitive behavioural therapy or motivational interviewing, and, in the absence of conclusive evidence, taking time to explore what matters to the patient may assist with a shared understanding of the realistic steps that can be taken to optimize blood pressure control, and this, combined with frequent follow-up, may be all that is required to reduce risk.

Resistant Hypertension

This can be defined as when a patient's hypertension remains unmanageable despite the use of three antihypertensives, one of which is a diuretic. Secondary hypertensive causes should be considered in patients presenting with resistant hypertension (see earlier, e.g. renal artery stenosis). It is also important to check the compliance of antihypertensive medication to ensure the measurements are an effect of the treatment provided. **Drugs** used for this include: spironolactone (adjunct, unlicensed indication), hydralazine and nitroprusside (see earlier).

Hypertensive Emergencies

Rapid Reduction in Blood Pressure

Occasionally, it may be necessary to reduce a very high blood pressure rapidly. Sodium nitroprusside (see earlier) is the drug of choice for initial treatment in this circumstance. However, great care must be taken when lowering a very high blood pressure, as a precipitous fall may cause renal failure or cerebral damage due to a sudden reduction of the blood supply to the kidney and brain. Therefore, the early stages of this treatment should be carried out in an intensive care unit if possible and the blood pressure monitored at frequent intervals. The aim of treatment should be to reduce the diastolic blood pressure slowly to around 100 mmHg. Thereafter, treatment for hypertension should be carried out in the normal way (see earlier).

If facilities for intensive monitoring are not available and if the clinical situation is less acute, bed rest and an α-blocker or slow-release nifedipine are satisfactory and should avoid a precipitous fall in blood pressure.

Hypertension in Pregnancy

Hypertension in pregnancy presents a special problem as occasionally it may progress to pre-eclampsia and eclampsia, with serious risk to both mother and child. Pharmacological treatment is required if blood pressure remains above 140/90 mmHg. Mild transient elevation of blood pressure occurring towards the end of pregnancy rarely needs drug treatment. More severe hypertension, particularly if the patient was hypertensive before the start of her pregnancy, may require medication to lower the blood pressure. Methyldopa has been found satisfactory in this situation and has been used for many years. β-Blockers (e.g. labetalol) are also used but may retard fetal growth. In severe hypertension, hydralazine orally or intravenously is effective. Diuretics, ACE inhibitors and ARB II should be avoided during pregnancy.

NURSING NOTE

Measuring blood pressure

Nurses frequently measure blood pressure. There are some key points to remember when treating hypertension. Refer to the local early warning score guidance for monitoring, frequency and escalation of blood pressure.

- The blood pressure should usually be recorded with the patient both lying and standing, as some antihypertensive drugs cause a much greater fall in blood pressure when the patient is standing than when lying down. In certain cases, it should also be recorded after exercise.
- Some patients are nervous when visiting the doctor and this may cause their blood pressure to rise, the so-called 'white coat' hypertension. Quiet reassurance and a rest period of 5 min are necessary before measuring the blood pressure.
- It is helpful to teach patients to take their own blood pressure, so a home record can be obtained, which will give a better idea of day-to-day fluctuations.
- Because smoking may alter blood pressure temporarily, patients should be asked to avoid it for 30 min before having their blood pressure measured.
- A well-applied and appropriately sized cuff are necessary for accurate readings.
- Measurements of blood pressure tend to show 'observer bias'. This may happen in trials of new drugs and it is necessary in these circumstances to use a special sphygmomanometer in which the blood pressure is recorded 'blind', so that the recording is not known by the observer.
- It is now possible to record patients' blood pressure as they go about their daily life (ambulatory BP recording), with an apparatus they can wear over a 24-h period. This gives a much better assessment of their overall blood pressure and is useful in evaluating white coat hypertension, responses to stress or the apparent failure of treatment. This approach is now the gold standard.

SUMMARY

- Blood pressure can be lowered by lowering: (1) total peripheral resistance; (2) cardiac output; and (3) blood volume and sodium stores.
- Patients can be fast or slow acetylators of medicines, which will affect the activity and duration of action of certain drugs (e.g. hydralazine).
- Hydralazine can cause arthralgia in high doses, but this is reversible on stopping the medicine.
- The actions of nifedipine and nicardipine are increased by cimetidine, a medicine used to treat gastric ulcers.
- Calcium channel blockers may be used alone or combined with other classes of antihypertensive medicines.
- β-Blockers are now rarely used for the sole treatment of hypertension but often used as an adjunct in treatment of other comorbidities which often present with hypertension such as heart failure. They are also used for the management of hypertension in pregnancy.
- Diuretics cause uric acid retention and can precipitate gout.
- In diabetes, diuretics decrease glucose tolerance and thus make control of the disease more difficult.
- In pregnancy, diuretics, ACE inhibitors and ARB II may damage the fetus and thus should be avoided.
- Diuretics cause impotence in about 20% of males. High dosage can lead to hypokalaemia, due to increased urinary loss of potassium. This is rare with low dosage but the blood potassium should be checked within 1 month after starting treatment.

DRUGS TO TREAT PERIPHERAL VASCULAR DISEASE

For many years, various drugs, which in normal subjects dilate arteries, were used in the treatment of patients with peripheral vascular disease in the hope that they would increase the blood supply to the ischaemic limb. Unfortunately, peripheral vascular disease usually affects the large arteries and these diseased arteries were poorly responsive to vasodilators and it is now accepted that this class of drug is of little value in this condition. They are, however, useful in the treatment of patients with Raynaud's disease, which is due to spasm in the small arteries of the hands and feet brought on by cold.

Treatment

Nifedipine, a calcium antagonist, used as for the treatment of hypertension, is the most useful drug. Other measures include keeping warm in cold weather. Do not forget that β-blockers, ergotamine and smoking make peripheral vascular disease worse.

DRUGS FOR PATIENTS IN SHOCK

During shock, the output of blood from the heart is acutely reduced, the blood pressure is low and circulation to the organs of the body is inadequate. Clinically, the patient is pale, sweating and confused, the pulse is rapid, the blood pressure low and the limbs cold; kidney failure may supervene. This state may occur for three main reasons:

- Sudden reduction of blood volume, usually due to bleeding, which is treated by replacing the lost fluid by infusion.
- Reduced pumping action of the heart (pump failure) following damage (e.g. after a myocardial infarct).
- Septic shock, usually due to infection with Gram-negative bacteria (see Chapter 26). This is commonly found in patients receiving steroids or cytotoxic drugs. Bacterial toxins such as lipopolysaccharide cause vasodilatation and leaking of fluid from the circulation, which reduces the blood volume, combined with a falling cardiac output. In addition to the usual measures to combat shock, rapid and vigorous (IV) treatment with the appropriate antibiotic is necessary, as the condition may prove fatal very quickly.

Drugs Commonly in Use for the Treatment of Shock

If the main underlying problem leading to shock is pump (heart) failure, known as cardiogenic shock, drugs can be given to increase the force of contraction of the heart muscle (positive inotropic effect) and thus improve cardiac output and raise the blood pressure. The most common cause of cardiogenic shock is myocardial infarction and the most effective intervention to reverse shock is early revascularization. The most commonly used drugs for the treatment of shock in heart failure are dopamine and dobutamine, treatment that requires careful monitoring, usually in an intensive care ward.

Please note, however, that digoxin is not effective in these circumstances and may precipitate a dangerous cardiac arrhythmia.

CLINICAL NOTE

Blood pressure is a part of the standardized track and trigger system used to recognize deteriorating patients. In the UK, the National Early Warning Scoring system has been endorsed by the Royal College of Physicians in 2012 and was revised to NEWS2 in 2017 (RCP, 2017). This tool provides a structured approach to monitoring clinical deterioration and care escalation. Cardiogenic shock is characterized by systolic blood pressure of <90, signs of hyperperfusion, e.g. altered conscious level poor capillary refill time, low urine output and elevated serum lactate (Thiele et al., 2015; RCP, 2017). See Chapter 8 for further information on resuscitation.

Dopamine

Dopamine is a naturally occurring substance, which is converted to noradrenaline in the body. However, it has actions of its own and is used to treat shock, which may follow cardiac infarction or major cardiac surgery.

Dopamine stimulates cardiac β_1 receptors, and also increases the release of noradrenaline in the heart, thus causing the heart muscle to contract more powerfully. In addition, dopamine stimulates receptors in the renal blood vessels, causing them to dilate and increase both renal blood flow and urinary output. This action is useful since shock often causes a decline in renal function.

Dopamine is given by continuous intravenous infusion (via a central line). It affects mainly the kidneys and is used to improve their function, often combined with a diuretic. Higher doses should not be used as the intense vasoconstriction that develops may cause gangrene of the extremities.

Drug interactions with dopamine: patients receiving monoamine oxidase inhibitors should be given one-tenth of the usual dose of dopamine. This is because MOA inhibitors potentiate the effect of dopamine and its duration of action.

Dobutamine

Dobutamine is similar to dopamine but has no effect on the kidneys. It is, however, less likely to cause cardiac arrhythmias.

Dopamine and dobutamine may be combined: a low dose of dopamine being used for its effects on the kidneys and dobutamine for its cardiac action.

Both dopamine and dobutamine should be infused via a central vein to minimize peripheral vasoconstriction.

In septic shock many different pharmacological approaches have been trialled to attempt to neutralize the effects of bacterial derived toxins and to date these have all failed to show any major clinical benefit. Early recognition of a patient becoming potentially septicaemic is very important with an urgent need to initiate systemic treatment with an appropriate antibiotic dependent on the organism(s) identified.

Another important type of shock is anaphylactic shock resulting from allergy to certain food products (e.g. peanuts or shellfish) and such patients are encouraged to carry an adrenaline autoinjector, e.g. an EpiPen® to allow self-administration of subcutaneous adrenaline at the first sign of problems, to increase blood pressure, reduce laryngeal oedema and to reduce bronchoconstriction. Adrenaline can also be used with or without an H1 receptor antagonist to treat the anaphylactic shock that occurs in patients sensitive to bee or wasp venom.

NURSING NOTE

Patients should be given essential patient education information relating to lifestyle and blood pressure reduction strategies (see Case History 6.1).

CASE HISTORY 6.1

Mr. Patel, a 55-year-old man, attended his GP practice for a routine NHS health check. He had an appointment with the nurse who asked questions about his lifestyle and family history. Mr. Patel discussed that, due to working long hours as a lawyer, he had not been successful in taking regular exercise and often resorted to grabbing a quick takeaway meal. He also smoked 10–15 cigarettes per day as he felt this was the only time he could relax and catch up with colleagues. He admitted to drinking 2 glasses of wine every night with his dinner. Mr. Patel was aware that he needed to make significant changes to his lifestyle, in particular as both his parents suffered from high blood pressure and his father had a heart attack at age 59. However, due to his busy work and homelife, as well as lack of symptoms, Mr. Patel had been unable to prioritize his health and felt motivated when he was invited for a health check.

The nurse measured his height and weight and calculated his body mass index (BMI), which was 29 kg/m^2. She proceeded to measure his blood pressure, which was raised at 160/98 mmHg and she followed this up with a couple of additional measurements, which showed similar values. They discussed at length about his possible lifestyle changes. During the conversation, the nurse discussed his alcohol intake and calorie consumption using an online drinkaware tracker tool, which provided useful guidance and he was surprised to see the calorie consumption from his drinking. She also gave him an information leaflet from the British Heart Foundation about hypertension, detailing treatment and important lifestyle changes for him to tackle. The nurse discussed the importance of smoking cessation and dietary aspects as well as weight reduction.

An ambulatory blood pressure check and a follow-up appointment with the GP for review was arranged. Mr. Patel's ambulatory blood pressure in day time averaged 154/94. Following this, a cardiovascular examination was conducted and investigations to look for end-organ damage ordered including:

- an ECG (to look for left ventricular hypertrophy)
- urine dip (to check for any proteinuria as an indicator for renal function)
- optician's review (to check for retinal haemorrhages).

The GP diagnosed essential hypertension. Additional blood tests were arranged to check if other risk factors needed to be addressed including a check for lipids, HbA$_{1c}$ (for the diagnosis of diabetes) as well as a baseline kidney function test. The GP also reinforced lifestyle interventions and discussed the importance of blood pressure control to prevent cardiovascular, cerebrovascular and renal complications. They discussed antihypertensive medication with either a calcium channel blocker or a diuretic for the patient and their possible adverse effects. Jointly it was agreed to start amlodipine (a calcium channel blocker), which was well tolerated by the patient and at follow-up, his blood pressure had normalized. Mr. Patel also started to tackle the suggested lifestyle interventions.

REFERENCES AND FURTHER READING

Alexis, O., 2009. Providing best practice in manual blood pressure measurement. Br. J. Nurs. 18 (7), 410–415.

BHF, 2019. What Are ACE Inhibitors and what Do They Do to Your Body. British Heart Foundation. https://www.bhf.org.uk/informationsupport/heart-matters-magazine/medical/drug-cabinet/ace-inhibitors.

Eldahan, K.C., Rabchevsky, A.G., 2018. Autonomic dysreflexia after spinal cord injury: systemic pathophysiology and methods of management. Auton. Neurosci. 209, 59–70.

Hwang, K., Aigbe, A., Ju, H., et al., 2018. Barriers to accurate blood pressure measurement in the medical office. J. Prim. Care Community Health 9, 2150132718816929.

Moon, S.J., Lee, W.Y., Hwang, J.S., et al., 2017. Accuracy of a screening tool for medication adherence: a systematic review and meta-analysis of the Morisky Medication Adherence Scale-8. PloS One 12 (11), e0187139.

Moore, N., Pollack, C., Butkerait, P., 2015. Adverse drug reactions and drug-drug interactions with over-the-counter NSAIDs. Ther. Clin. Risk Manag. 11, 1061–1075.

Nieuwlaat, R., Wilczynski, N., Navarro, T., et al., 2014. Interventions for enhancing medication adherence. Cochrane Database Sys. Rev. 11, CD000011.

Nishio, K., Kashiki, S., Tachibana, H., Kobayashi, Y., 2011. Angiotensin-converting enzyme and bradykinin gene polymorphisms and cough: a meta-analysis. World J. Cardiol. 3 (10), 329–336.

NICE, 2019. Hypertension in adults: diagnosis and management NICE guideline [NG136]. https://www.nice.org.uk/guidance/ng136.

RCP, 2017. National Early Warning Scoring 2, Standardising Assessment of Acute Illness Severity in the NHS. Royal College of Physicians. https://www.rcplondon.ac.uk/projects/outputs/national-early-warning-score-news-2.

Sato, A., Fukuda, S., 2015. A prospective study of frequency and characteristics of cough during ACE inhibitor treatment. Clin. Exp. Hypertens. 37 (7), 563–568.

Thiele, H., Ohman, E.M., Desch, S., et al., 2015. Management of cardiogenic shock. Eur. Heart J. 36 (20), 1223–1230.

USEFUL WEBSITES

BBC News: Inside Medicine: Pulmonary hypertension nurse. http://news.bbc.co.uk/1/hi/health/4762147.stm.

British and Irish Hypertension Society. https://bihsoc.org.

British Heart Foundation. https://www.bhf.org.uk.

Bupa. https://www.bupa.co.uk/health-information/heart-blood-circulation/high-blood-pressure-hypertension.

DrinkAware. https://www.drinkaware.co.uk.

NICE. Hypertension in adults: diagnosis and management [NG136]. https://www.nice.org.uk/guidance/ng136.

Nursing Times. https://www.nursingtimes.net/clinical-archive/assessment-skills/blood-pressure-1-key-principles-and-types-of-measuring-equipment-15-05-2020/.

Scottish Intercollegiate Guidelines Network (SIGN). https://www.sign.ac.uk/assets/sign149.pdf.

7 CARDIOVASCULAR SYSTEM 3
Atheroma and Thrombosis – Anticoagulants and Thrombolytic Agents

CHAPTER OUTLINE

LEARNING OBJECTIVES

At the end of this chapter, the reader should be able to:

- list the key stages of the coagulation cascade
- discuss the causes of thrombosis and its prevention and treatment
- give an account of the anticoagulants, their mechanisms, uses and dangers
- describe the causes and treatment of atheroma and arterial thrombosis
- discuss the use of cholesterol-lowering treatments
- list the drugs used to manage angina
- explain the causes and treatment of acute coronary syndrome
- list the drugs used for fibrinolysis
- discuss the use of 'antiplatelet' drugs

COAGULATION AND THROMBOSIS

Coagulation

When the wall of a blood vessel is damaged, the blood coagulates, and this arrests bleeding. Clotting is a complex process, which involves numerous enzymes and other chemicals called 'clotting factors'. Most are present in the blood plasma, some are released by platelets, and thromboplastin is released from damaged cells. When blood clots, each clotting factor is activated in sequence as part of a cascade of reactions, as shown in Fig. 7.1.

The key stages of this series of reactions are:

- The formation of factor Xa by the clotting cascade, which, when activated, converts prothrombin to thrombin.

- Thrombin forms fibrin strands from soluble fibrinogen, which then form a network over the damaged area.
- At the same time, platelets become activated, assisting in the clotting process and aggregate to form clumps, which become enmeshed in the fibrin network. The resulting clot plugs the defect in the blood vessel.

Thrombosis

Coagulation or thrombosis may sometimes occur in blood vessels that have not been injured and, in these circumstances, blockage of the vessel concerned may have serious consequences. There are two types of thrombosis:

- **venous thrombosis**
- **arterial thrombosis.**

Although both may result in obstruction to a blood vessel, they occur under different circumstances, have different mechanisms and differ in their treatment.

Venous Thrombosis

Patients immobilized in bed as a result of surgery, severe illness or trauma are at risk of venous thrombosis and pulmonary embolism. Overall, about 20% of untreated postoperative patients develop a thrombosis and about 1% have a fatal pulmonary embolus. Increasing age (over 60) or a past history of thromboembolism increase risk, as does pregnancy and the postnatal period. Persons who are immobile for hours during long distance flights are also at risk of venous thrombosis, particularly if they are obese, smokers or using the combined oral contraceptive. Malignancy also increases venous thrombosis risk.

Thromboses (clots) usually occur in the deep veins of the legs (DVT: deep vein thrombosis). There are genetic factors that predispose to thrombosis (*or thrombophilia*). The most common type of inherited thrombophilia is known as Factor V Leiden thrombophilia, but several other types of thrombophilia exist. The danger of deep venous thrombosis is that part of the clot may break off, forming an embolus, which passes via the heart to the lungs, where it blocks a branch of the pulmonary artery to cause pulmonary embolism, an event which can be fatal.

In atrial fibrillation, a thrombus may develop in the left atrium because of altered blood flow, and fragments can become detached, resulting in emboli to the brain and elsewhere. Anticoagulants, which interfere with the clotting (coagulation) of blood, can be used either to prevent the formation of thrombi or to treat an established venous thrombosis.

CLINICAL NOTE

All patients who are admitted to hospital must be assessed for venous thromboembolism risk. The nurse has a key role in such assessments. A number of assessment tools exist, such as the one developed by the Department of Health and endorsed by NICE (2010) and those at risk should be considered for DVT prophylaxis. Treatment includes low molecular weight heparin and compression (TED) stockings and optimizing mobility. This is discussed later in the chapter.

Anticoagulants are drugs that interfere with clotting and are used to prevent and treat venous thrombosis. They also have a role in preventing embolic strokes in patients with atrial fibrillation (AF). They include:

- **heparin and heparin-like compounds**
- **warfarin and the coumarins**
- **direct oral anticoagulants (DOACs).**

Heparin and Heparin-like Compounds

Heparin is a complex mixture of acidic polysaccharides and is extracted from pig mucosa or beef lung, where it occurs naturally in mast cells and basophils. It is a very potent anticoagulant.

Mechanism of Action of Heparin

The effects of heparin on the clotting mechanism are multiple and complicated. Briefly, heparin inhibits coagulation by binding to antithrombin III. Antithrombin III is part of the system that regulates clotting. It binds Factor Xa (see Fig. 7.1) and renders it inactive. When heparin binds to antithrombin III, this enhances antithrombin's reaction with these clotting factors considerably. The end result is a prolongation of the clotting time. The clotting time is the time taken for blood or plasma to coagulate under controlled laboratory conditions.

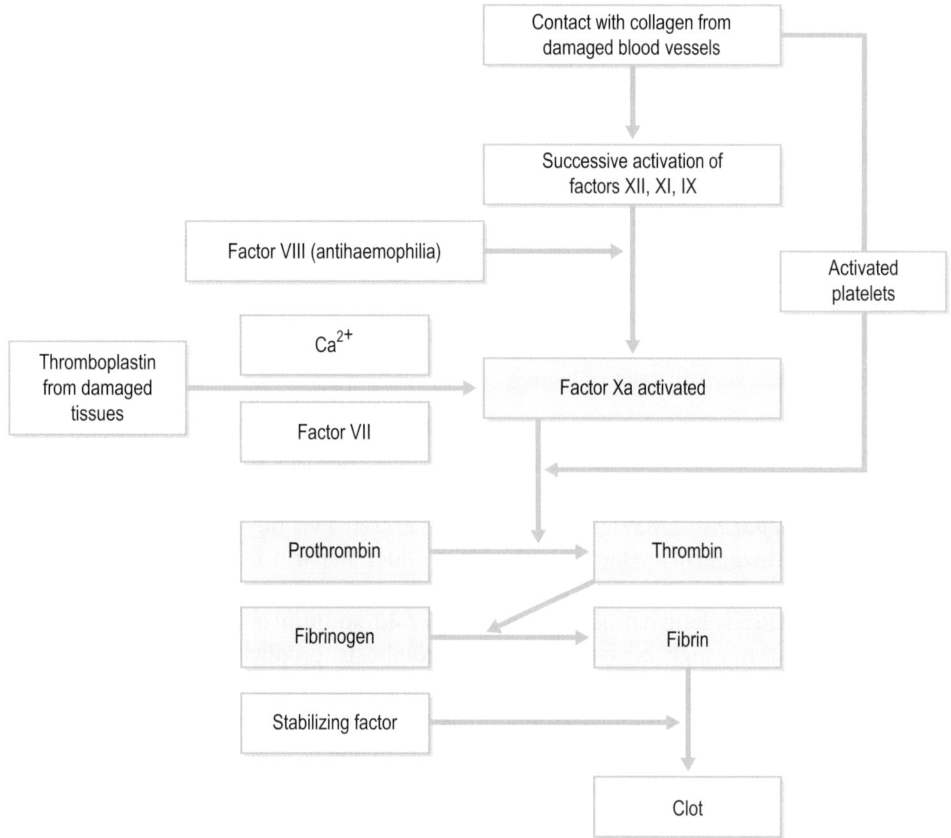

Fig. 7.1 ■ The clotting cascade.

Preparations of Heparin

There are two types of heparin:

- **unfractionated heparin**
- **low molecular weight heparins.**

Unfractionated Heparin. Heparin is a large molecule that can be broken down into a number of fragments or fractions, not all of which have anticoagulant properties. Those fragments that do have anticoagulant activity are known as low molecular weight heparins (LMWH). The use of unfractionated heparin has declined in the past 20 years, in favour of LMWH. It does still have a role in the management of acute coronary syndromes in patients with renal impairment and for angiograms and percutaneous coronary intervention.

ADMINISTRATION. Heparin is not absorbed by mouth and is given by intravenous infusion (unfractionated heparins) or subcutaneous injection (LMWH). The anticoagulant effect of unfractionated heparin is seen within 1–2 min of injection, but wanes within a few hours, which is why infusions are preferred. Heparin is often used at the beginning of anticoagulant treatment because its effects are so rapid. LMWHs are given once or twice daily by subcutaneous injection for maintenance anticoagulation and the dose can be calculated from the weight of the patient. When given by intravenous infusion, it is given via a syringe pump. The rate of infusion is monitored by measuring the kaolin cephalin time or activated partial thromboplastin time (APTT) 6 h after starting infusion and then at least once daily; these should be kept between 1.5 and 2.5 times the control value.

CLINICAL NOTE

An advantage of heparin is that its action is reversible with a slow injection of protamine sulphate within 3 h of the heparin-injection. A major unwanted effect of heparin is heparin-induced thrombocytopaenia (HIT) or low platelets (a major component of the clotting system). This adverse drug reaction affects 1%–5% of those prescribed heparin (Ahmed et al., 2007), and patients prescribed heparin for more than 5 days should have platelet levels monitored. In recent years, there has been a shift from heparin to low molecular weight heparin such as dalteparin and enoxaparin.

Low Molecular Weight Heparins. LMWH such as **enoxaparin, dalteparin or tinzaparin** are more highly purified heparins and reduce the risk of HIT and thrombosis. They have a relatively long half-life so can be given once daily and have a high bioavailability. While reversibility is more problematic than heparin, it is the preferred option for DVT prophylaxis and treatment. When used to prevent thrombosis, the preferred route of administration is subcutaneous. Other advantages include:

- LMWH are better than ordinary low-dose unfractionated heparin in preventing the venous thrombosis that may complicate surgery, particularly hip and knee replacement.
- Given subcutaneously, they are as effective as intravenous unfractionated heparin in the prevention and treatment of venous thrombosis and pulmonary embolism.
- As they do not cross the placental barrier, they can be used during pregnancy.
- Since their activity can be more consistently controlled during preparation, patients may not need the same degree of monitoring.
- The mechanism of anticoagulant action of active LMWH fragments is very similar to that of unfractionated heparin, but the effect is more prolonged than that of unfractionated heparin.
- Lower doses can sometimes be used, e.g. for prevention of thrombosis.

Heparin-like Compounds

A number of drugs have been developed that are structurally similar to heparin and have similar effects. There is also interest in the use of heparin-like drugs to treat inflammatory conditions.

Fondaparinux is a synthetic drug, which is identical to the polysaccharide sequence in unfractionated heparin that binds to antithrombin III, thus increasing the neutralizing effect on factor Xa to inhibit coagulation. Fondaparinux is administered daily subcutaneously, and has a significantly lower risk of thrombocytopaenia than that posed by heparin. It is used prophylactically in patients undergoing abdominal or major orthopaedic surgery and in the treatment of acute coronary syndrome. Fondaparinux is contraindicated in patients with impaired renal function, as it is excreted via the kidneys.

Older heparin-like drugs, referred to as heparinoids, are available, but their use has declined. **Danaparoid sodium** is occasionally used for deep vein thrombosis prophylaxis. The heparinoid **pentosan polysulfate sodium** is no longer used as an anticoagulant, but may be used to treat inflammatory conditions of the bladder.

Oral Anticoagulants

Warfarin and the Coumarins

Until recently, the only oral anticoagulants that were in clinical use were drugs in the class known as coumarins, of which **warfarin** is by far the most important (**phenindione**, **phenprocoumon** and **acenocoumarol** are similar agents, used in some countries).

Historically, this group of drugs were discovered when cows developed haemorrhage after eating spoiled sweet clover silage. Coumarin was identified as the active principle and warfarin is a chemical derivative of coumarin. These remain important drugs, although their use has declined in the past 10 years as DOACs have been introduced. Warfarin remains the anticoagulant of choice in patients with mechanical prosthetic heart valves. Coumarins are also used as rat poisons, and some patients may refer to warfarin as 'rat poison'.

Mechanism of Action of Warfarin and Other Coumarins

Warfarin interferes with the action of vitamin K, which is required for the synthesis of several important factors involved in clotting, namely factors VII, IX, X and XI. These clotting factors are called 'vitamin K-dependent clotting factors'. If they become depleted, clotting is delayed.

Administration. Warfarin is given orally in tablet form. The onset of action of warfarin is delayed, since it is only effective after the existing stores of the vitamin K-dependent clotting factors have been depleted. For this reason, anticoagulant therapy may be initiated with heparin, which acts immediately, and then warfarin is given, initially as a loading dose that is higher than the usual maintenance dose, which is then determined over several days by regular monitoring of the international normalized ratio (INR) (see later). Warfarin tablets are available in various strengths, which are usually colour coded to reduce the risk of dosing errors.

CLINICAL NOTE

Patients prescribed any anticoagulation must be monitored for signs of bleeding including, excessive bruising, nose bleeds, black stools and bleeding gums. Those prescribed warfarin therapy need to be carefully and regularly monitored for the levels of anticoagulant activity, since excessive activity can result in haemorrhage and insufficient activity can result in clotting. Both can be fatal. The monitoring blood test is known as the INR (International Normalized Ratio). The test can be undertaken in a hospital laboratory on venous blood or, more recently, on a finger prick sample using a near-patient testing machine. The INR should be measured before starting treatment, then daily, and the dose adjusted until the INR is stabilized. The dose is adjusted to keep the INR between 2.0 and 3.5 (depending on the clinical situation). Computer programmes are generally used to calculate the correct dose for a patient, depending on the current and previous INR measures and the target INR required. When stable, INR measures are still required every few weeks. Anticoagulant monitoring may have a significant impact on a patient's ability to go about their usual activities, and although warfarin is a very cheap drug, when the costs of monitoring it are factored in, the much more expensive DOAC anticoagulants (see later) may be more cost-effective, particularly when patient convenience is also factored in.

Precautions to be Taken when Prescribing Warfarin

- It is very important that strict accuracy is observed in the timing of doses.
- The patient's age and state of health must be taken into account. For example, patients with liver disease are more sensitive to oral anticoagulants, because these are inactivated in the liver.
- Poor nutrition, heart failure, previous surgery and concurrent drugs will increase the patient's sensitivity to warfarin and require smaller dosage.
- Contraindications: contraindications to the use of warfarin include active peptic ulcer, severe liver disease and renal failure.

Adverse Effects of Warfarin

The adverse effects are:

- haemorrhage
- teratogenic effects (fetal abnormalities).

Haemorrhage may result from overdosage and is the most important side-effect of the coumarin group of drugs, as with all anticoagulants. An INR of above 5 suggests a risk of dangerous bleeding. It is treated by temporary withdrawal of the drug. An INR >8 requires more urgent treatment. The effect of the anticoagulant can be reversed rapidly by an infusion of fresh frozen plasma. Alternatively, phytomenadione (vitamin K) intravenously can be given, but takes about 12 h to become effective. Large doses of phytomenadione interfere with further anticoagulation for some days.

Use in Pregnancy

Warfarin crosses the placenta and may cause fetal abnormalities if given in the first 3 months of pregnancy. If anticoagulation is required during pregnancy, LMWH can be used throughout, or used up to 16 weeks, warfarin from 16 to 36 weeks and then LMWH again until delivery. Patients can be taught to self-administer heparin injections.

Drug Interactions with Warfarin

Warfarin can interact with several other drugs and such interactions must be taken seriously as they can lead to clinically important increases or decreases in anticoagulant effectiveness, which may be dangerous. It is one of the most common adverse drug events resulting in hospital admission (Pirmohamed et al., 2004) and the action of warfarin is increased by a number of drugs including some antibiotics (quinolones, e.g. ciprofloxacin and penicillin), aspirin, alcohol, non-steroidal antiinflammatories (e.g. Ibuprofen) and antidepressants, e.g. citalopram. Conversely, the action of warfarin is decreased when prescribed with: carbamazepine, oestrogens (e.g. contraceptive pill), phenytoin and antacids.

CLINICAL NOTE

As a result of the many interactions between warfarin and other drugs and the narrow therapeutic range of the drug (see Chapter 1 for further explanation), patients on warfarin should be advised against taking any over-the-counter, herbal or complimentary medicines (see Case History 7.1). Healthcare professionals should be aware of drug–drug interactions and refer to a local drug formulary to check drug–drug interactions prior to prescribing or administering medication. The British National Formulary and similar drug handbooks are essential reference guides for building knowledge.

CASE HISTORY 7.1

Mrs. Y, a 70-year-old lady, was taken into the Accident and Emergency Department after collapsing at home, and after blood tests were taken, she was found to be very anaemic and was given 4 units of blood. When the history was taken, she reported that she was taking anticoagulant therapy with warfarin for stroke prophylaxis as she had AF. Initially, an overdose was suspected, although the INR had been monitored regularly. A careful medication history was taken, including health supplements and over-the-counter medications. It emerged that Mrs. Y had started taking garlic oil capsules and gingko biloba extract tablets from a health food shop. She had read about the evidence for the health benefits of these natural supplements (*and indeed there is some evidence to suggest they may be beneficial for some conditions*) and so had taken them as she felt she should take responsibility for maintaining her health. Unfortunately, both these substances affect the metabolism of warfarin and increase its effect and so had led to her INR increasing markedly since her last blood test a month previously. This had led to a gastrointestinal bleed. It is important to include natural and over-the-counter remedies when taking a drug history.

Direct Oral Anticoagulants

The inconvenience and potential dangers associated with the use of warfarin spurred a search for other anticoagulant drugs with reduced monitoring requirements and a better safety profile. At time of writing, a number of new drugs have become available and have become widely used in healthcare systems that are able to afford their considerable cost. Originally referred to as the 'New/Novel Oral Anticoagulants' (NOACs), they are now generally referred to as 'Direct Oral Anticoagulants' (DOACs), as they directly inhibit specific agents in the clotting cascade, rather than (as warfarin does) reducing the amount of them. In general, for most indications, the DOACs are as effective, or more effective, than warfarin and have a lower risk of serious haemorrhage.

None of the currently available DOACs are suitable for anticoagulation of patients with mechanical heart valves, for which warfarin should be used. Recently it has been recognized that there is an increased risk of recurrent thrombosis in patients with the antiphospholipid syndrome (a relatively common thrombophilic syndrome) when treated with some – possibly all – DOACs. Warfarin should be used for anticoagulation in these patients.

There are two main types of DOAC: Direct Thrombin Inhibitors and Direct Factor Xa inhibitors.

Direct Thrombin Inhibitors

Dabigatran. Unlike heparin and the other DOACs, dabigatran directly inhibits the activity of thrombin, a key part of the clotting cascade. It has a rapid onset of action and is commonly used for prophylaxis of venous thrombosis in joint replacement surgery, and also for anticoagulation after deep vein thrombosis or pulmonary embolus, and for stroke prevention in atrial fibrillation. The dose should be reduced when administered with verapamil or amiodarone. Renal function should be checked before starting and then annually, and the dose reduced if there is significant renal impairment. There are no monitoring blood tests available. Disturbances of liver function are common and may not be significant. Bleeding is the most serious side-effect. **Tinzaparin** is an intravenous direct thrombin inhibitor, occasionally used for prevention or treatment of venous thromboembolism.

Hirudin was originally obtained from leeches and has been recognized as an anticoagulant for many years. It is a direct thrombin inhibitor. **Bivalirudin** is a synthetic version of hirudin that can be given as an infusion in patients who need urgent angioplasty or coronary artery surgery.

Direct Factor Xa Inhibitors

Rivaroxaban, **apixaban** and **edoxaban** are all direct inhibitors of Factor Xa in the clotting cascade. They can be used for similar indications as dabigatran, although in the UK, some are not licensed for treatment of venous thrombosis or pulmonary embolus. In general, in UK practice, they are most commonly used for stroke prophylaxis in AF. Doses need to be reduced in renal impairment and starting doses depend on an estimate of renal function using the Cockcroft and Gault calculation for estimated creatinine clearance. No monitoring blood tests are available. Bleeding is the most serious side-effect.

Antidotes to DOACs

Until recently, no antidotes to the DOACs were available. It is now possible to reverse the effects of dabigatran in cases of severe haemorrhage by using the recombinant antibody **idarucizumab**, given by injection. **Andexanet alfa** is licensed in the USA for reversal of Direct Factor Xa inhibitors. It is extremely expensive at present.

CLINICAL NOTE

A major advantage of DOACs compared with warfarin is that it is not necessary to monitor clotting factors (INR). Bleeding is a major side-effect and long-term use can affect liver and renal function. Hence, renal and liver function should be monitored during treatment. As these drugs are relatively new to the market, any adverse drug events should be reported.

PREVENTION OF VENOUS THROMBOSIS (THROMBOPROPHYLAXIS)

There is an increased risk of venous thrombosis under the following conditions:

- immobility
- prosthetic heart valves
- established atrial fibrillation.

All patients being admitted to hospital should have an assessment made of their thromboembolism risk, using an approved checklist, and high-risk patients should receive thromboprophylaxis. Early mobilization of patients after surgery and care in maintenance of hydration are key nursing inputs that reduce thromboembolic risk. Oral contraceptives containing oestrogen are a risk factor and should be stopped 6 weeks before a major operation or any surgery involving the pelvis or hip.

Thromboprophylaxis can be mechanical or pharmacological, or a combination of both. Mechanical means include graduated compression stockings and intermittent pneumatic compression. These methods may be most appropriate when bleeding risk with anticoagulants outweighs the risk of thrombosis, and they should be continued until the patient is mobile or discharged from hospital. Pharmacological prophylaxis may be with heparins, most commonly low molecular weight or fondaparinux. Aspirin is sometimes used as a follow-on treatment. Rivaroxaban, dabigatran or apixaban are also sometimes used. The precise combination of treatment varies according to local policies and the reason for the thromboprophylaxis. The duration of treatment also varies locally and by indication for treatment.

Patients with **mechanical heart valves** require full anticoagulation with warfarin to prevent thrombosis on the valve. DOACs are not suitable for this indication. Thrombosis associated with mechanical valves is extremely dangerous, and it is vital to ensure the correct INR is maintained. Tissue heart valves, made from biological material, do not require anticoagulation (but do not last as long as mechanical valves).

In patients with **established atrial fibrillation**, anticoagulation with DOACs or warfarin substantially reduces stroke risk. Stroke risk can be estimated using scoring systems such as the CHA_2DS_2-VASc score. In practice, most AF patients receive anticoagulation. There is little evidence of benefit in using aspirin if anticoagulation is declined, or in low/moderate stroke risk patients, but some guidelines still suggest its use.

CLINICAL NOTE

Venous thromboembolism (VTE) is a common condition and affects 100–183/100,000 per year, and is common in people living with cancer (Heit, 2015). Thrombosis UK state that death from VTE is one of the leading causes of preventable death in hospital and the cost due to prolonged length of stay, treatment and litigation is significant. Routine screening for all patients admitted to hospital is essential and will save lives.

ANTICOAGULATION FOR VENOUS THROMBOSIS/PULMONARY EMBOLISM

Venous thrombosis may be treated with heparins of all types or fondaparinux and/or warfarin or DOACs. Treatment is normally commenced with a DOAC, but where warfarin is used, then LMWH or fondaparinux is used while the warfarin dose is established. Treatment duration is at least 3 months, but may be longer, or life-long in cases of recurrent venous thrombosis.

Anticoagulation therapy for pulmonary embolism is similar to treatment for venous thrombosis. However, pulmonary embolism is a medical emergency and supportive treatment with careful monitoring of vital signs is important. Other interventions, including surgery or fibrinolysis (see later) may also be required.

SUMMARY

- Low molecular weight heparins or fondaparinux are as effective as unfractionated heparin in most cases and do not require infusion.
- Overdosing with anticoagulants can cause serious haemorrhage.
- Protamine sulphate is an antidote to heparin.
- Oral anticoagulants, particularly warfarin, have a delayed onset of action.
- Patients on warfarin have to be monitored closely with the INR due to risk of underdosing or overdosing.
- Oral coumarin anticoagulants have many interactions with other drugs. It is important to discover what other drugs patients are on and know the health (e.g. liver function) of the patient.
- DOACs are increasingly replacing warfarin as oral anticoagulants.
- Long-term immobilization of patients in bed puts them at risk of venous thrombosis.
- All patients who are admitted to hospital should have their thromboembolus risk assessed.

ATHEROMA AND ARTERIAL THROMBOSIS

An atheroma is a mass or plaque of fatty or scar tissue on the inner lining of arterial walls. If atheroma is in a coronary artery then it can lead to ischaemic heart disease including myocardial infarction (heart attack). Atheroma in peripheral arteries can lead to peripheral vascular disease.

Causes of Atheroma

With increasing age, the lining (endothelium) of the arterial wall may become damaged by:

- mechanical stress on the endothelium due to raised blood pressure
- high levels of circulating low-density lipoprotein (LDL) cholesterol
- other factors, including toxins from tobacco smoke.

This damage to the endothelial wall leads to the patchy accumulation of cholesterol-containing lipoproteins and macrophages under the arterial endothelium, together with the deposition of platelet aggregates. The growth of the atheromatous area may lead to symptoms due to narrowing of the artery (see later). Ultimately, the patch may break down, leaving a rough area (atheromatous plaque) on which a thrombus (a platelet aggregate stabilized by fibrin) may form and block the artery. If this occurs in a coronary artery, it can lead to a heart attack, and if the thrombus detaches, it can then go on to lodge in other blood vessels such as the carotid and cerebral arteries to cause a stroke. Atheroma can be widely distributed throughout the vascular system, but it particularly affects:

- the coronary arteries, causing ischaemic heart disease
- the carotid and cerebral arteries, causing strokes
- the legs, causing claudication, which is pain in the calves on walking.

THE HYPERLIPIDAEMIAS AND CHOLESTEROL

The hyperlipidaemias are a group of disorders of metabolism in which there are increased amounts of various lipoproteins in the blood. Lipoproteins are substances that are composed of lipids (mainly cholesterol) and proteins and are produced by the liver. The concentration of blood lipoproteins is determined partly by the dietary intake of fats but mainly by metabolic processes within the body. Inherited genetic factors influence these processes. It is possible to lower the lipoprotein levels slightly by decreasing the intake or absorption of fats, but big changes require drugs that change the metabolism.

The most important lipid in lipoproteins is cholesterol, and there is strong evidence that a high level of cholesterol in the blood, especially in the form of LDL, is a cause of atheroma and cardiovascular disease. Conversely, high levels of high-density lipoproteins (HDL) protect against cardiovascular disease. The ratio of LDL to HDL (or the very similar total cholesterol/HDL ratio) is a strong predictor of cardiovascular disease risk, much more so than just total cholesterol.

Reducing blood cholesterol levels (even if not raised above the 'normal range') reduces the risk of cardiac death or disability in patients with established ischaemic heart disease (IHD) – including patients with chronic and acute coronary syndromes. It also reduces risk of death in patients with diabetes – who are at high risk of IHD, and it slows the progression of peripheral vascular disease.

Lowering cholesterol reduces cardiovascular risk even in subjects with normal cholesterol, and this effect is greater when cholesterol levels are raised in otherwise healthy people, as is common in the Western World. However, for many people, the size of the reduction in cardiovascular risk is too small to justify the use of medication to lower cholesterol. While lifestyle measures (particularly diet, exercise and smoking cessation) will offer some benefit to all, before suggesting that a healthy person should start cholesterol lowering drugs, their actual 10-year risk of developing cardiovascular disease should be calculated using a risk estimating algorithm. In the UK, the QRISK3 algorithm has been incorporated into clinical computer systems, while in the USA, the Framingham score has been developed for North American populations. Current UK guidance suggests that if a healthy person has a 10-year risk of having a cardiovascular event of 10% or more, then their risk factors should be aggressively managed – including drug treatment of cholesterol. The immediate aim of treatment is to reduce LDL cholesterol by 40%.

Reducing Plasma Cholesterol Levels

There are several complimentary approaches to lowering plasma cholesterol levels.

Diet and Weight Reduction

- Reduce total fat intake and decrease intake of saturated (mainly animal and dairy) fats relative to unsaturated (fish and some vegetable) fats.

A decrease in the total fat intake and the proportion of saturated (animal) fat to unsaturated/polyunsaturated (fish and vegetable) fat will reduce plasma cholesterol, particularly LDL, and should form part of a healthy diet. However, the saturated fats should not be replaced by refined carbohydrates such as sugars and white flour-based products, but with vegetables, minimally processed grains and nuts. Unsaturated fats include olive oil and rapeseed (canola) oil. Polyunsaturated fats include sunflower, corn and soya bean oils and omega-3-containing fish oils. There is much debate and misinformation about what constitutes the 'best' type of fat in the diet. Recently, some have advocated a return to dairy fats and the use of coconut-based oils. This advice seems to be based on a very selective interpretation of basic research. More research is needed, but on current evidence, polyunsaturated fats seem to have the most favourable effects on reducing LDL and cardiovascular events. However, there is insufficient evidence to support the use of fish oil supplements in capsule form to prevent cardiovascular events in people at increased risk of such events.

Many plant-based foods contain substances known as sterols and stanols. These prevent absorption of cholesterol by the gut and can help reduce cholesterol levels. A mixed plant-based diet is a good source, but yoghurt desserts and drinks, and margarines and spreads containing these substances are available in food stores. There is evidence that their use can reduce cholesterol levels, but it is not yet known whether this translates into reduced IHD risk.

A healthy diet is of vital importance to whole-person health. However, attempts to lower blood cholesterol using diet alone are often disappointing to patients and clinicians. At most, ~ 20% reduction is possible, but in real life, many only achieve a 3%–6% reduction in total cholesterol. In healthy people at relatively low risk, this is still useful, and the improved diet carries many other health benefits. In people at higher risk of IHD, and those with established IHD, drugs are almost always required.

CLINICAL NOTE

Not achieving adequate cholesterol reduction by lifestyle measures should not be presented as a failure on the patient's part. It is important to be positive about diet, but also to encourage realistic expectations about what it can achieve. The role of weight reduction, reduction in alcohol, increased exercise and smoking cessation cannot be overemphasized.

Drugs

Statins. The **statins** block the synthesis of cholesterol in the liver, lowering LDL cholesterol and often increasing HDL. They also appear to be a direct anti-inflammatory on the lining of blood vessels. This effect may be important and is why high intensity statin treatment is often recommended in people with coronary artery disease. They include:

- **atorvastatin**
- **simvastatin**
- **rosuvastatin.**

The earlier statins, **pravastatin** and **fluvastatin** are less potent and little used. **Pitavastatin** is available in some countries.

The side-effect profiles and tolerability of the statins as a group are very similar, although there are subtle differences that may be significant in individual patients. Atorvastatin and simvastatin are the most widely used of the inexpensive statins. Atorvastatin is more potent than simvastatin, and at doses that produce equivalent reductions in cholesterol, it may have fewer side-effects, particularly muscle pain (myalgia). Rosuvastatin is the most potent statin.

Statin prescribing has hugely increased over the past 30 years, and millions of people take the drugs. Much of the dramatic reduction in cardiovascular deaths seen throughout the world over the same period must be related to their use. Such widely prescribed drugs will not suit every person who takes them, and the Internet is full of scare stories about statins. However, the reality is that they are remarkably well-tolerated and effective drugs that cause no problems to the majority of people who take them. Their benefits and adverse effects have been extensively studied. They should not be taken during pregnancy. They may be slightly more effective when taken in the evening. It is possible that statin use may be beneficial in preventing some cancers and inflammatory diseases, but further research is required.

Adverse effects. Mild disturbances in liver function are common and are of no significance unless the changes are substantial. Liver function should be checked at 3 and 12 months after starting, but no further monitoring is required if the levels are stable.

The most common unwanted effect is myalgia (muscle pain), and rarely this may be severe enough to cause the release of muscle proteins into the blood (rhabdomyolysis). This can lead to kidney failure. Measurement of the muscle enzyme creatine kinase (CK) is helpful in patients with myalgia. If CK is normal or only slightly raised, patients can be reassured and encouraged to continue. It is also increased when statins are taken in combination with some other drugs. The most common of these are the macrolide antibiotics such as erythromycin and clarithromycin. Daily doses in excess of 5 mg of the antihypertensive drug amlodipine greatly increase the bioavailability of simvastatin and thus increase the risk of side-effects.

CLINICAL NOTE

Myalgia affects about 10% of people prescribed statins (Gitlin et al., 2018). If left unreported, in rare cases, this can progress to severe muscle damage, myopathy and rhabdomyolysis. The patient must be advised to see their doctor if they have muscle pain, weakness or tenderness. Patients should also be advised to avoid grapefruit juice when prescribed a statin because it competes with the enzyme that metabolizes statins, resulting in higher bioavailability of the statin and greater risk of side-effects.

Ezetimibe. Ezetimibe blocks absorption of cholesterol from the intestine and modestly reduces LDL cholesterol. It has a role as an adjunct to statin therapy if maximal statin dosing is ineffective or not tolerated. It can be used alone if statins are not tolerated at all.

PCSK9 Inhibitors. Sometimes known as PCSK9i, these represent a new application of biologic drugs (see Appendix: Biologic agents). They are monoclonal antibodies that inhibit the action of an enzyme known as PCSK9 that is involved in lipoprotein regulation. In people with very high LDL levels that do not adequately respond to statins, they can dramatically reduce the levels. Currently, **Evolocumab** and **Alirocumab** are available, with others being developed. They are given by injection, every 2 or 4 weeks. When compared to statin therapy, they are very expensive, although prices are coming down. Flu-like symptoms and muscle pain are the most common side-effects. Unless oral PCSK9i can be developed, or very long-acting injectable versions, their use is likely to be limited.

Other Drugs

Prior to the introduction of the statins, **bile acid-binding resins**, **nicotinic acid** and the **fibrates** were used for people with very abnormal cholesterol levels. They are difficult to take, have many side-effects and interactions and are much less effective than the statins. They have fallen out of use except in some rare familial disorders of cholesterol regulation.

SUMMARY

- Raised LDL cholesterol is an important cause of IHD.
- Cholesterol lowering is of proven value in preventing death in patients with established IHD.
- Healthy patients with raised cholesterol should have their 10-year cardiovascular risk estimated to aid decisions about whether to use drugs to lower cholesterol.
- Everyone benefits from a healthy diet, low in saturated fat, containing unsaturated fat, vegetables, grains and nuts.
- Diet alone will not reduce cholesterol sufficiently in most patients.
- Liver function tests should be carried out during the first year of treatment with statins.
- The aim of treatment should be to reduce LDL cholesterol by 40% – but any reduction is beneficial.

ISCHAEMIC HEART DISEASE

Advancing age, coupled with risk factors such as high blood pressure, smoking and raised plasma cholesterol levels lead to atheroma, which leads to narrowing of the coronary arteries – a process called *atherosclerosis*. Severe atherosclerosis can interfere with the blood supply to the heart muscle, which like all muscles, needs oxygenated blood supplied to it, in order to do its pumping work. The coronary blood flow is usually adequate when the patient is at rest, but, with effort, the increased demands of the heart muscle for oxygen cannot be met by the narrowed coronary arteries. This results in typical chest pain, often with radiation to the left arm and into the neck. It characteristically comes on with effort and is relieved by rest (angina, angina pectoris). In a few patients, the coronary artery may also be narrowed by spasm, which can also give rise to chest pain. This type of heart disease is now referred to as chronic coronary syndrome.

If a thrombus forms on a plaque of atheroma (coronary thrombosis), the blood supply to the area of heart muscle supplied by that artery is cut off and the muscle becomes ischaemic, is damaged and will die unless blood flow is rapidly restored. This is what underlies the acute coronary syndrome (ACS; see later).

Drugs Used in Chronic Coronary Syndrome

Chronic coronary syndrome (CCS) is a term now used in preference to older terms such as stable angina. This reflects the fact that CCS is not 'stable', but is a dynamic process involving atheroma and altered arterial function, and it is amenable to treatment.

For many patients, CCS is treated by coronary artery bypass grafting (CABG) or percutaneous angioplasty, with introduction of a vascular stent (PCI). All such patients will require some level of antiplatelet therapy lifelong (discussed later) and most will also continue on a β-blocker. Although such interventions have become increasingly common, there is little evidence that they decrease risk of death, or even have much effect on symptoms like angina. This is in marked contrast to the effectiveness of PCI and CABG in ACS. This may reflect the fact that in CCS, atheromas are relatively stable and unlikely to rupture, and also the fact that arterial function may be abnormal throughout the coronary arteries. Medication therefore remains very important, and some of the drugs listed here may be used:

- β-blockers
- calcium channel blockers
- the nitrates:
  - glyceryl trinitrate
  - isosorbide dinitrate
  - isosorbide mononitrate
- nicorandil
- ivabradine
- ranolazine.

Short-acting nitrates should always be prescribed to treat acute attacks. A β-blocker should be given as first-line therapy. A rate-limiting calcium-channel blocker is an alternative choice.

If a β-blocker alone fails to control symptoms adequately, a combination of a β-blocker and a calcium-channel blocker may be used. If this is ineffective or not tolerated, then a long-acting nitrate or nicorandil or ivabradine or ranolazine may be added. These can also be used in monotherapy in some circumstances.

All patients with angina require management of IHD risk factors, particularly blood pressure, cholesterol and smoking.

β-Blockers

β-Blockers (see Chapter 6) are first-line treatment of CCS, as well as being important in prevention of further cardiovascular events (secondary prevention). The rise in heart rate and heart work that occurs on exercise is partially brought about by the activity of the sympathetic nervous system (Fig. 7.2). By blocking this stimulating effect, the β-blockers protect the heart from overactivity and prevent the development of anginal pain.

Clinical Use. Most β-blockers have been used successfully in treating CCS. They may induce bronchospasm in asthmatics. **Nebivolol** is least likely to do this as it is most specific for the heart. The usual method of giving these drugs is to start with a small dose and increase it until a satisfactory control of symptoms is obtained.

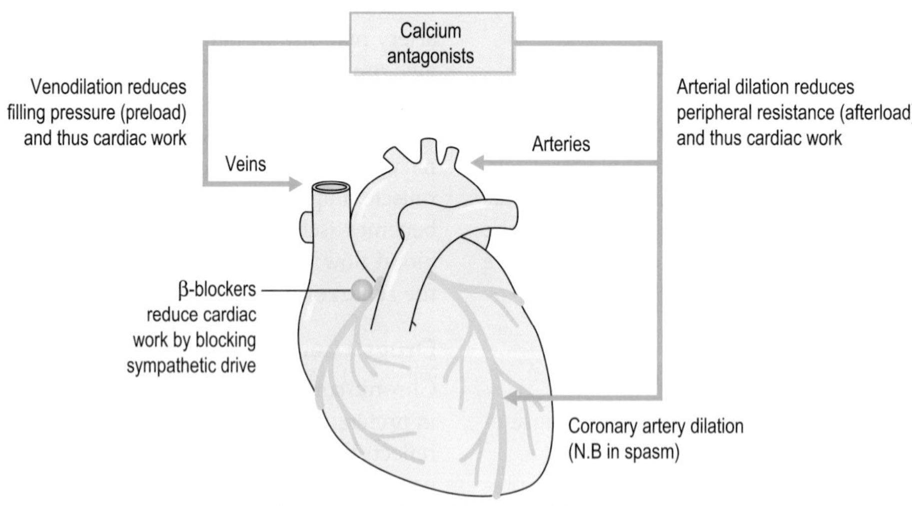

Fig. 7.2 ■ Action of drugs used in angina.

The drug is given regularly to prevent pain rather than to treat attacks.

Calcium Channel Blockers

The calcium channel blockers (see Chapter 6) are potent dilators of blood vessels and some also have a heart rate-limiting effect. The rate-limiting calcium channel blockers **verapamil** and **diltiazem** are used to treat CCS.

These drugs decrease cardiac work by dilating the peripheral blood vessels and reducing the heart rate. All are now available in modified release form to be taken once or twice a day.

Calcium-channel blockers that do not limit the heart rate have an additional effect of dilating the coronary arteries. This may be useful in the treatment of atypical angina caused by coronary artery spasm (Prinzmetal angina). **Amlodipine** or modified release forms of **nifedipine** may be used for this purpose.

Adverse Effects. Headache and flushing are common when first started, but generally pass. Lymphatic mediated swelling of the ankles is common, especially in hot weather, and may be troublesome. Constipation may be an issue, particularly in older people.

The Nitrates

These drugs act as vasodilators by relaxing smooth muscle in blood vessel walls. Nitrates relieve the pain of angina in two ways:

- by vasodilatation, which is their main action; this reduces the venous return of blood to the heart and thus reduces the heart work and lowers the demand for oxygen
- by dilating the coronary arteries, particularly if in spasm, so that the blood flow through these arteries is increased.

TABLE 7.1

Duration of Action of Nitrates

	Onset of Effect	Duration of Effect
Glyceryl trinitrate		
(sucked or chewed)	2 min	30 min
(patch)	1–2 h	up to 24 h
Isosorbide mononitrate		
(swallowed)	20 min	10 h
Isosorbide dinitrate		
(chewed)	2 min	2 h
(swallowed)	20 min	5 h
(modified release)	20 min	12 h

Some drugs in the nitrate group have powerful, but short-lived, actions; others act less powerfully, but over a longer period (Table 7.1).

Glyceryl Trinitrate. **Glyceryl trinitrate (GTN)** is an oily liquid. In its undiluted form it is a powerful explosive. It is prepared as tablets by dilution and mixing with an absorbent base. It is also prepared as a metered dose spray, impregnated skin patches or an intravenous infusion.

TABLETS. These are taken sublingually, the drug being absorbed from the mucous membrane of the mouth. If swallowed whole, it is not effective, because the drug is rapidly destroyed as it passes through the liver. Its effects start within a minute and last for 15–20 min. The tablets lose potency and should not be kept for more than 2 months, and they should be stored in a glass container and not exposed to light or cotton wool.

PUMP SPRAY. GTN can be given via a metered dose pump spray; this acts rapidly. It is sprayed under the tongue, and the mouth is then closed. The spray has a much longer shelf-life and has largely replaced the use of tablets.

IMPREGNATED SKIN PATCHES. GTN is also absorbed through the skin and impregnated patches are available for application to the skin. They release the drug slowly over 24 h, thus producing a prolonged effect. They have not proved particularly useful, as it is difficult to control dosage. Headaches can be troublesome and tolerance to the drug's action may develop. If this is suspected, the patches should be removed several times each day.

INTRAVENOUS INFUSION. GTN can be given by intravenous infusion. This approach is reserved for patients with severe chest pain, usually following myocardial infarction, when it may relieve the pain and also improve any complicating heart failure. It is best given in saline or 5% glucose by a syringe pump. PVC containers must not be used.

EFFECTS. GTN causes a marked general vasodilatation with a fall in blood pressure. It normally relieves angina pain within minutes, but headaches and faintness are common unwanted effects.

OTHER USES. GTN has also been formulated as an ointment to treat chronic anal fissures. The vasodilator effects of GTN are key to healing these common painful splits in the anal skin.

NURSING NOTE

All patients with angina should be counselled to use their GTN spray or tablets if they develop angina pain. If the patient develops angina pain they should be advised to stop what they are doing and take their spray under the tongue. If the pain is not relieved within 5 min, the dose may be repeated, but if the pain persists beyond 5 more minutes, they must seek emergency help (NHS UK, 2018).

Isosorbide Dinitrate and Isosorbide Mononitrate. **Isosorbide dinitrate** is similar to glyceryl trinitrate. It is broken down in the liver to **isosorbide mononitrate**, which is the active agent, and which is also available for clinical use. Isosorbide mononitrate is given twice daily, as its action is quite prolonged. Both the mononitrate and dinitrate are available for intravenous use.

Adverse Effects of Nitrates.

- Flushing
- Headaches
- Palpitations
- A fall in blood pressure, which can be particularly troublesome with long-acting preparations, when the patient may feel faint
- Rarely, large doses cause methaemoglobinaemias, leading to a cyanotic appearance.

Tolerance. Tolerance to the action of nitrates occurs with long-acting preparations or frequent dosage, but sensitivity is rapidly restored if the drug is stopped for a few hours. Intravenous infusions should not be given for more than 36 h without a break. The last dose of sustained-release or long-acting preparations should be taken with the evening meal and the patch removed overnight unless nocturnal angina is a problem. Glyceryl trinitrate is unlikely to produce tolerance, as it is so short-acting.

Nicorandil

Nicorandil is another vasodilator drug that activates potassium channels in the membrane of the vascular smooth muscle. It is used as an adjunct to other antianginal drugs. It should be used with caution in patients with cardiac failure or low blood pressure.

Adverse Effects. These include headache, flushing and nausea. These symptoms mainly pass. Rarely, nicorandil can cause serious skin, mucosal, genital and eye ulceration, including gastrointestinal ulcers.

Ivabradine

Ivabradine reduces heart rate by a different mechanism to that of other antianginal drugs. It thus reduces cardiac work and may help relieve angina as an adjunct to β-blockers. It also has a role in treating heart failure where the heart rate is >70 bpm. It should not be used in patients with disorders of the sinoatrial node or heart block or if they have a pacemaker fitted. It should not be used with macrolide antibiotics, verapamil or diltiazem, and the dose should be reduced when used with a number of other drugs.

Adverse Effects. Cardiac arrhythmias and heart block may be problematic. Dizziness, headache and hypertension are relatively common. A curious sensation of enhanced brightness of vision is common, but harmless and transient.

Ranolazine

Ranolazine reduces cardiac work via a direct action on cardiac muscle. The precise mechanism is unclear. It may be used as an adjunct to first-line drugs, and although it has similar drug interactions to ivabradine, it can be used with verapamil or diltiazem if its dose is reduced.

Adverse Effects. Headache, constipation and vomiting are all common. Many other side-effects have been reported, mostly minor.

ACUTE CORONARY SYNDROME

Acute coronary syndrome (ACS) is a blanket term for a number of related clinical conditions. It also includes the older term 'coronary thrombosis' and includes conditions that would be covered by the popular term 'heart attack'. All are related to a sudden partial or complete blockage of a coronary artery, by breakdown of an atheromatous area and some degree of platelet aggregation and thrombus formation.

ACS includes the conditions:

- Unstable angina
- Non-ST elevation myocardial infarction (NSTEMI)
- ST elevation myocardial infarction (STEMI)

The various conditions are diagnosed on the basis of symptoms, characteristic changes on the ECG and specific blood tests. All of these indicate some degree of damage to the heart muscle, with unstable angina being the least severe damage and STEMI being the most severe. Unstable angina can progress to NSTEMI or STEMI and the objective of treatment is keeping the patient alive while minimizing the degree of long-term damage to the heart muscle and then reducing the chance of future similar events. ACS is a medical emergency and time is of the essence in preventing further damage to the heart.

The drugs used in the treatment of ACS include anticoagulants (as previously discussed), thrombolytic agents and antiplatelet drugs. These will be discussed later, and the treatment of the various types of ACS will then be outlined. It is important to realize that treatment of these conditions will vary according to availability of drugs and the availability of prompt angioplasty and stenting (now more commonly known as percutaneous coronary intervention or PCI). Local protocols for treatment must be understood, especially as this is a fast-changing area of medical practice.

Thrombolytic Drugs

Fibrinolysis

Fibrinolysis is the end stage of the normal clotting cascade and is triggered in order to break down clots once they have served their purpose in preventing blood loss. Where a clot has formed in a coronary artery, drugs which trigger and increase the action of fibrinolysis can work to dissolve the clot and open up the artery. These so-called 'clot busting' or *thrombolytic* drugs can work to treat blood clots elsewhere in the body, such as in venous thrombosis or in thrombotic strokes. They work by activating a blood protein called plasminogen which binds to the fibrin in thrombi and is converted to an active protein which then destroys the fibrin. The greatest risk in their use is bleeding, which may in itself be fatal. Fibrinolytic drugs complement the use of anticoagulants, which prevent the formation of clots in the first place. Fibrinolysis is now mainly used in ACS where prompt access to PCI is not available (Fig. 7.3).

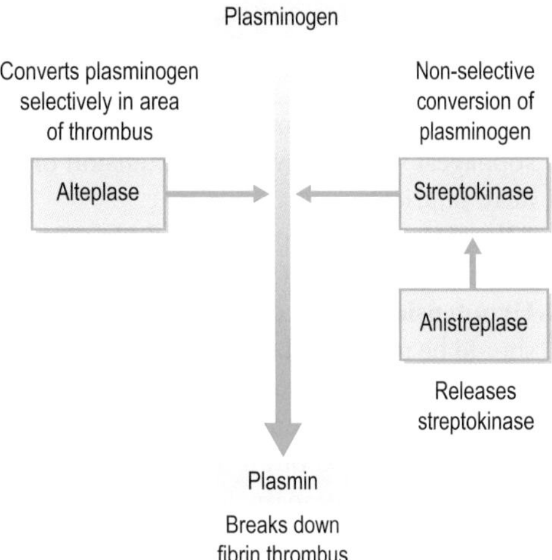

Fig. 7.3 ■ The action of thrombolytic drugs.

There are several fibrinolytic drugs available:

- **Streptokinase /anistreplase**
- **Tissue plasminogen activators**
- **Urokinase.**

Streptokinase/Anistreplase

Streptokinase is a protein isolated from β-haemolytic streptococci, which binds to plasminogen, thereby activating it. It was the first thrombolytic drug to be widely used and is relatively inexpensive. The use of tissue plasminogen activators is preferred, where available.

Therapeutic Use. **Administration** is by intravenous infusion. Patients may be pre-treated with chlorphenamine and hydrocortisone to reduce allergic reactions.

Adverse Effects.

- **Bleeding:** this is the main risk with streptokinase, and is particularly liable to occur at sites of recent trauma or invasive vascular procedures, which must be avoided if possible. It is contraindicated in those in whom it might precipitate bleeding (e.g. patients with peptic ulcers, oesophageal varices, severe hypertension or recent head injuries)

- **Allergies** are common and include fever, bronchospasm and rashes
- **Hypotension** can occur and the blood pressure should be monitored.

Contraindications. Patients develop antistreptokinase antibodies after about 4 days of treatment, and it should not be used again for at least 12 months to allow these antibody titres to fall, since the antibodies will neutralize the streptokinase and render it useless.

Anistreplase is a plasminogen–streptokinase complex that liberates streptokinase. It is therefore a prodrug. It is administered by intravenous injection over 4–5 min, and fibrinolytic activity is sustained for 4–6 h. It may have a role in treatment by clinicians or paramedics in remote areas with limited clinical facilities.

Tissue Plasminogen Activators

The tissue plasminogen activators are much more specific fibrin-bound plasminogen activators than streptokinase. Circulating streptococcal antibodies do not neutralize them; therefore they can be used in patients who have had streptokinase .

Alteplase has a short half-life and is therefore administered as an IV bolus, followed by an infusion. **Reteplase** and **Tenectaplase** may both be given as IV bolus injections. This may also be of value as a treatment option for clinicians or paramedics in remote areas. These drugs are all more expensive than streptokinase. Bleeding is the main unwanted effect.

Urokinase

Urokinase is not now used to treat ACS but is a fibrinolytic agent that activates plasminogen in a manner different to the other fibrinolytic drugs. It has been used for many years as an infusion to clear blocked intravenous and dialysis catheters. It is sometimes used to help reduce massive deep vein thromboses, and also to treat large pulmonary emboli.

CLINICAL NOTE

A major side-effect of thrombolytics is bleeding. Care should be taken to avoid intramuscular injections and obtaining central venous access post-administration. With streptokinase, it is likely to be ineffective if repeated after 4 days, therefore if a patient has a repeat thromboembolic event, an alternative such as alteplase or tenecteplase should be considered. With most of these drugs, heparin and aspirin are prescribed concomitantly to avoid further clotting.

Antiplatelet Drugs

Arterial thrombosis, such as occurs in ACS and strokes is partly due to an aggregation of blood platelets, which ultimately form small plugs in blood vessels. Certain drugs have been shown to reduce platelet 'stickiness' so that aggregation is less likely to occur. The main indications for the use of these *antiplatelet* drugs are:

- **ACS**
- **acute thrombotic stroke**
- **after coronary artery angioplasty and stenting**
- **after coronary artery bypass grafting**
- ***secondary prevention* of cardiovascular events in patients who already have established cardiovascular disease.**

Aspirin

Aspirin, by inhibiting the production of thromboxane in platelets, prevents them adhering to each other and to atheromatous plaques and so forming or extending a thrombus. Aspirin also has analgesic and antiinflammatory effects and may reduce the risk of certain cancers. It has a role in preventing eclampsia in pregnancy in women found to be at high risk of this condition. More than most drugs, its use has repeatedly fallen in and out of favour as research evaluates its risks and benefits.

Currently, it is not recommended for **primary prevention** (preventing disease in those who do not currently have it) of ischaemic heart disease or stroke as the risk of serious bleeding outweighs the benefits. Bleeding from the gastrointestinal tract is the greatest danger from regular aspirin treatment.

Aspirin is widely used for **secondary prevention** of cardiovascular events, particularly in patients who have had ACS, ischaemic stroke and PCI with stent placement, where it should be continued lifelong.

Dipyridamole

Dipyridamole prevents platelet aggregation by blocking the uptake of adenosine into platelets. It is less effective than other antiplatelet drugs and gastrointestinal and allergic reactions are relatively common. For these reasons it has generally fallen out of favour, although it may be used in its modified release form for secondary prevention of ischaemic strokes and transient ischaemic attacks.

Adenosine Diphosphate Receptor Antagonists – Clopidogrel, Ticagrelor, Prasugrel

Adenosine diphosphate (ADP) is a potent activator of platelet aggregation through the activation of P2Y12 receptors on platelets. A number of orally active antagonists for this receptor are in current use. They are often used in combination with aspirin for up to a year (and sometimes longer) in patients with ACS or after PCI. Aspirin is continued after they are discontinued.

Clopidogrel. Clopidogrel is widely used and relatively inexpensive. It is a prodrug and the onset of action is relatively slow. A loading dose is used to speed up the onset of action. Bleeding and bruising is the most common adverse effect. Rarely this may be a sign of dangerously severe depletion of platelets (thrombocytopaenic purpura).

Up to 14% of patients have a genetically mediated poor response to clopidogrel as they cannot metabolize it to its active form.

Ticagrelor. Ticagrelor acts more quickly than clopidogrel and its effects are reversed more rapidly. It does not have the same pharmacogenomic issues as clopidogrel. Its twice-daily dosage is a disadvantage. Shortness of breath is a relatively common side-effect of unknown cause. It can worsen heart block. It has a number of moderately important drug interactions.

Prasugrel. This has a more rapid onset of action than clopidogrel and is mainly used in combination with aspirin in patients with ACS who are undergoing urgent PCI.

Ticlopidine was the first of this class of drug to be developed. Its use is now limited because of adverse effects, particularly thrombocytopaenia. **Cangrelor** is an intravenous, rapidly-acting drug in this class. It is used for rapid antiplatelet activity in patients undergoing emergency PCI.

CLINICAL NOTE

Non-adherence to antiplatelet agents following PCI is associated with increased risk of stent thrombosis, acute myocardial infarction and death (Chen et al., 2015). Studies have suggested that younger patients and those with a history of depression are of greatest risk (Nordstrom et al., 2013; Zhu et al., 2011). The most effective interventions are those which are tailored to individual need and, therefore, healthcare professionals should seek a shared understanding with the patient about what matters to them and provide realistic treatment goals with regular follow-up.

Glycoprotein IIb/IIIa Receptor Antagonists

The final step in the clumping of platelets is the deposition of fibrin on the platelet surface, leading to the formation of a thrombus. This is due to the activation of a receptor called glycoprotein IIb/IIIa (GPIIb/IIIa) on the platelet surface. Drugs are now available which can block this receptor and thus prevent thrombus formation through a mechanism that is complementary to aspirin. They are used in patients undergoing PCI for ACS. **Eptifibatide** and **tirofiban** are used both used intravenously.

Abciximab is also used intravenously, but differs from the drugs above by being a monoclonal antibody. It thus belongs to the broad group of drugs known as 'Biologics' (see Appendix). Its effects last for up to 120 h. Thrombocytopaenia is a rare but serious unwanted effect.

TREATMENT OF ACUTE CORONARY SYNDROME

If a diagnosis of ACS is suspected, then first aid treatment should include giving the patient a 300 mg aspirin to chew and swallow, unless the patient is known to be allergic to aspirin. It is very unlikely that a single tablet will cause any harm, and early initiation of antiplatelet therapy may reduce cardiac damage significantly.

ACS will be confirmed on the basis of the history, ECG and biochemical evidence of cardiac damage. It will be categorized as unstable angina, NSTEMI or STEMI. Treatment approaches are similar but differ in some details. Local procedures and policies will vary and must be understood; the principles are outlined as follows:

- **Pain relief:** Pain and anxiety may be severe. GTN may be tried initially, but intravenous opiates are often used – commonly diamorphine or morphine, combined with an antiemetic drug as needed. Opiates may slow the absorption of oral antiplatelet drugs, although it is not known if this is of clinical significance.
- **Oxygen:** Oxygen is no longer routinely given to all ACS patients. It should be given if oxygen saturation on pulse oximetry is <94%. If pulse oximetry is not available, oxygen is best *not* given unless the patient has clinical signs of respiratory distress. Routine use of oxygen has been shown to increase the severity of cardiac damage in ACS.
- **Antiplatelet treatment:** After an initial loading dose of aspirin, as described previously, this should be continued indefinitely at 75 mg/day. If there is aspirin allergy, then clopidogrel may be used as an alternative. Dual antiplatelet therapy with aspirin and a P2Y12 receptor antagonist is usually given. Ticagrelor or prasugrel are often used in patients who are to undergo PCI. Dual antiplatelet therapy should be continued in all patients with confirmed ACS, for at least a year. High-risk patients may benefit from longer dual therapy, but bleeding risk needs to be assessed.
- Eptifibatide or tirofiban or abciximab may be used initially as intravenous antiplatelet treatment in patients with ACS who are likely to have urgent PCI.
- **Antithrombin (anticoagulant) treatment:** Patients with unstable angina and NSTEMI will usually be treated in hospital with some form of anticoagulation, unless their bleeding risk is high. Fondaparinux is often used in patients for whom urgent PCI is not anticipated. Unfractionated heparin is used if urgent PCI is anticipated. In STEMI patients undergoing PCI or fibrinolysis, unfractionated heparin is used.
- **Revascularization:** All patients with STEMI who present within 12 h of onset of symptoms should be offered revascularization as an urgent/emergency procedure. PCI is the treatment of choice, but if not available, fibrinolysis should be offered unless there are contraindications to this. In some cases (often failure of PCI), emergency CABG may be necessary, if available.
- Patients with unstable angina or NSTEMI should have their risk of death from future cardiovascular events estimated using an established tool such as the GRACE score (Global Registry of Acute Cardiac Events score). If they are found to be at intermediate or high risk, then they should be offered PCI during their hospital admission.
- **Other drugs:** As well as continuing antiplatelet therapy, most patients will be started on a β-blocker, such as bisoprolol, and an ACE-inhibitor, such as ramipril. Even in low doses, these drug classes are associated with improved outcomes in patients with ACS. The use of high-dose statin therapy has become usual. Other risk factors such as hypertension and diabetes may require further drug therapy. Some patients will have stable angina after ACS and drug treatment may be required. Most patients who have had an episode of ACS come out of hospital on many more drugs than they had previously. In most cases this is justified, but it should be remembered that the whole patient as a person needs to be considered, and not just their heart.

NURSING NOTES

- Careful explanation of the reasons for drug therapy will greatly increase the likelihood of patients continuing to take their drugs.
- It is important to enquire about side-effects of medication.
- Non-drug therapy is very important.
- Weight loss, exercise and smoking cessation are vital and nurses are well placed and trusted to help patients with these. Graded cardiac rehabilitation exercises can be very helpful.
- Many patients are very frightened by their experience of ACS and its treatment, and anxiety and depression are common sequels. It is important to enquire about how your patient feels and offer a sympathetic ear to their concerns.

STROKES

Strokes are an important cause of death and disability. Most of them (80%) are ischaemic, due to thrombi developing on atheroma, or emboli from atrial fibrillation blocking a branch of the cerebral circulation; the rest are due to haemorrhage.

For ischaemic strokes, fibrinolytic agents are increasingly used in centres that have access to suitable diagnostic and treatment facilities. The objective is to dissolve the thrombus in the brain before too much damage has been done. Alteplase is the preferred drug.

If the stroke is a consequence of emboli from the heart, as occurs in AF, then anticoagulation should be started. Ideally, stroke risk should be reduced by anticoagulation in most patients with AF.

For strokes or transient ischaemic attacks that are not a consequence of emboli from the heart, preventative antiplatelet treatment should be started in most cases. Clopidogrel 75 mg daily is the preferred drug, otherwise, a combination of aspirin and modified-release dipyridamole may be used. Aspirin alone is less effective but is better than no treatment.

Treatment of cardiovascular risk factors by medication and lifestyle measures is also very important.

Peripheral Vascular Disease

Peripheral vascular disease (PVD) is an important cause of limb loss, particularly in diabetics. In diabetics, both small blood vessels (microvasculature) and large blood vessels (arteries) are damaged and narrowed. In non-diabetics, it is mainly arteries that are narrowed. PVD can lead to leg pain on walking (claudication), but can also lead to gangrene and amputation. The main treatment is to make lifestyle changes (particularly smoking cessation), to encourage graded exercise, and (where possible), to surgically graft or stent narrowed arteries. Drug treatment of PVD mainly involves the treatment of the cause, plus the use of antiplatelet drugs. Clopidogrel 75 mg daily is the preferred drug.

In the past, drugs to dilate arteries have been developed and used in the hope of treating PVD. For the most part, they have proved to be ineffective and are little used today. **Naftidrofuryl oxalate** is the only drug currently recommended for use in UK practice. It may be used for a trial period in patients for whom revascularization is not appropriate or is declined. It should be discontinued if not effective. **Cilostazol**, **pentoxifylline** and **inositol nicotinate** are all vasodilator drugs that have been used to treat claudication, but none are currently recommended for use in the UK.

REFERENCES AND FURTHER READING

Ahmed, I., Majeed, A., Powell, R., 2007. Heparin induced thrombocytopenia: diagnosis and management update. Postgrad. Med. J. 83 (983), 575–582.

Chen, H.Y., Saczynski, J.S., Lapane, K.L., et al., 2015. Adherence to evidence-based secondary prevention pharmacotherapy in patients after an acute coronary syndrome: a systematic review. Heart Lung 44 (4), 299–308.

Gitlin, Z., Marvel, F., Blumental, R.S., Martin, S.S., 2018. Statin Safety and Adverse Events. Expert Analysis, American College of Cardiology. https://www.acc.org/latest-in-cardiology/articles/2018/12/12/07/23/statin-safety-and-adverse-events.

Heit, J.A., 2015. Epidemiology of venous thromboembolism. Nat. Rev. Cardiol. 12 (8), 464–474.

Kolandaivelu, K., Leiden, B.B., O'Gara, P.T., Bhatt, D.L., 2014. Non-adherence to cardiovascular medications. Eur. Heart. J. 35 (46), 3267–3276.

Lorie, E., 2016. The Warning Signs of Deep Vein Thrombosis. Nursing in Practice. https://www.nursinginpractice.com/cpd/the-warning-signs-of-deep-vein-thrombosis.

NHS UK, 2018. https://www.nhs.uk/conditions/angina/treatment.

NICE, 2010. Risk Assessment for Venous Thromboembolism (VTE). https://www.nice.org.uk/guidance/ng89/resources/department-of-health-vte-risk-assessment-tool-pdf-4787149213.

NICE, 2019. MI: Secondary Prevention. https://cks.nice.org.uk/mi-secondary-prevention.

NICE, 2020. Venous Thromboembolic Diseases: Diagnosis, Management and Thrombophilia Testing. NICE guideline [NG158] https://www.nice.org.uk/guidance/ng158.

Nordstrom, B.L., Simeone, J.C., Zhao, Z., et al., 2013. Adherence and persistence with prasugrel following acute coronary syndrome with percutaneous coronary intervention. Am. J. Cardiovasc. Drugs 13 (4), 263–271.

Pirmohamed, M., James, S., Meakin, S., et al., 2004. Adverse drug reactions as cause of admission to hospital: prospective analysis of 18 820 patients. BMJ 329 (7456), 15.

Zhu, B., Zhao, Z., McCollam, P., et al., 2011. Factors associated with clopidogrel use, adherence, and persistence in patients with acute coronary syndromes undergoing percutaneous coronary intervention. Curr. Med. Res. Opin. 27 (3), 633–641.

USEFUL WEBSITES

Anticoagulation Europe. https://www.anticoagulationeurope.org.

NHS UK. Angina: treatment. https://www.nhs.uk/conditions/angina/treatment.

NICE, Venous thromboembolism in over 16s: reducing the risk of hospital-acquired deep vein thrombosis or pulmonary embolism [NG89]. https://www.nice.org.uk/guidance/ng89.

Thrombosis UK. https://thrombosisuk.org.

8 RESUSCITATION

CHAPTER OUTLINE

LEARNING OBJECTIVES

At the end of this chapter, the reader should be able to:

- describe the ingredients and use of oral rehydration solutions
- describe the fluid compartments of the body
- describe the differences between crystalloids and colloids
- describe the differences between isotonic, hypotonic and hypertonic solutions
- list the main types of intravenous fluids and their uses
- outline the use of intravenous fluids in shock
- outline the use of intravenous fluids in maintenance therapy
- describe which drugs may be used in cardiopulmonary resuscitation
- outline the emergency treatment of anaphylaxis

BACKGROUND

Fluid and electrolyte balance, fluid replacement and fluid maintenance are a key part of medical and nursing management. A detailed description of all possible fluid replacement regimens is beyond the scope of this book; however, the principles are quite straightforward and aid in the understanding of the various regimens used in clinical practice. The most important principles are to understand that humans require a certain amount of water and electrolytes (mainly sodium and potassium) daily, to maintain normal fluid and electrolyte balance. The easiest way to achieve this is by normal oral intake of fluids and food. If this is not possible then fluids are given intravenously. If there are abnormal fluid and electrolyte losses then these need to be replaced using the most appropriate fluid, either orally or intravenously.

This chapter also briefly considers the use of drugs in cardiopulmonary resuscitation (CPR) and in the treatment of anaphylactic shock.

CLINICAL NOTE

Where intravenous (IV) access is not possible or impractical, moderate volumes of crystalloids may be given as fluid maintenance via the subcutaneous (SC) route. In an emergency, particularly in children, the intraosseous route may also be used for fluids and blood infusion (see later).

ORAL REHYDRATION SOLUTIONS

One of the most significant life-saving interventions of the 20th century was also one of the simplest. It was the development of oral rehydration solutions to replace water and electrolytes lost from diarrhoea or vomiting, particularly in children (Fig. 8.1). In many parts of the world, diarrhoeal illnesses still kill large numbers of children, and epidemics of cholera still occur, killing adults and children alike. Use of oral rehydration therapy (ORT) has reduced mortality by about 90%. Diarrhoea is, mainly, slightly salty water, and if lost in large amounts, dehydration and electrolyte imbalances occur and can lead to death. This abnormal fluid and electrolyte loss can be replaced by giving slightly salty water to drink, ideally with a little potassium and a weak alkali to counter metabolic acidosis. The most important additional ingredient is a small amount of glucose or other sugar. This key ingredient was first introduced by Dr Hemendra Nath Chatterjee in 1957. It has the effect of promoting active absorption of water by the intestines and so improves hydration and reduces stool volume. More recently, the recipe for ORT has been modified to make it slightly hypotonic. This reduces the stool volume further.

The current World Health Organization (WHO) recipe for ORT solution per litre of water is:

- 2.6 g salt (NaCl)
- 2.9 g trisodium citrate dihydrate
- 1.5 g potassium chloride
- 13.5 g anhydrous glucose.

In the UK, mixtures commonly have less sodium, as sodium loss tends to be less of an issue with diarrhoeal illnesses in higher income countries. The water should be clean, but if no clean water is available, it should be made up with whatever is available. This mixture is widely available in sachets to be made up with water. In an emergency, a reasonable ORT can be made up with half a **teaspoon** of salt (~1.5 g) and 2 **tablespoons** of sugar (~18 g) in a litre of water.

Oral rehydration solutions should be offered frequently and certainly after each loose motion. ORT is suitable for the treatment of mild to moderate dehydration. Severe dehydration, or if the person vomits all the ORT continuously, should be treated with intravenous rehydration.

CLINICAL NOTE

Oral hydration is a vital part of patient care in hospitals and nursing homes. The safest and most natural

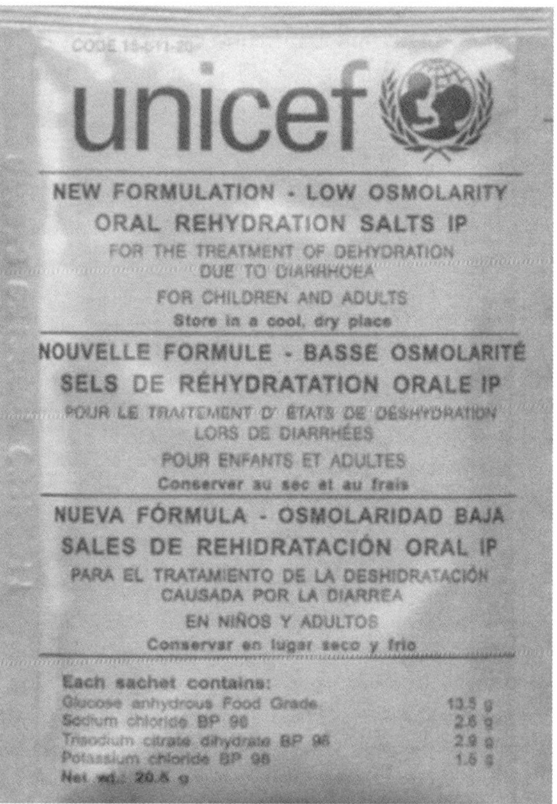

Fig. 8.1 ■ Oral rehydration sachet.

way of ensuring hydration is to ensure that patients have food and drink (if they can take them and their swallow reflex is intact) and are actually eating and drinking. Elderly and ill patients may need a lot of encouragement to drink, and on many occasions, frail people have struggled and failed to get the glass of water that has been placed just beyond their reach on the bedside table.

Oral potassium chloride supplements are sometimes used to treat or prevent low potassium (hypokalaemia), but with a decline in the use of antihypertensive drug regimens that could cause hypokalaemia, they are rarely needed today. **Oral sodium chloride** is very rarely required except in chronic sodium losing disorders. Most diets in upper- and middle-income countries already contain more sodium than is healthy.

INTRAVENOUS FLUIDS

There are some important concepts that need to be understood in order to grasp the principles of intravenous fluid therapy:

The Fluid Compartments of the Body

The human body is overall about 60% water, some tissues having more and some less (Fig. 8.2). This water is found in the three major fluid compartments of the body:

- Intravascular
- Interstitial
- Intracellular.

The **intravascular** compartment contains water within the blood vessels of the body. This water is in the form of blood, made of plasma and red and white blood cells. Plasma contains, among other things, ***solutes*** in the form of sodium and potassium, and proteins, mainly albumin. In an adult man the intravascular volume is ~3.5 litres (~**1/9** of total body water).

The **interstitial** compartment is water that is outside of the blood vessels, but not inside the cells. It is divided from the intravascular compartment by the endothelial cells that make up capillaries, and from the intracellular compartment by the cell walls of individual cells. It contains solutes in a similar concentration to blood, but little protein and far fewer cells. In an adult man, it is ~10.5 litres (~**2/9** of total body water).

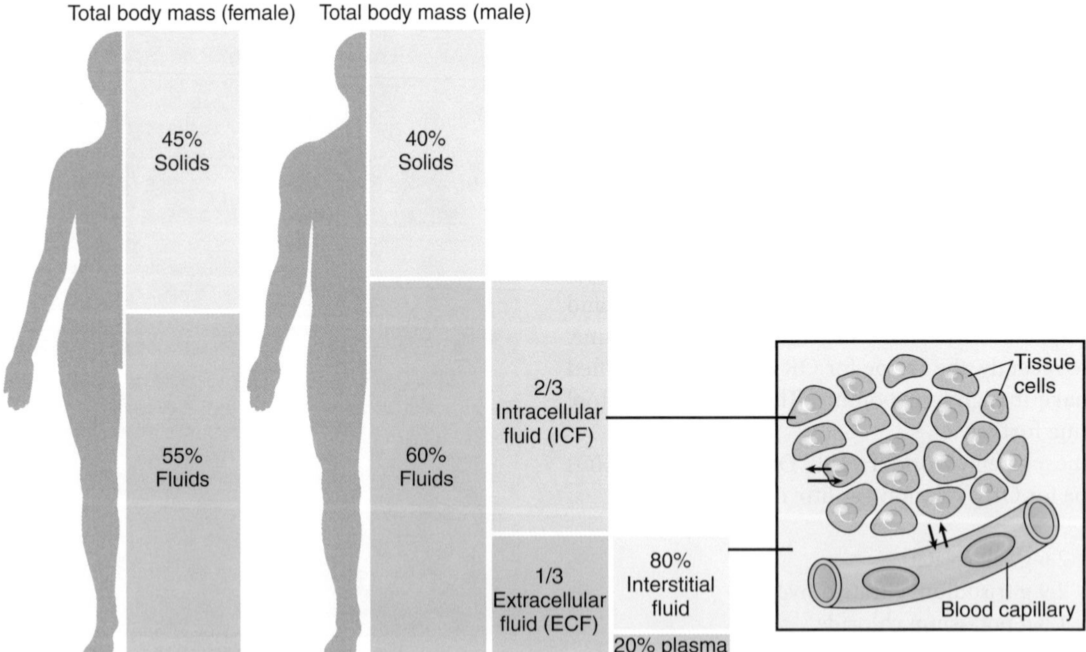

Fig. 8.2 ■ Volume of body fluid in the different body compartments. (From Sharma Y. Fluid, electrolyte, and acid-base homeostasis. http://www.slideshare.net/dryuktisharma/chapter-27-37583036. John Wiley & Sons.)

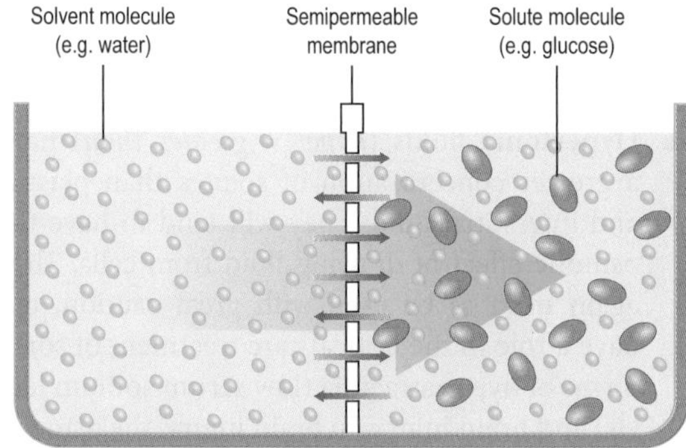

Fig. 8.3 ■ Osmosis: The arrows show solvent flow across a semipermeable membrane from an area of low solute concentration to an area of high solute concentration.

The **intracellular** compartment contains water that is inside the cells of the body, kept there by a ***semi-permeable*** **cell membrane** that is also able to actively move substances into and out of the cells. In consequence the concentration and composition of solutes dissolved in the intracellular water is very different to that outside the cells. In an adult man it is ~28 litres (**~2/3** of total body water).

The importance of understanding the fluid compartments is that the concentration and constituents of intravenous fluids can have a major influence on the water content of individual compartments.

Osmotic Pressure and Oncotic Pressure

Osmotic pressure is measure of the pressure generated by the flow of water across a semipermeable membrane from an area of low concentration of a solute to an area of high concentration of solute (Fig. 8.3).

This process is called *osmosis*, and the semipermeable membrane is the key item here. Conceptually it is a membrane with holes in it that are large enough to be fully permeable to water molecules, but small enough to obstruct the passage of larger molecules of solutes, such as sodium ions or glucose molecules. If there are more solute molecules on one side of a semipermeable membrane than the other, then water will tend to pass across the membrane in the direction of the higher solute concentration. In humans, the semipermeable membranes are the cell membranes, which separate the intracellular and interstitial fluid compartments. If the solute concentration outside the cell is less than

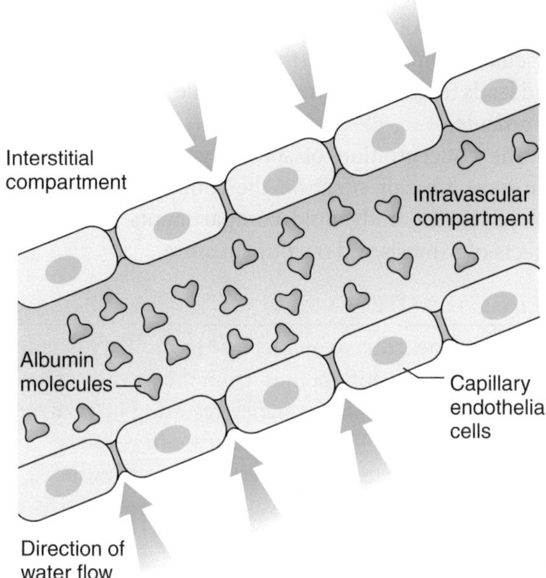

Fig. 8.4 ■ Oncotic pressure: water flowing into a capillary that contains large albumin molecules, from the interstitial space.

that inside the cell, then water will tend to flow into the cell, causing it to expand. If too much water enters the cell it may burst, which is what happens when red blood cells *haemolyse* when placed in a hypotonic solution (see later). If the solute concentration outside the cell is greater than inside the cell, then water will flow out of the cell, causing them to shrink, shrivel and ultimately die.

Oncotic pressure is a closely related idea and may also be called *colloid osmotic pressure*. This is the pressure generated by the flow of water **into** a capillary from the outside of the capillary (which is interstitial fluid with little protein), to the inside of the capillary, which is intravascular fluid and contains large plasma proteins (mainly albumin) in solution (Fig. 8.4). Here, it is the concentration of these plasma proteins that determines the pressure generated. The capillary wall is analogous to the semipermeable cell membrane, but in this case, it is fully permeable to water and electrolytes, but acts like a sieve, keeping the plasma proteins inside. These large intravascular proteins are often referred to as *colloids* (see later). If the concentration of albumin in the plasma falls (due to some kinds of kidney disease, or even malnutrition), then the oncotic pressure is reduced, and fluid moves from the intravascular compartment to the interstitial compartment, and leads to the development of tissue swelling, known as *oedema*.

The concentration of solutes given intravenously can have a major effect on the concentrations of the solutes in the body fluid compartments due to the effects of osmosis and oncotic pressure.

CLINICAL NOTE

In septic shock, due to an increase in capillary permeability there is a 'shift' of fluid from the intravascular to the interstitial compartments, resulting in 'relative' hypovolaemia resulting in an increase in respiratory rate, heart rate, reduction in blood pressure and increased risk of cardiovascular collapse. Early identification and management is crucial for survival from this and guidance published from the European Intensive Care Society (Rhodes et al., 2017) provides a standardized approach to treatment and management.

ISOTONIC, HYPOTONIC AND HYPERTONIC FLUIDS

Any fluid used in intravenous therapy may be isotonic, hypotonic or hypertonic, although the vast majority of fluids given are isotonic. 'Tonic' refers to the tonicity of a fluid and is an indicator of the concentration of solutes in that fluid relative to some other fluid. In medical practice it is normally the concentration of solutes in an intravenous fluid relative to the concentration of solutes in blood plasma and interstitial fluid.

- **Isotonic** fluids (*iso = the same*) have approximately the same concentration of solutes in them as blood plasma and interstitial fluid, so there is no osmotic effect on the cells in the blood; 0.9% sodium chloride solution is a typical isotonic intravenous fluid.
- **Hypotonic** fluids (*hypo = less than*) have a lower concentration of solutes than plasma and interstitial fluid. They will tend to have an osmotic effect on cells that can be useful in rehydrating them in very severe dehydration. They need to be used with great caution, however, and in most cases isotonic infusions are preferred; 0.45% sodium chloride solution is a typical hypotonic intravenous fluid.
- **Hypertonic** fluids (*hyper = greater than*) have a greater concentration of solutes than plasma and interstitial fluid. They will tend to have the osmotic effect of drawing fluid from cells. They again need to be used with great caution, but have a role in the critical care treatment of some forms of hyponatraemia (low serum sodium levels) and brain injury. In brain injury, the osmotic effect of hypertonic fluids may help reduce the dangerous swelling of brain cells that can occur; 3% and 5% solutions of sodium chloride are typical hypertonic solutions.

CLINICAL NOTE

Intravenous infusion of a hypertonic **mannitol solution** is also used in the same way as hypertonic saline, in the treatment of brain injury.

Infusions of moderately hyper- or hypotonic solutions can be irritant and painful and should be given slowly.

It is worth noting that it is not only intravenous fluids that can be iso-, hypo- or hypertonic. As noted previously, the slightly hypotonic nature of oral rehydration solutions means that water tends to be drawn by osmosis from the gut lumen into the interstitial fluid compartment and so reduces the volume of diarrhoea.

CRYSTALLOIDS AND COLLOIDS

The final key concept is the distinction between colloids and crystalloids in intravenous fluid therapy. Crystalloids are solutions of small atoms and molecules such as sodium, chloride and glucose. They may be isotonic, hypotonic or hypertonic. Crystalloids are by far the most widely used intravenous fluids.

Colloids are solutions of large molecules in water. The water may also contain small molecules in solution. Colloids may be natural, such as the albumin in plasma, which can also be extracted and used as infusion, or they may be synthetic such as gelatin or dextrans. Colloids generate a positive oncotic pressure that draws water into capillaries and thus maintains the circulating volume in the intravascular compartment.

The most important examples of crystalloids and colloids are as follows:

Crystalloids

Sodium chloride ('saline'; NaCl): Sodium chloride is the main electrolyte in blood and is a mainstay of intravenous fluid therapy. An isotonic solution is 0.9% and is often referred to as **normal saline.** It contains 150 mmol/L of Na^+ and Cl^-. It is used for fluid resuscitation and for maintenance provision of water and sodium. Hypertonic and hypotonic solutions are occasionally used, as noted earlier.

Potassium chloride 0.3% with sodium chloride 0.9% is used to provide maintenance quantities of potassium in the form of potassium chloride (KCl). One litre (1 L) contains 40 mmol of K^+, 150 mmol of Na^+ and 170 mmol of Cl^-. **Potassium chloride 0.15% with sodium chloride 0.9%** contains 20 mmol of K^+ per litre and is also often used.

Glucose 5% ('Dextrose') solution in water is used to provide maintenance quantities of water. The glucose makes it an isotonic or only mildly hypotonic solution, which means it is not irritant when given by a peripheral vein and does not cause haemolysis. However, the glucose is rapidly metabolized, leaving only water. The amount of glucose is insufficient to provide nutrition for patients, but is sufficient to prevent the body switching into 'starvation mode' and producing acidic ketone bodies. Higher concentrations of glucose are used as part of parenteral nutrition regimens.

Potassium chloride 0.15% and glucose 5% is used for maintenance of daily requirements for potassium and water and contains 20 mmol/L of K^+. This is also available with 3% potassium chloride, containing 40 mmol/L of K^+.

Sodium chloride with glucose ('dextrose saline') is an isotonic mixture that is available in various proportions of sodium chloride to glucose. **Sodium chloride 0.18% with glucose 4%** is much used in the UK for maintenance therapy, as for the average 3 L/day regimen, it provides the daily sodium requirement (see later) spread out over the whole day. Dextrose saline is also available with added potassium for maintenance therapy. For the above regimen, each litre bag should contain 20 mmol of potassium, and the correct way of writing this prescription would be: **Potassium chloride 0.15%/glucose 4%/sodium chloride 0.18%.**

CLINICAL NOTE

Although the correct way of writing the prescription is shown here, this combination is very often referred to as just 'dextrose saline' or 'dextrose saline and potassium'. Various concentrations of sodium chloride and glucose could all be referred to informally as 'dextrose saline'. Always ensure that you know exactly what combination is required and do not be afraid to challenge ambiguous prescriptions. When writing prescriptions ensure that they are not ambiguous.

CLINICAL NOTE

You will note that the descriptions of solutions containing potassium always have the potassium chloride component written first. This is good practice, as overdose of potassium is dangerous and it should be absolutely clear how much potassium is required. In the past it was common practice to inject strong potassium chloride solution into bags of crystalloids to make up the correct potassium concentration. Many dangerous dose errors have occurred and potassium chloride should **never** be added to fluid bags.

Lactated Ringer's solution (Hartmann's solution; compound sodium lactate) or Acetated Ringer's solution: These are all related compounded mixtures of crystalloids. They all comprise an isotonic mixture of potassium chloride, sodium chloride and a buffering mixture, which is metabolized to alkaline bicarbonate ions. There are slight differences in composition between these solutions in different countries, but the most important distinction is between lactated Ringer's solution (*which is normally known as Hartmann's solution in the UK*) and acetated Ringer's solution. In one, the buffer is calcium chloride and sodium lactate and in the other, it is calcium chloride and sodium acetate. Acetated Ringer's solution is preferred in Scandinavian countries, but there are no overwhelming reasons to choose one buffer over the other. In the UK, Hartmann's solution contains 131 mmol/L Na^+, 111 mmol/L Cl^-, 5 mmol/L K^+ and

29 mmol/L HCO_3^- (bicarbonate ions). This composition is very close to that of the electrolytes found in plasma and means that Hartmann's/Ringer's solutions are an ideal solution for replacing plasma loss. They are the crystalloids of choice for immediate fluid resuscitation in hypovolaemic shock. However, although they have a 'physiological' composition, they are not suitable on their own for maintenance fluids. If 3 L of Hartmann's solution were given in a day, it would provide 3 times too much sodium and not enough potassium.

CLINICAL NOTE

There is an emerging fashion for the use of slightly different buffered crystalloid solutions, e.g. *Plasma-Lyte 148*. These are physiologically balanced solutions similar to Ringer's solutions, and are used widely across the UK and Europe, yet with a paucity of evidence on their effectiveness (Weinberg et al., 2016). When fluid resuscitation is required, the key principles are the right fluid at the right time at the right rate, that is to say, it is based on individual response and physiological parameters.

Sodium bicarbonate (Na HCO_3) is used intravenously to treat severe metabolic acidosis, especially if this is caused by bicarbonate loss from kidneys or gut; **1.26% sodium bicarbonate** infusion can be given over a few hours, with careful monitoring of other electrolytes and pH; 50 mL of a hypertonic 8.4% solution may be given as a bolus in cardiac arrest where severe metabolic acidosis may develop, but is no longer routinely given and is not included in current Resuscitation Council Guidelines (Resuscitation Council, 2015). Sodium bicarbonate may also be given by mouth to treat chronic acidosis.

Colloids

Intravenous colloids were extensively used as 'plasma expanders' to treat hypovolaemic shock; however, over the last 20 years they have fallen out of favour, as research has shown that crystalloids are generally safer and more effective than colloids in the immediate treatment of blood loss. The reasoning behind the use of colloids was that as they remained in the intravascular compartment, they rapidly replaced circulating volume and restored blood pressure. However, it became apparent that they also tended to dilute circulating clotting factors and may have made it more difficult to stop blood loss. It has also become clear that in many cases, rapidly restoring normal blood pressure may actually also worsen bleeding. Colloids still have a role, however, particularly in patients with poor cardiac reserve who may develop fluid overload if aggressively resuscitated with crystalloids, but their use has declined markedly. The most important colloids are:

Albumin solution is prepared from whole blood and is therefore a relatively scarce and expensive resource. It contains physiological amounts of electrolytes as well as plasma proteins – mainly albumin. It can be used in acutely ill people to correct an intravascular fluid deficit, but it is wasteful to use it to correct hypovolaemia in most other circumstances. A concentrated (20%) solution is sometimes used in severely ill fluid overloaded patients.

Gelatin is a large protein that is slowly metabolized and acts as a colloid. The solutions also contain physiological amounts of electrolytes and a lactate buffer; the amounts of electrolytes vary slightly between individual brands. It is used to replace circulating plasma volume in hypovolaemic shock due to bleeding (but see earlier). It is used to increase plasma volume in hypovolaemic shock due to septicaemia or burns, but should not be used over extended periods.

Dextrans are a family of large polysaccharide macromolecules, that are used in the same way and for the same indications as gelatin. They are used in some countries, but not in the UK, except as an iron–dextran infusion that is occasionally used to treat severe iron deficiency.

Hydroxyethyl starch (tetrastarch) are also part of a family of large polysaccharide macromolecules (including hetastarch, pentastarch and hexastarch). They were much used from the 1960s onwards, but have severely fallen out of favour, as evidence of serious harms arose, and it became apparent that much of the evidence for their safe use was probably false and the result of scientific fraud. Tetrastarch may only be used in the UK to correct hypovolaemia from bleeding when crystalloids are insufficient. It must not be used in severely ill patients.

CLINICAL NOTE

During resuscitation, the current recommendations are to use crystalloid instead of colloids and only to use colloids if crystalloids are no longer effective. A recent Cochrane review noted no difference in outcomes when using colloid vs crystalloid (Lewis et al., 2018) and a second meta-analysis called for clear guidance of when to transition from crystalloid to colloid solutions in critical care and resuscitation (Martin and Bassett, 2019).

INTRAVENOUS FLUID TREATMENT

Intravenous Fluids in Shock

The basic elements of the treatment of shock with fluids are outlined here. There are many possible variations on this, depending on the type of patient and their presenting complaint. It is important to follow local guidelines and to obtain expert advice early.

In treating shock, it is important to identify and control the cause as soon as possible, thus bleeding needs to be controlled or infection treated. If a patient is shocked due to bleeding, then the most effective fluid replacement is whole blood. However, cross-matching blood takes time and blood is not available to paramedics outside of hospital. Hypovolaemic shock can also be due to other causes such as infection or dehydration. In most cases, the initial treatment should be a rapid infusion of a bolus of a crystalloid. Hartmann's solution is ideal, but 0.9% sodium chloride solution is satisfactory. An initial bolus of 500 mL is given over 15 minutes or less, and the response is assessed. In normally healthy adults, the bolus can be repeated up to a total of 2000 mL of fluid, but in children and the elderly and those with cardiac and renal problems, the volumes will be less (often much less) and expert advice is needed sooner. Colloids may be necessary in some of these cases. An estimation of the fluid deficit is required to guide further fluid replacement. It is increasingly recognized that when treating shock due to bleeding, *permissive hypotension* may be allowed. This is where, rather than aiming for a normal blood pressure, a systolic blood pressure of around 80 mmHg is the aim. It has been shown that, **except for traumatic brain injury**, this target leads to better outcomes. When the cause of the shock is treated and the patient is stabilized, they will require maintenance intravenous fluids until they are able to drink and eat normally.

Maintenance Intravenous Fluids

Maintenance fluid regimens are based upon a person's daily fluid and electrolyte requirements plus any additional requirements due to abnormal losses of fluids and electrolytes. A wide variety of crystalloids can be used if they provide these requirements. In people who are generally healthy, with normal cardiac and renal function, who are perhaps 'nil by mouth' pre- or post-operatively, absolute precision in prescribing maintenance fluids is not needed as normal kidneys can cope with a little too much water or salt. Children, ill and frail people need a great deal of care in determining their fluid requirements.

- The hourly water requirement in a person with no abnormal losses is 1–2 mL/kg per h.
- The daily sodium requirement is 1–2 mmol/kg per 24 h.
- The daily potassium requirement is 0.5–1 mmol/kg per 24 h.

The range in values here allows for variation dependant on the patient's fluid status, frailty and their electrolyte (U&E) results. In most cases, the upper end of the ranges shown will be safe. Thus, e.g. for a 70 kg person with no other fluid losses, who is not eating or drinking, the amounts per day would be:

- Water: ~3 L
- Na: ~140 mmol
- K: ~70 mmol.

This could be achieved by giving 1 L of 0.15% potassium chloride and 0.9% sodium chloride and 2 L of 0.15% potassium chloride and 5% glucose. This regimen, sometimes referred to as '*one salty and two sweet*' is a reasonable basis for fluid maintenance, but many other variations are possible. This regimen will provide 3 L of water, 150 mmol Na and 60 mmol K over 24 h. Recent guidelines have suggested reducing the daily sodium requirement to around 1 mmol/kg per 24 h and the average fluid volume to 2.5 L.

Additional fluid requirements: It is important to realize that intravenous fluid maintenance needs to account for abnormal losses of fluids and electrolytes. In addition to the normal fluid requirements, an estimate of additional daily requirements will be needed. This will be based on the previous day's measured (ideally) or estimated (less ideally) volumes of fluid loss and a calculation of their electrolyte content. Abnormal fluid losses include vomit, diarrhoea and nasogastric aspirate. Tables are available that give the electrolyte content of these fluids, but most of these fluids have an electrolyte mix similar to plasma, so Hartmann's solution is a good replacement in most cases. Pyrexia also increases fluid loss through sweating and faster breathing (known as *insensible loss*), which should be replaced with 5% glucose solution. Abnormal polyuria is also an abnormal loss which needs to be replaced, but in general, careful charting of urine output is a good indicator of a patient's state of hydration and whether fluid replacement is adequate. A urine output of 0.5–1 mL/kg per hour is often regarded as normal for the average adult.

CLINICAL NOTE

Intravenous fluid replacement can seem something of a 'black art', but the key clinical messages are that careful attention to charting fluid balance is essential in order to plan for adequate replacement, and that where possible, patients should be taking their fluids orally rather than intravenously.

DRUGS USED DURING CARDIOPULMONARY RESUSCITATION

Basic Life Support

No drugs are used in basic life support. *Basic life support* is the term used to describe the initial attempts at resuscitation following cardiac or respiratory arrest.

Basic life support starts once it has been established that a patient is unconscious and unresponsive.

Action takes three parts and consists of:

- *Airway*: the patient's airway must be cleared and kept open.
- *Breathing*: if the patient is not breathing, then their lungs should be ventilated using mouth-to-mouth, or other techniques as appropriate.
- *Circulation*: if there is no pulse, then cardiac massage is started.

CLINICAL NOTE

This brief account of basic life support is not intended to supplement or replace the training that is given, but is presented to show that drugs are of secondary importance. Clinicians should have their mandatory training for basic life support in line with current recommendations.

Advanced Life Support

Once equipment and drugs appropriate for resuscitation become available, as would happen in any hospital, then *advanced life support* is started. These are outlined in Fig. 8.5.

Drugs Used During Resuscitation

Adrenaline (epinephrine) is widely used during CPR. It has several useful effects: it elevates the blood pressure generated during chest compressions and so increases coronary artery perfusion; it improves myocardial contractility and heart rate; it increases the vigour of ventricular fibrillation and makes it easier to terminate by defibrillation; and it helps to redirect blood flow to the brain. It is given in a large dose immediately a diagnosis of asystole is made, or if attempts at defibrillation fail to terminate ventricular fibrillation or ventricular tachycardia. Thereafter, it is given at regular intervals during CPR, whatever the cardiac rhythm, until resuscitation is ended.

SAFETY NOTE

Adrenaline is also known as **epinephrine** in many countries.

Do not confuse **epinephrine** with **ephedrine**, which is another sympathomimetic medicine used to raise blood pressure, particularly for the treatment of hypotension associated with general anaesthesia and with the use of epidural and spinal anaesthesia.

NURSING NOTE

A drug concentration oddity: You may still hear adrenaline described as '1 in a 1000' (1:1000) or '1 in 10,000' (1:10,000):

1 mg of adrenaline is contained in 1 mL of '1 in 1000' adrenaline (epinephrine) or 10 mL of '1 in 10,000' adrenaline (epinephrine).

This information is important to know during CPR. It is unfortunate that the concentration of adrenaline (epinephrine) is still given in such a curious manner; '1 in 1000' means one gram in 1000 millilitres (1 g in 1000 mL). The concentration of no other drug is indicated in this way.

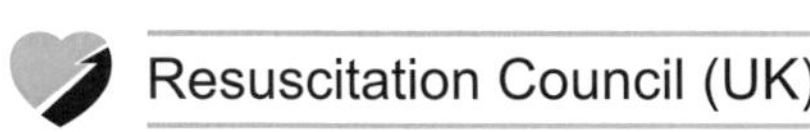

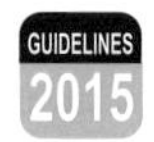

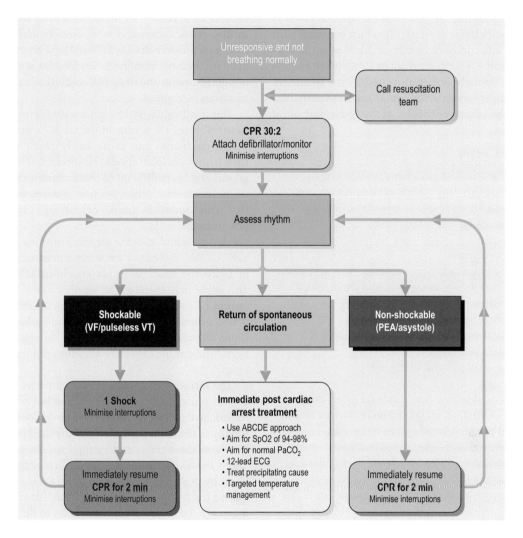

Adult Advanced Life Support

Fig. 8.5 ■ Adult advanced life support. *CPR*, Cardiopulmonary resuscitation; *$PaCO_2$*, partial pressure of carbon dioxide; *PEA*, pulseless electrical activity; *SpO_2*, oxygen saturation; *VF*, ventricular fibrillation; *VT*, ventricular tachycardia. (Resuscitation Council. http://www.resus.org.uk/resuscitation-guidelines/adult-advanced-life-support.)

Amiodarone is an effective and relatively safe antiarrhythmic drug that is given to patients with ventricular fibrillation if the first three attempts to terminate this rhythm by defibrillation fail. It is given as a single quick bolus during CPR, which contrasts with the slow infusion over 20 min to 2 h that is the normal method of giving the drug in patients not requiring CPR. Amiodarone is also used in the treatment of several peri-arrest arrhythmias such as ventricular tachycardia, supraventricular tachycardia and atrial fibrillation.

CLINICAL NOTE

Current resuscitation guidelines recommend the use of only these two drugs. Additional drugs are used to treat potentially reversible causes, commonly called the 4 Hs and 4 Ts. which stand for:

- Hypoxia
- Hypovolaemia
- Hyperkalaemia, hypokalaemia, hypoglycaemia, hypocalcaemia, acidaemia and other metabolic disorders
- Hypothermia
- Thrombosis (coronary or pulmonary)
- Tension pneumothorax
- Tamponade – cardiac
- Toxins.

Oxygen and intravenous fluids are given as standard treatment during cardiac arrest, and blood and blood products will be given if there are signs of major haemorrhage. Other drugs that are used are *intravenous calcium chloride* to treat hyperkalaemia, hypocalcaemia and calcium channel blocker overdose. If there is a history of toxic overdose, antidotes may be administered and will be in accordance with the drug or toxin that has been ingested. Further information on this is in Chapter 33.

Route of Administration of Drugs During Cardiopulmonary Resuscitation

Drugs can be administered by the following routes:

- intravenous (IV)
- endotracheal tube
- intraosseous
- intracardiac.

The most common route of administration of medicines during CPR is through a **peripheral vein** since this is usually the most easily and safely established form of IV access. The circulation will be slow during cardiac resuscitation and it is therefore essential that each injection of a drug is followed by a generous flush of 20 mL of normal saline or 5% glucose, so that there is a good chance the drug will reach the heart, where its action is required.

The ideal route is through a cannula placed in a **'central' vein**, i.e. a vein in the neck or groin, from where medicines can more easily reach the heart than from a peripheral vein. However, it is more dangerous and more difficult to place cannulas into these veins in an emergency, so it is not recommended that this route is tried, except by experienced practitioners.

Lidocaine and atropine are also absorbed fairly reliably via the respiratory route (by inhalation) if given in twice the usual dose via an **endotracheal tube**. This route may therefore be worth using if IV access cannot be established. However, it is doubtful if sufficient adrenaline (epinephrine) is absorbed by this route, although it is sometimes used during resuscitation. Amiodarone cannot be administered through the lungs.

The **intraosseous route** is as effective as the intravenous route. It involves a specialized but not difficult technique that inserts a stout needle into bone marrow, usually in the tibia. It is generally only used in children in whom the bone is soft enough for the technique. There are no exceptions to the medicines that can be given by this route (there used to be a few exceptions quoted but it is now accepted that there are none) and it can also be used for administration of fluid and the transfusion of blood.

Finally, the intracardiac route, using a long needle inserted through the chest wall directly into the heart, is no longer used. It is far too unreliable and dangerous.

NURSING NOTE

During CPR and emergency situations, do not discard any medicine ampoules, vials, syringes or tablet packages. This is important for review and assessment of the emergency situation. Often medicines are verbally ordered during these times and a clearly documented record of verbal prescription, verbal orders and administration may not be possible without having the containers to check human memory against.

Drugs Used in Anaphylactic Shock

Anaphylaxis is an acute, life-threatening allergic reaction. It may occur in reaction to even small amounts of an allergen in people previously sensitized to that allergen. Many foods are potentially allergenic and peanuts are the most common food-related cause of acute anaphylaxis. Bee or wasp venom may provoke anaphylaxis and many drugs can also do so, particularly protein-based drugs, such as some vaccines and some biologic drugs. Penicillins quite frequently lead to allergic reactions and anaphylaxis has occurred, particularly with IV use. It is important that people with known anaphylactic reactions to substances carefully avoid the substance, but also that they carry auto-injectors of adrenaline (epinephrine) with them.

The first aid treatment of anaphylaxis is to administer **intramuscular (IM) adrenaline** as soon as possible, repeated in a different site after 5 min, if there is no improvement. Any clinician who administers drugs or vaccines should be familiar with the treatment of anaphylaxis and be competent to give the injection in an emergency.

The adrenaline dose is:

- Adult 500 micrograms (μg) IM (0.5 mL)
- Child >12 years: 500 μg IM (0.5 mL)
- Child 6–12 years: 300 μg IM (0.3 mL)
- Child <6 years: 150 μg IM (0.15 mL).

When the patient responds to adrenaline, they should be admitted to hospital overnight, as anaphylaxis often returns. To reduce the likelihood of this happening, they may also be treated with IV **hydrocortisone** and IV **chlorphenamine**, or similar drugs. If oxygen is available it should be administered, and a bolus of intravenous crystalloid to restore blood pressure.

SUMMARY

- Fluid and electrolyte balance are most effectively maintained by feeding your patient and ensuring they have enough to drink (where they are able to do so).
- Oral fluid and electrolyte replacement are lifesaving in childhood diarrhoea.
- Intravenous fluid replacement involves providing maintenance volumes of fluid and electrolytes, plus replacing abnormal losses.
- Isotonic fluids are most commonly used.
- Crystalloids are used far more frequently than colloids.
- Colloids can be used to replace intravascular fluid loss (from bleeding), but should be used cautiously.
- Blood is the most effective fluid to replace blood loss.
- It is important to know the electrolyte content of commonly used fluids.
- Hartmann's/Lactated Ringer's solutions have an electrolyte content similar to plasma and are useful in emergency resuscitation.
- 0.9% sodium chloride is used to replace sodium and water.
- 5% glucose (dextrose) is used to replace water.
- Potassium is also required but should never be added to a bag of fluid – instead use pre-made solutions.
- Fluid and electrolyte maintenance therapy requires a calculation of the daily fluid and electrolyte requirements of the patient.
- Abnormal fluid losses must be replaced.
- Basic life support in cardiac arrest does not require the use of drugs, and prompt defibrillation is life-saving.
- Adrenaline (epinephrine) is the most important drug for use in cardiac arrest and in anaphylaxis.

REFERENCES AND FURTHER READING

Lewis, S.R., Pritchard, M.W., Evans, D.J.W., et al., 2018. Colloids versus crystalloids for fluid resuscitation in critically ill people. Cochrane Database Syst. Rev. 8, CD000567.

Martin, G.S., Bassett, P., 2019. Crystalloids vs. colloids for fluid resuscitation in the intensive care unit: a systematic review and meta-analysis. J. Critical Care 50, 144–154.

Resuscitation Council, 2015. Guidelines: Adult Advanced Life Support. http://www.resus.org.uk/resuscitation-guidelines/adult-advanced-life-support.

Rhodes, A., Evans, L.E., Alhazzani, W., et al., 2017. Surviving Sepsis Campaign: International guidelines for management of sepsis and septic shock: 2016. Intensive Care Med. 43 (3), 304–377.

Weinberg, L., Collins, N., Van Mourik, K., et al., 2016. Plasma-Lyte 148: a clinical review. World J. Crit. Care Med. 5 (4), 235–250.

9 THE RESPIRATORY SYSTEM

CHAPTER OUTLINE

LEARNING OBJECTIVES

At the end of this chapter, the reader should be able to:

- define what is meant by asthma and COPD
- classify the severity of asthma exacerbation
- list the treatments available for asthma and COPD
- understand that the reasons for coughing is multifactorial
- list cough suppressant drugs and their effectiveness
- explain the term 'respiratory failure'

ASTHMA

There are two main inflammatory conditions of the respiratory tract, *asthma and chronic obstructive pulmonary disease* (COPD). The pathogenesis of these two conditions was thought to be very different, although the drugs used to treat these diseases have considerable overlap. It is now felt that a significant number of patients can present with features of both asthma and COPD.

Starting with asthma, the disease is characterized by recurrent bouts of coughing, wheeze, shortness of breath and chest tightness. A key point in asthma is the **variability** of expiratory airflow limitation, which can occur on a daily and seasonal basis. These symptoms are caused by an underlying chronic inflammatory response of the airways associated with eosinophils and a marked increase in the irritability of the airways. Patients with asthma have an inherent sensitivity of the bronchi that is probably inherited and many patients also have allergy. Asthma attacks are precipitated by trigger factors such as respiratory tract infection, exercise, exposure to environmental triggers such as cold air, pollutants, cigarette smoke and in allergic subjects, various allergens such as house-dust mite faeces and animal dander. Asthma attacks can also be triggered by a number of psychological factors such as stress and laughter. Much of our understanding of the mechanisms of an asthma attack come from studying patients with allergic asthma. When an allergic asthmatic patient encounters an appropriate antigen they are allergic to, this causes the activation of cells in the lung, called 'mast cells', which triggers the release of substances in the bronchial wall (particularly histamine and leukotrienes), causing spasm of the airway smooth muscle and triggering airway inflammation. Asthma is a common disorder that causes considerable morbidity and some mortality, occurring predominantly in younger people. The attack of asthma, with its characteristic wheeze, is due to narrowing of the bronchi by spasm of the circular airway smooth muscle in the bronchial wall and inflammation with oedema of the bronchial mucosa.

The diagnosis of asthma is made from a combination of clinical history, physical examination (expiratory polyphonic wheeze) and objective tests. Objective available tests for asthma include the widely used *spirometry*, in which the results of the FEV1/FVC ratio of <70% is a positive test for obstructive disease. Subsequent bronchodilator reversibility is important in asthma, which should be an improvement in FEV1 of >12%, together with an increase in volume of 200 mL. Peak flow variability monitoring over 2 weeks provides an effective diagnostic tool and a 20% variability is a positive test. Although fractional exhaled nitric oxide (FeNO) could be considered for helping diagnose asthma, its availability currently is restricted within primary care in the UK. These objective tests are not suitable for use in children under the age of 5, due to logistical challenges and therefore accuracy of asthma diagnosis in children under 5 years is also limited due to the presence of other respiratory illnesses in this age group.

Treatment of Asthma

NURSING NOTE

Your patient will know their asthma symptoms well, and their exacerbation triggers.

The main treatment aims for asthma control are as per NICE (2017):

- No daytime symptoms
- No night-time waking due to asthma
- No requirement of rescue medication
- No asthma attacks
- No limitation of activity.

The correct use of drugs, given either regularly to prevent an attack or intermittently to relieve one, plays an important part in the management of asthma. Several classes of drugs are used:

- Bronchodilators (relievers)
- Corticosteroids (preventers)
- Maintenance and reliever therapy (MART)
- Sodium cromoglycate and nedocromil sodium (preventer)
- Leukotriene modifiers (preventer)
- Xanthines (preventer)
- Biologics (preventer).

Bronchodilators

Bronchodilator drugs play an important part in the treatment of asthma. There are several pharmacological classes of bronchodilators used in the treatment of asthma:

- inhaled β_2 agonists
- oral β_2 agonists
- methylxanthines
- anticholinergic drugs (muscarinic receptor antagonists).

Inhaled β_2 Agonists. These drugs are the most widely prescribed bronchodilators for the treatment of asthma. They are usually given by inhalation to treat a developing attack or to prevent an attack when it seems likely (e.g. prevention of exercise-induced asthma). Their regular use alone as a preventive is not encouraged without concomitant use of an antiinflammatory drug (i.e. inhaled corticosteroid, ICS), as they do not control the inflammatory component of asthma and there is some evidence that their regular use can lead ultimately to more severe and sometimes fatal attacks, although this is rare.

The usage of a short-acting β_2 agonist such as salbutamol can be used as a guide by the patient of how well they are controlling their asthma. If the requirement for β_2 agonist increases to greater than

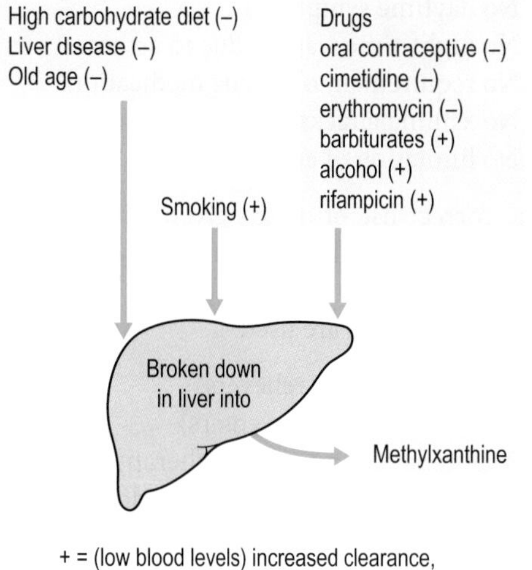

Fig. 9.1 Factors affecting the blood level and activity of methylxanthines.

three times a week, this is probably a sign that the asthma is inadequately managed. If regular use of a β_2 agonist is required to control asthma, an inhaled corticosteroid (see later) should be added to the regimen, so as not to increase the use of the β_2 agonist. The most widely used short-acting β_2 agonist for the relief of asthma symptoms is **salbutamol** which has a 4–6 h half-life. It produces the relaxation of airway smooth muscle by acting as an agonist at β_2 receptors on these cells, leading to the elevation of the signalling molecule cyclic-AMP (cAMP) in the muscle cells (Fig. 9.1).

Longer-acting inhaled selective β_2 agonists (LABAs) are approved, which can be used either twice a day (**salmeterol** and **eformoterol**) or once daily (**vilanterol** and **indacaterol**; the latter is licensed for COPD only). These drugs are recommended to be given with an inhaled corticosteroid, often in a combination inhaler (see later).

CLINICAL NOTE

Patients should be encouraged to keep a diary of their peak flow measurements or have an awareness of their normal peak flow measurement, so as to easily identify a decrease. Patient education relating to asthma control is essential.

Oral and IV β_2 Agonists. Oral salbutamol is not very widely used, as it has largely been succeeded by the introduction of inhaled LABAs that provide prolonged bronchodilation with fewer side-effects. IV β_2 agonists are sometimes administered for the treatment of severe asthma attacks in a hospital setting (see later).

Corticosteroids

Corticosteroids (steroids) reduce the inflammatory and allergic aspects of asthma by inhibiting the recruitment and activation of inflammatory cells such as eosinophils. Regular use of inhaled steroids leads to an improvement in airway irritability and, over time, a reduction in asthma attacks. The preferred route of administration for steroids is by inhalation because if steroids enter the blood they can profoundly affect other body systems such as the endocrine system, leading to potentially serious adverse effects (e.g. suppression of the hypothalamic/pituitary axis that can ultimately lead to stunted growth). The first inhaled corticosteroid (ICS) was beclomethasone diproprionate. Other examples include budesonide, ciclesonide, mometasone, fluticasone propionate and more recently, the introduction of the once daily fluticasone furoate. ICSs have a much improved safety profile compared with orally active steroids such as prednisone, but they can cause occasional candida infections of the oropharynx, as high doses of the ICS are deposited in the back of the throat, which can cause local immunosuppression; occasionally a hoarse voice develops due to weakening of the vocal cords and this can be particularly troublesome in professional singers. These effects usually disappear if the drug is stopped or the dose reduced, and can be minimized by rinsing the mouth out after inhalation.

Patients receiving inhaled corticosteroids generally do not experience the side-effects seen after chronic use of tablets or injections, although children on high doses of inhaled corticosteroids may show a reduced growth rate; thus it is useful to discuss this with the parents in initiation of an ICS prescription. One of the major challenges with ICS is adherence to the drugs as ICS do not produce acute bronchodilation and there are significant numbers of patients who are 'steroid phobic' confusing corticosteroids with the side-effects of anabolic steroids. However, it is important that patients are encouraged to maintain their ICS treatment because this results in improved lung function and improvement in asthma control. To help this situation, there are now a number of 'fixed dose combination inhalers' containing a LABA and an ICS, which are highly effective in the treatment of the majority of patients with mild to moderate asthma (see later). It is important to note that switching patients from ICS to monotherapy with inhaled β_2 agonists such as salbutamol could destabilize their asthma and lead to treatment failure with the latter drug.

An acute asthma exacerbation usually requires oral prednisolone at the minimal effective dose and is usually used for just a few days to bring the asthma under control. Following treatment of the acute exacerbation, an overview of their chronic asthma management should also be undertaken.

CLINICAL NOTE

Patients who are prescribed inhaled corticosteroids may be susceptible to oral thrush. To reduce the risk of this, patients should be advised to take their inhalers before brushing their teeth, or to rinse their mouth out after using inhalers. If patients do experience a burning sensation in their mouth or notice white plaques on their oral mucosa, they should contact their primary care provider for further advice. Recent research suggests that people with COPD receiving corticosteroid inhalation therapy may be at greater risk of pneumonia (Mkorombindo and Dransfield, 2020).

ICS/LABA Fixed Dose Combination Inhalers

A number of fixed dose combination inhalers are now in routine clinical use for the treatment of patients with mild to moderate asthma. These include the combination of fluticasone propionate and salmeterol and the combination of budesonide and formoterol which can be administered twice daily. More recently, a once daily fixed dose combination has been approved containing *fluticasone* and *vilanterol*. These fixed dose combinations increase adherence to taking the medication and improve the chances of the patients receiving regular ICS.

Leukotriene Receptor Antagonist

The leukotriene receptor antagonist, *montelukast*, is a once-a-day tablet used in the treatment of patients with mild asthma. It is usually used as an add-on therapy in adults. This drug blocks the action of substances called 'leukotrienes' on airway smooth muscle; leukotrienes are some of the substances released from inflammatory cells during an asthma attack. Montelukast is considered reasonably safe, but does not have the overall effectiveness of ICS. Zileuton is a drug that works by inhibiting the release of leukotrienes from inflammatory cells by inhibiting an enzyme called 5-lipoxygenase. Montelukast can be given orally (via tablets, chewable tablets or granules) and is approved for use in children. At present, it is used as a continuous treatment for mild-to-moderate asthma and may reduce the need for other drugs. It is also useful in preventing exercise-induced asthma and aspirin-induced asthma (aspirin-induced asthma can affect up to 20% of the asthma population).

Methylxanthines

This group of drugs inhibits a family of enzymes called 'phosphodiesterases' in the bronchial smooth muscle (PDE3 and 4), causing them to elevate the levels of a signalling molecule cAMP that leads to the muscle relaxing and thus relieves the bronchospasm. They are structurally related to the naturally occurring xanthines caffeine (in coffee) and theobromine (in tea and chocolate).

Aminophylline and Theophylline

The most widely used xanthines are *aminophylline* and *theophylline*, although another related drug is *doxofylline*. They are mainly used as oral drugs for the maintenance treatment of asthma, but can be used IV for the treatment of acute severe asthma attacks. They are very effective but they require careful use, as there is a very narrow therapeutic window, i.e. there is only a small difference between the therapeutic plasma level and the concentrations that will elicit significant side-effects (traditionally 10–20 μg/mL plasma levels have been desired for bronchodilation, with plasma levels above 20 μg/mL leading to a range of side-effects) (see later). More recently, the recommended plasma levels are in the range of 5–15 μg/mL for maintenance treatment, given data showing that theophylline can also have antiinflammatory effects at lower plasma levels. In addition, the rate of elimination of xanthines depends on a number of factors, including weight, sex, age, concurrent disease and other medication, and may vary considerably.

Aminophylline can be given slowly IV to terminate an acute attack of asthma. It can also be given as a loading dose followed by an infusion by pump or micropipette. If the infusion is prolonged, then plasma levels should be measured at intervals as a guide to dosage. High plasma levels may result if oral and IV administration are combined and this can be dangerous. Therefore, before giving IV aminophylline, always ask if the patient is already taking a methylxanthine orally.

NURSING NOTE

Refer to local administration and preparation policies prior to giving IV medicines.

CLINICAL NOTE

Taken orally, aminophylline and theophylline can cause nausea, but this can be overcome by using slow-release preparations, which require 12-hourly administration. This avoids peaks in plasma levels of these drugs, and is less likely to cause side-effects. Slow-release preparations must be swallowed whole to avoid interfering with the slow delivery system. Because of interindividual variation, fixed-dose regimens are not ideal and it is better to control dosage by measuring blood levels to obtain optimal results. Patients who continue to smoke while on theophylline may require higher doses of the drug; this is because nicotine induces the metabolism of theophylline, resulting in less of the drug available for action (Goseva et al., 2015).

Available slow-release oral preparations include:

- Phyllocontin Continus – contains aminophylline
- Slo-Phyllin – contains granules that can be sprinkled on food for easier administration.

Adverse effects are dose-related and include nausea, anxiety, tachycardia and arrhythmias, and convulsions.

Interactions are common and effects are increased by cimetidine, erythromycin and oral contraceptives.

Anticholinergic Drugs

A number of muscarinic receptor antagonists are used by inhalation to treat patients with asthma, including ipratropium bromide and oxitropium bromide. These are both short-acting drugs used to relieve symptoms of bronchospasm. They are usually used in the treatment of more severe asthma in addition to β_2 agonists and indeed are sometimes used in the same inhaler. Longer-acting inhaled muscarinic receptor antagonists such as tiotropium bromide are licensed for the treatment of severe asthma, and were widely used to treat the symptoms of COPD (see later). By topically administering the anticholinergic drugs by inhaler or nebuliser, a local action against muscarinic receptors on airway smooth muscle and mucous glands is achieved, but avoiding the unwanted side-effects of atropine, as these inhaled drugs are designed to be poorly absorbed into the blood. Ipratropium bromide should be used for those patients who have not responded to β_2 agonists. The bronchodilator effect of ipratropium bromide begins after about 45 min (i.e. is slower in onset than β_2 agonists) and lasts for 3–4 h; it may be combined with a β_2 agonist or corticosteroids. Nebulised ipratropium bromide could be given with β_2 agonists in patients with severe or life-threatening asthma in order to provide greater bronchodilation. Adverse effects associated with this drug are an unpleasant taste and a dry mouth due to blocking the muscarinic receptors that control salivation.

Other Drug Classes Used to Treat Asthma

Sodium Cromoglycate and Nedocromil Sodium

Sodium cromoglycate and nedocromil sodium are used by inhalation for the prophylaxis of allergic asthma. They are thought to work by stabilizing the action of inflammatory cells and preventing the release of substances that can cause spasm of airway smooth muscle and airways inflammation. They are not to be used in acute attacks of asthma, as they do not cause bronchodilation and only work if patients take them prior to exposure to an offending antigen. They have to be administered several times a day and with the introduction of ICS they have largely fallen out of favour. However, *sodium cromoglycate* in particular is a very safe drug that has been widely used in children with asthma.

Biologics

The last few years has seen the introduction of drugs for the treatment of a number of diseases, including asthma, called 'biologics'. These drugs are monoclonal antibodies that are administered by injection for patients with more severe disease and, being antibodies, have a very long half-life, meaning they can be administered every 2–3 weeks. The first of these for use in the treatment of asthma was the anti-IgE monoclonal antibody omalizumab, which has been shown to reduce the need for steroids in more severe asthma patients and to reduce the need for hospitalization. More recently, a monoclonal antibody against an inflammatory substance called IL-5 (mepolizumab) has been introduced for treatment exacerbations of severe asthma.

Management of Chronic Asthma

The management of patients with asthma is not easy in spite of the number of remedies available and the various guidelines drawn up to advise on which therapy should be used. It is important that the management involves a partnership between the patient (or for children, including the parents) and the health professional, e.g. health visitor and district nurse. Drug therapy will depend on the age of the patient and the severity and pattern of attacks. The use of drugs in chronic asthma may be approached in stages, with the patient starting at the appropriate level and moving up or down according to the response to treatment. For adults and older children, the following programme is widely used:

- **Stage 1:** The patient has occasional episodes of wheezing. These can be treated with an inhaled bronchodilator (usually a short-acting β_2 agonist such as salbutamol). Bronchodilators can also be used as a preventative before some known precipitating trigger, e.g. exercise. Using the bronchodilator more than three times a week requires proceeding to the next stage.
- **Stage 2:** Regular inhaled low-dose steroid or sodium cromoglycate is given and a β_2 agonist used as required. If this fails to prevent attacks, treatment should proceed to stage 3.
- **Stage 3:** The use of fixed dose inhaler combinations containing a LABA and an ICS are now the preferred treatment at this stage, rather than increasing the dose of the ICS. If these treatments do not control the asthma then proceed to stage 4.
- **Stage 4:** At this stage, it is often necessary to use high-doses of ICS, alongside a LABA and other bronchodilators such as a leukotriene receptor antagonist or muscarinic receptor antagonist or a xanthine. These patients should then be referred to specialist care for further assessment and management.
- **Stage 5:** For severe asthma that often requires recurrent hospitalizations, oral steroids are added to the regimen, alongside one of the biologics to reduce the long-term need for steroids.

As well as stepping up therapy to ensure adequate control of asthma, similar consideration should be given to patients to step down their therapy if their asthma has been well-controlled and if they remain asymptomatic for at least 3 months.

The combined use of ICS and steroids is illustrated in Case History 9.1.

Management of Acute Asthma

An 'asthma attack' otherwise known as an asthma exacerbation can be classified into moderate, acute-severe and life-threatening (see Table 9.1). Peak-flow measurement comparisons to the individual's baseline values or that predicted for their age, sex and height can be used to help categorize the patient into these grades and can be useful goalposts for monitoring treatment and the need for escalation, e.g. for hospitalization.

Table 9.1 shows the parameters for the grades of exacerbation for adults. If the patient has clinical features of an exacerbation grade which is worse than, e.g. their peak-flow percentage, then more caution should be observed as the patient may deteriorate more quickly.

Usually moderate asthma can be managed in the community and acute–severe and life-threatening exacerbation needs closer monitoring in the hospital, but initial treatment should be started as soon as possible.

The immediate treatment in severe asthma:

- Oxygen is administered as required to maintain oxygen saturation between 94%–98%.
- Use bronchodilators such as salbutamol by nebuliser (may require 'back-to-back' nebuliser) or, in very severe attacks, methylxanthines.

CASE HISTORY 9.1

Andrew was diagnosed as having atopic asthma at the age of 4 years following several admissions to the hospital during acute attacks with wheeze and respiratory distress. These were treated by nebulised β agonists such as salbutamol (*Ventolin*), or the atropine-like drug ipratropium (*Atrovent*), both of which dilate the bronchi, and both intravenous and oral steroids, which suppress the immune response. During his annual asthma reviews, a personalized asthma action plan was given, which helped his parents judge how well he was and what to do when his asthma deteriorated. At a follow-up review, it was discovered he was using his salbutamol inhaler more than twice a week, for symptomatic relief of his cough and wheeze. He was subsequently stepped up for his asthma therapy by initiation of an inhaled steroid, beclomethasone, using a spacer device. This was beneficial and his parents noted that he had to use his β agonists infrequently while using the inhaled steroid, usually when he had a respiratory infection. He was also advised to avoid any allergic stimulus known to precipitate his problem. Unfortunately, as with up to one-half of childhood asthma cases, his problem persisted into his adulthood. He was strongly advised not to smoke and to avoid aspirin and other non-steroidal antiinflammatories such as ibuprofen. β-Blockers (non-selective) as a drug group must also be avoided, since, as explained in the text, they will block the action of the bronchodilators on β receptors. Due to osteoarthritis in his hands in late adulthood, he was maintained on a selective β_2 agonist and a corticosteroid given by an Autohaler (breath-actuated pressurized metered dose inhaler), as he was not very coordinated when using a pressurized inhaler. Over time he failed to attend his routine asthma follow-up appointments and this resulted in frequent acute asthma exacerbations requiring oral steroids. Unfortunately, this caused osteoporosis, which was detected by arranging bone scans.

- Hydrocortisone, given IV, or prednisolone orally, is given to reduce inflammation.
- Corticosteroids, even if given IV, however, take several hours to be effective.
- No sedative drugs should be given due to the risk of respiratory depression.

TABLE 9.1 The Parameters for the Grades of Exacerbation for Adults

Asthma Exacerbation	Peak Flow % Best/Predicted	Clinical Signs
Moderate	50%–75%	Normal speech
Acute severe	33%–50%	Respiratory rate >25, pulse rate of 110 beats/min. Inability to complete sentences, using accessory muscles. Oxygen saturation >92% on air
Life-threatening	<33%	Oxygen saturation <92% on air; altered consciousness, exhaustion, poor respiratory effort, cyanosis, silent chest, hypotension, arrhythmia

- Chest infection frequently complicates the attack and is treated with antibiotics such as amoxicillin.
- Occasionally, patients who respond poorly will require mechanical ventilation.

SPECIAL POINTS FOR PATIENT EDUCATION

It is very important that the patients learn to manage their own disease as far as possible, and, for children, the parents should be fully involved. This means that they should be taught to:

1. Modify their lifestyle as far as possible to avoid attacks. This includes identifying and managing possible asthma triggers, stopping smoking in the household, avoiding obesity and increasing exercise to build a good pulmonary reserve.
2. Understand the use of their drugs whether they are for an acute attack or used prophylactically (i.e. preventer vs reliever medication).
3. Understand the care and maintenance of their home nebuliser if they use one.
4. Learn to monitor their own disease by means of a peak flow meter and adjust their treatment accordingly. It is useful to give patients a written action plan to aid this (e.g. as available on Asthma UK).
5. Recognize the signs of dangerous deterioration in asthma. A rapid pulse (>110 per min), rapid respiration (>25 per min), exhaustion and inability to complete a sentence requires urgent medical attention and is likely to require hospital admission.

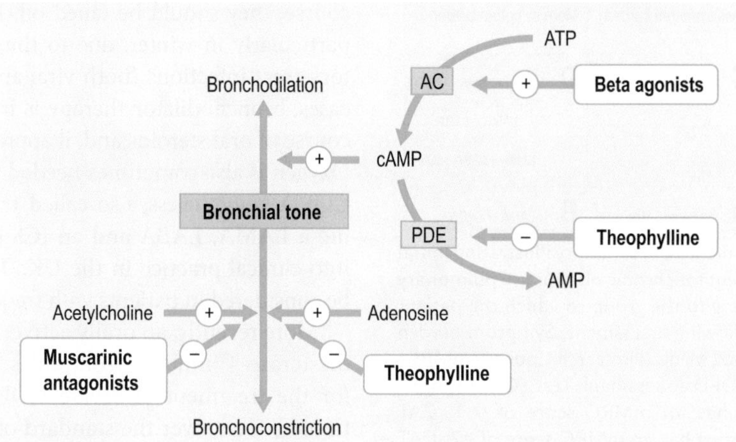

Fig. 9.2 ■ Bronchodilation is promoted by cyclic adenosine monophosphate (cAMP). Intracellular levels of cAMP can be increased by β-adrenoceptor agonists, which increase the rate of its synthesis by adenylyl cyclase (AC); or by phosphodiesterase (PDE) inhibitors such as theophylline, which slow the rate of degradation. Bronchoconstriction can be inhibited by muscarinic antagonists. *ATP*, Adenosine triphosphate; *AMP*, activated protein kinase. (With permission from Katzung, B., Trevor, A., 2015. Basic and Clinical Pharmacology, 13th ed. McGraw-Hill Education, New York.)

CHRONIC OBSTRUCTIVE PULMONARY DISEASE

Chronic obstructive pulmonary disease (COPD) is a common disease that differs from asthma in that it is progressive rather than intermittent, predominantly affects older people and is more clearly related to smoking and exposure to air pollution such as cooking over wood smoke. COPD is used as an umbrella term covering several phenotypes which, in the past, were described as patients with typical 'chronic bronchitis' symptoms and those with more progressive destruction of the alveolar air spaces who had emphysema. In patients with COPD, the small bronchi are obstructed by inflammation that is usually neutrophilic and they have excess mucus production (chronic bronchitis). In some patients, there is the additional problem of emphysema, which reduces the total surface of the respiratory membranes available for gas exchange.

Unlike for asthma, current treatment of COPD is not very satisfactory and is aimed at improving quality of life, minimizing progressive lung destruction and treating/reducing acute exacerbations as they arise. It is essential that the patient gives up smoking and avoids other forms of air pollution as far as possible. Smoking cessation should be encouraged and supported through offering nicotine replacement therapy, as stopping smoking helps slow the decrease in FEV1 in COPD. Pulmonary rehabilitation should also be offered to patients who find themselves functionally disabled by COPD. An annual influenza vaccine and a one-off pneumococcal vaccination should be considered to help reduce the number of serious COPD exacerbations in patients. COPD also often exists with other comorbidities including cardiovascular disease, which can make assessment of symptoms a challenge. Lung cancer is also a leading cause of death in patients with COPD and so must be considered when assessing patients with frequent exacerbations.

NICE (2018) and GOLD guidelines are useful in the management of COPD. The GOLD (2020) update provided an ABCD assessment tool, which has been developed over time to include symptom burden and prevent COPD exacerbation with appropriately targeted therapies according to the group that the patient falls under (Fig. 9.2).

Bronchodilators are widely used in the treatment of patients with COPD. A short acting β_2 agonist (SABA), e.g. salbutamol, or a short-acting muscarinic antagonist (SAMA), e.g. ipratropium are first-line treatments of COPD. If a patient remains symptomatic and has no asthmatic features or steroid responsiveness, then a long-acting β_2 agonist (LABA) (e.g. salmeterol) + long-acting muscarinic antagonist (LAMA)

COPD exacerbation in the previous year	Less symptom burden	More symptom burden
≥2 in community or ≥1 hospital admission	**C** LAMA	**D** LAMA or LAMA + LABA or LAMA + LABA + ICS
≤1 in community	**A** SABA or SAMA	**B** LAMA or LABA

Fig. 9.3 ABCD Assessment Tool summary illustrating initial pharmacological treatment for chronic obstructive pulmonary disease (COPD) according to the group to which the patient has been categorized following assessment. Symptom burden is calculated using modified Medical Research Council (mMRC) dyspnoea scores and COPD Assessment Test (CAT) scores. Less symptom burden has an mMRC score of 0–1, CAT <10; more symptom burden has an mMRC score of ≥2, CAT ≥10. *ICS*, Inhaled corticosteroid; *LABA*, long acting β_2 agonist; *LAMA*, long acting muscarinic antagonist; *SABA*, short acting β_2 agonist; *SAMA*, short acting muscarinic antagonist. (Adapted from GOLD 2020. Please refer to GOLD 2020 for details on calculating mMRC and CAT scores.)

(e.g. tiotropium) should be offered. If a LAMA is initiated, then the SAMA must be discontinued but a SABA can be continued long term, to be used as required. If the patient has features of asthma or steroid responsiveness and remains symptomatic while using SABA or SAMA, then they should be considered for a LABA + ICS. A number of studies have shown that the blood eosinophil counts predict the positive effect for a patient using an ICS. An eosinophil count of <100 cells/μL in patients indicates that ICS containing regimens have little or no effect (GOLD 2020).

The longer-acting muscarinic receptor antagonist (LAMA), tiotropium bromide can be administered once daily by inhalation and is used as a maintenance treatment for COPD. Other examples include glycopyrronium, aclidinium bromide and umeclidinium, which are all inhaled. Increasingly LAMAs are administered in fixed dose combination inhalers with a LABA for 'dual bronchodilation', which appears to provide improved lung function when compared with use of a single class of bronchodilator. Examples now approved include tiotropium and formoterol, umeclidinium and vilanterol, and glycopyrrolate and indacaterol.

While inhaled or systemic steroids are worthy of a trial in patients with COPD, there remains considerable controversy as to the value of these drugs for this disease, as there are many reports of an increased risk of pneumonia in patients taking these drugs regularly. Thus, if there is little or no improvement over a short course, they should be tailed off. Exacerbation occurs, particularly in winter, due to the presence of respiratory tract infections (both viral and bacterial). In such cases, bronchodilator therapy is increased, alongside a course of oral steroids and, if appropriate, an antibiotic. Oxygen is also sometimes needed to treat patients with COPD. Nonetheless, a so-called 'triple inhaler' containing a LAMA, LABA and an ICS has been introduced into clinical practice in the UK. Triple therapy should be considered in patients with frequent exacerbations.

More recently, an orally active, once daily phosphodiesterase-4 inhibitor, roflumilast, has been approved for the treatment of severe COPD to provide additional benefit over the standard of care described previously. This drug is an antiinflammatory drug that, by inhibiting the phosphodiesterase-4 enzyme found in inflammatory cells, reduces the degree of neutrophilic inflammation in the lung, and when used for up to a year can reduce exacerbations. However, this drug has a very narrow therapeutic window and can produce significant gastrointestinal side-effects in a proportion of patients. Furthermore, there is some suggestion that it can also cause unexplained weight loss when used chronically in some patients.

Some recent studies have supported the use of some antibiotics continuously to help with reduction of exacerbation risk; an example of this is azithromycin. However, it can cause prolongation of QTc and therefore an ECG should be undertaken prior to initiation, as well as regular monitoring of liver function blood tests.

INHALATION DELIVERY SYSTEMS

Inhalation is a useful and effective way of giving some of the drugs used to treat asthma and other airways diseases such as COPD.

There are various delivery systems for inhalation:

- Pressurized metered dose inhalers (MDIs)
- Breath-activated inhalers – MDIs and dry powder inhalers
- Nebulisers
- Delivery systems for children.

Pressurized Metered Dose Inhalers and Breath-activated Inhalers

These are the most convenient systems for routine use by patients. A standard MDI is the most widely used inhaler. The drug is dissolved or suspended in a propellant gas and on pressing the plunger, a standard amount is released in the form of fine particles measuring 2–5 μm.

Breath-activated inhalers (also known as dry powder inhalers) are triggered to release the medication by breathing in through the mouthpiece and do not require pressing a canister on top as that required for the standard MDIs, therefore they can be more useful in patients who may find coordination of standard MDI more challenging. These include easyhalers, accuhalers and turbohalers.

It is essential that the patient is taught the technique of using their inhaler if the treatment is to be effective.

CLINICAL NOTE

A recent systematic review suggested that regular reminders of inhaler technique was important (Klijn et al., 2017) Repeated instruction in the use of inhalers, particularly children and the elderly, are of particular importance. Inhalers containing a placebo are available for teaching, using visual aids, video instruction and regular follow-up and checks on technique are important to maintain effective symptom control (Román-Rodríguez et al., 2019).

For standard MDIs:

1. Remove the cap from the mouthpiece and shake the inhaler.
2. Breathe out slowly but not fully.
3. Place the mouthpiece in the mouth and close the lips around it.
4. Breathe in slowly and at the same time depress the plunger, thus releasing the drug.
5. Hold the breath for at least 10 seconds and longer if possible.
6. If a second inhalation is required, wait for 1 minute.
7. Following steroid inhaler use ensure mouth is rinsed.

Spacers

A spacer is a reservoir between the aerosol and the mouthpiece. There are varying brands available and are to be used with MDIs. Pressing the plunger releases the drug into the reservoir, following which it may be inhaled. There is a valve at the mouthpiece, which allows the drug to remain in the spacer until the patient breathes in, the valve closes again on breathing out. Spacers allow a better delivery of the drugs to the lungs and therefore can improve clinical symptom control, especially in patients who may otherwise find coordinating MDIs difficult. Another potential benefit of using spacers is that they can help to reduce the side-effects from the drugs due to better delivery of the drug to the lungs. They are particularly useful, as facemasks are attached to some spacers, which allows them to effectively be used for young children.

Nebulisers

Nebulisers are used to deliver drugs to patients with more severe asthma and COPD and enable a larger dose to reach the airways. Air, or oxygen, is driven through a solution of the drug and the resulting mist is inhaled via a mask. It is important to have the correct particle size, which is best obtained by using an airflow rate of 6–8 L/min, depending on the type of nebuliser. Piped air or oxygen may be used; various mechanical compressors are available, which allows some patients to use them at home. It is important that these are cleaned regularly to prevent bacterial contamination. There is now an increasing number of highly portable nebulisers becoming available for delivering drugs to the airways as alternatives to MDIs and breath-activated inhalers.

Other drugs used in the treatment of asthma and COPD that can be delivered in a nebuliser are: corticosteroids, sodium cromoglycate and ipratropium bromide.

Delivery Systems for Children

Asthma is a common disease in childhood, affecting about 10% of children and is not usually diagnosed until the child is about 5 years old. It usually disappears in adolescence. Drug treatment with inhalers may be required but may be difficult to administer and can be very dependent on an individual's ability. As described previously, use of spacers with or without facemasks can help in effectively managing asthma in children.

COUGH REMEDIES

The Coughing Reflex

Cough is a reflex, although one can cough deliberately as well. The stimulus to cough may arise from inflammation or foreign material in the pharynx, larynx, trachea or bronchial tree. It may also be provoked by stimuli arising in the pleura. It is therefore advantageous to aid the removal of foreign material from the respiratory passages, and increase the secretion of the bronchial glands, thus 'loosening' the sputum. The cough reflex can also be activated inappropriately by respiratory inflammation or by neoplastic growth in the tract and is therefore often a symptom of inflammatory airways diseases such as asthma and COPD, as well as lung cancer. In addition, it can commonly present in patients suffering with gastritis. Cough is one of the most common symptoms leading patients to seek medical advice, as most over-the-counter (OTC) remedies available to treat cough are not very effective. The following details some of the drugs used to treat coughs.

Expectorants and Decongestants

Expectorants and mucolytics are drugs that loosen the sputum and thus facilitate expectoration from the bronchial tree. While mucolytic drugs such as N-acetyl cysteine have successfully been used to reduce exacerbations of COPD, there is little, if any, hard evidence that expectorants in the doses commonly prescribed or available in OTC remedies have any useful effects in reducing cough and in general, their use should be discouraged. Among the ingredients that may be found in such cough mixtures are ammonium chloride, ipecacuanha, guaifenesin and squill, and many can be bought OTC.

One of the symptoms of the common cold in addition to cough is excessive nasal secretions and many OTC remedies for cough also contain a vasoconstrictor to reduce nasal blood flow and thus reduce secretions. Commonly, the vasoconstrictor is phenylephrine, which is an alpha 1 agonist that mimics the action of adrenaline. It needs to be noted that while such remedies may be useful in acutely reducing secretions in the treatment of the cold-plus-cough case, it must be remembered that those remedies containing vasoconstrictors must not be used by patients taking monoamine oxidase inhibitors (MAOIs), since this may greatly enhance the activity of sympathomimetic drugs.

Some remedies available OTC also contain an antihistamine, usually one of the older sedating H1 receptor antagonists that can cross the blood–brain barrier, such as chlorpheniramine. However, there is little evidence that this class of drug has any clinically meaningful benefit in reducing secretions or cough (see later), although the sedative effect may help patients to sleep.

Cough Suppressants (Antitussive Drugs)

Under certain circumstances it is advantageous to suppress a cough that is tiring the patient and serving no useful purpose. However, undue suppression of a cough can lead to sputum retention and thickening, and antitussives should not be used in patients with chronic bronchitis, bronchiectasis or for cough associated with asthma or COPD. It is also debatable whether cough remedies actually work. A study published in the *British Medical Journal* found *no significant efficacy* for most cough remedies available OTC (Schroeder and Fahey, 2002).

Demulcents

Cough arising from irritation of the mucous membranes of the mouth and throat may be suppressed through the soothing action of syrup, which forms a protective film over the inflamed tissues. These syrups are called 'demulcents'. **Simple linctus**, which is essentially flavoured syrup, is satisfactory but should be avoided in patients with diabetes, as it contains sugar. A sugar-free substitute is available. The WHO recommends the use of honey in this case.

Opioids

For many years, the only really effective cough-supressing drugs were those derived from the opioid group, which include morphine, heroin and codeine. These drugs were included in many cough mixtures and, by virtue of their action within the cough centre in the brain (the nucleus tractus solitarius), they are valuable antitussives, particularly in supressing the cough associated with lung cancer. Opioids should be used with caution due to issues of tolerance and addiction associated with their prolonged use.

Codeine, the most widely used opiod in the treatment of cough is often used as linctus codeine (BPC). This linctus, although widely used, has been found not to be very effective unless given in doses above those usually recommended, which will often cause constipation.

Dextromethorphan is related in structure to levorphanol, which is a synthetic narcotic analgesic. A number of OTC preparations for cough, colds and influenza contain dextromethorphan. It is about as potent as codeine as a cough suppressant and, like codeine, can cause constipation, depending on the dosage and frequency of use.

Pholcodine is closely related to codeine and depresses the cough centre. On a weight-for-weight basis, experimental results suggest it is more active than codeine, although the side-effects are probably similar. Its action lasts 4–6 h. It is included in various mixtures, including linctus pholcodine (BPC). In terminal care, morphine or diamorphine (heroin) may be required to relieve a distressing cough.

Antihistamines

These drugs have some antitussive effect, partly perhaps by a local antihistamine action, but their antitussive action is more likely to be through a sedative effect on the nervous system as any antitussive effect has only been demonstrated with older sedating H1 receptor antagonists.

INHALATIONS AND MUCOLYTIC AGENTS

Mucolytic agents are those that are used to try and liquefy mucus. In the past, various drugs were inhaled, particularly in the treatment of chronic lung infections, although with the advent of antibiotics, this treatment has been largely superseded. **Steam** itself is, however, a very good expectorant, as it liquefies the sputum and thus enables it to be coughed up. Other approaches include the use of the mucolytic drugs N-acetyl cysteine and carbocysteine. In COPD, mucolytic agents may help to reduce exacerbations and it is worth a trial of these treatments to see if it has a positive benefit for the individual.

Benzoin Tincture

Benzoin tincture is one of the balsams that contain resins and volatile oils. A tincture is a plant extract in alcohol. When it is added to hot water, the volatile oil is given off and may be inhaled; it exerts a mildly soothing effect on the bronchial mucous membrane and is frequently used in acute bronchitis. Menthol and eucalyptus inhalation can be used in a similar way and produce a considerable outpouring from the bronchial glands and a transient vasoconstriction of the respiratory mucous membrane with clearing of the air passages. Menthol is often found as an ingredient in OTC remedies for the treatment of coughs and colds, such as in vapours and rubs and there is some evidence that menthol can reduce coughing.

SAFETY POINT

Great care must be taken when patients are inhaling these drugs so that they do not spill the hot water over themselves or severe burns may occur. Particular care is needed with the very young and the elderly.

CLINICAL NOTE

Non-pharmacological options for supporting people with a cough should also be considered, such as maintaining adequate hydration levels, encouraging mobility and deep breathing. In the hospital environment to minimize severe respiratory complications postoperatively, chest physiotherapy may be effective. Reviewing medications that may induce a cough, e.g. angiotensin-converting enzyme inhibitors, and considering alternatives, e.g. angiotensin receptor blockers may be beneficial.

Pulmonary Surfactants

Natural surfactants allow the surfaces of the pulmonary alveoli to separate so that the lungs can expand and function immediately after birth. In premature infants, this factor may be lacking, so the lungs do not function properly and respiratory distress syndrome develops. This is treated by mechanical ventilation and the inhalation via an endotracheal tube of **colfosceril palmitate**, a synthetic surfactant. However, it is now standard practice to try and provide steroids antenatally 24–48 h prior to a premature delivery (if a delay in delivery can be achieved) to help with lung maturity.

RESPIRATORY FAILURE

Respiratory failure occurs when the lungs are unable to maintain an adequate exchange of oxygen and carbon dioxide. There are two types.

Type I

In type I respiratory failure, the balance between circulation and ventilation of the alveoli is disturbed. This results in a reduction of oxygen in the blood, but normal levels of carbon dioxide. It may occur in heart failure, pneumonia and shock lung. Oxygen may be given freely and the underlying disorder should be corrected if possible.

Type II

Type II respiratory failure occurs in obstructive airways disease, usually associated with COPD, which results from damage to the alveoli of the lungs. This reduces the surface area for O_2 and CO_2 exchange and in severe cases, the patient becomes breathless. The disease may be due to a combination of advancing age, chronic bronchitis and smoking. The essential abnormality is underventilation of the alveoli, resulting in a low blood oxygen concentration and a raised level of carbon dioxide. Hypoxaemia can be relieved by the inhalation of oxygen, but this may lead to decreased respiration with a further fall in alveolar ventilation and an increased blood concentration of carbon dioxide, which causes the patient to become disorientated and, finally, comatose. This can be avoided to some extent by giving **low** concentrations of oxygen, which will not reduce alveolar ventilation. In addition, physiotherapy helps to remove retained bronchial secretions, antibiotics are used to treat complicating bronchial infections and bronchodilators relieve spasm.

CLINICAL NOTE

People living with COPD and type II respiratory failure will tolerate lower levels of oxygen saturation and it may well be more problematic to give excessive amounts of oxygen. This is reflected in early warning illness severity track and trigger systems, e.g. NEWS2 (Tirkkonen et al., 2019) that adopts a lower threshold for oxygen saturations for people with type II respiratory disease. Discussing treatment goals and parameters with the clinician managing the patient is vital for effective management of these cases.

Respiratory Stimulant Drugs

Respiratory stimulant drugs have limited use in these circumstances. Given intravenously, they increase ventilation for a short period.

Doxapram is the most effective respiratory stimulant and is given by intravenous infusion. The dose is adjusted depending on response. This treatment requires careful monitoring and every effort should be made to remove retained secretions in the respiratory tract, by physiotherapy. In overdose, doxapram can cause convulsions.

SUMMARY

- Do not give cough suppressants (which cause sputum retention and thickening) to patients with chronic bronchitis, bronchiectasis or cough associated with asthma.
- Cough syrups containing sucrose must not be given to diabetics.
- Codeine and pholcodine may constipate the patient.
- In type II respiratory failure lower oxygen saturations may be acceptable and thus oxygen may be used in lower concentrations in patients with type II respiratory failure.

REFERENCES AND FURTHER READING

Bacharier, L.B., Guilbert, T.W., 2012. Diagnosis and management of early asthma in preschool-aged children. J. Allergy Clin. Immunol. 130 (2), 287–298.

GOLD, 2020. Pocket Guide to COPD Diagnosis, Management and Prevention. A Guide for Health Care Professionals. 2020 Report. Global Initiative for Chronic Obstructive Lung Disease (GOLD).

Goseva, Z., Gjorcev, A., Kaeva, B.J., et al., 2015. Analysis of plasma concentrations of theophylline in smoking and nonsmoking patients with asthma. Open Access Maced. J. Med. Sci. 3 (4), 672–675.

Holmes, L.J., 2017. Nurses' role in improving outcomes for patients with severe asthma. Nursing Times 113 (4), 22–25 [online].

Klijn, S.L., Hiligsmann, M., Evers, S.M.A.A., et al., 2017. Effectiveness and success factors of educational inhaler technique interventions in asthma & COPD patients: a systematic review. NPJ Prim. Care Respir. Med. 27 (1), 24.

Mkorombindo, T., Dransfield, M.T., 2020. Inhaled corticosteroids in chronic obstructive pulmonary disease: benefits and risks. Clin. Chest Med. 41 (3), 475–484.

Montag, S., 2018. Asthma medication update. Nurs. Made Incred. Easy 16 (1), 26–32.

NICE, 2017. Asthma: Diagnosis, Monitoring and Chronic Asthma Management [NG80].

NICE, 2018. Chronic Obstructive Pulmonary Disease in over 16s: Diagnosis and Management [NG115].

Román-Rodríguez, M., Metting, E., Gacía-Pardo, M., et al., 2019. Wrong inhalation technique is associated to poor asthma clinical outcomes. Is there room for improvement? Curr. Opin. Pulmonary Med. 25 (1), 18–26.

Schroeder, K., Fahey, T., 2002. Systematic review of randomised controlled trials of over the counter cough medicines for acute cough in adults. BMJ 324, 329–331.

Tirkkonen, J., Karlsson, S., Skrifvars, M.B., 2019. National early warning score (NEWS) and the new alternative SpO2 scale during rapid response team reviews: a prospective observational study. Scand. J. Trauma Resusc. Emerg. Med. 27 (1), 111.

Yawn, B.P., Han, M.K., 2017. Practical considerations for the diagnosis and management of asthma in older adults. Mayo Clin. Proc. 92 (11), 1697–1705.

Zakrisson, A., Hagglund, D., 2010. The asthma/COPD nurses experience of educating patients with COPD in primary health care. Scand. J. Caring Sci. 24 (1), 147–155.

USEFUL WEBSITES

Asthma UK and British Lung Foundation Partnership. https://www.asthma.org.uk.

Global Initiative for Chronic Obstructive Lung Disease (GOLD). https://goldcopd.org.

NHS. https://www.nhs.uk.

RightBreathe. https://www.rightbreathe.com.

10 DRUGS AFFECTING THE GASTROINTESTINAL SYSTEM

CHAPTER OUTLINE

LEARNING OBJECTIVES

At the end of this chapter, the reader should be able to:

- explain how to prevent and treat specific oral infections
- list the treatments for acid reflux and describe how acid and pepsin are produced
- understand the causes of peptic ulcer and aims of treatment
- discuss the antacids and the problems associated with their use
- give an account of the drugs used to treat chronic inflammatory bowel disease
- list the various classes of laxatives and appreciate the dangers associated with their inappropriate use
- describe how to diminish peristaltic activity with drugs
- discuss the significance of the liver in the use of drugs
- understand what is meant by the vomiting centre and chemoreceptor trigger zone (CTZ)
- describe how they are stimulated
- give an account of the emetics and the classes of antiemetic drugs

THE MOUTH

Salivation

A proper flow of saliva is necessary to keep the mouth fresh and free from infection. Salivary flow will be diminished in fever and dehydration and also by certain drugs, notably those of the phenothiazine group and the tricyclic antidepressants. Antimuscarinic drugs such as atropine will also diminish salivation. Severe oral infection may supervene if salivary flow is markedly decreased. This was a frequent complication in very ill patients in former times when dehydration was not adequately corrected and measures to ensure oral hygiene not practised. Patients receiving cytotoxic drugs are especially at risk, as their resistance to infection is lowered and some cytotoxic drugs cause ulceration of the mouth.

Prevention of Oral Infection

- **Avoid oral infection during surgery**
- **Avoid dehydration**

Before **major surgery** or any other procedure with a special risk of oral infection, the mouth should be inspected and infected gums or teeth treated via a dentist. **Dehydration** must be avoided and several topical treatments are available.

Mouthwashes

Mouthwashes are not routinely recommended for periodontal disease as they do not have significant effect on established plaques and do not stop periodontitis from progressing (NICE, 2018).

Artificial Salivas

If dry mouth is a special problem, various artificial salivas are available, instead of, or as well as, mouthwash solutions. These include *Glandosane* and *Luborant*. In unconscious patients, the mouth should be cleaned regularly. Sodium hydrogen carbonate one-quarter teaspoonful in 50 mL is particularly valuable for clearing mucus. (Note that sodium bicarbonate is also called sodium hydrogen carbonate and has the chemical formula $NaHCO_3$.)

Hydrogen Peroxide

In some hospitals hydrogen peroxide is used to remove debris from ulcers, etc. In seriously ill patients, the care of the mouth is a particularly important aspect of nursing care. Hospitals often use different regimens and nurses will have to draw their own conclusions as to the most effective treatments.

CLINICAL NOTE

In oral infection, oral mouth care is the most important care that can be provided. Recognition that it is a potential problem is important, as it can cause considerable discomfort to the patient. Some patients will need assistance with oral hygiene and this should be maintained at all times; ensure regular mouth washes, teeth cleaning, denture removal and if needed, application of artificial saliva and lip moisturizer. Documentation of oral hygiene needs is also essential so that holistic care for the patient can be maintained.

Oral Infections and Ulceration

In spite of care, some patients will develop infections in the mouth; those receiving cytotoxic drugs are at special risk. The main infections are:

- *Candida*
- oral herpes simplex/herpes labialis (cold sores)
- non-specific stomatitis with/without ulceration
- aphthous ulceration
- infections of the pharynx and tonsils.

Candida

This is a common oral infection and is commonly treated by **nystatin drops**, an antifungal, which is not absorbed from the intestine. Nystatin is dissolved in the mouth four times daily after food. Some patients find the taste unpleasant. Treatment should be continued for 48 h after symptoms have resolved.

In young children, miconazole gel smeared around the mouth is easier. However, as per the British National Formulary (BNF), the drug is not licensed for children under 4 months old. If used off-licence it must be discussed and documented in the clinical notes. The restriction is mainly due to risk of choking, but it is an effective drug for use in treatment of infants with oral *Candida* infection. If treating infants for oral *Candida* who are breastfed, it is important to also treat the mother with topical antifungal (applied to the nipples) simultaneously to prevent reinfection. However, this should not be with the use of miconazole gel due to the choking risk.

Oral Herpes Simplex/Herpes Labialis (Cold Sores)

The herpes simplex virus (HSV) is classified as HSV-1 and HSV-2. HSV-1 is largely responsible for cold sores and blisters around the mouth. HSV-2 primarily causes genital herpes.

NICE (2016) recommends not to prescribe topical antiviral preparations such as aciclovir or penciclovir, which are available for people to purchase over-the-counter if they find them helpful. In a large majority of people the infection is mild and self-limiting. Prescription of oral prophylactic aciclovir should be considered if the patient has six or more episodes in 1 year, persistent or severe recurrent episodes or if associated with erythema multiforme. Gaining a specialist review in challenging circumstances is helpful to investigate other underlying organic problems that may cause persistent blistering, e.g. immunocompromise.

Stomatitis with/without Ulceration

- Dehydration, if present, should be corrected.
- Chlorhexidine mouthwashes may be used.
- Hydrogen peroxide can be used to cleanse ulcers.
- Benzydamine mouthwash (*Difflam*), which acts as a local anaesthetic, is extremely effective in relieving the discomfort of oral ulceration. The mouth should be rinsed out every 2–3 h with the undiluted solution. If this causes stinging, a 50:50 diluted solution should be used.
- Choline salicylate (*Bonjela*) is a mild local anaesthetic in gel form that may be applied before meals and at night.
- Trying to elicit the underlying cause is also important, e.g. fungal/viral infection, trauma, drugs, iron deficiency, etc.

Aphthous Ulceration

These small, painful, recurrent oral ulcers are common, even in healthy people. The cause is unknown, but may be related to stress, and treatment is only partly effective. **Hydrocortisone** oro-mucosal tablets dissolved in the mouth four times daily are often trialled as first-line treatment. Topical lidocaine or **tetracycline** mouthwashes can also be used.

Infections of the Pharynx and Tonsils

Infections of the pharynx and tonsils are very common and are usually viral. Most of them require no specific treatment, since recovery is rapid. Many people use gargles, although there is little evidence that they do any good. Compound thymol glycerin, a mild antiseptic, is popular and does no harm. Soluble analgesia can also be used as a gargle.

Bacterial throat infections require the use of the appropriate antibiotic, governed by local guidelines, to be given systemically and there is little indication for the topical use of antibiotics in these circumstances. Using the FeverPAIN or Centor criteria (see later) can help to identify people who are more likely to benefit from an antibiotic in whom the cause of infection is likely streptococcal. FeverPAIN criteria allows a maximum score of 5, increasing likelihood of isolating streptococcus with increasing score, i.e. a score of 4 or 5 is associated with positive culture in 62%–65% of individuals. Similarly, using the Centor criteria in which the maximum score is 4; a score of 3 or 4 is associated with a 32%–56% likelihood of isolating streptococcus.

- FeverPAIN criteria:
  - Fever (in the previous 24 h)
  - Purulence (pus on tonsils)
  - Attend rapidly (within 3 days onset of symptoms)
  - Severely inflamed tonsils
  - No cough or coryza.
- Centor criteria:
  - Tonsillar exudate
  - Tender anterior cervical lymphadenopathy/lymphadenitis
  - Fever over 38°C
  - Absence of cough.

THE OESOPHAGUS AND STOMACH

The stomach is a hollow organ receiving food from the oesophagus and passing it on to the intestines after a variable interval of between 4 and 6 h. It is concerned with the mechanical breaking down of the food to render it more easily digested and more easily absorbed. Its muscular walls are capable of powerful waves of peristalsis, which mix and macerate the food. The mucosa lining the stomach secretes hydrochloric acid and pepsin, which together initiate the digestion of proteins. Inflammation may occur at the lower end of the oesophagus, which is usually due to reflux of acid from the stomach, and may be associated with a peptic ulcer. Antacids and drugs that block the release of gastric acid can relieve this.

Dyspepsia and Peptic Ulcers

Dyspepsia, which is commonly called indigestion, is discomfort or pain in the abdomen or lower chest after eating. It may be accompanied by nausea and vomiting and is usually ascribed to disordered digestion.

Peptic ulcers are lesions of the lining (mucosa) of the stomach (gastric ulcer), the duodenum (duodenal ulcer) or of the oesophagus (oesophageal ulcer). One or a combination of the following may cause ulcers:

- **excessive secretion of hydrochloric acid and pepsin**
- **breakdown of the protective mechanism of the mucosa**
- **a microorganism, *Helicobacter pylori*.**

Hydrochloric acid, which is produced to excess in duodenal, but not in gastric ulcers, is responsible for the pain, and for many years, the use of antacids was the mainstay of treatment. The whole approach to the healing of ulcers has changed with the discovery that infection of the stomach lining by the organism *H. pylori* is a major cause of them.

Infection of the lower part of the stomach (the antrum) increases acid production. This acid passes to the duodenum and the combined effect of acidity and damage to the mucosa gives rise to duodenal ulceration and prevents healing. Infection of the body of the stomach is a frequent cause of gastric ulcers and may also lead to gastritis and gastric carcinoma. Eradication of this infection (see later) usually results in healing of the ulcer.

Other factors may be involved, the most important being the resistance of the lining of the stomach to acid and pepsin. Prostaglandin E_2, which is formed in the stomach, reduces acidity and helps in the secretion of a layer of mucus, which coats and protects the gastric lining. If the production of prostaglandin E_2 is inhibited by non-steroidal antiinflammatory drugs (NSAIDs), the protection is lost and ulcers are liable to develop (see later). For this reason, NSAIDs may cause gastric bleeding and ulceration and must be used with care.

CLINICAL NOTE

Holistic approach must also be applied in management of dyspepsia in patients including offering lifestyle measures to lose weight, avoiding trigger foods, such as caffeinated drinks or spicy food, smoking cessation and reducing alcohol intake to within the recommended limits. Stopping or reducing drugs that may cause an exacerbation is also important. Non-steroidal Antiinflammatory Drugs (NSAIDs) are commonly associated with dyspepsia and considering alternative drugs such as paracetamol or codeine, may alleviate symptoms. Alternatively, advising the patient to take NSAIDs with or after food or considering prescribing an antacid, H_2 receptor antagonist or proton pump inhibitor during treatment, may alleviate symptoms.

The Production of Acid and Pepsin

Acid secretion is a complex process. There are two ways in which it can be provoked (Fig. 10.1):

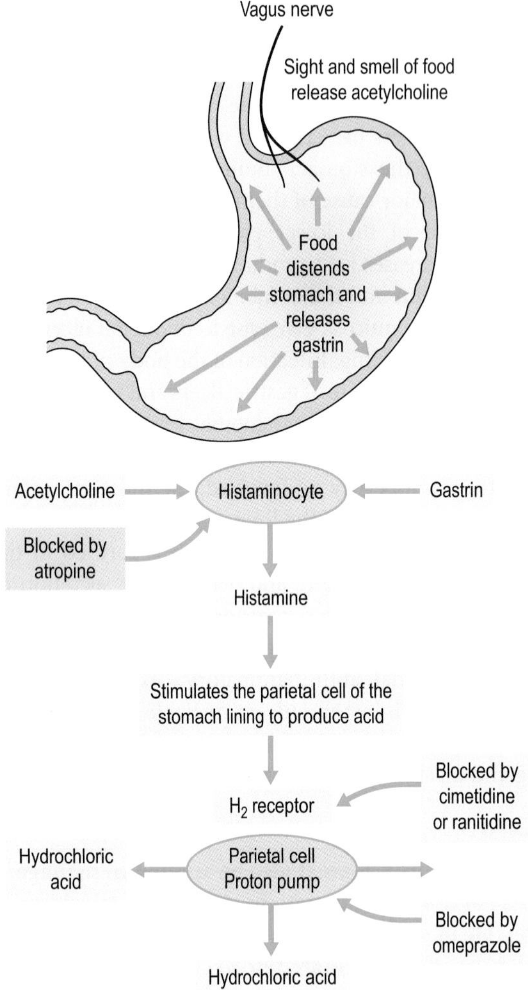

Fig. 10.1 The mechanisms involved in the secretion of acid into the stomach and the effect and site of action of H_2 blockers.

- Stimulation of the vagus nerve innervating the wall of the stomach leads to the release of acetylcholine and thus to increased secretion of acid. In healthy people with an intact gastric mucosa, this is brought about by the thought, sight or smell of appetizing food. Adequate acid and pepsin are thereby produced to start the digestion of food when it arrives in the stomach. However, in patients with ulcers, the acid causes the typical pain, particularly if the hoped-for food is delayed.
- Distension of the stomach (for instance by food) causes the production of the hormone gastrin, and this in turn stimulates the stomach to produce acid.

The common factor in acid production by both these mechanisms is the release in the stomach wall of histamine from cells called *histaminocytes*. Histamine in turn stimulates the proton pump in the parietal cells, which causes the release of acid in the stomach. The secretory effect of histamine on the stomach is mediated by H_2 receptors.

Treatment of Peptic Ulcers and Dyspepsia

Approach to the Treatment of Peptic Ulcers

Reducing acidity and protecting the ulcer from acid will relieve the pain of duodenal ulcer, and will heal the majority of ulcers, but relapse within a year is very common (75%) unless the associated *H. pylori* infection is eradicated (see later). It is probably advisable, as demonstrated by Case History 10.1, to always test early for the presence of *H. pylori*. Reducing acidity and eliminating infection is achieved by reducing acid secretion (usually by a proton pump inhibitor (PPI) such as omeprazole) and using a combination of antibacterials (see later). This will cure the majority of patients, but a few will require further treatment.

For gastric ulcers, the initial treatment may be either with H_2 blockers or the eradication of infection, if present. After the treatment of gastric ulcers, repeat endoscopy is essential to eliminate the possibility that the ulcer may be malignant. Ulcers due to NSAIDs usually respond to a PPI, e.g. omeprazole. For patients who are: at a high risk of developing an ulcer, e.g. the elderly; those with a previous history of an ulcer; or those taking high-dose NSAIDs, PPIs may be co-prescribed. This approach is summarized in Fig. 10.2.

Aims of Treatment

- To reduce acidity, which relieves pain and also helps the healing process
- To protect the ulcer from further damage by acid
- To eradicate *H. pylori* infection
- To discourage the use of NSAIDs.

Drugs for Reducing Acidity

- Antacids
- Proton pump inhibitors

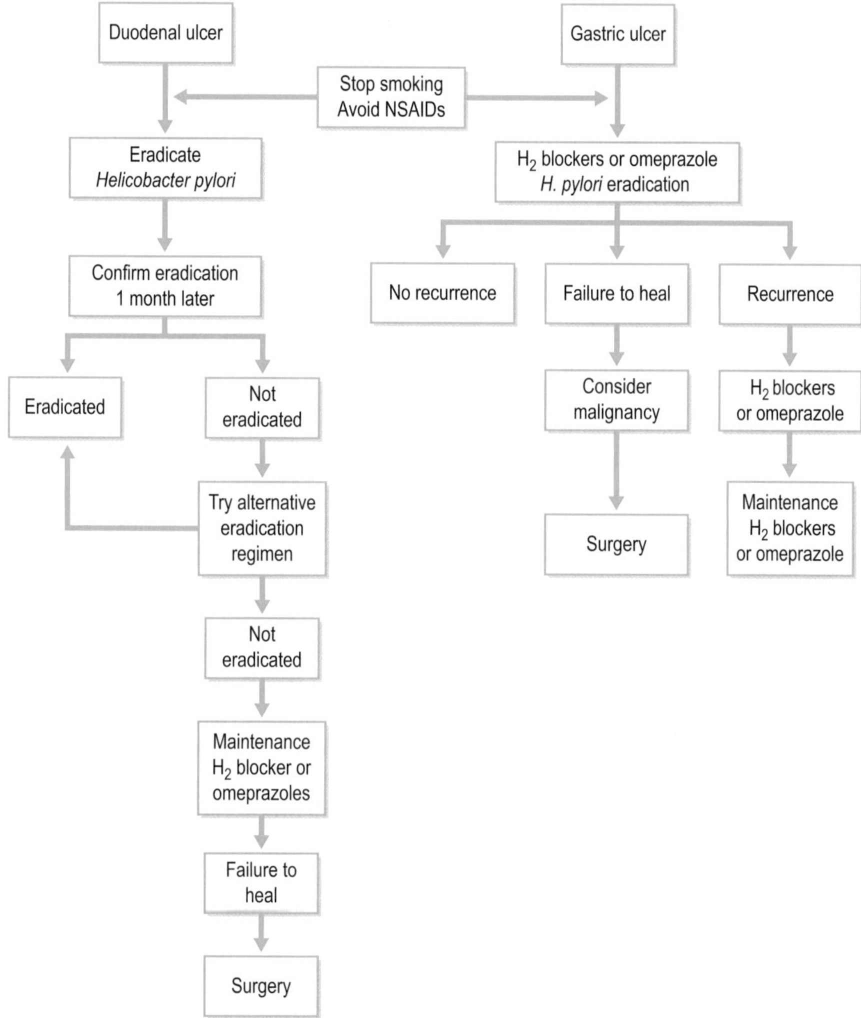

Fig. 10.2 ■ Flow diagram of the management of gastric and duodenal ulcers.

- Histamine H_2 receptor blockers
- Sucralfate
- Prostaglandins.

Antacids

Antacids were once widely used in the treatment of peptic ulcers and other forms of dyspepsia. They act by reducing the acidity in the stomach and they also reduce pepsin activity. They are very effective at temporarily relieving the pain from an ulcer, but, unless used intensively, do not accelerate healing. They are also used in various minor gastric upsets. Magnesium or aluminium salts are the most popular. Magnesium is available as magnesium oxide, magnesium hydroxide or magnesium trisilicate.

Magnesium trisilicate is a white, gritty powder, usually prescribed as a mixture that contains sodium hydrogen carbonate and magnesium carbonate. Magnesium salts are very poorly absorbed from the gut and can cause diarrhoea.

Aluminium hydroxide is a white powder, insoluble in water and usually given as a mixture or a tablet, which is sucked to prolong its effect. In addition to reducing gastric acidity, aluminium salts inactivate gastric pepsin. This antacid is slightly astringent (causes cells to shrink by precipitating proteins from their surface) and can also cause constipation.

The frequency of dosage of antacids is important. They are usually given 1 hour after meals throughout the day and at bedtime. This produces a moderate reduction in acidity and keeps symptoms at bay. To accelerate healing, however, larger than usual doses must be given more often.

Antacid Mixtures. There are many antacid mixtures available. They contain a variety of antacids, sometimes combined with substances that protect the mucosa, including anticholinergic drugs or local anaesthetics. **Gaviscon** is a combination of an antacid with alginates, which float on the gastric contents; if reflux occurs, they protect the mucosa of the lower oesophagus. **Alginates/antacids are useful for short-term use only.**

Antacids in Renal Failure and Other Disorders. Although the amount of magnesium or aluminium absorbed is very small and harmless in patients with normal renal function, accumulation can occur in patients with renal failure. Some antacids contain fairly large amounts of sodium and cause fluid retention and oedema in patients with cardiac, renal or hepatic failure, and also in pregnant women and in infants under 6 months of age. Some antacids contain magnesium, and this ion may be dangerous in patients with arrhythmias.

Drug Interactions. Antacids may interfere with the absorption of digoxin, tetracycline, iron salts, indomethacin and isoniazid.

Blocking Gastric Acid Secretion

Gastric acid secretion is reduced in two ways:

- **by blocking the action of histamine at the H_2 receptors**
- **by inhibiting the proton pump.**

Proton pump inhibitors are now first-line medical therapy for the management of dyspepsia in adults in the UK.

Histamine Receptor (H_2) Blockers

The H_2 blockers are:

- cimetidine
- famotidine
- nizatidine
- ranitidine.

These drugs block the action of histamine on H_2 receptors in the stomach wall and thus reduce the excretion of acid by about 70%. They are given orally, although injections of cimetidine and ranitidine are also available.

Ulcer symptoms usually disappear within a week and about 85% of duodenal ulcers heal in a month; gastric ulcers may take rather longer. Unfortunately, about half the patients will develop a recurrence of symptoms after treatment is stopped.

H_2 blockers can also be used in the treatment of reflux oesophagitis or to prevent the development of ulcers in patients under severe stress.

There is little to choose between these drugs; cimetidine and ranitidine have been in use the longest. Adverse effects are a little more troublesome with cimetidine.

Adverse Effects. These are rare, but with cimetidine they include gynaecomastia (enlargement of the breasts in the male) and male impotence due to interfering with the action of testosterone. Cimetidine can also sometimes cause confusional states in elderly patients.

Drug Reactions. Cimetidine interacts with various drugs by interfering with their metabolism in the liver. Drugs whose action may be prolonged are phenytoin, morphine, warfarin, methadone, theophylline, labetalol, propranolol, diazepam and metoprolol.

These effects have not been reported with the other H_2 blockers. MHRA (2019) sent out alerts about ranitidine due to concerns about unacceptable NMDA levels and all formulations are anticipated to be out of stock with no date for resupply in the UK.

Proton Pump Inhibitors

Proton pump inhibitors (PPIs) form the mainstay of treatment for dyspepsia. Examples of PPIs include:

- **lansoprazole**
- **omeprazole**
- **pantoprazole.**

These drugs inhibit gastric acid secretion more powerfully than the H_2 blockers and are combined with antibiotics to eliminate *H. pylori*. They are also used to treat reflux oesophagitis and in the rare Zollinger–Ellison syndrome in which there is gross oversecretion of acid.

Adverse Effects. These include headache, nausea, diarrhoea and rashes. The lowest dose for the desired effect should be used.

CLINICAL NOTE

Long-term use has also been linked to osteoporosis in the elderly due to reduced calcium absorption. There is some evidence to suggest that patients and clinicians are reluctant to stop medication due to fear of symptoms returning. Qualitative literature suggests that patients are willing to reduce treatment provided that they have a strategy should symptoms return (Thompson et al., 2018). Furthermore, empowering older people through a structured education programme prior to a medicines review may optimize medicines management (Turner et al., 2018).

Ulcer Protection

In addition to reducing acid, ulcer healing can be encouraged by drugs that protect the ulcer and increase the resistance of the gastric and duodenal lining to acid. Drugs used include:

- sucralfate
- prostaglandins, e.g. misoprostol.

Sucralfate is a compound of aluminium and sucrose that coats the base of an ulcer, protecting it from pepsin and allowing healing to take place.

Prostaglandins exert some protective effect on the gastric mucosa and this is the reason why drugs that inhibit prostaglandin production (e.g. NSAIDs) can cause peptic ulcers. **Misoprostol**, which is a prostaglandin analogue, has been shown to reduce the risk of gastric ulcers in patients at special risk (e.g. the elderly and those with a history of ulcers) who are taking NSAIDs.

Eradication of *H. Pylori*

NICE (2019) has reviewed 12 randomized controlled trials and concluded that *H. pylori* eradication was more effective than placebo at reducing dyspepsia symptoms. Furthermore, eradication rates of 80%–85% were achieved using triple therapies. Urea breath tests and stool antigen tests are accurate with about 95% sensitivity in detecting the presence of *H. pylori*. To reduce false-negative results, PPIs should be avoided for 2 weeks and antibiotics for 4 weeks prior to testing.

Various triple-drug combinations that are effective include:

- 7-day triple therapy with PPI with amoxicillin and clarithromycin or metronidazole
- If penicillin allergic: PPI with clarithromycin and metronidazole
- If first-line is ineffective, then second-line treatment can be tried as per local antibiotic protocols/BNF.

The use of triple treatment is illustrated in Case History 10.1. Diarrhoea may complicate all these treatments.

CASE HISTORY 10.1

Mrs. K was in her early 30s when she noticed that she developed indigestion after spicy meals and a little too much alcohol. Initially, this was controllable with over-the-counter antacids when necessary. She then began to notice more pain, especially at night and also a couple of hours after eating. As the antacids were no longer sufficient, she went to her local surgery for further advice. Suspecting that the patient's problem might be caused by a *Helicobacter pylori* infection of the stomach, which can often be the underlying cause of duodenal/gastric ulcers, the GP sent a stool antigen check for *H. pylori*, which confirmed the diagnosis. She was advised on lifestyle changes, including safe limits of alcohol as well as dietary changes. Mrs. K was started on a 1-week course of triple therapy to eradicate the bacteria, which consisted of the proton pump inhibitor lansoprazole, combined with amoxicillin and clarithromycin.

CLINICAL NOTE

Long-term use of OTC antacids and other gastric medication should be avoided and used only as directed. If the pain and indigestion persists, then a medical opinion should be sought. When admitting a patient for care the nurse should ask about use of OTC preparations specifically for gastric reflux and other gastric problems.

SUMMARY

- Stop NSAIDs in patients with peptic ulcers.
- Discourage smoking in patients with peptic ulcers.
- Prescribe antacids with care in patients with renal problems.
- Do not prescribe antacids for patients taking digoxin, tetracycline, iron salts, indomethacin or isoniazid, as antacids interfere with their absorption from the gastrointestinal tract.
- Cimetidine is a histamine H_2 receptor blocker that can reduce fertility in men.
- Proton pump inhibitors are preferred over H_2 blockers.
- Misoprostol should be considered for at risk patients who need to be taking NSAIDs.
- PPIs and antibacterials are usually co-prescribed in a triple regimen to eradicate *H. pylori* and reduce acid and pepsin secretion.

Non-ulcer Dyspepsia

Non-ulcer dyspepsia may also be associated with *H. pylori* infection, but the link is less clear-cut. Patients should be screened for infection. Patients aged 55 and over should also be considered for an urgent endoscopy to exclude upper gastrointestinal cancer (in those with dysphagia, weight loss and any of the accompanying symptoms: upper abdominal pain, reflux, dyspepsia). In patients with evidence of an infection for *H. pylori*, eradication (as detailed earlier) can sometimes produce an improvement, although it may be delayed for some months. Those without infection are usually treated with short-term antacids or PPIs.

SPECIAL POINTS FOR PATIENT EDUCATION

1. Special diets are no longer popular. Patients should be advised to take regular meals (not too widely spaced), avoiding irritating foods and alcohol.
2. Patients should stop smoking.
3. Drugs such as NSAIDs (including aspirin) and antiplatelets make ulcer bleeding and perforation more likely, particularly in elderly patients. Steroids in high doses may cause ulcers to develop and make their complications more dangerous. These classes of drug should be avoided, if possible, in patients with a history of peptic ulcers.

Carminatives (Flatus-relieving)

Carminatives are substances which, when taken by mouth, produce a feeling of warmth in the stomach. They cause relaxation of the cardiac sphincter and allow the 'belching up' of wind and may thus relieve gastric distension. Examples in common use are the oils of ginger and peppermint.

THE INTESTINES

After food has been partially digested in the stomach, it passes into the small intestine, where the digestion of proteins, carbohydrates and fats is completed and absorption occurs.

The passage of food through the small intestine takes about 12–24 h and the residue then enters the colon, where further absorption, largely of water, takes place and the intestinal contents become semi-solid. The filling of the rectum produces the characteristic sensation of the 'call to stool' and the bowels are then emptied by a complicated mechanism, partially voluntary and partially involuntary.

The passage of food through the intestines is brought about by peristalsis, which consists of a wave of contraction preceded by a wave of relaxation. Parasympathetic stimulation increases peristaltic activity and sympathetic stimulation decreases it.

Enemas and Suppositories

The wall of the rectum contains nerve receptors, which respond to pressure when needing to defecate but may also be stimulated by various substances that can be introduced into the rectum as suppositories or micro-enemas to initiate the evacuation of the bowel. Larger-volume enemas distend the rectum and lower bowel, causing contraction, and also have some washout effect.

Enemas

Enemas may be used to soften the stool and include arachis oil or docusate sodium (see later). To promote evacuation of the bowel, a phosphate enema, run into the rectum, is useful, e.g. before sigmoidoscopy. An alternative is to use a micro-enema such as *Micolette*. This is given rectally and acts as a colon stimulant.

Enemas can also be used to treat conditions of the bowel. In ulcerative colitis, corticosteroids (e.g. prednisolone) can be introduced into the rectum and retained if possible for at least 1 h. A certain amount of corticosteroid is absorbed into the circulation and so both local and systemic therapeutic effects result (see later).

Suppositories

Glycerol suppositories, one or two moistened with water and inserted into the rectum, are quite satisfactory. Other suppositories are available but, in general, offer no advantage.

Laxatives (see later) are also used to prepare the bowel before colonic surgery or colonoscopy. Various regimens are used, but essentially a low-residue diet is taken for a few days and one sachet of sodium picosulfate in water is given in the morning and one in the afternoon on the day before the procedure.

THE TREATMENT OF CHRONIC INFLAMMATORY BOWEL DISEASE

Inflammatory bowel disease (IBD) is any inflammation of the bowel and includes Crohn's disease and ulcerative colitis. These are chronic autoimmune diseases, in which the immune system attacks the tissues in the absence of any foreign invader. Both Crohn's disease and ulcerative colitis are inclined to run a relapsing course. Crohn's disease is a chronic inflammatory disease of the bowel and may affect any part of the gastrointestinal tract (from mouth to anus), but commonly affects the small bowel (terminal ileum) and colon. Ulcerative colitis is confined to the colon and rectum. The cause of these diseases is not fully known, but many studies support the concept that inflammatory bowel disease (IBD) results from a dysregulated response by the mucosal immune system to the microbiota that reside within the intestinal lumen (Snapper and Abraham, 2019). It is thought that patients with IBD have alteration in the composition and function of intestinal microbiota. Thus, new therapeutic developments are targeting these areas.

The usual pattern of treatment is to bring the acute attack under control and then keep the patient in remission. In addition to the use of drugs, other aspects of management include the maintenance of nutrition and electrolyte balance, correcting anaemia (if present), and occasionally surgery to deal with complications or intractable disease. Crohn's and colitis can increase the risk of bowel cancer (except for patients with a history of proctitis alone), therefore the patients are also advised to have surveillance colonoscopies 8–10 years following diagnosis, to help detect cancer early, which in turn should improve survival rates. Other investigations may also be required earlier, which will be assessed according to the disease flares.

Drugs currently used in the treatment of chronic inflammatory bowel disease include:

- Corticosteroids
- Aminosalicylates: mesalazine and sulfasalazine
- Immunosuppressants: azathioprine or methotrexate (second-line)
- Biologic therapy, e.g. infliximab and adalimumab.

Corticosteroids

Corticosteroids are used to induce remission in inflammatory bowel disorders. In ulcerative colitis, they may be used for induction of remission if aminosalicylates are ineffective or not tolerated. **Budesonide** is a glucocorticoid, which can be administered as a foam/enema to have local effects, particularly for ulcerative colitis affecting the sigmoid colon/rectum, or can be given orally for mild to moderate Crohn's disease affecting the ileum or ascending colon. Alternatively, in mild ulcerative colitis, if it is confined to the descending colon, prednisolone enemas may be used instead. Oral prednisolone is the next step if topical steroids do not induce remission and this is normally done in a reducing regimen. Corticosteroids are also used in the treatment of Crohn's disease, as illustrated in Case History 10.2. The adverse effects of corticosteroids are covered in Chapter 17 (see also Fig. 17.2).

CASE HISTORY 10.2

Mr. H, aged 22 years, began to experience lower right abdominal pain associated with diarrhoea and fever. He initially self-treated with anti-diarrhoeal agents bought over the counter but, as his symptoms persisted and he started to lose weight and needed time off work, he visited his GP. Blood tests showed an iron deficiency anaemia and stool cultures did not show any infections. A colonoscopy was performed, showing narrowing and ulceration of the affected bowel, and a diagnosis of Crohn's disease affecting the ileo-caecal junction was made following this. He was started on high-dose oral steroids (prednisolone) 40 mg daily. The symptoms improved rapidly, but on reducing the dose of prednisolone there was a relapse and a 5-aminosalicylic acid-containing drug (*Pentasa*), more frequently used for ulcerative colitis, was added; however, the relapse persisted and, to be able to reduce the steroid dose below 10–15 mg daily, the immunosuppressant azathioprine was added. This required regular blood tests since azathioprine affects blood cell production. He was maintained for 2 years in a stable condition, but a further relapse and fistula formation led to a bowel resection of the affected area. The patient was informed that there is up to a 50% relapse rate after surgery in the first 10 years.

Mesalazine

Mesalazine (a 5-aminosalicylic acid) is also available and has fewer side-effects than sulfasalazine, but is more expensive. In mild to moderate flare of distal ulcerative colitis, the first-line treatment is rectal aminosalicylates; if this does not have the desired response then oral aminosalicylates should be added. Typically a period of 4 weeks is used to assess treatment response in patients with mild to moderate disease. Asacol is a delayed-release preparation of mesalazine, which is useful in the treatment of distal disease.

Sulfasalazine

Sulfasalazine can also be started to keep the patient in remission. Sulfasalazine is a combination of 5-aminosalicylic acid and sulfapyridine, and is broken down in the bowel to release 5-aminosalicylic acid, which is the active component. Its action is largely antiinflammatory. Sulfasalazine is effective in maintaining a remission in ulcerative colitis and in colonic Crohn's disease.

Adverse Effects. These include headache, nausea, rashes and, rarely, blood disorders. Male fertility may be temporarily reduced as sulfasalazine can decrease sperm count and motility which is reversible on stopping the drug.

Immunosuppressants

Immunosuppressants reduce the activity of the immune system, which is important in causing the inflammation of autoimmune diseases such as inflammatory bowel disease. Immunosuppressants reduce inflammation by inhibiting the production of immune cells and/or by interfering with their production of inflammatory proteins (cytokines). However, immunosuppressive drugs weaken the immune system and make the patient prone to infection, but the benefits obtained are often considered sufficient to outweigh the risks.

Azathioprine

Azathioprine, which is also used in the treatment of rheumatoid arthritis (see Chapter 13), another autoimmune disease, is sometimes used combined with corticosteroids so that the steroid dose can be reduced to minimize the side-effects that are common with corticosteroids. This approach to therapy is illustrated in the Case History 10.2.

Methotrexate

This immunosuppressant drug was originally introduced for the treatment of cancer, but is now widely used to treat autoimmune diseases such as rheumatoid arthritis (see also Chapter 13) and second-line treatment in inflammatory bowel disease.

BIOLOGIC THERAPY

Infliximab

Infliximab (*Remicade*) is one of a group of newer drugs, called **biologics** (see also Appendix), that block the action of a powerful inflammatory substance called tumour necrosis factor alpha (TNF-α) that is produced by the cells of the immune system. Monoclonal antibodies that inhibit TNF-α are now widely used to treat autoimmune diseases and their effects can be dramatic.

Mechanism of Action. Infliximab binds to and inactivates TNF-α.

Administration. Infliximab is given by intravenous infusion and the patient is usually admitted to a day-bed for the procedure. Patients may suffer a relapse within 3 months after the first infusion, but this is generally prevented if the infusion is repeated thereafter at regular intervals, usually every 8 weeks. After the disease is brought under control, patients can be maintained on other orally active immunosuppressants such as azathioprine.

Effects. The beneficial effects in Crohn's disease can be very rapid and dramatic, especially in patients who do not respond to other treatments. The drug is also effective in healing anal fistulae associated with Crohn's disease, which are generally unresponsive to other treatments.

Adverse Effects. This type of treatment is relatively new, and data about the adverse effects are still being gathered. During the infusion, the patient may complain of nausea, shortness of breath or chest pains, and these symptoms usually disappear if the infusion is stopped. Since infliximab is a large molecule, it can cause an immune response and patients may develop fever, a worsening of the Crohn's disease and 'flu'-like symptoms. These immune reactions may be severe enough to warrant treatment with other immunosuppressants. Infliximab has been reported to allow dormant tuberculosis (TB) to reappear in some patients and is therefore contraindicated in patients who have had TB. Patients should be tested for TB before receiving infliximab. It is also contraindicated in patients with cancer and in patients with existing infections such as abscesses, urinary tract infections or pneumonia.

Adalimumab

Adalimumab is another biologic that is used in the treatment of inflammatory bowel disease. It also binds to TNF-α and interferes with the binding to TNF-α sites and subsequent cytokine-driven antiinflammatory process (Lichtenstein, 2018).

Administration. Induction therapy is given subcutaneously and is available through the use of single-use prefilled pen or in a single-use prefilled syringe. Therapeutic drug monitoring for it includes the measurement of drug trough levels, to allow the prescribers to decide if dose increase or switching to an alternative drug is required. In addition to this, markers for disease monitoring (e.g. C-reactive protein/erythrocyte sedimentation rate and faecal calprotectin, increases in which demonstrates mucosal inflammation) are also recommended.

Contraindications to using anti-TNF therapy includes an active infection (including latent TB), heart failure and demyelinating disease.

CLINICAL NOTE

In view of the risk of a suppressed blood count with sulfasalazine, mesalazine, methotrexate or infliximab, patients taking any of these should be warned to report to a healthcare professional if they develop a sore throat, fever, bruising or bleeding, as rapid deteriorating and acute illness may occur. The patients should be closely monitored and consideration given to withholding or stopping treatment. Nurse-led interventions to support people living with inflammatory bowel disease appears to be cost-effective, and improve both patient satisfaction and their quality of life (Linedale et al., 2020).

Diet

In addition to the drugs detailed previously, an elemental diet which contains the essential constituents for nutrition (e.g. carbohydrates, amino acids, fats and vitamins in pure form) given for 2 weeks has a specific therapeutic effect in Crohn's disease, but not in ulcerative colitis.

THE TREATMENT OF CONSTIPATION

Before making a diagnosis of constipation, it is important to realize that there is considerable natural variation in the frequency with which people open their bowels. The majority vary between twice daily and once every other day.

Constipation has two main causes:

- Delayed passage of faeces through the colon
- People neglecting responding to the body's signal to defecate.

Causes of Delayed Stool Passage

Causes of delayed passage are:

- low-fibre diet
- lack of exercise
- various drugs, including opioids, antidepressants and verapamil
- local lesions of the bowel
- disorders that interfere with bowel muscle function, such as hypercalcaemia or myxoedema
- pregnancy
- old age
- depression
- weakness of the abdominal muscle.

Neglecting the Body's Signal to Defecate

This cause of constipation may occur for social reasons or may be due to illness, surgery or some painful lesion of the anus such as a fissure. As a result, the rectum becomes used to distension of its walls by faeces and loses its ability to contract and empty.

In patients who are ill and who have been constipated for a few days, *Senokot* tablets at night followed by a glycerin suppository the next day are often sufficient.

In chronic constipation the object of treatment is to re-educate the intestines so that a normal bowel habit is restored. This can be achieved by increasing the bulk of the faeces either by a high fibre content in the diet, i.e. bran or similar substances, or by the use of bulk laxatives such as methylcellulose. A reasonably high fluid intake and exercise are also helpful. This should be combined with regular habits and may require the use of some laxatives such as *Senokot* at night until a normal rhythm is regained.

Constipation is a common problem in the elderly, especially those who are housebound or in care homes. It is due to poor diet, inadequate muscle tone and immobility. If faecal impaction occurs, it can be relieved by a retention enema of docusate sodium. If this fails or rapid evacuation of the bowels is required, manual removal may be necessary.

Long-term management needs dietary advice, as much exercise as is practicable, regular habits and the use of a laxative as required. Senna or bisacodyl are cheap and probably as effective as the more expensive preparations.

Laxatives

Laxatives are commonly used drugs to treat constipation when lifestyle factors have failed such as increasing the fibre in the diet as well as drinking plenty of fluids with regular exercise. Bowel habits vary considerably, and many people need to open their bowels less frequently. For these people, there is nothing to be gained by trying to attain a more frequent bowel action with laxatives.

Even more dangerous is the indiscriminate use of laxatives for all types of abdominal pain. In many acute abdominal diseases, the use of such drugs aggravates the condition, a classic example being the rupture of an acutely inflamed appendix following a laxative. Therefore they should not be given to patients with undiagnosed abdominal pain.

Bowel evacuation may be achieved using orally administered **laxatives** or by the use of **enemas** and **suppositories**.

Laxatives may work in different ways and there are several types:

- bulk laxatives that are high-residue foods, e.g. bran, ispaghula husk
- stimulant laxatives, e.g. senna, bisacodyl
- faecal softeners, e.g. docusate sodium and glycerol suppositories
- osmotic laxatives, e.g. magnesium sulphate, lactulose, macrogols.

The bulk laxatives increase the contents of the bowel and thus stimulate peristalsis. The stool-softening laxatives aid the passage of faecal material by their lubricating action. The stimulant laxatives increase peristalsis and thus the intestinal contents pass more rapidly through the bowel and remain more fluid.

Bulk Laxatives

High-residue foods contain a high proportion of cellulose, which is not digested or absorbed and thus increases the bulk of the intestinal contents. Common examples are green vegetables, fruit and wholemeal bread.

Bran. Bran, which is a by-product of milling, contains about 30% fibre made up of celluloses, pectins and lignins, substances which are not absorbed from the intestine and which swell as they take up water and thus increase the bulk of the faeces. The initial dose is one tablespoonful, combined with fluid, daily and this is increased at weekly intervals until a satisfactory result is achieved. The main side-effect is wind (flatulence).

Methylcellulose. Methylcellulose is available in a number of preparations either as granules or tablets. It is an effective bulk laxative.

Ispaghula Husk. Ispaghula husk is of plant origin and swells on contact with water, thus acting as a bulk laxative. Combine with plenty of water.

SAFETY POINT

Patients must be warned **not** to take granular preparations that swell in water without first mixing with water. There have been fatalities due to the ingestion of dry granules that swell in the throat and cause asphyxiation.

Bulk laxatives depend on the ability of the colon to respond to distension and may not be effective in elderly patients.

Stool Softeners

Liquid Paraffin

Liquid paraffin has been in use for many years and has been heavily used, especially by elderly patients, who took it chronically and regularly. It is odourless, tasteless and facilitates evacuation of the bowels in the chronically constipated patient. It is, however, associated with potentially serious adverse effects if taken for long periods. It may cause:

- leaking via the anal sphincter
- lipoid pneumonia in the very young and very old
- interference with the absorption of vitamins A, D and K.

Liquid paraffin should therefore not be used for long periods.

Docusate Sodium

Available as tablets or syrup, docusate sodium acts by softening the stools, which may be sufficient to relieve constipation, particularly if a painful condition such as piles or anal fissure is interfering with bowel evacuation. It may be combined with a stimulant laxative as it takes 2 or 3 days to be effective. It can also be used as a micro-enema in the management of faecal impaction, when docusate in solution is injected into the rectum.

Osmotic Laxatives

Saline Laxatives

The most commonly used saline laxative is magnesium sulphate (*Epsom Salts*). It is poorly absorbed from the intestinal tract. Originally it was thought to make the intestinal contents more fluid, but it is now considered that its laxative effect is a response to magnesium ions reaching the intestine.

A saline laxative should be given on an empty stomach (before breakfast is a good time) so that it passes rapidly through the stomach and into the intestine. If it is held up in the stomach, it may not be effective. It is given dissolved in water and the concentration should not exceed 8 g of magnesium sulphate to 120 mL of water, as a more concentrated dose may cause closure of the pyloric sphincter and delay the drug leaving the stomach. These drugs are usually effective within 1–2 h.

Fruit salts usually contain some sodium hydrogen carbonate and tartaric acid. When these are mixed with water, sodium tartrate is formed with the liberation of carbon dioxide. The sodium tartrate acts as a mild laxative.

Lactulose

Lactulose is a sugar that is broken down by bacteria in the large bowel with the production of various acids. These act as osmotic laxatives, rendering the bowel contents more fluid, and as mild irritants, both of which produce a laxative effect. Lactulose is given in liquid, which can take 48 h to act and may cause a certain amount of flatulence and distension. For these reasons, it is not a particularly good laxative, but is sometimes used in the long-term treatment of constipated elderly patients and for those receiving opioids for intractable pain when constipation may be a problem. It also has a limited use in patients with severe liver disease to reduce the absorption of toxic substances from the bowel.

Stimulant Laxatives

The anthracene group of laxatives all contain the anthraquinone emodin, which is the chief active constituent of the group; the varying properties of the anthracene laxatives depend on the ease with which this active constituent is released. After liberation in the intestine, emodin is absorbed into the bloodstream and acts on the large intestine, causing increased peristalsis. All members of this group of drugs therefore take about 8–12 h to act and are best given at bedtime. They may occasionally cause griping (severe abdominal pain) and should be avoided during pregnancy.

Senna

Senna (available OTC in the UK as *Senokot*) is a proprietary preparation that contains the purified principles called 'sennoside A and sennoside B'. It is highly satisfactory and can be used either as granules, tablets or syrup.

Bisacodyl

Bisacodyl is a preparation that stimulates activity of the colon when it comes in contact with the wall of the bowel. It can be used either orally or as a suppository.

Co-danthramer

Co-danthramer is a mixture of a stool softener and a stimulant laxative (dantron). Unfortunately, it has been shown to produce tumours in rodents with high and prolonged dosage, although there is no evidence that this occurs in humans. Its use is therefore restricted to palliative patients whose constipation is due to opioid analgesics.

Sodium Picosulfate

Sodium picosulfate is a very powerful bowel stimulant used for preparation before surgery or bowel preparation prior to radiological investigation or endoscopy (e.g. Picolax) and is not for the long-term treatment of constipation.

Laxative Abuse

Some patients become dependent on laxatives because they believe that these drugs wash away poisons from the body. If carried to extremes, this can lead to serious electrolyte depletion and damage the bowel, with dilation of the colon. In severe electrolyte depletion, intravenous replacement may be required, but for the majority of patients the oral route is satisfactory and preparations containing sodium, potassium, glucose and water in the optimum concentrations are available.

Adverse Effects of Laxatives

- Diarrhoea with loss of fluids and electrolytes
- Dependence on laxatives with chronic use
- Systemic absorption of laxatives
- Lipoid pneumonia with liquid paraffin
- Damage to the bowel
- Abdominal pain
- Dangers associated with the use of stimulant laxatives in pregnancy.

SUMMARY

- Never give laxatives to patients with undiagnosed abdominal pain.
- Proper diet containing roughage and exercise are important complementary strategies in addition to laxatives.
- Bulk laxatives that swell in water must be mixed with water before oral use.
- Powerful stimulant laxatives should be avoided in pregnancy.
- Saline laxatives such as magnesium sulphate should be taken on an empty stomach.
- Liquid paraffin should not be used for long periods.
- A trial of stopping the laxatives can be considered once a regular pattern of evacuation is achieved but may need continuing particularly when co-prescribed to counteract adverse effects of other drugs (e.g. opioids).

CLINICAL NOTE

Any laxatives should be prescribed alongside lifestyle advice such as eating a diet rich in fruit, vegetables and fibre, minimizing ingestion of processed foods and taking regular exercise. Drinking plenty of fluids will also prevent and reduce the risk of constipation.

INTESTINAL 'SEDATIVES'

Several drugs may diminish the peristaltic activity of the intestines.

Anticholinergic Medicines

The anticholinergic drugs (muscarinic receptor antagonists) decrease the tone of the gastrointestinal smooth muscle by blocking the contractile action of acetylcholine (ACh) released from parasympathetic nerves innervating the gut wall. They are particularly useful in the treatment of colon spasm.

Opioids

Opioids actually increase gut tone, but reduce peristalsis. They are useful in the treatment of severe pain. The most widely used weak opiate is codeine phosphate, which has an adverse effect of causing constipation.

Co-phenotrope (Lomotil)

This preparation is a combination of the muscarinic receptor antagonist atropine and diphenoxylate hydrochloride. The latter drug is related to the narcotic analgesics. Co-phenotrope is widely used in controlling diarrhoea, but it must be remembered that it is dangerous in overdose, particularly in children, as it can cause depression of respiration due to the action of the opioid.

Loperamide

Loperamide decreases large-bowel motility and therefore useful for treating diarrhoea (once infection and acute colitis has been excluded). Toxicity is relatively low. It is available for adults and older children OTC, without prescription.

PANCREATIC SUPPLEMENTS

As a result of pancreatic disease (usually cystic fibrosis or chronic pancreatitis), the pancreatic enzymes may be deficient, leading to a failure to digest fat and protein, malabsorption and loose fatty stools (steatorrhoea). The missing enzymes may be given orally, but they are broken down by the acid in the stomach and thus rendered ineffective. This may be circumvented by combining the enzyme with an H_2 blocker to reduce gastric acidity or by using preparations that are coated to protect them against acid.

Available preparations include:

- ***Pancrex***, which is supplied as a powder, capsules or tablets, is given before or with meals. The capsules should be broken and mixed with water or milk.
- ***Creon*** capsules containing coated pellets may be swallowed whole or opened and the pellets mixed with food. They must not, however, be chewed, as they will lose their protective coating. The dose is very variable and is best judged by observing the nature of the stool.

CLINICAL NOTE

Patients should maintain a reasonable fluid intake. Some high-strength pancreatic supplements have been associated with bowel strictures. The development of new abdominal symptoms should be reported.

GALLSTONES

Gallstones are a common finding, although they do not always cause symptoms. They are usually removed surgically either by 'keyhole' surgery (laparoscopic cholecystectomy) or by endoscopy (if the stones are located in the bile ducts). There are, however, drugs that dissolve cholesterol-rich gallstones and they are used to treat selected patients.

Ursodeoxycholic Acid

Most gallstones are largely composed of cholesterol. Ursodeoxycholic acid reduces the concentration of cholesterol in the bile and makes it more soluble so that cholesterol-containing stones are slowly dissolved.

Only small stones are suitable for this treatment. It may take from 6 to 18 months for the stones to disappear. Relapse is liable to occur when the treatment is stopped. Because of the relatively few patients suitable for this method of treatment and the lengthy supervision required, it is not widely used.

DRUGS AND THE LIVER

The liver plays an important part in regulating the effect of many drugs as it is the major organ involved in metabolizing and detoxifying drugs. It is therefore an important part of pharmacology to understand the role of the liver when administering drugs for the following reasons:

- Most orally ingested drugs pass first through the liver via the hepato-portal circulation that is normally involved with absorption of materials from food from the gastrointestinal tract. So-called

'first pass metabolism' of drugs means that much of the dose of an orally ingested drug does not reach the systemic circulation as many drugs are inactivated by the liver (see Chapter 1).
- Liver disease (e.g. cirrhosis or chronic hepatitis) may reduce the ability of liver enzymes to inactivate drugs, resulting in drug toxicity.

Care must be taken when administering combinations of drugs metabolized by the cytochrome P450 enzymes in the liver to prevent drug–drug interactions, which can lead to loss of effectiveness of toxicity.

- Some drugs can cause liver damage, e.g. alchohol.
- Drugs are used to treat certain diseases of the liver.

Drugs pass through the liver, either via the portal system after absorption from the intestine or, if the drug has been injected, via the systemic circulation. Many drugs are inactivated by the liver, being either broken down or combined with some substance which renders them inactive.

If the liver cells are damaged by disease or if the portal circulation partially bypasses the liver, as in cirrhosis, the elimination of drugs may be reduced and they will accumulate and produce toxic effects. It is therefore important to consider this possibility whenever drugs are given to patients with liver disease and in the elderly, and to adjust the dose as necessary.

A comprehensive list of drugs to avoid or use with care is given in the BNF.

Some drugs can cause liver damage. This may be either dose-related or idiosyncratic, although the distinction is not always easy. Such drugs include:

- paracetamol
- phenothiazines (chlorpromazine)
- methotrexate
- isoniazid
- rifampicin
- pyrazinamide
- halothane.

Recovery usually occurs when the drug is stopped, but in a few cases (e.g. paracetamol overdose) the damage can be severe and fatal. The use of antioxidants such as N-acetyl cysteine can be used to try and reduce paracetamol toxicity.

Chronic Viral Hepatitis

Viral hepatitis B and C present a serious and widespread health hazard that is likely to increase in incidence. Intravenous drug abuse, sexual promiscuity and exposure to contaminated blood or blood products can transmit hepatitis B virus. The majority of patients clear the virus and make a complete recovery but in about 5%, the infection continues and becomes chronic active hepatitis. Hepatitis C infection is also associated with intravenous drug abuse and the injection of contaminated blood and blood products. In about 30% of infected subjects, the disease progresses as a very slow and indolent hepatitis. Some of these patients will remain as asymptomatic carriers of the virus, but some may develop cirrhosis and a few will develop hepatocellular carcinoma.

Interferons

The only specific treatment for viral hepatitis available at present are the interferons (see also Chapter 27). The interferons are peptides that are produced by cells infected with virus. These drugs stimulate immunity and also have an antiviral action. The interferons are active against a wide variety of viruses, but a particular interferon will be effective only in the species that produced it. There are three types of interferon: namely, interferon alpha from white blood cells, interferon beta from fibroblasts, and interferon gamma from lymphocytes. The course of treatment is prolonged, but in about 50% of those with hepatitis B and 25% of those with hepatitis C, the progress of the disease is halted. Interferons may be combined with other antiviral agents.

Adverse Effects. These include depression, flu-like symptoms and lethargy, and may be very severe.

Vaccines

For those exposed to the risk of infection with the hepatitis B virus, a vaccine is available, and there is also a specific hepatitis B immunoglobin ('HBIG') when rapid protection is required. The BNF lists individuals at high risk of infection and healthcare professionals are particularly at risk. A combined hepatitis A and B vaccine is also available.

CLINICAL NOTE

People living with hepatitis C often find adherence to treatment regimens challenging. Factors associated with medicines adherence are psychological factors, motivation and provider support. Building a therapeutic relationship with these clients will optimize adherence and improve outcomes and quality of life (Williams, 2018).

EMETICS

Mechanism of Vomiting

Vomiting is a complex series of actions involving the stomach, oesophagus and pharynx with the voluntary muscles of the chest and abdomen, and results in the ejection of the stomach contents. A vomiting centre in the medulla of the brain coordinates these actions. This centre can be stimulated:

- Directly from the labyrinth of the ear in conditions such as motion sickness or vertigo.
- By gastric irritation or distension.
- By mental activity (e.g. being sick with fright; imagining something extremely unpleasant).
- Via the chemoreceptor trigger zone (CTZ) which lies close to the vomiting centre in the brainstem and which is stimulated by a number of circulating substances, including certain drugs.
- By stimulation of the 5-hydroxytryptamine (5-HT; serotonin) receptors in the CTZ. Circulating cytotoxic drugs (particularly cisplatin; see Chapter 29) release 5-HT from nerve endings, and this activates the CTZ receptors. From the CTZ, impulses travel to the vomiting centre and activate it by acting on muscarinic ACh receptors.

The stimulation of vomiting outlined is summarized in Fig. 10.3.

Before the act of vomiting occurs, stimulation of the vomiting centre produces a sensation known as nausea, which is often associated with increased secretion by the salivary and bronchial glands. Drugs that provoke vomiting are called **emetics**.

Emetics are rarely used in medical practice except in cases of poisoning. They may be divided into two types:

- **reflex emetics**, e.g. ipecacuanha
- **central emetics**, e.g. apomorphine.

Reflex Emetics

This group of drugs produces vomiting by irritating the stomach. The only one in common use is ipecacuanha, a plant extract, which is dispensed as ipecacuanha emetic mixture, and vomiting should occur in 15–30 min after ingestion. Ipecacuanha may be used as a first-aid treatment for overdose or poisoning provided that:

- the patient is fully conscious
- overdose is not of corrosive substances or petroleum products, when inhalation of vomit could be fatal.

Ipecacuanha can be used up to 1 h after ingestion of poison and longer for some substances, such as tricyclic antidepressants and salicylates, when gastric emptying is delayed. It is not as effective as a stomach washout, but is particularly useful in children, when the upset caused by the process of lavage should be avoided if possible, and in removing such objects as berries, which cannot be washed out of the stomach. In general, the use of emetics in poisoning is decreasing because there is little evidence that, even if used soon after ingestion of poison, they usefully reduce absorption.

Central Emetics (those Acting on the Brain)

Apomorphine stimulates dopamine receptors in the CTZ. It is closely related to morphine but has none of its analgesic effects. Apomorphine has, however, a very powerful emetic action and also produces some cerebral depression. It was formerly used as an emetic but because of its depressant action **it should not be used in treating patients who have taken an overdose**. At present its use is confined to patients with resistant Parkinson's disease (see Chapter 21).

ANTIEMETICS

Cautionary Note

Antiemetics should not be taken if the cause of the vomiting is unknown, as they may hinder diagnosis. Vomiting may be the result of, e.g. drug overdose or diabetic ketoacidosis, which should be diagnosed and treated appropriately.

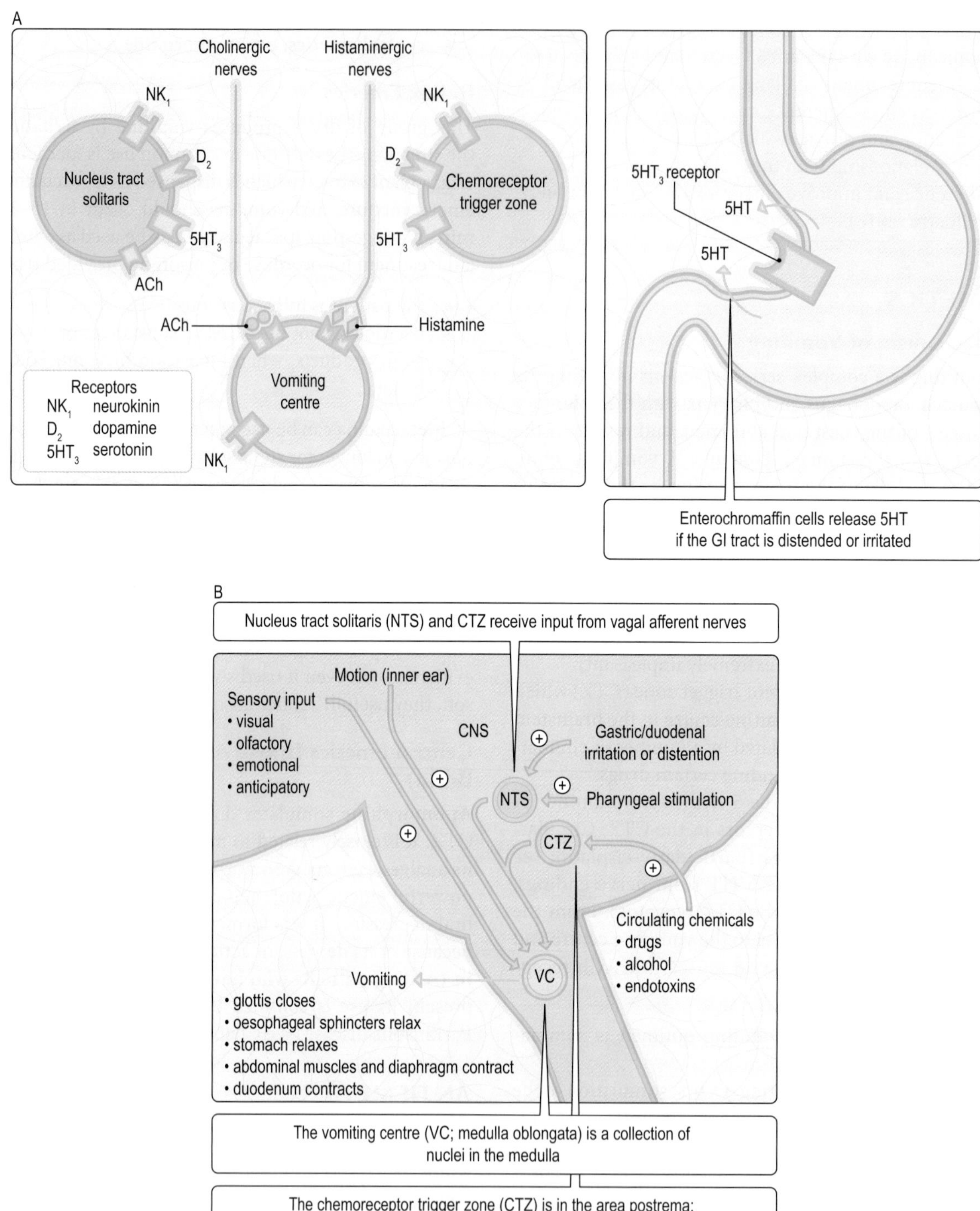

Fig. 10.3 (A) Physiology of nausea and emesis. (B) Receptors involved in nausea and emesis. *ACh,* Acetylcholine, *CNS,* central nervous system, *GI,* gastrointestinal. (With permission from Dom Spina (ed.), 2008. Flesh and Bones of Medical Pharmacology. Figs 3.20.1 and 3.20.2. Philadelphia, Elsevier.)

TABLE 10.1

The Management of Vomiting – There are Several Causes of Vomiting and Specific Drugs are Effective for Different Types

Types of Vomiting	Effective Drug	Comment
Vomiting of pregnancy	Promethazine	Dietary management if possible. Keep drugs to a minimum in early pregnancy, owing to risk of fetal deformity. Promethazine appears to be safe, cyclizine is also sometimes used first-line
Motion sickness	Hyoscine	Dry mouth. Blurred vision. Some sedation. Short journey
	Cinnarizine	Preferred for longer journey
Vertigo	Prochlorperazine	
	Cinnarizine	
	Betahistine	Ménière's disease
Opioids	Haloperidol	Less sedating. Long-acting
	Metoclopramide	
	Domperidone	
Cytotoxic medicines	Domperidone	Not sedative
	Metoclopramide	High doses required
	Ondansetron	
	Dexamethasone	
Migraine	Metoclopramide	Risk of extrapyramidal disorders. Limit to short-term use (up to 5 days)
Post-anaesthetic (often opioid)	Prochlorperazine	
	Cyclizine	
	Ondansetron	Can cause headache

It is believed that acetylcholine, histamine, dopamine and 5-HT act as intermediate transmitters in the CTZ and vomiting centre. By blocking the action of these substances on their receptors, it is possible to prevent or diminish vomiting (Table 10.1).

The classes of antiemetic drugs are:

- Muscarinic receptor antagonists
- H_1 receptor antagonists
- dopamine receptor antagonists
- 5-HT receptor antagonists
- miscellaneous antiemetics.

Muscarinic Acetylcholine Receptor Antagonists

Hyoscine blocks the action of acetylcholine in the vomiting centre and is useful for the short-term control of motion sickness. It is administered orally or as a transdermal patch. The patch is applied behind the ear for maximum absorption for 6 h before starting a journey. Drowsiness and blurring of vision, due to paralysis of ocular accommodation, can occur.

Antihistamines (H_1 Receptor Antagonists)

Antihistamines commonly used as antiemetics include:

- Cyclizine
- Promethazine
- Cinnarizine.

H_1 receptor antagonists block the action of histamine on H_1 receptors, but most of the antihistamines useful as antemetic drugs also block muscarinic receptors. H_1 receptor antagonists can be classified as those that are able to cross the blood–brain barrier and those that do not. The most useful antihistamines for the treatment of emesis are those able to cross the blood–brain barrier and interact with H_1 receptors in the CNS such as **cyclizine** and **promethazine**, which occasionally have a place in severe vomiting of pregnancy. **Cinnarizine** is an antiemetic, which has found particular favour among yachtsmen and others at risk from seasickness, but it can also be used in other types of vomiting, especially that associated with Ménière's disease. Sedation is not usually a problem.

Dopamine Antagonists

Several of the phenothiazine drugs (see Chapter 22) are powerful antiemetics due to their action in blocking the effects of dopamine on the CTZ. Some do not act only on dopamine receptors, i.e. they are relatively non-specific in action, and therefore have side-effects; e.g. they may be sedatives (see Table 10.1). Among those used as antiemetics are:

- prochlorperazine
- chlorpromazine
- haloperidol
- levomepromazine
- domperidone
- metoclopramide.

Prochlorperazine suppresses opioid-induced vomiting. It can be given orally or by intramuscular, but not by subcutaneous, injection. If given intravenously, it must be well diluted before use. **Chlorpromazine** is similar in action to prochlorperazine. **Haloperidol** is also similar but is longer-acting and less sedating. **Levomepromazine** is used, particularly in terminal care, to control vomiting and reduce agitation.

Domperidone is less sedative than chlorpromazine and less liable to produce dystonic reactions (muscle spasms of the face, neck, shoulders, limbs and the trunk) than metoclopramide (see later) because its action on the nervous system is confined to the CTZ. It also enhances gastric emptying. Unfortunately, only about 15% of the oral dose reaches the circulation and a parenteral preparation is not available. It can be used to suppress the vomiting that accompanies long-term treatment with the opioids, levodopa and with the mildly emetic cytotoxic drugs.

Metoclopramide increases gastric tone and dilates the duodenum. This causes the stomach to empty more quickly. In addition, it has some central action on the vomiting centre. It is a fairly effective antiemetic and is administered orally or by intramuscular injection. It is used in postoperative and opioid-induced vomiting and in migraine. In very large doses, it also blocks 5-HT receptors and is used to prevent vomiting due to cytotoxic drugs.

CLINICAL NOTE

Adverse reactions with metoclopramide are rare, but even with normal doses, patients may develop dystonia of the facial and neck muscles. This is more common in young people. The spasms pass off within a few hours of stopping the drug and can be controlled by diazepam. Prolonged use of metoclopramide has been reported to cause tardive dyskinesia (involuntary repetitive movements of muscles of the face, mouth and upper trunk, brought on by repetitive use of certain drugs, especially antipsychotic drugs; see Chapter 22). Metoclopramide is used in caution in the elderly because of risk of increase in parkinsonian side-effects (BNF, 2020)

5-HT Antagonists

Ondansetron and **granisetron** block the 5-HT receptors associated with the central connections of the vagus nerve in the brainstem in close proximity to the CTZ. They are used to prevent vomiting in patients receiving highly emetic cytotoxic drugs for the treatment of cancer, such as cisplatin.

Miscellaneous Antiemetics

Cannabinoids

Cannabinoids are derivatives of *Cannabis sativa* (marijuana); they have an antiemetic action and have been used with some success in controlling vomiting in patients receiving cytotoxic drugs. They also produce some sedation and occasionally confusion. Cannabis cannot be prescribed at present, but **nabilone**, a derivative, is available.

Betahistine

Betahistine differs from other antiemetics in that its use is confined to the treatment of Ménière's disease in which vertigo and vomiting are due to a disturbance in the labyrinth of the inner ear. The drug is believed to lower pressure in the inner ear and thus relieve symptoms.

Dexamethasone

The corticosteroid dexamethasone has proved useful as an antiemetic during cancer chemotherapy.

SUMMARY

- Do not use an emetic if the patient is not fully conscious.
- Do not use any emetic if the ingested material is corrosive or a petroleum product.
- It is generally better to pre-treat with an antiemetic *before* administering an emetic stimulus.
- Do not administer a muscarinic antagonist such as hyoscine if that patient is to drive or operate heavy machinery after taking the drug.
- Cinnarizine is favoured for seasickness.
- Antiemetics are of major importance in treating the nausea and vomiting associated with cancer chemotherapy.

NURSING NOTE

Antiemetics have the best result if they are given at least half an hour before the emetic stimulus.

REFERENCES AND FURTHER READING

BNF, 2020. *Helicobacter pylori* Infection. NICE/BNF treatment summary. https://bnf.nice.org.uk/treatment-summary/helicobacter-pylori-infection.html.

Lichtenstein, G.R., 2018. Treatment of Crohn Disease in Adults: Dosing and Monitoring Tumor Necrosis Factor-Alpha Inhibitors. UpToDate. https://www.uptodate.com/contents/treatment-of-crohn-disease-in-adults-dosing-and-monitoring-of-tumor-necrosis-factor-alpha-inhibitors.

Lindsay, J., Chipperfield, R., Giles, A., et al., 2013. A UK retrospective observational study of clinical outcomes and healthcare resource utilisation of infliximab treatment in Crohn's disease. Aliment Pharmacol. Therapeut. 38 (1), 52–61.

Linedale, E.C., Mikocka-Walus, A., Gibson, P.R., Andrews, J.M., 2020. The potential of integrated nurse-led models to improve care for people with functional gastrointestinal disorders: a systematic review. Gastroenterol. Nurs. 43 (1), 53–64.

Luthra, P., Camilleri, M., Burr, N.E., et al., 2019. Efficacy of drugs in chronic idiopathic constipation: a systematic review and network meta-analysis. Lancet Gastroenterol. Hepatol. 4 (11), 831–844.

Maes, M.L., Fixen, D.R., Linnebur, S.A., 2017. Adverse effects of proton-pump inhibitor use in older adults: a review of the evidence. Ther. Adv. Drug Saf. 8 (9), 273–297.

MHRA, 2019. Press Release. MHRA Drug Alert: Recalls for 13 Over-the-counter Ranitidine Medicines. https://www.gov.uk/government/news/mhra-drug-alert-recalls-for-13-over-the-counter-ranitidine-medicines.

NICE, 2016. Scenario: Herpes Labialis (Cold Sores) and Gingivostomatitis. https://cks.nice.org.uk/topics/herpes-simplex-oral/management/herpes-labialis-gingivostomatitis.

NICE, 2018. Scenario: Gingivitis and Periodontitis. https://cks.nice.org.uk/topics/gingivitis-periodontitis/management/gingivitis-periodontitis.

NICE, 2019. Gastro-oesophageal Reflux Disease and Dyspepsia in Adults: Investigation and Management [CG184]. https://www.nice.org.uk/guidance/cg184.

Snapper, S.B., Abraham, C., 2019. Immune and Microbial Mechanisms in the Pathogenesis of Inflammatory Bowel Disease. UpToDate. https://www.uptodate.com/contents/immune-and-microbial-mechanisms-in-the-pathogenesis-of-inflammatory-bowel-disease.

Thompson, W., Black, C., Welch, V., et al., 2018. Patient values and preferences surrounding proton pump inhibitor use: a scoping review. Patient 11 (1), 17–28.

Turner, J.P., Richard, C., Lussier, M.-T., et al., 2018. Deprescribing conversations: a closer look at prescriber-patient communication. Ther. Adv. Drug Saf. 9 (12), 687–698.

Williams, S., 2018. Impact of nursing interventions on medication adherence during hepatitis C treatment: state of the science. Gastroenterol. Nurs. 41 (5), 436–445.

11 VITAMINS, IRON AND TREATMENT OF ANAEMIA

CHAPTER OUTLINE

LEARNING OBJECTIVES

At the end of this chapter, the reader should be able to:

- give an account of the sources, symptoms of deficiency and preparations of the vitamins
- describe the use of antioxidants
- describe the use of iron preparations for treatment of iron deficiency anaemia
- explain the association between anaemia and vitamin B_{12} deficiency, and describe how it is treated

VITAMINS

Vitamins are substances that are present in certain foods, but which humans cannot manufacture for themselves. They are necessary for the proper functioning of many body tissues, and a deficiency of vitamins in the diet leads to a number of diseases specific to each particular vitamin. Many of the vitamins exert their action by taking part in the complex chemical reactions that occur within the cell.

It is important to realize that provided a sufficiency of vitamins is taken, which should be provided by a good mixed diet, there is no advantage to be gained by taking further large doses of the various vitamins, unless there is some form of malabsorption. In fact, the taking of excessive amounts of certain vitamins, e.g. vitamin A, can even be harmful. At present, there is no good evidence that extra vitamins protect against cancer and heart disease and indeed, there is some evidence that antioxidant vitamin supplements may be harmful in cancer.

The vitamins in detail:

- vitamin A (retinol) and retinoids
- vitamin B group
- vitamin C (ascorbic acid)
- vitamin D (calciferol)
- vitamin E (tocopherol)
- vitamin K (phytomenadione).

Vitamin A (Retinol)

Occurrence

Retinol is a fat-soluble, oily liquid. It is present in dairy products such as milk, butter and cream, and in fish-liver oils. Beta-carotene, a substance which is closely allied to retinol and can be converted to retinol by the body, is found in carrots, green vegetables and liver.

Absorption, Function and Deficiency

The absorption of retinol is helped by the presence of fat and bile salts in the intestine. Retinol is concerned with maintaining the health of epithelium. Deficiency leads to keratinization of the epithelium of the nose and respiratory passage and to changes in the conjunctiva and in the cornea that may lead to blindness. Retinol is also concerned with the mechanism of dark adaptation by the retina and deficiency leads to night blindness.

Therapeutic Use

Retinol should be given in cases of deficiency causing night blindness or epithelial changes. The minimum human requirements in the adult are 2250 IU (international units) daily. The therapeutic dose is 50,000 IU.

Toxicity

Overdosage with retinol can produce liver damage, headache and vomiting. Fatalities have been reported. Pregnant and breastfeeding women are advised to avoid vitamin A supplements or liver products, as there is some evidence that excessive intake is associated with fetal defects.

Retinoids

These substances are related to vitamin A but are used for their effect on the skin.

Therapeutic Use of Retinoids

Retinoids are used mainly in the treatment of psoriasis and acne. **Isotretinoin** (*Roaccutane*), given orally, is used to treat severe acne. It dries and irritates the skin and mucous membranes, and in many countries including the UK, may only be prescribed by certain specialists. **Acitretin, alitretinoin (and also isotretinoin)**, given by mouth, cause some desquamation of the skin (the process in which the outer layer of the epidermis is removed by scaling). Their main indication is for severe psoriasis, but they are also used for keratinization disorders such as ichthyosis and Darier's disease (keratosis follicularis). **Tazarotene** is a retinoid in gel form that can be used for mild to moderate psoriasis. Skin irritation is common and may prevent continuation. **Tretinoin** and **adapalene** are retinoids that are used topically for the treatment of acne.

Adverse Effects and Precautions

Topical Application. Both tretinoin and adapalene may cause peeling of the skin and reddening when first used, but this effect usually disappears after a few days. All retinoids for topical use should be used sparingly and applied thinly to the skin. They should not be smeared over large areas of skin, especially if the acne is severe. Contact with broken or sunburned skin, mucous membranes, mouth, nose and eyes should be avoided, and patients who apply these should protect their skin from direct sunlight and not use ultraviolet (UV) lamps. In the UK, the drug licences require the use of highly effective contraception (progesterone only contraception not being considered adequate) for these drugs to be used. Research evidence does not support such a high risk of teratogenicity for topical use, but non-medical prescribers should respect drug licence restrictions, and pregnancy should be avoided, and the discussion of this with the patient should be recorded in the patient notes.

Oral Use. Patients taking retinoids orally should have regular tests of liver function and blood lipid concentrations. Patients taking retinoids orally may experience effects on epithelial tissues, such as sticky palms, cracked and dry lips, paronychia (whitlows), which is a painful swelling of the nail folds, and hair thinning. These are reversible effects. Neuropsychiatric reactions have been reported, and a history of depression is an important relative contraindication to using these drugs.

CLINICAL NOTE

Acne vulgaris is most common in the adolescent population and side-effects are reported to be the most common reason for non-adherence to treatment. Commonly reported side-effects are irritation, itching, erythema, scaling and stinging. These symptoms are common with acne and often patients discontinue treatment because they believe symptoms are worsening. The adolescent population should therefore be encouraged to report these symptoms, allowing alternatives to be considered if necessary.

Contraindications

Retinoids alter cell division and are teratogenic (cause fetal malformations). They must not therefore be used in pregnancy or during breastfeeding, especially when used orally, as the danger of possible teratogenicity can persist for years after stopping oral treatment with retinoids. With acitretin, for example, whose main indication is for psoriasis, it is recommended that patients with childbearing potential should cease taking the drug for 3 years before a planned pregnancy. In the UK and other countries, the regulations regarding the use of these drugs restrict their prescription to accredited specialists and require frequent and regular pregnancy tests before doses and after treatment has finished.

Vitamin B Group

The vitamin B group comprises:

- thiamine (vitamin B_1)
- riboflavin (vitamin B_2)
- nicotinic acid (niacin, nicotinamide, niacinamide)
- pyridoxine (vitamin B_6)
- cyanocobalamin (vitamin B_{12}).

Thiamine (Vitamin B_1)

Occurrence. Vitamin B_1 is a white crystalline solid, soluble in water. It is obtained from wheat germ, yeast, egg yolk, liver and some vegetables.

Function and Deficiency. Vitamin B_1 is essential for certain stages of carbohydrate metabolism. Deficiency of this vitamin leads to a nervous system disorder known as ***beriberi***. This deficiency may not only result from an inadequate intake of vitamin B_1, but may also occur in disturbances of metabolism in which requirements of vitamin B_1 are higher than normal, a good example being chronic alcoholism. Beriberi is characterized by heart failure and polyneuritis. The ***Wernicke–Korsakoff syndrome***, characterized by ataxia, vision changes and impaired memory and mainly seen in chronic alcoholics, is caused by thiamine deficiency. If not suspected and detected, it has a 20% mortality and 75% of survivors have permanent brain damage.

Therapeutic Use. Beriberi responds rapidly to vitamin B_1. Severe cases will require up to 100 mg daily by intramuscular injection; in milder cases, oral administration is satisfactory. Vitamin B_1 is also used in high doses in the polyneuritis of chronic alcoholism and in the Wernicke–Korsakoff syndrome. The minimum human requirement for adults is 2 mg daily. The normal therapeutic dose is 50 mg orally or intravenously daily.

Adverse Effects. Patients given parenteral thiamine should be observed afterwards in case of an anaphylactic reaction.

CLINICAL NOTE

People with excessive alcohol use, who are admitted to hospital should be prescribed thiamine either orally, or intravenously (NICE, 2010). When given intravenously it should be diluted in either saline or dextrose and given over 30 minutes. This reduces the incidence of adverse effects.

Vitamin B_2 (Riboflavin)

Occurrence. This vitamin is found in high levels in fish, egg yolks, cheese, meat, milk, poultry and whole grains.

Function and Deficiency. Vitamin B_2 is necessary for antibody production, red cell formation, cell respiration and growth. Deficiency in humans causes several symptoms, including cracking and fissures at the corner of the mouth and a sore tongue and skin lesions. The syndrome is called *ariboflavinosis*.

Therapeutic Use. Vitamin B_2 may be given in doses of 2 mg daily. Some sources recommend an increased intake of this vitamin when taking oral contraceptives or during periods of strenuous exercise. Vitamin B_2 is destroyed by light, alcohol and antibiotics.

Nicotinic Acid

Nicotinic acid is also called *niacin*. Some sources refer to it as vitamin B_3.

Occurrence. Nicotinic acid is found in high concentrations in brewer's yeast, dairy products and beef liver.

Function. Nicotinic acid is a derivative of pyridine, from which the pyridine nucleotides, building blocks of DNA and RNA, are derived. Nicotinamide is the amide of nicotinic acid and is a component of the ubiquitous coenzyme NAD (nicotinamide adenine dinucleotide). It is therefore vital for the proper functioning of many enzymes in the body. It is important in the production of hydrochloric acid in the stomach and is involved in the normal secretion of gastric and bile fluids. It has been claimed to lower cholesterol and aid circulation. It is needed for proper synthesis of the sex hormones and is important for normal operation of the nervous system.

Deficiency. Deficiency of nicotinamide leads to a disorder known as pellagra, which may occur in alcoholism and renal failure, as well as with deficient diets. This disease is characterized by the '3Ds' – namely, diarrhoea, dermatitis and dementia.

Therapeutic Use. Nicotinamide is available both in a 50 mg tablet and in cream form. The cream is used topically as a mild antiinflammatory for use in eczema and the tablets are used to treat nicotinamide deficiency.

Adverse Effects. It is worthwhile remembering that nicotinamide is also a vasodilator; thus, if it is taken in large doses, flushing and tingling of the face may occur. High doses can cause liver damage if taken for prolonged periods. Pregnant women and those suffering from diabetes, liver disease, gout, glaucoma or peptic ulcers should use nicotinic acid with caution and in any event should take medical advice before taking it.

Vitamin B_6 (Pyridoxine)

Occurrence. Pyridoxine occurs in all foods. High levels are found in brewer's yeast, walnuts, carrots, poultry, eggs, fish, meat, peas (not well cooked), wheat germ and sunflower seeds.

Function. Pyridoxine is involved in very many metabolic processes. It is required for normal functioning of the nervous system, including the brain. It is involved in red blood cell formation and for that of DNA and RNA. It is important in immune function and is part of the body's mechanisms to prevent atherosclerosis. It is required for healthy heart function since it blocks the formation of homocysteine, a toxic chemical that promotes the deposition of cholesterol around heart muscle.

Deficiency. Deficiency of pyridoxine causes:

- dry and flaking skin
- nausea and vomiting
- headache
- sore, shiny tongue (*atrophic glossitis*)
- cracked, sore angles of the mouth (*angular cheilitis*)
- Central nervous system symptoms, e.g. convulsions, difficulty with concentration, weak memory.

Other symptoms sometimes seen include acne and oily skin, anorexia, fatigue, hyperirritability, depression and impaired wound healing. Deficiency may be caused by use of some antidepressants, oral contraceptives and other oestrogen therapy. Severe deficiency may lead to a sideroblastic anaemia.

Therapeutic Use. Pyridoxine tablets for oral use are available and the dose for pyridoxine deficiency is 20–50 mg up to three times daily. It is sometimes used in the treatment of vomiting of pregnancy or following radiation. It can be used in doses of 10–20 mg daily to prevent the polyneuritis which rarely complicates the use of high-dose isoniazid, and it has been tried with varying success in the treatment of the premenstrual syndrome.

Adverse Effects. There is some evidence that high doses of pyridoxine can damage peripheral nerves and such doses should be avoided, particularly when pyridoxine is being used as a food supplement and not for a specific medical purpose.

Although the deficiency of vitamins in the B group have been discussed separately, it is common to find that deficiencies are often mixed and in treating patients who show evidence of vitamin B deficiencies, it is worth giving all the vitamins of the group. The vitamin B group are available in tablet form universally labelled as vitamin B complex. An inspection of the ingredients will reveal a much larger list than might be expected. Other ingredients include inositol, choline, para-aminobenzoic acid and pantothenic acid, often called vitamin B_5. Deficiency of these substances is very rare, and it is not clear if there is any benefit in adding them to the vitamin B complex tablets.

CLINICAL NOTE

High dose vitamin B complex is an important part of the management of patients with severe alcohol dependence, who are frequently very vitamin B deficient and have increased requirements for it.

Vitamin B_{12} is considered later, in the section on anaemias.

Vitamin C (Ascorbic Acid)

Occurrence and Function

Vitamin C is a crystalline solid, soluble in water. It is found in fresh fruits, particularly citrus fruit and blackcurrants, tomatoes and green vegetables. It is important to remember that vitamin C is relatively unstable and it is destroyed by boiling, especially in an alkaline solution. Vitamin C is not stored in the body and excess is excreted by the kidney. The implication of this is that regular intake is required, and megadoses (as are advocated by some health faddists) will be flushed down the toilet without any benefit. Vitamin C is necessary for the formation and maintenance of the connective tissue proteins, which literally hold organs together. Deficiency leads to a disorder known as scurvy.

Scurvy

Scurvy has been recognized for hundreds of years. It was particularly liable to attack mariners, who in the days of sailing ships were away from land for long periods and were thus deprived of fresh food and vegetables. Infants and children are also susceptible.

Scurvy is rarely seen in the UK at the present time, although it is occasionally found in people who for, *supposed* medical reasons, have been living on a self-imposed very restricted diet.

Scurvy is characterized by a tendency to bleed, due to increased capillary fragility. Haemorrhages occur into the skin and mucous membranes; sponginess and haemorrhage around the gums may be found in those with teeth. Bleeding also occurs under the periosteum of bones and into joints, producing great pain and tenderness; in time anaemia occurs. If vitamin C is not given, the disease is fatal.

Therapeutic Use

Scurvy is cured by giving vitamin C, the dose for adults being 500 mg daily. The bleeding is arrested and the anaemia, which is not entirely secondary to haemorrhage, is relieved. Vitamin C is also used in a number of other disorders, where it is of doubtful value; it does appear, however, to be useful in promoting the healing of wounds in those who, although showing no evidence of scurvy, have a mild degree of deficiency.

Very high doses of vitamin C are sometimes taken to treat colds. The balance of evidence suggests this to be ineffective. Requirements are, however, increased with prolonged exercise and illness.

Minimum Human Requirements

- Children 100 mg daily
- Adults 50 mg daily
- Pregnancy 200 mg daily
- Lactation 150 mg daily
- Therapeutic dose 500 mg daily.

Vitamin B and C Combination

The B vitamins and vitamin C have been combined into preparations to give emergency replacement after malabsorption due to, e.g. alcohol poisoning, postoperatively, after acute infection or in certain psychiatric conditions.

Pabrinex contains high doses of B and C vitamins and is given intravenously or intramuscularly. Rarely, it can cause a severe allergic reaction and infusion should be over at least 10 min, and facilities should be available for treating an acute allergic reaction.

Vitamin D

Occurrence and Function

This fat-soluble vitamin is found in fish-liver oils and dairy produce, but the main source is from the skin on exposure to sunlight. In summer, it is suggested that around 10–30 min of sunlight on the face and arms is sufficient to provide adequate amounts of vitamin D. The vitamin is most concerned with calcium

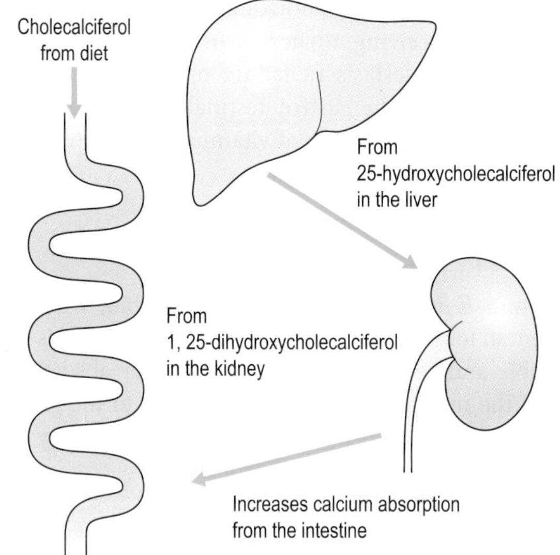

Fig. 11.1 ■ The changes undergone by cholecalciferol (vitamin D) in the body.

metabolism and bone formation. After absorption, it is modified in the liver to form 25-hydroxycholecalciferol, and undergoes further change in the kidney to form 1,25-dihydroxycholecalciferol (Fig. 11.1). This substance is highly active in facilitating calcium absorption from the gut and the laying down of calcium and phosphate during bone formation. The vitamin D receptor is widespread in the body, and it appears that vitamin D has many other varied effects, including immunomodulation and control of inflammation.

Deficiency

A deficiency of vitamin D leads to inadequate calcification of the bones, resulting in them becoming soft and easily deformed. When this disorder occurs in children it is known as rickets and these children with their bowed legs and deformed chests were a familiar sight in former times. With the arrival of cheap milk, cod liver oil and better care of young children it has now become rare, although there has been a reappearance of the disease in some ethnic groups. In adults, prolonged deprivation of vitamin D gives rise to a disorder similar to rickets. People with restricted diets and those who are not exposed to sunlight – particularly the housebound and people who cover their whole bodies while outside – are at risk of severe deficiency. People with dark pigmented skin are also more likely to be deficient in vitamin D. Minor degrees of insufficiency seem to be almost ubiquitous in populations living above 37 degrees North or below 37 degrees South of the equator. What, if any, effects these minor deficiencies have, and what, if any, benefit arises from correcting them, is uncertain. Several studies are underway attempting to answer these questions.

Vitamin D deficiency can also result from poor absorption from the intestine, as in coeliac disease, and from resistance to the action of vitamin D, which is found in renal failure, leading to stunting in children (renal rickets). Dietary recommendations have been set for at-risk groups, and currently the UK department of Health recommends low-dose daily supplementation for everyone through the autumn and winter.

Therapeutic Use

In therapeutic use, the term 'vitamin D' covers a range of substances that share the same essential properties. They include **ergocalciferol** (calciferol, vitamin D_2), **cholecalciferol** (vitamin D_3), **dihydrotachysterol**, **alfacalcidol** (1α-hydroxycholecalciferol) and **calcitriol** (1,25-dihydroxycholecalciferol). Because there are several different agents all sharing similar properties, but with differing potencies, it is often helpful to consider them in terms of their standardized biological activity, as International Units (IU) of activity. Cholecalciferol is the most commonly prescribed form of vitamin D.

Patients at risk of deficiency can be given 1 tablet containing 400 IU of vitamin D daily; 5000 IU of vitamin D daily is adequate for the treatment of established rickets.

As vitamin D is fat soluble and therefore stored in the body, deficiency can be treated by giving 3 capsules of 20,000 IU once a week for 6 weeks, to restore the body stores before low dose daily supplementation is started.

In coeliac disease, very large doses of vitamin D may be required at first, but these requirements diminish as the disease is controlled by diet. In chronic renal failure, vitamin D in the form of alfacalcidol is used. Active vitamin D in the form of **calcitriol cream** and the vitamin D analogues **calcipotriol** and **tacalcitol** are useful and well-tolerated topical treatments for mild to moderate psoriasis. Because of their vitamin

D-like effects and considerable systemic absorption, the total amount used each day needs to be controlled (see Chapter 24).

Adverse Effects

Overdose with vitamin D is rare, as the body is capable of storing large amounts of the vitamin. Long-term overuse leads to deposition of calcium in the kidneys and other organs and the production of some types of kidney stone. Patients receiving high doses of vitamin D over long periods should have their plasma calcium measured periodically.

Minimum Human Requirements

- Young children – 600 IU daily
- Adults – 400 IU daily
- Pregnancy and lactation – 1000 IU daily.

Alfacalcidol (1α-hydroxycholecalciferol) is closely related to vitamin D and is used to treat various disorders in which there is a resistance to the action of vitamin D – this is principally caused by kidney failure.

CLINICAL NOTE

Vitamin D supplementation has been linked to falls prevention in the elderly population living care facilities, and treatment should be considered in this population (Cameron et al., 2018).

Vitamin E (Tocopherol)

Occurrence and Function

Vitamin E is found in nuts, wheat germ, cold-pressed vegetable oils, dark-green leafy vegetables and brown rice. The daily requirements have not been fixed with certainty but are estimated to be in the region of 3–20 mg daily. It is an antioxidant, and on this basis, it has been suggested that it may reduce the incidence of cancer and vascular disease, prevent cell damage by inhibiting the oxidation of fats, and prevent the formation of free radicals. A number of other claims have been made, but following extensive investigation, the benefits of vitamin E and other antioxidants have not been established. One large trial of antioxidant supplements (including vitamin E) in patients with cancer was stopped when there was excess mortality in the group of patients receiving antioxidants, when compared to a group receiving a placebo. In children who have congenital cholestasis (a failure of normal amounts of bile to reach the gastrointestinal tract), there may be abnormally low levels of vitamin E associated with neuromuscular abnormalities.

Vitamin K (Phytomenadione)

Occurrence and Function

Vitamin K is a precursor of prothrombin, which is essential for the coagulation of blood. Vitamin K is fat-soluble and requires bile salts for proper absorption from the intestine. It is also synthesized in the gut by bacteria. After absorption, this vitamin is used by the liver for the synthesis of prothrombin.

Deficiency

Deficiency of vitamin K will lead to bleeding and may result from insufficient uptake due to various intestinal diseases or to deficient utilization following liver disease or anticoagulant drugs. In the newborn, there is a lack of vitamin K because it has not been synthesized by the gut bacteria and this may lead to bleeding (vitamin K deficiency bleeding (VKDB), previously known as haemorrhagic disease of the newborn). It is rare; about 1 in 10,000 births and can occur from birth up to a few months of age. About 30% of babies who develop it are left with mental impairment due to an intracranial bleed, and about 7% of babies with VKDB will die. It is more common in premature babies and in breastfed babies, as formula feeds contain vitamin K. It can be prevented by giving an injection of vitamin K at birth, which is the preferred method. Oral vitamin K can be given but is a course of 3 treatments required over 6 weeks and is therefore less likely to be completed. In the 1990s, an association was reported between the use of vitamin K injection in the newborn and an increased risk of later childhood leukaemia. This association has been extensively investigated and the conclusion is clear – **vitamin K injections do not cause childhood leukaemia**.

Trace Elements

Certain elements, including zinc, manganese, boron, cobalt and copper, exist in very small amounts in the body. They are essential for some important metabolic processes and deficiency can cause or contribute to several disorders. Adequate amounts are present in a full, normal diet but insufficiency can arise in those whose diet is severely restricted, or with malabsorption. Patients who are on total parenteral nutrition are especially at risk of deficiency and trace elements may be added to their intravenous infusion.

Patients who are poorly nourished and are about to undergo surgery may be given dietary supplements before operation. **Zinc** is thought to be of particular importance in aiding wound healing and improving immunity to infection. There is reasonable quality evidence that zinc supplements reduce the duration of the common cold, although there is uncertainty as to the ideal dose.

CLINICAL NOTE

Vitamin K is given either orally or intramuscularly; the intravenous route can cause anaphylaxis and hypotension. The effect of treatment should be monitored with prothrombin time measurements. People with vitamin K deficiency are at high risk of bleeding and blood products may be required in the event of a bleed.

Antioxidants

Antioxidants include some vitamins and other compounds, which are not usually classified as vitamins but are considered to be important constituents of the diet. Oxidation is a metabolic activity occurring in nearly all tissues and is necessary for life. It can, however, produce substances called 'free radicals', which are chemically very active and can damage constituents of cells. They are believed to play a part in the development of vascular diseases, cancer and, possibly, some other diseases. Antioxidants suppress the formation of free radicals and might, therefore, be expected to protect against these conditions.

Antioxidants are found in fruit and vegetables, and should form part of a healthy diet, but the consensus of research at present does not support the use of antioxidant supplements.

IRON DEFICIENCY ANAEMIA

Iron is an essential constituent of haemoglobin, which is contained in the erythrocytes in blood. Haemoglobin is concerned with the transport of oxygen from the lungs to the tissues. When the red cells break down, the

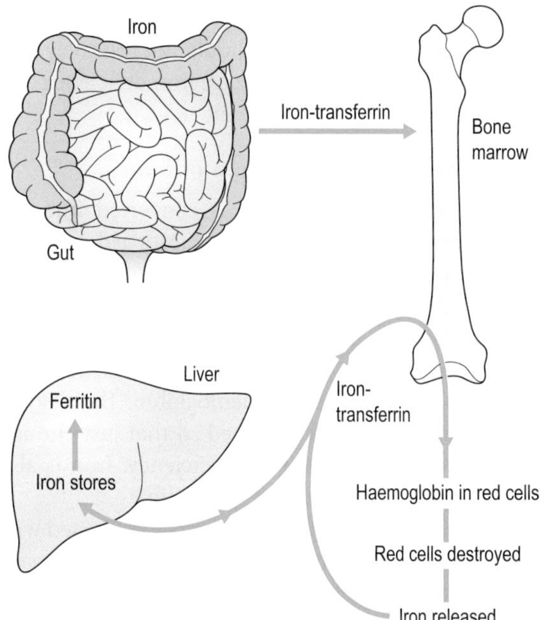

Fig. 11.2 ■ Metabolism of iron.

iron is retained by the body and built up again into further haemoglobin molecules. There is very little iron held in storage depots, the major portion being constantly in use (Fig. 11.2). A little iron, probably about 2 mg/day or less, is lost by desquamation of cells by the skin and gut, but the chief drain of iron from the body occurs in the various forms of blood loss, mostly menstruation or giving birth, or due to chronic bleeding, usually from the gastrointestinal tract. In pregnancy, the growing fetus requires a certain amount of iron, and during lactation, iron is lost in the mother's milk.

It can be seen, therefore, that although the average diet, which supplies about 25 mg of iron a day, is sufficient for most people, if there is any prolonged iron loss, a deficiency will occur. The result is anaemia, since not enough haemoglobin is produced. Typically, the blood count will show small red blood cells (*microcytosis*) with low intracellular haemoglobin (*hypochromic*). Measures of iron stores, such as ferritin, will be low. It is not unusual for women with relatively heavy periods to develop **iron deficiency anaemia**, and they may benefit from regular iron supplements. However, iron deficiency anaemia in men, and women who are not menstruating, requires further investigation to determine the cause – which may sometimes be serious, such as bowel cancer. Too much iron is harmful, leading to iron deposition in the liver, which may lead to liver damage. Most people should not routinely take iron supplements unless they have iron deficiency or a proven tendency for this to occur.

Absorption and Metabolism of Iron

Iron, when taken by mouth, is converted into the ferrous form in the stomach. It is absorbed from the upper part of the small intestine, forming a loose compound with a protein in the intestinal wall, which is called transferrin; in this form it is transported across to the bloodstream, where it is carried to the bone marrow for the synthesis of haemoglobin. The absorption of iron is carefully regulated so that just enough is absorbed to make good any deficiency. Iron is also stored in the liver in the form of ferritin.

Iron deficiency anaemia is sometimes associated with deficient secretion of hydrochloric acid by the stomach and this leads to a failure of release of ferrous iron from the diet. It can occur as a result of diseases of the intestine, which interfere with iron absorption. If a deficiency of iron occurs, less haemoglobin is synthesized and the amount of haemoglobin in the erythrocytes decreases.

Iron Preparations

Iron is given to correct a deficiency. It is usually given orally. The rise in blood haemoglobin level should be at least 0.7 g/dL per week and treatment should be continued for 4 months after the blood haemoglobin level has returned to normal to replace depleted iron stores. It is also given during pregnancy when the iron requirements increase.

Ferrous sulphate tablets are a satisfactory way of giving iron to most people. Ferrous salts are rapidly changed to ferric salts in the air and thus ferrous salts are given as coated tablets. The therapeutic dose is 200 mg, three times a day. In sensitive patients, ferrous sulphate may cause gastric discomfort and nausea or diarrhoea, or sometimes constipation. **Ferrous gluconate** is another ferrous salt. It is less irritating to the stomach than most ferrous salts. Ferrous glycine sulphate is a complex of ferrous sulphate and the amino acid glycine. It causes less gastrointestinal disturbances and is useful in sensitive patients.

Liquid preparations are also available, **sodium feredetate** (*Sytron*) and a **polysaccharide–iron complex** (*Niferex*) are satisfactory and do not stain the teeth. Although slow-release iron preparations can be used, they may be less effective, as iron absorption takes place in the upper small intestine, whereas these preparations release it lower down the gut.

Iron can also be given by intramuscular injection in those who are not absorbing iron satisfactorily. Before injecting iron, oral iron should be stopped for at least 72 h, as this appears to reduce the chances of a reaction after injection.

Iron sorbitol is an iron preparation for intramuscular injection. It is rapidly absorbed from the injection site. It contains 50 mg of iron/mL of solution. Side-effects appear slight, but shock-like reactions can occur and care must be taken when giving the injection, to prevent leakage along the needle track and subsequent staining of the skin.

CLINICAL NOTE

For maximum effect, iron supplements should be taken before food. As mentioned earlier, iron can cause constipation so advice to eat plenty of vegetables and fluids are important. Iron supplements may turn the stool black but this is a harmless side-effect. Iron supplements are dangerous in overdose. Children have suffered fatal overdose from eating shiny ferrous sulphate tablets, thinking them to be sweets. Parents should be warned to keep these supplements away from children, as they would with other drugs.

DRUGS USED TO TREAT OTHER ANAEMIAS

Cobalamins (Vitamin B_{12})

Source

There are several factors required for the proper maturation of the red cells. The best known of these is **cyanocobalamin** (vitamin B_{12}). It works together with folic acid to regulate the formation of red blood cells and promotes the utilization of iron. The principal dietary sources are milk, eggs, clams, herring, liver and kidney. Brewer's yeast is also rich in vitamin B_{12}.

Absorption of Vitamin B_{12}

In the normal person, a factor (the intrinsic factor) is produced by the stomach and is necessary for the

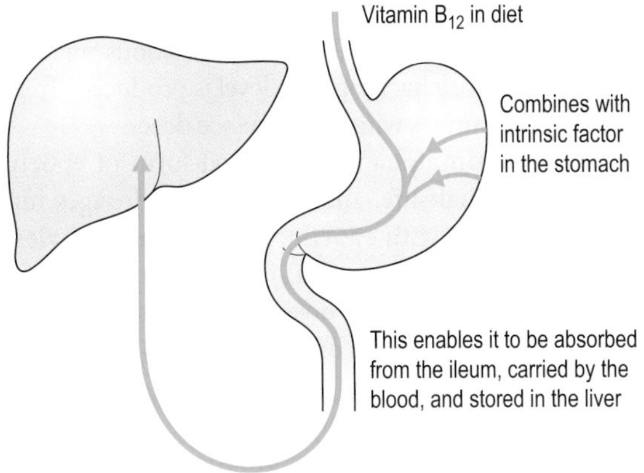
Vitamin B_{12} in diet
Combines with intrinsic factor in the stomach
This enables it to be absorbed from the ileum, carried by the blood, and stored in the liver

Fig. 11.3 ■ Absorption of vitamin B_{12}.

absorption of cobalamin in the intestine (Fig. 11.3). Intrinsic factor enables the stomach to actively absorb vitamin B_{12}, even when present in small amounts.

Deficiency of Vitamin B_{12}

Deficiency of vitamin B_{12} leads to a failure in production of erythrocytes. There is, therefore, a decrease in the number of circulating erythrocytes and those which do manage to mature appear abnormal, being large (*macrocytosis*) and irregular in shape and size. Primitive red blood cells may also appear in the blood.

In addition to the change in the blood, deficiency in cobalamin leads to glossitis (inflammation of the tongue) and degenerative changes in the nervous system. The anaemia produced by cyanocobalamin deficiency is known as **pernicious anaemia**. This deficiency is believed to be due to a failure to absorb cobalamin from the intestine as a result of a lack of the intrinsic factor. Failure to absorb cobalamin can also result from diseases of the intestine, and in those who have had ileostomy. Pernicious anaemia is common, and fatal if untreated. The most severe form of nervous system damage caused by vitamin B_{12} deficiency is known as *subacute combined degeneration of the cord*. It causes both sensory and motor changes, and at its worst can cause permanent paralysis. It can also occur in vitamin E deficiency and copper deficiency. It may be triggered by anaesthesia with nitrous oxide, in people with borderline vitamin B_{12} deficiency. It used to be thought that in combined B_{12} and folic acid deficiency (see later), the B_{12} deficiency should be treated first to prevent the precipitation of subacute combined degeneration. This is probably not the case, but treatment with folic acid may mask some of the symptoms of B_{12} deficiency and allow neurological damage to progress. It is important therefore, to check for and, if necessary, treat, both B_{12} and folic acid deficiency.

Treatment

The usual treatment is to give cobalamin by injection. **Hydroxocobalamin** is the only cobalamin in routine use, it is stable being highly bound by the plasma proteins so that it is excreted slowly and thus its action is prolonged. The use of an injection bypasses the stomach with its defective active absorption. An alternative approach is to give high doses of oral **cyanocobalamin** (1000 μg a day). Passive absorption through the stomach mucosa provides adequate concentrations of vitamin B_{12}. While effective, this regimen is rarely used and is not licensed in the UK.

Therapeutic Use

For pernicious anaemia and other macrocytic anaemias without neurological involvement, the BNF recommends 1 mg IM three times weekly for 2 weeks followed by 1 mg every 3 months. For pernicious anaemia and other macrocytic anaemias *with* neurological involvement, it recommends 1 mg on alternative days until there is no further improvement, followed by 1 mg every 2 months.

The lesions in the nervous system also respond to cobalamin, but it may be many months before the full effect of treatment is seen.

Vegans may develop vitamin B_{12} deficiency due to a shortage in the diet. Fortification of foods, or oral supplements are necessary.

Folic Acid

Sources

Folic acid (often called **folate**) is obtained from animal and vegetable sources and is also synthesized by gut bacteria. It is necessary for the maturation of red cells, and deficiency will produce changes in the blood similar to those found in pernicious anaemia.

Deficiency

The common causes of deficiency in this country are malabsorption syndromes such as coeliac disease and pregnancy. People on limited diets, particularly the housebound elderly, may develop folate deficiency.

Some women do not absorb folic acid in the later months of pregnancy and thus become anaemic. In addition, folic acid taken in the 3 months before pregnancy and for the first 3 months of pregnancy has been shown to reduce the incidence of neural tube defects, such as spina bifida. Iron deficiency is also common in pregnancy and both folic acid and iron supplements are often given throughout pregnancy.

Preparations

- Folic acid tablets
- Ferrous fumarate/folic acid tablets (*Pregaday*)

Therapeutic Use. Folic acid can be given orally in doses of 15 mg daily. Larger doses may be required in malabsorption states. Tablets containing both iron and folic acid are available for use in pregnancy. *Pregaday* contains ferrous fumarate equivalent to 100 mg of ferrous iron plus folic acid 350 µg, the dose being 1 tablet daily.

CLINICAL NOTE

If possible, a woman considering pregnancy should start taking folic acid (400 µg daily) before conception and for the first 3 months of pregnancy, to minimize the risk of neural tube defects, which occur very early in pregnancy. If a previous pregnancy resulted in a child with a neural tube defect, a dose of 5 mg of folic acid daily should be used, and continued for the first 3 months of pregnancy. There is also some evidence that the addition of folic acid to the diet reduces the incidence of cardiovascular disease.

Epoetins

Erythropoietin is a hormone manufactured by the kidney, which is necessary for erythrocyte formation. If the kidneys fail, the level of erythropoietin in the blood may fall, with resulting anaemia. Some cancer chemotherapy can also lead to anaemia and some epoetins are licensed to treat this problem. Use of epoetins in cancer patients not receiving chemotherapy is associated with increased risk of mortality, and should be avoided.

Preparations and Therapeutic Use

Epoetin is an analogue of erythropoietin. It is synthesized by recombinant DNA technology and four forms, alpha, beta, theta and zeta, are available commercially. They are very similar, but dosing frequency varies. In patients with renal failure and anaemia, epoetins alpha is given three times weekly by subcutaneous or intravenous injection until a satisfactory haemoglobin level is produced. Treatment then continues with maintenance doses.

Darbepoetin alpha is a modified form of epoetin with a longer half-life, and less frequent dosages may be required than with epoetin. **Methoxy polyethylene glycol-epoetin beta** (*Mircera*) is another modification that needs less frequent dosing. All these drugs are expensive, some are very expensive.

Adverse Effects. Hypertension is fairly common and may be severe. The blood pressure should be measured every week in the initial stages of treatment and then at 6-weekly intervals. Thrombosis and flu-like symptoms occasionally occur. Severe and dangerous skin reactions can occur, very rarely. Patients should be warned to stop treatment and seek advice if skin reactions occur. It is important to not overcorrect the haemoglobin level, as this may lead to thrombosis and other cardiovascular problems. Pure red cell aplasia can also occur, and so regular monitoring of full blood count is essential.

CLINICAL NOTE

Blood urea and phosphate and potassium concentrations need to be monitored during treatment, which will be standard monitoring practice in people with kidney disease. Rises in levels should be reported and acted upon.

Blood Growth Factors

Blood growth factors that stimulate the growth of white blood cells are now available and are especially useful in patients whose white cells have been depressed by cancer chemotherapy, immunosuppression or treatments associated with HIV infection:

- **Human granulocyte colony-stimulating factor (filgrastim, lenograstim, lipegfilgrastim and pegfilgrastim)**, given by subcutaneous or intravenous injection, increases the production of neutrophils.

The use of these factors has considerably improved the treatment of a wide range of serious diseases in which it is necessary to suppress, temporarily, the white blood cell count to achieve a satisfactory therapeutic effect. They accelerate the recovery of the bone marrow and thereby decrease the risk of serious infection that accompanies leukopenia.

SUMMARY

- Vitamin A overdose can be toxic, and even fatal.
- Retinoids are teratogenic and potentially toxic and should be used only under the supervision of a specialist.
- It is advisable to wait at least 3 years after taking retinoids such as acitretin before a planned pregnancy.
- High doses of pyridoxine may cause damage to peripheral nerves.
- Always check for both B_{12} and folate deficiency, and treat both deficiencies.
- Vitamin C is destroyed by heat; vegetables, especially leafy vegetables, should be eaten raw or very lightly cooked.
- Iron sorbitol: shock-like reactions can occur when giving iron sorbitol citrate intramuscularly, and care must be taken when giving the injection, to prevent leakage along the needle track and subsequent staining of the skin.
- Folic acid taken early in pregnancy reduces the incidence of neural tube defects.

NURSING NOTE

All vitamin and over-the-counter preparations should be documented within the patient notes to ensure there is a full medication history and drug–drug interactions can be identified early. All allergies to over-the-counter preparations should also be documented.

REFERENCES AND FURTHER READING

Cameron, I.D., Dyer, S.M., Panagoda, C.E., 2018. Interventions for preventing falls in older people in care facilities and hospitals. Cochrane Database Syst. Rev. 9, CD005465.

Critical Care Nursing, 2009. Anaemia, Iron Deficiency. Nursing Times [online]. https://www.nursingtimes.net/archive/anaemia-iron-deficiency-06-02-2009.

Diez-Sampedro, A., Olenick, M., Maltseva, T., Flowers, M., 2019. A gluten-free diet, not an appropriate choice without a medical diagnosis. J. Nutr. Metab. 2019, 2438934.

Heinlein, C., 2013. Teaching Patients about Vitamin and Mineral Supplements. American Nurse Today. https://www.myamericannurse.com/teaching-patients-about-vitamin-and-mineral-supplements.

Kolli, S.S., 2019. Topical retinoids in acne vulgaris: a systematic review. Am. J. Clin. Dermatol. 20 (3), 345–365.

NICE, 2010. Alcohol-use Disorders: Diagnosis and Management of Physical Complications [CG100]. https://www.nice.org.uk/guidance/cg100/chapter/recommendations#wernickes-encephalopathy.

Ortet-Walker, A., Ponsford, A., McIntosh, B., 2019. Communicating with patients using a new vitamin B12 deficiency leaflet. Br. J. Nursing 28 (22), 1450–1454.

Sevimli Dikicier, B., 2019. Topical treatment of acne vulgaris: efficiency, side effects, and adherence rate. J. Int. Med. Res. 47 (7), 2987–2992.

USEFUL WEBSITES

BNF. Treatment summary: Anaemia, iron deficiency. https://bnf.nice.org.uk/treatment-summary/anaemia-iron-deficiency.html.

Clinical Knowledge Summaries: Anaemia – B12 and folate deficiency. https://cks.nice.org.uk/topics/anaemia-b12-folate-deficiency.

Clinical Knowledge Summaries: Anaemia – iron deficiency. https://cks.nice.org.uk/topics/anaemia-iron-deficiency.

NetDoctor. Vitamins and minerals: functions, benefits and doses. https://www.netdoctor.co.uk/healthy-eating/a10801/vitamins-and-minerals-what-do-they-do.

12 DRUGS AFFECTING THE KIDNEY

CHAPTER OUTLINE

LEARNING OBJECTIVES

At the end of this chapter, the reader should be able to:

- give a definition of diuretics
- list the factors that cause fluid retention
- describe the basic sites of diuretic action in the nephron
- list the main classes of currently used diuretics
- explain the mechanism of action and uses of the diuretic drugs
- enumerate the risk factors associated with diuretics and potassium loss
- state the three examples of potassium-sparing diuretics
- explain the dangers associated with diuretic use in patients with liver cirrhosis and in elderly patients

INTRODUCTION TO DIURETICS

Diuretics are drugs that cause increased urine production. They are useful in patients who are suffering from retention of water and sodium chloride (salt), which usually accumulates in the tissue spaces, and is called 'oedema'. Peripheral oedema commonly causes swollen ankles, feet and legs. Note that diuretics are not used in patients who cannot empty their bladders; this is called 'urinary retention'. This is treated through the use of a urinary catheter which is passed through the urethra and placed into the patient's bladder. The catheter is attached externally to a urine bag or a catheter valve to collect or drain the urine from the body.

Oedema

Oedema occurs most commonly in heart failure, nephrotic syndrome (severe loss of protein in the urine) and cirrhosis of the liver. Ankle oedema may also develop in individuals sitting with their legs dependent, a common example being elderly people who are confined to their chairs for long periods. It can also complicate the use of calcium channel blockers (see Chapter 6). Blood clots and infection can also present with peripheral oedema. Therefore, a thorough clinical assessment should be undertaken to elicit the cause of the oedema prior to initiating the treatment.

Factors Causing Fluid Retention

The factors that cause fluid retention are various and depend on the underlying disease. They include:

- **Lowered cardiac output** and underfilling of the vascular system (hypovolaemia), which activates the renin–angiotensin system with subsequent increased secretion of aldosterone by the adrenal cortex, leading to salt and water retention by the kidney. This occurs in patients with heart failure, cirrhosis of the liver or the nephrotic syndrome.
- **Raised pressure in the veins and capillaries.** This leads to increased exudation of fluid from the blood into the tissue spaces, and occurs in patients with heart failure, liver cirrhosis, or oedema due to prolonged immobility with legs dependent.
- **Low plasma proteins.** This is found in patients with the nephrotic syndrome, where it is due to protein loss in the urine, and in patients with cirrhosis of the liver, where there is a failure to make protein.

Renal Function

The role of the kidney is to excrete the waste products of metabolism, drugs, etc. and maintain the correct amounts of water and electrolytes in the body by getting rid of any excesses that may be absorbed or produced by the body. This happens in two stages (Fig. 12.1):

- Glomerular filtration
- Tubular reabsorption.

Glomerular Filtration. At the glomeruli, water, along with soluble substances, is filtered from the blood. The volume of this filtrate is about 100 L of water per day and it contains glucose, electrolytes, urea and other substances.

Tubular Reabsorption. In the renal tubules a selective reabsorption occurs. Glucose is normally completely reabsorbed. Water and electrolytes (including sodium, potassium, chloride and hydrogen carbonate) are partially reabsorbed, whereas urea is almost entirely excreted. The exact amount of each substance finally excreted in the urine is carefully controlled, so that the composition of the body fluids remains constant.

DIURETIC DRUGS

All diuretic drugs produce their effect by decreasing the reabsorption of water and electrolytes by the renal tubules and thus allowing more water and electrolytes

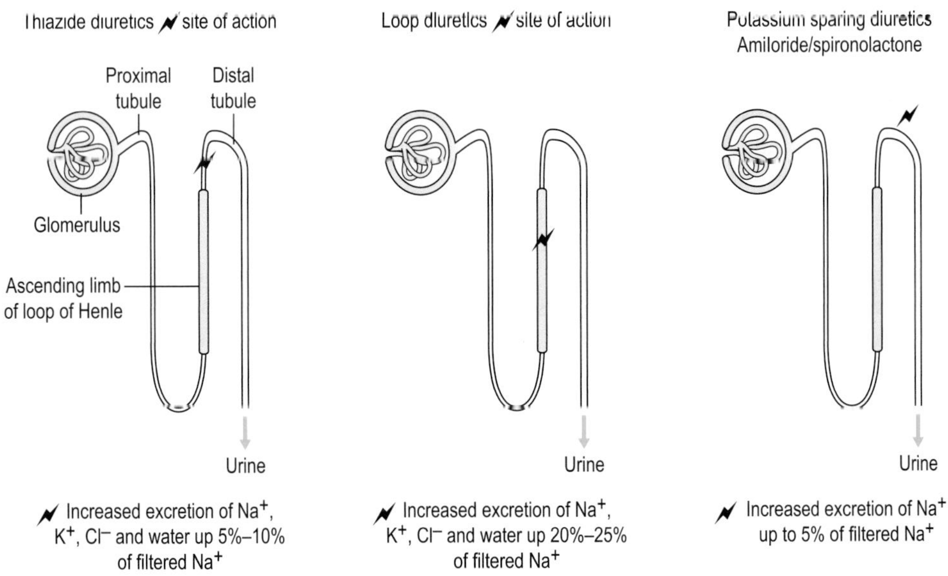

Fig. 12.1 ■ Sites of action of diuretics.

to be excreted. The diuretic drugs fall into various classes, depending on their site and mechanism of action:

- Osmotic diuretics
- Thiazide diuretics
- Loop diuretics
- Potassium-sparing diuretics.

Water

It is common experience that, in a normal person, increased ingestion of water results in an increased urine flow. When water is absorbed, it causes the plasma to become more dilute and this in turn decreases the release of antidiuretic hormone (ADH) by the posterior lobe of the pituitary gland (see Chapter 14). Less ADH reaches the kidney and this causes the tubules to reabsorb less water, so that more is excreted as the urine. In patients with fluid retention, e.g. in heart failure, the normal response to water disappears and so it is of no use as a diuretic under these circumstances.

Osmotic Diuretics

Any substance that passes through the glomeruli and is not reabsorbed by the renal tubules will increase the concentration of the urine within the tubules. This prevents the reabsorption of sodium chloride and water from the tubules back into the blood, and the water is then passed out to produce a diuresis. A commonly used example is **mannitol**.

Mechanism of Action. The osmotic diuretics are filtered by the glomerulus and increase the osmotic pressure in the tubules. This inhibits the passive reabsorption of water from the tubules. Water is normally able to pass back into the body from the proximal tubule, the descending limb of the loop of Henle and from the collecting ducts, which are therefore the sites of action of the osmotic diuretics. Some sodium is lost as well, but not enough to make the osmotic diuretics useful in conditions associated with salt retention.

The osmotic diuretics must meet certain criteria for use:

- They must be otherwise pharmacologically inert
- They must be freely filterable by the glomerulus
- They must not be reabsorbed from the tubules.

Mannitol

Administration and Therapeutic Uses. Mannitol and other osmotic diuretics are usually given intravenously and are sometimes used:

- During cardiovascular surgical procedures when urine flow through the kidneys needs to be maintained
- To lower raised intracranial pressure after a head injury or in a patient with a cerebral tumour
- To reduce the intraocular pressure in patients with glaucoma.

Adverse Effects. These include headache, nausea and vomiting. Osmotic diuretics can cause pulmonary oedema or heart failure in patients who are unable to produce urine.

CLINICAL NOTE

Repeated doses of mannitol can result in urea and electrolyte imbalances and frequent monitoring of levels is important if this diuretic is prescribed. Please refer to local protocols for guidance on frequency of monitoring.

Thiazide Diuretics

Thiazide diuretics comprise:

- **Bendroflumethiazide**
- **Indapamide**
- **Metolazone**
- **Xipamide**
- **Chlortalidone.**

There are several diuretic drugs in this group. Although there are marginal differences in their actions, the general pattern of their effects is the same and they will be described together. They are all absorbed from the intestinal tract and are therefore effective after oral administration. Drugs containing hydrochlorothiazide are now not commonly used following MHRA advice (November 2018) as they are associated with an increased risk of non-melanoma skin cancer development particularly in long-term use (MHRA, 2018).

Mechanism of Action

The actions of thiazide diuretics on the kidney are:

- They interfere with the reabsorption of salt and water by the early distal tubules, by binding to, and inhibiting a sodium chloride pump: thus, less sodium chloride is reabsorbed and the salt together with accompanying water passes out of the tubules and causes a diuresis.
- There is an increased excretion of potassium by the kidney (see more on potassium secretion later). This takes place because sodium is normally reabsorbed in the collecting ducts in exchange for potassium; therefore, the more sodium is presented to the collecting ducts, the more will be exchanged for potassium, which is then excreted.

Therapeutic Uses

The therapeutic uses of thiazide diuretics are in the treatment of:

- Mild cardiac failure
- Hypertension
- Cirrhosis of the liver with ascites (accumulation of fluid in the peritoneal cavity)
- Nephrotic syndrome
- Prevention of renal stone formation in idiopathic hypercalciuria.

Mild Cardiac Failure. The thiazides are used to treat the oedema associated with cardiac failure. They are not very powerful diuretics and their use is usually confined to mild failure. They are given in the morning as the diuresis lasts throughout the day.

Hypertension. The thiazides also have some blood pressure lowering action and therefore may be used for this purpose, either alone or with other hypotensive drugs. This is not only due to their diuretic action; they also act as mild vasodilators. For this purpose, small doses of thiazides, e.g. bendroflumethiazide, may be used. Potassium supplements are not usually required. In the chronic treatment of hypertension with thiazides, blood pressure stays down even after the diuretic action ceases, and this may be due, at least in part, to the vasodilator action of the thiazides. Indapamide and chlortalidone are the preferred diuretic choices in the treatment of hypertension.

Cirrhosis of the Liver with Ascites. The thiazides will produce a diuresis in patients with this condition, with reduction in the ascites and oedema. Care is required, however, as their use may be followed by mental changes with disorientation, which it is believed is due to the potassium deficiency produced by these drugs.

Nephrotic Syndrome. The thiazides can be used to treat the oedema associated with this condition. Frequently, however, a more powerful diuretic will be required, e.g. a loop diuretic such as furosemide (see later).

Prevention of Renal Stone Formation in Patients with Idiopathic Hypercalciuria. The term *idiopathic* refers to a condition, the cause of which is unknown and which may arise spontaneously. Hypercalciuria is elevated calcium excretion, and calcium salts may be deposited in the kidney as stones that need to be dissolved and flushed out.

Chlortalidone is very similar to the other thiazides in terms of onset and site of action, but it has a more prolonged action. **Metolazone** is a thiazide, which generally has no advantage over others in the group, but it can produce a significant diuresis when other thiazides have become ineffective. It may be combined with a loop diuretic (see later), particularly in patients with impaired renal function. As a result of a profound diuresis, particularly in combination with a loop diuretic, the patient would require close monitoring.

Adverse Effects

Generally speaking, the thiazide diuretics are well-tolerated, have a high therapeutic index, and adverse effects are relatively uncommon. These may include:

- hyperglycaemia
- metabolic alkalosis
- in diabetics, thiazides can actually reduce urine flow
- potassium loss: thiazides have in the past been prescribed together with potassium chloride
- increased uric acid secretion and can induce gout

- photosensitivity: patients on thiazides should consider using a sun block when in direct sunlight.

Loop Diuretics

The loop diuretics are the most powerful of the diuretics. They are called 'loop diuretics' because they act on the ascending limb of the loop of Henle (see Fig. 12.1). The main examples are:

- **furosemide**
- **bumetanide**
- **torasemide.**

Mechanism of Action

This group of diuretics is far more powerful than the thiazides. The loop of Henle is impermeable to water, but is anatomically where much of the sodium chloride is usually reabsorbed into the body. Loop diuretics therefore interfere to a greater extent, than do the thiazides, with the reabsorption of salt and water and are the most powerful of all the diuretics. They are sometimes referred to as 'high ceiling' diuretics. Like thiazides, these diuretics also increase renal excretion of potassium. This is because a lot of sodium is presented to the collecting ducts, where sodium is normally reabsorbed in exchange for potassium.

Administration, Distribution and Metabolism

The loop diuretics are well absorbed from the gastrointestinal tract and can therefore be given orally; they can also be administered IV. These drugs will act within 1 h after oral administration and their diuretic effect will peak within 30 min following IV injection. The duration of action of the loop diuretics after oral administration is relatively short (3–6 h). **Torasemide** is the longest acting and is taken orally once a day.

In the blood, loop diuretics are strongly bound to plasma proteins. This prolongs their action because only the unbound fraction of the drug can be metabolized in the liver. They are not filtered by the glomerulus and reach their site of action in the ascending loop by being pumped into the tubular lumen in the proximal tubule, and after exerting the diuretic action, are excreted in the urine. The fraction of drug not secreted into the lumen is ultimately metabolized in the liver.

Clinical Use of Loop Diuretics

Loop diuretics are used in the treatment of:

- salt and water overload due to:
  - oedema caused by chronic heart failure
  - nephrotic syndrome
  - renal failure
  - hepatic cirrhosis complicated by ascites
- resistant hypertension, especially in patients with renal impairment
- acute treatment of hypercalcaemia.

Furosemide

Furosemide is probably the most commonly used loop diuretic and is especially useful in the treatment of patients with:

- Acute left ventricular failure with oedema of the lungs. Given intravenously, furosemide rapidly clears the oedema and pulmonary congestion. In these circumstances, it also has a vasodilating action that relieves the load on the heart.
- Patients with congestive heart failure that is no longer responding to other diuretics.
- Oedema associated with the nephrotic syndrome, especially if there is some degree of renal failure. In these cases, very large oral doses are sometimes used.
- Large doses may be given when acute renal failure is developing, to try and jolt the kidneys into resuming normal function.

Bumetanide

This powerful diuretic is similar to furosemide in its pharmacological action, although it is distinct chemically. It is given orally and produces a rapid diuresis lasting about 3 h. For an even more immediate effect it may be given intravenously. Its therapeutic uses and adverse effects are similar to those of furosemide.

When a patient's kidney function is *normal* a 40 mg dose of furosemide is equivalent to 1 mg bumetanide and 20 mg of torsemide. However, this dose equivalence changes when there is *impaired* kidney function, to 20 mg furosemide to 1 mg bumetanide, due to an increase in bumetanide clearance (Brater and Ellison, 2019).

Adverse Effects of Loop Diuretics

Some of these adverse effects are similar to those of the thiazides:

- Hypokalaemia (decreased plasma potassium) due to increased potassium loss by the kidneys; it is more marked with high doses of diuretics (see later)
- Sodium depletion: with large doses of loop diuretics, particularly when given intravenously. The patient's blood volume may be reduced rapidly, causing hypotension and collapse. This can also occur with prolonged oral treatment
- A large and rapid diuresis can precipitate acute urine retention in those with prostatic enlargement
- Large doses of furosemide can cause transient deafness
- Furosemide has been reported to cause photosensitivity.

Drug Interactions that can Occur when Treating with Thiazides and Loop Diuretics

Thiazides and loop diuretics can exhibit a number of drug interactions including:

- Non-steroidal antiinflammatory drugs (NSAIDs) and steroids reduce the efficacy of these diuretics
- lithium retention (see Chapter 22)
- renal damage when combined with gentamicin
- increased digoxin toxicity due to hypokalaemia
- hypotension when used with angiotensin-converting enzyme (ACE) inhibitors.

CLINICAL NOTE

Adverse drug reactions in the elderly as a result of diuretics are common. In one study of 106 adverse drug reactions, it accounted for 30% and was the most frequently reported (Ognibene et al., 2018). These can be minimized by maintaining the patient on the lowest possible dose for greatest therapeutic effect. If an elderly person taking diuretics develops diarrhoea and/or vomiting it is sometimes wise to stop the diuretic temporarily to prevent undue water and salt loss. This may reduce the incidence of hospital admission and adverse events due to diuretics.

Diuretics and Potassium Depletion

Both the thiazides and loop diuretics cause loss of potassium through the kidneys and if the plasma potassium is lowered excessively (>3.0 mmol/L) there is a risk of dangerous cardiac arrhythmias. This rarely occurs in patients receiving small doses of diuretics for the treatment of hypertension or heart failure and usually the plasma potassium level is checked within 2 weeks after the start of treatment. Note that indapamide does not appreciably affect potassium or uric acid excretion.

Risk Factors

The following risk factors may require more careful monitoring and some form of potassium replacement:

- large doses of diuretics
- poor diet, especially in the elderly
- concurrent use of digitalis – the toxicity of digitalis is increased by potassium deficiency
- immediately following myocardial infarction – low plasma potassium is associated with an increased risk of dangerous arrhythmias
- patients with cirrhosis of the liver are particularly sensitive to potassium depletion
- concurrent use of steroids increases potassium loss.

In all these patients, the plasma potassium should be monitored and replacement started if depletion occurs. This may be achieved using:

- potassium supplements
- potassium-sparing diuretics (see later).

Potassium supplements should be given in the form of potassium chloride. Unfortunately, this substance can cause nausea and can cause ulceration of the gut if given in tablet form. It is therefore formulated as:

- effervescent potassium chloride tablets (*Sando-K*)
- slow-release potassium chloride tablets (*Slow-K*).

Potassium can also be given by IV infusion if depletion is severe. This can be a dangerous procedure, however, as hyperkalaemia from too rapid infusion can cause cardiac arrest. Careful monitoring of plasma potassium is therefore mandatory.

Potassium-sparing Diuretics

Triamterene and Amiloride

These drugs increase the excretion of salt and water without producing appreciable potassium loss. Neither drug is a potent diuretic, and they are usually given with a reduced dose of a more potent diuretic that does cause potassium loss.

Mechanism of Action. It is thought that potassium sparing diuretic drugs work by a direct action on the renal tubules. Amiloride antagonizes the action of aldosterone on the renal tubule by binding to the sodium channels where aldosterone, the salt-retaining hormone, exerts its actions (see Chapter 17). This increases sodium and water excretion with some potassium retention. Triamterene may have the same mechanism of action.

Administration and Absorption. Both triamterene and amiloride are administered orally. Triamterene is well absorbed from the gastrointestinal tract, whereas amiloride is poorly absorbed. The effect of triamterene is evident within 2 h, and lasts up to 15–16 h, whereas that of amiloride is evident within 6 h, and lasts about 24 h.

Clinical Use. A thiazide or a loop diuretic can be combined with a potassium-sparing diuretic in 1 tablet to prevent potassium loss. *Co-Amilofruse* is an example of a preparation available in the UK, which is a combination of furosemide and amiloride hydrochloride.

Adverse Effects. Hyperkalaemia can occur in patients with impaired renal function and those taking ACE inhibitors or supplemental potassium. These preparations are effective and reduce potassium loss, but it must be remembered that the combination drugs have the potential to elicit the adverse effects of both pharmacologically active constituents. In the case of co-amilozide, both sodium depletion and potassium retention can occur, particularly in elderly patients.

Spironolactone

Spironolactone is an antagonist of aldosterone at its receptor site inside the tubule cell. Aldosterone is released from the cortex of the adrenal gland in response to a fall in blood volume and in emergency situations such as blood loss resulting from haemorrhage (see also Chapter 17). It is a sodium-retaining hormone at the expense of potassium, and if sodium is retained, then water is retained with it. Therefore, if aldosterone is blocked, sodium is lost, taking water with it, and less potassium is excreted.

Administration, Absorption and Clinical Use. Spironolactone is given orally and is well absorbed from the gastrointestinal tract. It has a very short half-life in the circulation (about 10 min), but is converted into an active metabolite called **canrenone**, which has a half-life of about 16 h. Therefore, spironolactone is a prodrug. The diuretic effect has a very slow onset, and may not be observed for some days after administration. **Potassium canrenoate** has been prepared and is administered by injection, it is indicated for oedema in heart failure and in ascites in neonates and children. However, it is not licensed for use in the UK. Spironolactone, when used, is often combined with other diuretics.

Adverse Effects. These are rare, but may include:

- *Hyper*kalaemia, especially if spironolactone is used on its own. Spironolactone should be discontinued in the presence of hyperkalaemia, which is to prevent serious cardiac arrhythmias. To help reduce this complication, e.g. in the use of resistant hypertension (unlicensed use) NICE (2019) recommends a low dose spironolactone only if the blood potassium level is below 4.5 mmol/L. Potassium supplements should also be avoided in patients taking spironolactone to reduce the risk of hyperkalaemia
- Metabolic acidosis
- Risk of carcinogenicity if used in the long term (e.g. in treating hypertension)
- Skin rashes
- Oestrogenic effects, e.g. gynaecomastia (breast enlargement in the male), testicular atrophy and menstrual disorders.

Drug Interactions

Supplementary potassium or potassium-sparing diuretics should not normally be combined with ACE inhibitors, as this causes potassium retention by the kidneys and can be dangerous.

CLINICAL NOTE

All clinicians should be aware of the categories of diuretics. These medications affect patients' blood results, blood pressure and observations. Knowledge of these categories makes it easier to assess a patient and be aware of interventions that may be needed when caring for a patient on a diuretic. Frequent review of medicines considering whether it is necessary to continue is important as frequently they can be stopped with no adverse effects (van Kraaij et al., 2000).

Diuretics in Patients with Cirrhosis of the Liver

In such cases, diuretics carry serious risks of hypokalaemia and hypotension, leading to renal failure. It is best to start with spironolactone and then add a thiazide or loop diuretic cautiously a few days later. All drugs causing fluid retention (e.g. NSAIDs) should be avoided in such patients.

Diuretics in Elderly Patients

For various reasons, not always sound, one in five people over 65 take diuretics, and they are possibly the commonest cause of adverse reactions in elderly people. These adverse effects are the same as those that occur in younger subjects, but are more severe and may have serious consequences. The most important is sodium depletion, which leads to a marked fall in blood pressure, particularly on standing, causing faints, falls and confusion. As in other age groups, disturbances of potassium and uric acid metabolism also occur.

CLINICAL NOTE

Swollen ankles in the elderly do not necessarily call for a diuretic – they may be due to sitting in a chair all day. Patients who have sat with their legs in one place should be encouraged to mobilize or wear pressure stockings as required.

The best way to monitor the efficiency of a diuretic is to weigh the patient regularly; if strict fluid monitoring is needed, weighing the patient daily at the same time is essential. Fluid balance charts are not always accurate, but can be improved with the cooperation of the patient. Before leaving the hospital, the timing of diuretic dosage must be tailored to the patient's daily programme.

Acetazolamide

As a diuretic, acetazolamide is largely of historical interest only. Acetazolamide suppresses the activity of the enzyme carbonic anhydrase, which is present in the renal tubule and the eye. In the kidney, this prevents the reabsorption of sodium and water from the tubules, and thus causes a diuresis. It is a poor diuretic, as its effect is short-lived and it is not now used for this purpose. Acetazolamide increases hydrogen carbonate excretion and thus creates a metabolic acidosis. This limits its action, as the body reacts by limiting hydrogen carbonate loss and the diuretic action of acetazolamide is lost.

Other Uses of Acetazolamide

In the eye, acetazolamide reduces the formation of aqueous humour through the inhibition of carbonic anhydrase, and it is useful in lowering the intraocular pressure in glaucoma (see Chapter 31). Acetazolamide will also help relieve mountain sickness. Hyperventilation, which occurs at high altitude, 'washes out' carbon dioxide from the lungs and causes increased alkalinity of the blood. By increasing the excretion of hydrogen carbonate (alkali) by the kidneys, acetazolamide helps to correct this disorder.

MAKING URINE ALKALINE

It may be necessary to render the urine alkaline (e.g. to enhance aspirin excretion after overdosage; see also Chapter 33). Sodium citrate is the substance most commonly used to make the urine alkaline and is usually given every 2 or 4 h. Sodium hydrogen carbonate is often combined with sodium citrate and acts in a similar fashion.

SUMMARY

- Diuretics are not used to treat urinary retention caused by, e.g. benign prostatic hyperplasia.
- Swollen ankles, especially in the elderly, are not always due to oedema.
- Osmotic diuretics are of little or no use in conditions associated with salt retention.
- Osmotic diuretics can be dangerous in patients who are unable to produce urine.
- Thiazides can inhibit urine flow in diabetic patients and may induce hyperglycaemia.

- Patients on thiazides and loop diuretics should avoid bright sunlight or wear sunglasses and apply sunblocks.
- Diuretics such as thiazides and loop diuretics can cause cognitive disturbance in patients with liver cirrhosis, due to potassium loss.
- Potassium loss due to diuretics can increase the toxicity of digoxin.
- Check elderly patients carefully for adequate diet when prescribing potassium-losing drugs.
- Potassium loss is increased if patients are on antiinflammatory steroids.
- Patients with impaired renal function taking ACE inhibitors or those on supplemental potassium can develop hyperkalaemia (raised plasma potassium), which is dangerous, especially in patients with heart conditions.
- Spironolactone can cause oestrogenic effects, and there is risk of carcinogenicity with prolonged use.
- Weight measurement is useful in monitoring patients on diuretics.
- It may be prudent to stop diuretics temporarily, especially in elderly patients, if diarrhoea or vomiting occurs, to limit salt and water loss.

REFERENCES AND FURTHER READING

Brater, C., Ellison, D.H., 2019. Loop Diuretics: Dosing and Major Side Effects. UpToDate. https://www.uptodate.com/contents/loop-diuretics-dosing-and-major-side-effects.

Burgess, S., Abu-Laban, R.B., Slavik, R.S., et al., 2016. A systematic review of randomized controlled trials comparing hypertonic sodium solutions and mannitol for traumatic brain injury: implications for emergency department management. Ann. Pharmacother. 50 (4), 291–300.

Estridge, K.M., Morris, D.L., Kolcaba, K., Winkelman, C., 2018. Comfort and fluid retention in adult patients receiving hemodialysis. Nephrol. Nurs. J. 45 (1), 25–60.

MHRA, 2018. Hydrochlorothiazide: risk of non-melanoma skin cancer, particularly in long-term use. https://www.gov.uk/drug-safety-update/hydrochlorothiazide-risk-of-non-melanoma-skin-cancer-particularly-in-long-term-use.

NICE, 2019. Hypertension in Adults: Diagnosis and Management [NG136]. https://www.nice.org.uk/guidance/ng136.

Ognibene, S., Vazzana, N., Giumelli, C., et al., 2018. Hospitalisation and morbidity due to adverse drug reactions in elderly patients: a single-centre study. Intern. Med. J. 48 (10), 1192–1197.

Psaty, B.M., Lumley, T., Furberg, C.D., et al., 2003. Health outcomes associated with various antihypertensive therapies used as first-line agents: a network meta-analysis. J. Am. Med. Assoc. 289 (19), 2534–2544.

Redman, A., McClelland, H., 2006. Chronic kidney disease: risk factors, assessment and nursing care. Nurs. Stand. 21 (10), 48–55.

Seo, W., Oh, H., 2010. Alterations in serum osmolality, sodium, and potassium levels after repeated mannitol administration. J. Neurosci. Nurs. 42 (4), 201–207.

Stolt, M., Suhonen, R., Puukka, P., et al., 2012. Foot health and self-care activities of older people in home care. J. Clin. Nurs. 21 (21/22), 3082–3095.

van Kraaij, D.J.W., Jansen, R.W.M.M., Gribnau, F.W.J. et al., 2000. Diuretic therapy in elderly heart failure patients with and without left ventricular systolic dysfunction. Drugs Aging. 16, 289–300.

USEFUL WEBSITES

Kidney Research UK. https://kidneyresearchuk.org.

MHRA. Hydrochlorothiazide: risk of non-melanoma skin cancer, particularly in long-term use. https://www.gov.uk/drug-safety-update/hydrochlorothiazide-risk-of-non-melanoma-skin-cancer-particularly-in-long-term-use.

National Institute for Health and Care Excellence (NICE). https://www.nice.org.uk.

Nursing Times. https://www.nursingtimes.net.

13 DRUGS USED FOR THE TREATMENT OF RHEUMATOLOGICAL CONDITIONS

Treatment of Arthritis and Gout

CHAPTER OUTLINE

LEARNING OBJECTIVES

At the end of this chapter, the reader should be able to:

- describe the basic features of the acute inflammatory process and immune responses
- list the important NSAIDs
- explain the differences between non-selective and COX-2-selective NSAIDs and give examples of each
- explain the principles to be followed in NSAID treatment
- state the main aims in the treatment of rheumatoid arthritis (RA)
- list the main classes of drugs used for RA and examples of each
- explain the meaning of the acronym DMARDs
- describe the newer 'biologic' treatments for RA and other rheumatological conditions and how they are administered
- explain what gout is and the drugs used to treat it and to prevent it

Certain key events of the inflammatory process and of the immune response should be known in order to understand the mechanism of the antiinflammatory drugs in diseases such as rheumatoid arthritis, lupus and gout.

THE ACUTE INFLAMMATORY REACTION

The acute inflammatory reaction is the body's defence mechanism against invading pathogens such as bacteria, cells infected with viruses, parasites and fungi. The reaction consists of:

- innate, non-specific and non-immune responses
- acquired specific immune responses (antibody response).

Innate Response

The innate response is a 'general purpose' reaction, involving the release of proteins and other chemicals known as 'inflammatory mediators' at sites of tissue injury or in response to invading pathogens. Different mediators elicit different aspects of the inflammatory response, such as prostaglandins and bradykinin (pain to warn of a problem), histamine, prostaglandins and bradykinin (vasodilation that produces the classic redness associated with an acute inflammatory response, and increased leakage of the vascular endothelium lining the post-capillary blood vessels, causing oedema due to the leaked proteins and fluid). In addition, various chemotactic substances are released that 'call' leukocytes, such as neutrophils, into extravascular tissues where they can phagocytose invading microorganisms. These substances include C5a, generated by activation of the complement system, Leukotriene B4, and various cytokines and chemokines. Inappropriate activation of the innate inflammatory response produces many of the symptoms of inflammatory diseases. Non-steroidal antiinflammatory drugs (NSAIDs) such as naproxen (see later) target the cyclooxygenase enzymes (COX) that synthesize prostaglandins (PGs) such as PGE_2, thus reducing the redness and pain associated with acute inflammation. Knowledge of the cytokines involved in the innate inflammatory response has led to the introduction of powerful new 'biologic treatments' (see later).

Acquired Response (Antibody Response)

The acquired specific immune response involves components of the immune system that are able to recognize as foreign, specific proteins presented on invading organisms, or on neoplastic cells, and lead the B-lymphocytes to make specific **antibodies** against them. A common example of the clinical use of exploiting the acquired immune response is in the use of vaccines as prophylaxis of certain diseases. However, in other situations the acquired immune response is wrongly directed against normal proteins/tissues in the body leading to **autoimmune** diseases, such as rheumatoid arthritis, lupus, type 1 diabetes and hypothyroidism, while in other diseases, the acquired immune response is directed against innocuous foreign substances such as grass pollen or house dust, leading to allergic rhinitis and asthma. Several of the disease-modifying antirheumatic drugs (DMARDs; see Case History 13.1) are drugs that target cells involved in the acquired immune system.

CASE HISTORY 13.1

The patient, an 82-year-old woman, was brought to hospital by her neighbour, who had found her on the floor in the kitchen of her house. The patient remembered making a cup of tea and feeling dizzy and light-headed. She had sustained bruising to her forehead and left arm. For the preceding 3 weeks, she had experienced increasing fatigue and had noticed that whenever she arose from a sitting or lying position she temporarily felt light-headed. This sensation would last for 1–2 min, during which she would support herself on any furniture to hand.

She was previously a fit and active person. Over the last 3 months she had been treated by her GP for swelling, pain and stiffness of her left knee, with naproxen 250 mg twice daily. The patient reported that these symptoms had been attributed to osteoarthritis. After routine tests, a preliminary diagnosis of gastric ulceration secondary to non-steroidal antiinflammatory drugs was made. The patient was admitted to the medical assessment unit and transfused 4 units of blood. She was placed 'nil by mouth' and given 40 mg of omeprazole intravenously. The following morning, she underwent an oesophagogastroduodenoscopy (OGD), which confirmed the presence of an ulcer in the gastric antrum. The ulcer was not actively bleeding. Tests for *Helicobacter pylori* or an underlying malignancy proved negative. The patient returned to the ward and was prescribed paracetamol 1 g four times a day and omeprazole 20 mg once a day. Two further haemoglobin concentrations were normal, as was her blood pressure over the next 4 days. The patient also noted resolution of her postural symptoms and she was discharged.

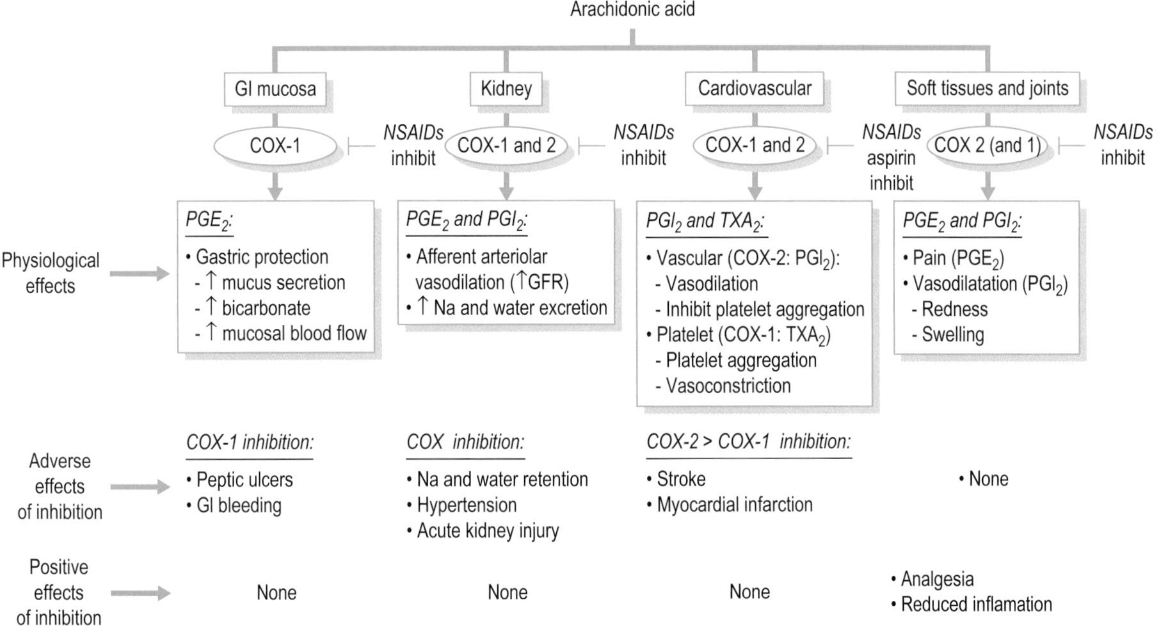

Fig. 13.1 ■ COX enzymes: physiological effects and positive and adverse effects of inhibition in different tissues. *COX,* Cyclooxygenase; *GFR,* glomerular filtration rate; *GI,* gastrointestinal; *NSAIDs,* non-steroidal antiinflammatory drugs; *PGE,* prostaglandin; *PGI,* prostacyclin; *TXA2,* thromboxane A2.

NON-STEROIDAL ANTIINFLAMMATORY DRUGS

The NSAIDs comprise:

- salicylates (and paracetamol)
- non-selective COX inhibitors
- selective COX-2 inhibitors (the COX-2 inhibitors presently used are not completely selective for the COX-2 enzyme).

This is a large group of drugs used to treat mild to moderate pain and to control the pain, stiffness and inflammation associated with rheumatic disorders and osteoarthritis. Paracetamol (acetaminophen) has some similarities to NSAIDs and is also discussed here. Most of the NSAIDs have three major therapeutic actions:

- analgesic (pain relief)
- antipyretic (temperature reduction)
- antiinflammatory (reduce acute symptoms of inflammation).

Mechanism of Action of NSAIDs

NSAIDs act by inhibiting COX enzymes, thus suppressing the formation of prostaglandins (PGE_2 and PGI_2) and thromboxane A2 (TXA_2) from arachidonic acid within the peripheral tissues. Fig. 13.1 presents some functions of these agents and the positive and adverse effects of inhibiting them in different tissues. One of the actions of PGE_2 is to trigger the sensation of pain, and PGI_2 activity contributes to many of the features of acute inflammation (i.e. swelling and redness). They also have a role in homeostasis, including control of body temperature by the hypothalamus in the brain. At least two enzymes are concerned with the formation of prostaglandins: cyclooxygenase-1 (COX-1) and cyclooxygenase-2 (COX-2). Prostaglandins produced by COX-2 are responsible for pain and inflammation, whereas those from COX-1 have a protective effect on the stomach lining and have effects on platelet function and in the renal tract. Most NSAIDs block both COX-1 and COX-2 and, although they relieve pain and inflammation, may cause serious gastric bleeding and peptic ulcers. Some NSAIDs inhibit COX-2 preferentially (see later) and are somewhat less likely to cause stomach ulceration, but these drugs are associated with an increased risk of heart attacks, with long-term use, particularly in patients at high cardiovascular risk. A third enzyme, COX-3, has been discovered, but it is not yet clear what role it plays in humans.

NSAIDs and the Kidney

NSAIDs rarely damage the kidneys in normal patients. However, in patients with heart failure, cirrhosis of the liver, renal disease, or who are taking diuretics, they can occasionally precipitate renal failure. This is believed to be due to an alteration of blood flow through the kidneys, which follows inhibition of prostaglandin production. It usually recovers on stopping the drug, but, rarely, NSAIDs cause irreversible renal damage. When these groups of patients are given regular treatment with NSAIDs, their renal function should be checked after a short period of treatment.

CLINICAL NOTE

NSAIDs interact with many common medicines and it is important that, when prescribing or administering these medicines, interactions are checked with the patient's existing treatment. This is particularly important for people who have multiple comorbidities and who may be living with one or more conditions (e.g. heart failure, liver or renal disease). While the over-the-counter dose does not pose too many issues in relation to side-effects, prescription strength doses are more problematic. The most common side-effect of NSAIDs is gastric bleeding, which is aggravated when given with certain medicines such as selective serotonin reuptake inhibitors (SSRIs), steroids and anticoagulants; alcohol intake should also be moderated when treatment is prescribed.

The Salicylates

Aspirin (Acetylsalicylic Acid)

History: Aspirin was the first widely available synthetic analgesic not derived from opiates. Since ancient times, the pain relieving, antiinflammatory and antipyretic effects of the bark of the willow tree was known and used clinically. The active substance, salicylic acid (from *Salix*, the willow), was identified in the 19th century, and efforts were made to synthesize it in a form that could be easily absorbed. This was acetylsalicylic acid. By 1899, Bayer had devised an improved way of manufacturing it and sold it under the brand name Aspirin around the world.

Aspirin is a prodrug, rapidly absorbed orally.

Modes of Action

Unlike other NSAIDs, aspirin **irreversibly** inhibits COX-1 and modifies the activity of COX-2. This means that some of its effects are particularly prolonged. This leads to its particularly troublesome problems of gastric irritation and bleeding, but also leads to its prolonged inhibition of platelet aggregation, as COX enzymes are involved in the production of thromboxane A2 in platelets, leading to platelets becoming 'sticky' and clumping together. (This property of aspirin is used for secondary prevention of coronary disease and is discussed further in Chapter 7.) Aspirin has at least three other modes of action that combine to produce its antiinflammatory and other effects.

Therapeutic Uses

Aspirin has moderate analgesic activity and in higher doses, it has moderate antiinflammatory activity. High-dose aspirin (3 adult tablets ~1000 mg) is effective treatment for many migraine attacks. However, it is now mostly used as an adjunct in the secondary prevention of cardiovascular disease (CVD). For this, it is generally given as a low daily dose of 75 mg. Regular use appears to reduce the risk of some cancers, particularly colon cancer. It remains first-line treatment for rheumatic fever, and in children, *Kawasaki's disease* – one of the few times it is recommended for use in children (see later). Low-dose aspirin is moderately effective in the prevention of pre-eclampsia in women at high risk of developing this condition in pregnancy.

Side Effects

The principal unwanted effect is gastric irritation and bleeding. Slight bleeding occurs in ~70% of regular users and may lead to iron deficiency anaemia. Severe bleeding occurs occasionally and may be fatal. Gastric ulceration may also occur. The presence or absence of gastric pain (dyspepsia) is a poor predictor of gastric ulceration or severe bleeding. Although aspirin has many beneficial effects, this side-effect outweighs its benefits for most people, which is why it has fallen from favour for primary prevention of CVD in healthy people. It is generally recommended that aspirin (and other NSAIDs) be given with food, although it is not clear if this actually reduces the likelihood of gastric side-effects.

Aspirin should not routinely be used in children and adolescents, as it may very rarely precipitate the dangerous and often fatal *Reye's syndrome*. This is a rapidly progressive encephalopathy with associated liver damage. In the UK, it is recommended that children under the age of 16 should not normally take aspirin.

Aspirin can trigger skin rashes, including urticaria (hives) and rarely can trigger dangerous allergic skin rashes, such as the *Stevens Johnson syndrome*.

Aspirin should not be used to treat gout, as in standard doses it reduces the excretion of uric acid by the kidneys and may therefore worsen the attack.

Around 7% of people with asthma notice a worsening of their symptoms after taking aspirin. This may sometimes be severe, and aspirin and other NSAIDs should be avoided if this has ever been noticed. This does not represent allergy, but rather, a hypersensitivity to the effects of aspirin.

High doses of aspirin can induce tinnitus.

Treatment of Aspirin Poisoning. In aspirin poisoning, patients suffer acidosis and should receive gastric lavage and forced alkaline diuresis, provided renal and circulatory functions are adequate.

Drug Interactions. Aspirin may increase the effects of anticoagulants and some oral hypoglycaemic drugs, partly by displacing them from their plasma-binding sites.

CLINICAL NOTE

Aspirin is a widely used medicine, and has similar side-effects to NSAIDs. It is important when treating patients receiving aspirin that they are monitored for signs, e.g. gastric reflux black bowel movements or excessive bruising. If these symptoms occur, treatment may be reviewed and an alternative treatment considered. If a patient has been fitted with a drug eluting coronary artery stent, they should continue low dose aspirin for life and should not stop this without discussion with a cardiologist. Stopping aspirin in these circumstances is associated with a high risk of stent thrombosis.

Paracetamol

Paracetamol (called acetaminophen in the USA) is a widely used minor analgesic and antipyretic. Although it has some general cyclooxygenase inhibiting properties, this action is very weak in the peripheral tissues and it has practically no antiinflammatory action. It has recently been discovered that it inhibits the action of COX-3, but it is not clear if this is what leads to its analgesic effects in humans. Its analgesic effect does seem to be mediated by some action on the central nervous system, which is not yet understood. Its main advantage is that, unlike other NSAIDs, it does not cause indigestion or gastric bleeding and is widely used for its antipyretic effects. Arguably, paracetamol should be regarded as a **simple analgesic** rather than an NSAID.

Therapeutic Use

Paracetamol is given orally in tablet form. It is well absorbed, and peak plasma concentrations are achieved usually well within 60 min. It is partly bound to plasma proteins and inactivated by metabolism in the liver. Paracetamol is the preferred mild analgesic and antipyretic for children under 12 years old, as it does not cause Reye's syndrome. In this age group, it is frequently given as an oral suspension. The child should be over 3 months old, except for post-immunization pyrexia, when 2 months is acceptable. Paracetamol is not very useful in inflammatory arthritis and is inferior to NSAIDs in the treatment of back pain. It is available in suppository form, which may be useful in febrile, vomiting children.

Adverse Effects

Adverse effects are uncommon at normal dosage but in overdose, it causes dangerous liver damage. The margin of safety is relatively low, and doses as low as two to three times the maximum therapeutic dose can cause fatal liver failure (see Chapter 33).

CLINICAL NOTE

Postoperative pain is often managed with intravenous paracetamol and a Cochrane review noted that in around 36% of cases, pain was managed well. This review also reported that when IV paracetamol was compared to morphine, there did not appear to be a difference in pain relief (McNicol et al., 2016).

Analgesic Mixtures with Aspirin or Paracetamol. There are many analgesic mixtures in which aspirin or paracetamol is combined with a small dose of a weak opiate. These combinations are little stronger than aspirin or paracetamol alone but are more dangerous in overdose and have more side-effects. Except for some preparations of co-codamol and co-dydramol, where the codeine/dihydrocodeine dose is high (with concurrent increased risk of opiate side-effects and dependence), there is little reason to prescribe these combinations. Nevertheless, they are very popular, and some are available over-the-counter. The higher doses of codeine or dihydrocodeine may affect the ability to drive or operate machinery safely and prescribers should ensure that patients understand this.

Among those in common use are:

- **Co-codaprin** tablets (available without prescription): 8 mg codeine phosphate and 400 mg aspirin. This is also available in a dispersible form.
- **Co-codamol** tablets: codeine phosphate and paracetamol. In the UK, this is available with 8 mg, 15 mg or 30 mg of codeine with 500 mg of paracetamol. The codeine dose must be specified when prescribing.
- **Co-dydramol** tablets: dihydrocodeine tartrate and paracetamol. In the UK, this is available with 10 mg, 20 mg or 30 mg of dihydrocodeine with 500 mg of paracetamol. The dihydrocodeine dose must be specified when prescribing.

Note: Co-proxamol tablets (dextropropoxyphene and paracetamol) was a very popular analgesic, despite it being little more effective than paracetamol alone. However, it is very much more dangerous in overdose than paracetamol alone. In consequence, it has been withdrawn from most world markets. In the UK, deaths from attempted suicide fell after co-proxamol was withdrawn.

Non-selective NSAIDs

Many, but by no means all, of the NSAIDs (including selective COX-2 inhibitors) are listed in Table 13.1, with their major adverse effects.

There are large numbers of non-selective NSAIDs available for use in reduction of pain and inflammation. They are very useful drugs but are also potentially dangerous and need to be used carefully. They are used to reduce the inflammatory element in rheumatoid and osteoarthritis; however, it seems likely that long-term use may accelerate cartilage breakdown in osteoarthritis. It also appears that use of NSAIDs may delay healing in bone fractures. However, they are useful treatment for the pain of bony metastases in palliative care. NSAIDs should not be used to treat non-prostaglandin mediated pain, such as neuropathic pain or the pain of tendinopathies (which are degenerative but not inflammatory in nature).

Prostaglandins can cause contraction of the uterus and are important in the initiation of labour. NSAIDs, by modifying prostaglandin formation, are useful in reducing period pains (dysmenorrhea) and also reduce the volume of bleeding in menstrual periods by about 20%, which can help in the treatment of dysfunctional uterine bleeding. NSAIDs have also been used to prevent premature labour. NSAIDs are used to stimulate closure of a patent ductus arteriosus in new-born babies. The ductus arteriosus should close spontaneously at birth, but in some infants, particularly premature infants, this does not happen. Modification of prostaglandin formation by use of NSAIDs will often stimulate closure of the ductus arteriosus.

Phenylbutazone is included in Table 13.1, as it still has a role in the treatment of refractory ankylosing spondylitis (and is widely used in horse veterinary medicine, from whence it has sometimes found its way into the human food chain). Its distinctive adverse effect is dangerous or fatal blood dyscrasias, and it is not available in many countries. **Azapropazone** is not shown, as it is not available in many markets, and has very marked typical NSAID side-effects without offering any particular advantages.

CLINICAL NOTE

Some NSAIDs, including ibuprofen, ketoprofen and piroxicam, are available without prescription, as gels for topical application. Small amounts penetrate to deeper tissues and they produce some improvement in soft-tissue injuries and arthritis. They should be rubbed in gently over the affected area, and the hands washed after application or gloves should be worn. Occlusive dressings should not be used. Occasionally, excessive application can cause systemic adverse effects. When patients are admitted and need medication assessment, they should be asked about topical NSAIDs, as these can have adverse reactions with other medications that may be prescribed. Some NSAIDS, including diclofenac, are available in suppository form.

TABLE 13.1

The NSAIDs: A Small Selection of the Available Types

Drug	GI risk	CVD risk	Notes
Non-selective NSAIDs			
Diclofenac	+ +	+ +	Relatively COX-2 specific. CVD risk raised, but does not inhibit aspirin's antiplatelet activity if doses separated. Injection available
Etodolac	+	+ +	Relatively COX-2 specific. CVD risk raised
Felbinac	+ +	+	This is the active metabolite of fenbufen. Fenbufen has been withdrawn in most markets due to hepatotoxicity
Fenoprofen	+ +	+	More side-effects than ibuprofen
Flurbiprofen	+ +	+	May be slightly more potent than naproxen, but more GI side-effects
Ibuprofen (and dexibuprofen)	+ +		CVD risk is raised in doses over 1200 mg a day (ibuprofen). Generally well-tolerated, but antiinflammatory effects weaker than naproxen
Ketoprofen (and dexketoprofen)	+ +	+	More side-effects than ibuprofen
Meloxicam	+	+ +	Relatively COX-2 specific. CVD risk raised
Nabumetone	+ +	+ (?)	As potent as naproxen. Relatively COX-2 specific. CVD risk uncertain
Naproxen	+ +		Better antiinflammatory than ibuprofen. Lowest CVD risk
Piroxicam	+ + +	+	More side-effects than most NSAIDs but once daily dosage may be useful
Sulindac	+ +	+ (?)	Similar in tolerance to naproxen
Indometacin	+ + +	+ +	Serious skin reactions, bone marrow disorders and many other side-effects reported
Ketorolac		N/A	IM/IV injection for short -term use in postoperative pain. Also eye drops
Tolfenamic acid	+ + (?)	+ (?)	Licensed in the UK for short-term treatment of migraine
Tiaprofenic acid	+ +	+	May trigger severe cystitis; use with caution in bladder disorders
Phenylbutazone	+ +	(?)	High risk of severe bone marrow suppression. Only used for ankylosing spondylitis in the UK
Mefenamic acid	+ +	+	Often used for menstrual pain. No more effective than other NSAIDs and more side-effects, particularly gastrointestinal
COX-2 selective NSAIDs			
Celecoxib	+	+ +	Does not inhibit aspirin's antiplatelet activity
Etoricoxib	+	+ +	Does not inhibit aspirin's antiplatelet activity. Licence in the UK includes treatment of acute gout. Not available in the USA
Parecoxib	N/A	N/A	IM/IV injection; licensed for postoperative pain relief only. Not available in the USA

Notes: Bold indicates NICE recommended first-line choice. + + +, + + and + indicate best estimate of degree of risk. (?) indicates no elevated risk found in most studies. *COX*, Cyclooxygenase; *CVD*, cardiovascular disease; *GI*, gastrointestinal; NSAIDs, non-steroidal antiinflammatory drugs.

Drug Interactions of the Non-selective COX Inhibitors

These drugs may:

- antagonize the actions of diuretics and blood pressure drugs
- increase the effects of warfarin
- decrease the excretion and increase the effect of lithium.

Selective COX-2 Inhibitors

Examples of these drugs are:

- **celecoxib**
- **etoricoxib** (not in the USA)
- **parecoxib** (not in the USA).

A few years ago, there were several others on the market, but most have been withdrawn, when it became apparent that they did not offer the protection against gastric ulceration and bleeding that had been hoped for, but also, quite unexpectedly, showing an increased risk of CVD events such as myocardial infarction. These risks became clear in the routine post-marketing surveillance that is undertaken with all new medications. In some cases, skin reactions or liver toxicity also contributed to the decisions to withdraw the drugs.

It was known that the COX-1 enzyme was involved in protecting the stomach from acid attack, and that the COX-2 enzyme was involved in pain and inflammation. Quite rationally, it was hoped that selective inhibition of COX-2 would relieve pain without leading to the gastric problems. Unfortunately, this was not the case. COX-2 inhibitors do reduce gastric problems and may be more appropriate for people at higher risk of ulceration, but the risk is still there and gastric protection with other drugs is still often a wise course. The unexpected increased CVD risk is not fully explained, but it would appear that protection against thrombosis is mediated by a balance of the activity of the products of the COX-1 and COX-2 enzymes, and over inhibition of one of the enzymes seems to lead to an imbalance that leads to an increase in thrombotic risk in the coronary arteries.

COX-2 inhibitors do not antagonize the antiplatelet activity of aspirin to the same degree as other NSAIDs, so may have a role in short-term treatment of pain and inflammation in patients taking aspirin for its cardioprotective action.

Adverse Effects of all NSAIDs

These are similar for all COX inhibitor drugs and mainly apply to long-term use for:

- Dyspepsia (indigestion). Dyspepsia does not strongly predict bleeding or ulceration, which may occur without preceding dyspepsia.
- Gastric bleeding, ulceration and perforation are a substantial risk. They are particularly common in elderly patients (see Case History 13.1) and are believed to be due to the inhibition of the gastric protective action of prostaglandins. These drugs should not be given to patients with peptic ulcers or bleeding disorders. Most patients on long-term NSAID treatment should be prescribed gastric protection (see later).
- Salt and water retention can occur and lead to oedema.
- NSAIDs increase the risk of heart failure and can worsen pre-existing heart failure.
- NSAIDs may worsen renal function (see earlier).
- Most NSAIDs increase CVD risk with prolonged use.
- NSAIDs that are not selective for COX-2 inhibit the antiplatelet effects of aspirin. This may be particularly important in patients with coronary artery stents, which may block if aspirin is not working.
- NSAIDs may trigger bronchospasm and worsen asthma, as with aspirin.
- Urticaria (hives) is a relatively common side-effect of NSAID treatment. Allergic rashes can occur and are sometimes serious.

Clinical Use of all NSAIDs

Consideration of Table 13.1 and knowledge of the side-effects of this class of drug lead to a number of important principles that should guide NSAID treatment:

- Long-term use of NSAIDs should be avoided if possible, and simple analgesics like paracetamol, along with non-drug treatments, should be used where appropriate.
- Long-term use of NSAIDs in patients with renal impairment or risk factors for this should be avoided.

- All NSAIDs including COX-2 inhibitors may lead to dangerous gastric bleeding or ulceration.
- The risk of gastric bleeding is less with COX-2 inhibitors.
- All patients on long-term NSAIDs should be considered for gastric protection with a PPI or H2 blocking drug (see Chapter 10). This is particularly important in middle-aged and older patients.
- NSAIDS are generally less suitable for older patients, although these patients are often prescribed them because alternative drugs are either less effective or otherwise problematic.
- Increased risk of CVD is associated with the use of more COX-2 selective NSAIDs, and this increased risk begins to become apparent in the first month of use.
- **Ibuprofen and naproxen** are associated with no increased CVD risk in normal doses and on balance are the NSAIDs of choice in most cases. Naproxen may be a more potent antiinflammatory than ibuprofen
- The antiplatelet effects of aspirin are antagonized by concurrent use of most NSAIDs. Selective COX-2 inhibitors are the best choice for concurrent use, but not long term, in view of the overall increase CVD risk of COX-2 inhibitors.
- It is recognized that patient responses to NSAIDs can be idiosyncratic, and if one does not work, it is worth trying an alternative NSAID.
- There is no value in giving two different NSAIDs simultaneously.
- Topical forms of NSAIDs are effective for localized pain and inflammation and are generally safer.

SUMMARY

- NSAIDs inhibit the COX enzymes that produce prostaglandins.
- Aspirin and other NSAIDs should not be given on an empty stomach.
- Long-term use of NSAIDs should be avoided, if possible.
- All NSAIDs, including COX-2 selective, can cause gastric bleeding.
- Do not use aspirin in children of 15 years and under.
- Paracetamol is the preferred analgesic for children under 12 years old.
- Paracetamol is not antiinflammatory and is therefore of little or no use in rheumatoid arthritis.
- Paracetamol is toxic to the liver at doses not far above therapeutic.
- Analgesic mixtures are not proven to be more effective than either aspirin or paracetamol alone and are less suitable for prescribing.
- Some NSAIDs can be applied topically to the skin.
- Naproxen and ibuprofen appear to have the best overall safety profile of the NSAIDs, but interfere with the antiplatelet action of aspirin.
- COX-2 inhibitors are preferred where low dose aspirin is being used in CVD, but not for long-term use.
- Most NSAIDs, in particular COX-2 inhibitors, increase CVD risk with prolonged use.

RHEUMATOID ARTHRITIS (AND OTHER RHEUMATIC DISORDERS)

Rheumatoid arthritis (RA) is a fairly common disorder affecting small and medium-sized joints causing chronic pain. In many patients it can lead to considerable deformity and disability. Although the exact cause is unknown, RA is an example of an autoimmune disease, in which the immune system attacks soft tissues in the joints and inflames and damages them, ultimately destroying them. The inflammation in the joints is due to prostaglandins and other chemical mediators, which give rise to pain and swelling, and to cytokines, which are responsible for progressive damage to the joints, leading to deformity. RA is one of a considerable number of rheumatic (or *connective tissue*) diseases, each of which have a different autoimmune basis, and which attack different tissues, although there is a fair degree of overlap in their symptoms. Examples include systemic lupus erythematosus, psoriatic arthritis, ankylosing spondylitis and Behçet's disease. It is important to realize that all of the rheumatic diseases are, to a greater or lesser extent, systemic diseases, which affect many organs and systems in the body. They can cause a wide variety of symptoms and morbidity from them can be very severe. Some may be fatal if untreated, and most decrease life expectancy. We mainly consider the treatment of RA here, but the principles and drugs (with some variations), apply to most rheumatic disorders.

Treatment of Rheumatoid Arthritis

The treatment of patients with RA involves:

- slowing the rate of degenerative change and tissue damage, and delaying or preventing deformity of the hands and feet
- controlling the symptoms of pain, stiffness and swelling of the joints
- preventing the progression of associated systemic disease, such as CVD or lung fibrosis
- other rheumatic diseases may have specific symptoms, such as rashes or ulcers, which also require treatment.

Although NSAIDS have a role in the treatment of pain and inflammation in RA, they do not affect the production of cytokines and so do not reduce joint damage. They are, at best, an adjunct to other treatment. The consensus today is that a **c**onventional disease modifying antirheumatic drug (cDMARD) (usually methotrexate), should be introduced very early on in the course of the disease. If necessary, corticosteroids may also be used, to settle the initial disease or treat flares. If cDMARDs do not work reasonably quickly, then **t**argeted **s**ynthetic DMARDs (tsDMARDs) or **b**iologic DMARDs (bDMARDs) are the preferred next step in treatment. The treatment strategy is 'treat to target' – either complete remission, or low disease activity, if remission cannot be achieved.

Case History 13.2 illustrates the use of this principle of treatment. This approach has become established since effective and relatively safe DMARDs became available. Only a few decades ago, the most effective DMARDs were gold salts (see later). Their toxicity and monitoring requirements made them very much second-line treatment, and patients would already be badly disabled by their disease before receiving them.

Drugs used in the treatment of RA comprise:

- NSAIDs (discussed earlier)
- antiinflammatory steroids
- DMARDs – cDMARDs tsDMARDs and bDMARDs.

CASE HISTORY 13.2

Shortly after the birth of her second child, Mrs. M began to have severe pain in both wrists. She woke up feeling stiff in the mornings and the stiffness could persist all day. She took paracetamol tablets for a while, but the pain and stiffness did not go away. She went to her GP, who referred her to a rheumatologist, who undertook blood tests, ordered X-rays and diagnosed rheumatoid arthritis. He explained that she had developed an autoimmune disease: the body's immune system begins to regard the soft tissues of the joints as foreign and attacks them, causing inflammation, pain and destruction of the tissues. The doctor prescribed a short course of prednisolone to reduce the inflammation, celecoxib (Celebrex), an NSAID, to help with the stiffness and pain, and methotrexate, a DMARD, by once-weekly injection to start the disease-slowing process. Appointments were made for regular blood tests because of the methotrexate treatment.

Antiinflammatory Corticosteroids

The antiinflammatory corticosteroids have been available for over 60 years and are synthetic analogues of the body's own antiinflammatory steroid, cortisol (see Chapter 17), which is synthesized by the adrenal cortex. These steroids are not only antiinflammatory but are also immunosuppressant. They therefore have a two-pronged action, since rheumatic diseases such as RA and lupus are autoimmune in origin. Hailed as miracle drugs when they were first introduced, they proved to be a two-edged sword because of the side-effects associated with the prolonged use of these drugs in comparatively high doses when administered orally. They are, nevertheless, still very occasionally used in lower doses long term, as an adjunct to DMARDs in patients with very severe disease, and on a short-term basis to deal with flare-ups. Treatment may be oral – often with prednisolone, or intramuscular with methylprednisolone or triamcinolone, or intraarticular, injected directly into the inflamed joint, again using methylprednisolone or triamcinolone. In flares, the dose should be as low as possible, and for the shortest period of time needed for effect. Corticosteroids have a role in the treatment of other rheumatological conditions and some autoimmune conditions, often combined with azathioprine (see later).

Disease-modifying Drugs (DMARDs)

Many of the DMARDs are used to treat other autoimmune diseases and diseases suspected to be of autoimmune cause. They may be used in dermatology, in particular. Their main use is in the treatment of rheumatological disorders. They are classified as: conventional (c), targeted synthetic (ts) and biologic (b) DMARDs.

Conventional (Non-biologic) DMARDs

- cDMARDs may take 2–3 months to have clinical benefit, and corticosteroids may be useful as bridging treatment.
- cDMARDs and tsDMARDs used in the treatment of RA include:
  - **methotrexate** – first-line in RA
  - **leflunomide** – first-line in RA
  - **sulfasalazine** – first-line in RA
  - **hydroxychloroquine** (mainly for palindromic RA)
  - **baricitinib** – tsDMARD – second-line treatment
  - **tofacitinib** – tsDMARD – second-line treatment.

Older cDMARDs such as sodium aurothiomalate (gold), ciclosporin and penicillamine are rarely used today, as newer treatments are more effective, less toxic and require less onerous monitoring. There are a few patients for whom only these drugs work. They require highly specialized management and regular monitoring. For instance, gold injections can require weekly full blood counts and dipstick testing of urine for proteinuria. Ciclosporin and penicillamine are sometimes used in the treatment of other rare autoimmune disorders, under highly specialized supervision.

cDMARDs and tsDMARDs used to treat other rheumatological conditions include:

- **methotrexate**, **leflunomide** and **sulfasalazine** – all used in the treatment of psoriatic arthritis (and there is a degree of overlap between the treatments for most rheumatic disorders)
- **azathioprine** – may be used to enable a reduced dose of corticosteroid in the management of very severe RA, psoriatic arthritis and other rheumatological and autoimmune conditions
- **hydroxychloroquine** (and occasionally, **chloroquine**) – are used to treat systemic and discoid lupus erythematosus
- **apremilast** – tsDMARD used to treat psoriatic arthropathy and psoriasis – as second-line treatment
- **mepacrine** – usually used to treat the parasitic disease *giardiasis*, is also used to treat discoid lupus erythematosus. It does not have a UK licence for this indication. It can worsen psoriasis.

Monitoring of DMARDs

All cDMARDs require careful monitoring of effects and side-effects. They are powerful drugs, in some cases originally developed to treat cancer, and treatment will usually be shared between secondary and primary care, as specialized knowledge and experience is needed to manage them effectively and safely. Clinical nurse specialists have an increasingly important role in this. It is important to ensure that patients are well-educated about their treatment and are given written information about it. In the UK, patients are provided with their own treatment booklets for methotrexate therapy, into which the results of blood and other tests are entered.

It is important to be aware of drug interactions when patients are prescribed cDMARDs and to be aware that serious toxicity can occur with some of these drugs if a patient develops renal impairment or sepsis.

cDMARDs affect immune responses and many of them can increase the risk and severity of infections. Patients should be offered routine vaccinations, especially influenza and pneumococcal vaccines, and there should be a lower threshold for prescribing antibiotics than in patients not on these drugs. Live vaccines should not be given.

All patients taking cDMARDs (apart from hydroxychloroquine), require regular blood tests. In most cases, these should be full blood counts, liver function tests and renal function tests. The precise blood tests and the frequency of them depends on the drug, and with some drugs, urine testing for protein is also required.

Both the absolute values of blood parameters, and any trends in them, are very important. For instance, a stable platelet count that is a little less than the lower value of the normal range is much less concerning than a rapidly declining trend in the platelet count, even if it remains in the normal range. If in doubt, the drug should be withheld, and the patient discussed with a senior clinician.

CLINICAL NOTE

Prescribers should familiarize themselves with the monitoring regimes for individual drugs and they should ensure that patients are being monitored before they issue a prescription for one. Blood dyscrasias may manifest as unexplained bruising, bleeding or sore throats that do not rapidly settle. The *British Medical Journal* published an excellent review of managing people with arthritis which advocates the need for shared support across hospital and community practice and rheumatology specialists should guide changes to treatment (Ledingham et al., 2017).

The most important cDMARDs are as follows:

Methotrexate

Methotrexate is the most commonly used first-line cDMARD in RA. Chemically, it is an antagonist of folic acid and is cytotoxic (destroys cells by blocking cell division). It was originally introduced for the treatment of cancer, but was found to slow disease progression in RA in terms of joint and bone damage, probably by inhibiting lymphocyte activity. It acts more rapidly than many cDMARDs and, if given in relatively low doses, toxicity is acceptably low provided renal function is normal. The drug is taken orally or by subcutaneous injection **once a week**.

Adverse Effects. The main adverse effects are gastrointestinal (GI) upsets and decreased white blood cell counts. GI upsets may be severe, and a sore mouth may be the first sign of this. Other bone marrow suppression can occur and can be quite sudden in onset. Liver cirrhosis has been reported, and pneumonitis and pulmonary fibrosis can occur and may be more common in patients with RA. Folic acid, given once a week on a different day to the methotrexate, reduces GI side-effects and may reduce the chance of liver damage. Regular blood counts and liver function tests are necessary, and a chest radiograph and lung function tests if a patient develops a persistent cough or dyspnoea. Methotrexate is teratogenic and effective contraception is required for men and women during, and for 6 months after, treatment.

CLINICAL NOTE

The once weekly dosing regimen for methotrexate when used as a DMARD is a potential cause of serious drug errors. Accidental overdose of methotrexate should be regarded as a '**Never Event**'. It should never be prescribed unless systems exist to ensure it is prescribed safely. Patient education is key, but it is also good practice to only prescribe and dispense one strength of methotrexate (usually 2.5 mg tablets) and to indicate clearly on the prescription and label how many the patient should take and on which day of the week they should take it.

Sulfasalazine

Sulfasalazine was developed specifically to treat RA. Chemically, it is a combination of an antibacterial sulphonamide with a salicylate. Originally, it was thought that infection was an underlying cause of RA. This is not the case, but the drug has significant DMARD activity, although exactly why is not known. It is somewhat less effective than methotrexate and takes longer to work, but may be better tolerated. Bone marrow suppression is a rare but serious side-effect, and regular blood tests are required when initiating treatment. When stable, annual full blood counts and liver function tests are required. It should not be prescribed if patients are allergic to salicylates or sulphonamides. Sulfasalazine is an important treatment for inflammatory bowel disease (Chapter 10).

CLINICAL NOTE

Sulfasalazine has been confused with sulfadiazine; ensure the correct drug is prescribed and dispensed. Prior to starting treatment the patient should be screened specifically for an allergy to aspirin; as explained previously, sulfasalazine contains salicylate, a chemical also found in aspirin.

Leflunomide

Leflunomide was introduced in the early 2000s. It inhibits an enzyme involved in DNA and RNA synthesis and thus particularly affects rapidly dividing cells, such as lymphocytes, which are of particular importance in RA. It is a prodrug, and has a long half-life in the body, requiring a 'wash-out' procedure with oral activated charcoal or cholestyramine for 11 days, with blood levels monitoring, before introducing another DMARD. It requires similar blood monitoring to methotrexate, but blood pressure should also be monitored.

Adverse Effects. The adverse effects are similar to those with methotrexate, but diarrhoea is particularly common. Potentially fatal liver damage has been reported in the first 6 months of treatment. Pulmonary fibrosis has been reported. Use with methotrexate increases the risk of liver damage, but the drugs are sometimes used together. Increased blood pressure has been reported. If significant side-effects occur, then the drug should be discontinued and a 'wash out' procedure instituted. Leflunomide is teratogenic and effective contraception is required during and after treatment, for up to 2 years in women and 3 months in men.

Hydroxychloroquine (and Chloroquine)

Hydroxychloroquine was derived from the antimalarial drug chloroquine, which was found to be useful in some rheumatic disorders. Hydroxychloroquine itself may be used to treat certain types of malaria. Hydroxychloroquine is of value in the treatment of lupus erythematosus, and used in *palindromic RA* where the symptoms of RA flare up and then settle. It may reduce the frequency of flares and possibly prevent progression to true RA. It is used because of its relative lack of toxicity (but see later). Its mechanism of action is not fully understood, but involves blocking the activity of specific receptors on messenger cells in the innate immune system, thus reducing inflammation, particularly inflammation associated with autoimmunity to DNA.

Adverse Effects. The most important adverse effects are related to the eye. Vision disorders are more common than previously thought and involve corneal oedema and opacities and, more seriously, retinal damage, particularly to the macula. Macular damage may be irreversible and severely affect sight.

Specialist eye examination is required at, or shortly after, initiation of treatment and should be repeated annually after 5 years of treatment. Visual disturbances – haloes, loss of acuity or colour perception – should be enquired of at each medication review with the patient.

Azathioprine

Azathioprine is a long-established immunosuppressive drug used in many diseases, mainly as an adjunct to corticosteroid therapy, in order to reduce the steroid dose required. It disrupts the synthesis of DNA and RNA in cells, and so reduces the activity of rapidly dividing cells, such as those involved in inflammatory reactions. In RA, it is not used in combination with other DMARDs and in general, it is used more in other inflammatory conditions than in RA, and as immunosuppressive treatment in kidney and liver transplants. It is orally active and requires regular blood monitoring, particularly of blood counts.

Adverse Effects. The most important adverse effect is a dose-dependant suppression of bone marrow function, which is why patient education and regular blood tests are required. Nausea is a common initial side-effect that usually settles; however, hypersensitivity reactions such as diarrhoea, dizziness, severe fatigue or rashes require the drug to be discontinued. Azathioprine is classified as a carcinogen, although the evidence for this is mixed. Skin cancers are known to be substantially more common in transplant patients, many of whom receive azathioprine. In general, the risk of all adverse effects, including cancers, seem to be greater when higher doses are given for long periods and also seem to be more prominent when azathioprine is given for GI disorders or transplantation rather than RA. Azathioprine is potentially teratogenic, but should not be stopped if a transplant patient becomes pregnant.

CLINICAL NOTE

Healthcare professionals are advised to handle uncoated azathioprine tablets with gloves and adhere to cytotoxic drug policy when prescribing and administering this medication.

Baricitinib and Tofacitinib

These relatively recently introduced orally administered second-line DMARDs are known as 'targeted synthetic DMARDs' (tsDMARDs) because they were designed to inhibit a specific enzyme target and are a product of rational design and development of new synthetic medications.

They are members of a large group of new drugs known as 'tyrosine kinase inhibiters', mainly used as targeted cancer treatments. Baricitinib is a specific inhibitor of subtypes of the tyrosine kinase enzyme, known as JAK1 and JAK2. Tofacitinib inhibits the JAK1 and JAK3 subtypes. This results in a reduction in the production of inflammatory mediators. Both are licensed for use with methotrexate (or alone, if methotrexate is not tolerated), to treat moderate to severe RA that has not responded to first-line treatment, and as an alternative to biologic therapy. These are currently expensive drugs.

Adverse Effects. This is a relatively well-tolerated group of drugs, although they may cause a rise in blood pressure and hyperlipidaemia, and require blood monitoring, as they can, rarely, lead to a drop in the white cell count. The risk of potentially serious infections seems greater with this group than other cDMARDs, and patients should be assessed for latent TB and chronic hepatitis before starting treatment, as these may become active. Baricitinib seems to be better tolerated than tofacitinib, about which there have been some concerns about possible carcinogenesis in some patient groups. The risk of pulmonary embolism may also be increased with tofacitinib treatment. Baricitinib is a more recent drug, and other adverse effects of its use may also become apparent as time progresses.

Apremilast

The orally administered tsDMARD apremilast is a second-line treatment for psoriatic arthritis and psoriasis. By inhibiting the enzyme PDE4 in various inflammatory cells, this drug reduces the activation of many of the cell types implicated in the underlying mechanisms of psoriasis. This is a moderately expensive drug.

Adverse Effects. It is generally well-tolerated, but it is possible it may worsen or trigger depression and suicidal thoughts. It should be used with caution in patients with a past history of depression, and mood should be enquired about at reviews. Weight loss has also been noted and weight should be monitored. There are no specific blood monitoring requirements.

CLINICAL NOTE

Patients usually take DMARDs long term and they must be aware of possible adverse effects, and the importance of regular check-ups, and of reporting symptoms associated with bone marrow depression, liver, lung and eye damage. If a patient is on a continuous medication regimen, a yearly medication assessment should be carried out to ensure the current treatment is being used and adhered to.

Biologic DMARDs

Biologic drugs, and 'biosimilar' drugs are a new development in therapeutics, that do not fit comfortably into conventional pharmacology. First introduced to treat RA, as bDMARDs; they are now used to treat many different and often seemingly unrelated conditions. In many of the indications for biologic treatment, the underlying issue is autoimmunity, but this is not always the case. There is now a bewildering array of biologics and biosimilars, and more will surely appear. Characteristically, they are large biological protein molecules, often monoclonal antibodies, produced using recombinant DNA technology from living organisms. This is why they are referred to as 'biologics', and also explains the typical 'ab' (for 'antibody') at the end of many of their unusually unpronounceable generic names. (The Appendix discusses biologics and biosimilars in more detail.)

Monitoring of bDMARDs

As with cDMARDs, many bDMARDs require monitoring, most commonly blood counts and liver function. The frequency of monitoring bloods is less than with many cDMARDs, and when stable, twice-yearly checks will suffice in many cases. It is generally advised to check lipids 1–2 months after starting. Some biologics do not require blood monitoring. It is important to be familiar with the monitoring requirements for individual agents when prescribing them. When reviewing patients, it is important to be alert for infections and for reactivation of TB (cough, haemoptysis or weight loss).

Before starting a bDMARD, all of the previously mentioned tests should be performed, as well as screening for chronic hepatitis, HIV infection and latent TB, particularly if patients are at increased risk of these diseases.

bDMARDs in Rheumatoid Arthritis and Other Rheumatological Disorders. These agents have revolutionized the treatment of RA and other rheumatological disorders. The first bDMARDs, introduced at the end of the 20th century, were the agents that blocked the action of the inflammatory cytokine TNF-α. These include:

- adalimumab
- certolizumab pegol
- etanercept
- golimumab
- infliximab.

Since then, bDMARDs have been introduced for use in RA, acting against other inflammatory pathways. Among these pathways are: T cell co-stimulation blockade, IL-6 receptor inhibition, B-cell depletion, and interleukin-1 inhibition. Examples of these agents include:

- abatacept
- anakinra
- belimumab
- ixekizumab
- rituximab
- secukinumab
- tocilizumab
- ustekinumab.

Administration and Therapeutic Effects. These drugs, being proteins, have to be injected. Infliximab and rituximab are given by slow intravenous infusion that needs to be done in hospital. Adalimumab is administered by subcutaneous injection on alternate weeks. Etanercept is administered twice weekly by subcutaneous injection. Many of the more recent bDMARDs may be given by intravenous infusion or by subcutaneous injection. Patients are often able to self-administer the injections at home, although around 50% of patients are unable or unwilling to do so.

CLINICAL NOTE

Drugs administered by infusion, especially large molecules such as peptides and proteins, which have the potential to produce anaphylactic shock, must be administered in clinical environments such as hospitals and clinics where facilities and trained personnel are on hand for rapid resuscitation procedures. A systematic review published in 2017 reported the greatest risk when giving these medicines is that of serious infection (Ramiro et al., 2017).

Results of controlled trials and a good deal of clinical experience suggest that in many cases, these drugs work faster and stop or slow degenerative changes better than cDMARDs. Combination of a bDMARD with methotrexate is the norm, although around 30% of patients are unable to tolerate the methotrexate, in which case monotherapy with a bDMARD is used. There is currently insufficient evidence in most cases to recommend one bDMARD as markedly more effective than other, and so the choice is made on the basis of acceptability of route of administration, cost and availability. On this basis, one of the TNF-α blockers is generally the first choice. There is evidence that TNF-α blockers may worsen multiple sclerosis and so they should not be used in patients with this disease. If treatment with the first TNF-α blocker is not adequately effective, it would seem rational to change to a bDMARD with a different mode of action, but research evidence suggests that changing to an alternative TNF-α blocker may be equally effective. Adding a new bDMARD without stopping the original one does not appear to increase effectiveness, but may increase adverse events.

Adverse Effects. The reported adverse events vary from agent to agent; however, most bDMARDs can trigger skin reactions and can cause bone marrow suppression in a similar manner to cDMARDs. Lung fibrosis has been reported. Some agents can cause liver damage and tocilizumab treatment has occasionally been associated with liver failure. This drug has also been associated with lower intestinal perforation and should be used with caution in patients with diverticulosis. Some bDMARDs can adversely affect lipid profiles, which should be checked after initiation of treatment and may require lipid lowering treatment. This is important, as patients with RA are already at increased risk of CVD.

There has been conflicting evidence regarding cancer risk with bDMARDs, but the current consensus is that they do not increase the risk of any type of tumour. However, these are new drugs and surveillance continues.

While there were initial reports that infliximab (and possibly other TNF-α blockers) might trigger or worsen heart failure, a recent review of the evidence does not strongly support this possibility. Licence restrictions should be followed for individual drugs, but TNF-α blockers appear to be safe to use in patients with mild to moderate (New York Heart Association class I or II) heart failure. For patients with worse heart failure, other types of bDMARD are more appropriate.

bDMARD treatment does increase the risk of infections, probably to a greater degree than cDMARDs. Reactivation of latent TB has occurred and seems to be a more marked issue with the TNF-α blockers. It is important to appropriately screen for chronic viral infections and latent TB before initiating bDMARDs.

Concurrent Care

Concurrent care of patients with RA includes physiotherapy to strengthen muscles and prevent deformity, sometimes rest, occasionally surgery, the treatment of complications and advice and counselling. It is important to remember comorbidities, and to manage cardiovascular risk. Patients with long-term poorly-controlled RA may have special difficulties. In severe cases, they cannot open drug containers or hold even quite light objects such as bottles, and can also have trouble opening doors. Health professionals who work with these patients need to be acutely aware of these problems. The occupational therapist is particularly important in this respect.

SUMMARY

- After diagnosis of RA, prevent disease progression with DMARDs.
- An important aim is to try to induce remission and to treat to this target.
- Oral corticosteroids are used in RA, in lower doses, to treat flares and cover initiation of DMARDs.
- Patients should have their eyes examined before starting on hydroxychloroquine and should report any disturbance of vision while on the drug.
- Methotrexate is given with folic acid and patients must have regular blood tests.
- Biologic drugs are important DMARDs, generally regarded as second-line therapies.
- Biologic drugs have idiosyncratic side-effects and require blood test monitoring.
- Any immunosuppressive drug increases risk of infections.
- Anti-TNF-α DMARDs may lead to reactivation of latent TB.
- Patients with RA need concurrent care, such as physiotherapy and special equipment at home.

GOUT

Gout is a metabolic disorder that tends to run in families. In gout, there is an increase in the amount of uric acid in the body, probably due to increased production, and this precipitates in and around joints (particularly the big toe), producing an acute and extremely painful arthritis. If untreated, it gradually resolves, but may recur, sometimes frequently. In long-standing cases, uric acid may also accumulate in other parts of the body. Although the caricature of a person with gout is an elderly man who overindulges in (purine rich) food and drink, particularly port wine, the reality is that gout occurs in young people too, and that diet only plays a modest role in precipitating attacks. Dehydration is a more common trigger. However, the treatment of gout should include advice regarding weight loss, exercise, diet, alcohol consumption and fluid intake. The incidence of gout appears to be increasing, for currently unknown reasons.

CLINICAL NOTE

A recent study published in *The Lancet*, reported improved patient outcomes when patients were treated by a nurse for gout compared to a doctor. Uptake and adherence levels (96% vs 56% $P<0.0001$) were better in the nurse-led group and urate concentrations were lower (Doherty et al., 2018). This was attributed to better education and counselling in the nurse-led group. Given that gout is the most common rheumatological condition it appears that time spent educating patients on gout and pathophysiology and treatment has a positive effect on outcomes.

Drug Treatment of Gout

Acute attacks of gout can be treated with:

- NSAIDs
- Colchicine.

Either treatment is effective and the choice depends on patient preference and previous experience of side-effects, other medications and morbidities, as well as renal function (as colchicine dose should be reduced with renal impairment and not used if the eGFR is <10). However, overall, NSAIDs are probably the safer first choice of treatment. If NSAIDs are used, then the maximum licensed dose should be given and continued for 1–2 days after the attack has settled. While indometacin has historically been the first choice, there is little evidence that it is superior to other NSAIDs and its side-effect profile is considerably worse. A PPI should be prescribed concurrently. COX-2 inhibitors may be better tolerated for short-term high dose use.

Colchicine is a natural alkaloid obtained from the 'flame lily', 'autumn crocus' or 'meadow saffron'. Colchicine is not an analgesic in the strict sense of the word because it relieves only one type of pain, namely that associated with an acute attack of gout. It reduces inflammation through several mechanisms, including inhibition of cellular microtubule formation. This prevents mitosis and also the migration of inflammatory cells such as neutrophils

Therapeutic Use

Colchicine has been used to treat gout since ancient times, and may also be used to prevent gout flares when starting gout-preventing treatment. It is also used to treat the ulcers of Behçet's disease, and to treat familial Mediterranean fever, although in many countries, these are not licensed indications. It is administered orally in tablet form and is well absorbed. It was formerly used in relatively high doses to treat acute gout, but lower doses appear to be effective and better tolerated; 500 µg 2–4 times a day can be given, up to a total dose of 6 mg, with the course not then repeated for 3 days. Lower doses can be used for prophylactic treatment.

Adverse Effects. Although widely used and effective, colchicine is very toxic in overdose and has a narrow therapeutic window. It has many drug interactions, some of which increase the likelihood of serious toxicity. It should, for instance, be used with caution in patients taking statins, and concurrent use of macrolide antibiotics should be avoided. Colchicine treatment is generally less suitable for older people because of the risk of side-effects. These are largely in the GI tract, and diarrhoea and nausea and vomiting are common. In older people, lower doses may be effective, with reduced side-effects. Alopecia, myopathy and peripheral neuropathy can occur and may sometimes be severe. Long-term use may cause blood dyscrasias (abnormalities).

If neither NSAIDs nor colchicine are tolerated or effective, then a short course of oral **corticosteroids** or an intraarticular injection of a corticosteroid are sometimes used.

Canakinumab is a monoclonal antibody that can be given by injection to treat acute attacks of gout that do not respond to conventional therapy. It selectively inhibits interleukin-1 beta receptor binding, and must not be given more frequently than 3 monthly. All the adverse effects common to biologics can occur.

Prevention of Gout. For younger patients, and patients who have more than two acute attacks of gout a year, or if they have evidence of joint damage, kidney stones, kidney impairment or urate deposition in other tissues, preventative treatment should be considered. This is a daily treatment to reduce the likelihood of an attack of gout. Most commonly, patients are offered drugs to reduce the synthesis of uric acid. In specialist care, drugs that increase uric acid excretion are sometimes also used. These are referred to as *uricosuric* drugs.

Drugs Preventing the Production of Uric Acid: Allopurinol and Febuxostat

Allopurinol slows the production of uric acid by inhibiting an enzyme (xanthine oxidase), which is concerned with the synthesis of uric acid within the body. It reduces the frequency and severity of attacks of gout, and will usually need to be continued for the rest of the patient's life.

Therapeutic Use

Allopurinol is given orally. It is a prodrug, and is converted into the active metabolite, alloxanthine, which in turn inhibits the enzyme that produced it.

It is excreted via the kidneys and the dose should be reduced in renal impairment and in the elderly. When starting allopurinol (or febuxostat), flares of gout are common. The drugs should ideally be started when the gout is quiescent, but if this is not possible or if attacks are frequent, then low dose colchicine may be given daily for up to 6 months. Allopurinol should be started at a low dose and gradually increased after 4 weeks, depending on the serum uric acid level. The aim of treatment is to have the uric acid level in the mid or lower part of the normal range, and for the frequency and severity of attacks to be tolerable.

Adverse Effects. Allopurinol is generally well-tolerated, however skin rashes are common, and the drug should be stopped and then reintroduced if a rash occurs. If the rash recurs, then allopurinol should not be used again, as dangerous skin reactions can occur. Serious blood dyscrasias can occur, but these are rare. Renal and liver function should be checked before starting treatment, and monitoring of renal function should occur annually. A blood count is needed if bleeding, bruising or unusual infections occur. There are many drug interactions, the most important of which are with azathioprine and 6-mercaptourine, both of which are metabolized by xanthene oxidase and which can accumulate dangerously if given with allopurinol (or febuxostat).

Febuxostat is a relatively new, second-line gout prophylactic treatment, for use when allopurinol is contraindicated or not tolerated. It is important to note that hypersensitivity to allopurinol and/or the presence of renal disease, increases the likelihood of hypersensitivity to febuxostat. It reduces uric acid production by xanthene oxidase inhibition, like allopurinol, and should be started in a similar manner to allopurinol. It may be used in elderly people and in mild/moderate kidney disease without dose reduction. The dose should be reduced in liver disease, and liver function should be checked before starting. It should not be used in IHD or heart failure, and there is evidence that all-cause mortality is greater in patients treated with febuxostat, compared with allopurinol – although it may be that this is because it is more likely to be given to sicker patients than allopurinol. It is generally well-tolerated, but rashes are relatively common, and dangerous hypersensitivity reactions have occurred, although rarely.

Uricosuric Drugs. Uricosuric drugs increase the excretion of uric acid by the kidney. They are not commonly used today and only when allopurinol or febuxostat are ineffective or not tolerated. The primary uricosuric drugs are **sulfinpyrazone**, **probenecid** and **benzbromarone**. Sulfinpyrazone is the only one of these used to any great degree. Benzbromarone is no longer available in most countries. Probenecid is not often used in gout, but does have the effect of increasing plasma levels of some drugs, including penicillins, and this is sometimes of clinical use. Aspirin antagonizes the effect of uricosuric drugs and should not be used to treat gout.

CLINICAL NOTES

1. Uricosuric drugs and allopurinol may cause an acute attack of gout in the first few months of treatment, probably because deposits of uric acid are mobilized, and should therefore be combined with colchicine or a NSAID during this period.
2. If uricosuric drugs are used, the patient should be advised to maintain a high fluid intake to prevent the formation of uric acid crystals in the renal tract.
3. Diuretics and pyrazinamide can cause attacks of gout.

SUMMARY

- Do not use aspirin in patients with gout.
- Patients with frequent attacks of gout need preventative treatment, commonly allopurinol.

REFERENCES AND FURTHER READING

Doherty, M., Jenkins, W., Richardson, H., et al., 2018. Efficacy and cost-effectiveness of nurse-led care involving education and engagement of patients and a treat-to-target urate-lowering strategy versus usual care for gout: a randomised controlled trial. Lancet 392 (10156), 1403–1412.

Ledingham, J., Snowden, N., Ide, Z., 2017. Diagnosis and early management of inflammatory arthritis. BMJ 358, j3248.

McNicol, E.D., Ferguson, M.C., Haroutounian, S., et al., 2016. Single dose intravenous paracetamol or intravenous propacetamol for postoperative pain. Cochrane Database Sys. Rev. 5, CD007126.

Moore, N., Pollack, C., Butkerait, P., 2015. Adverse drug reactions and drug-drug interactions with over-the-counter NSAIDs. Ther. Clin. Risk Manag. 11, 1061–1075.

NICE, 2007. Adalimumab, Etanercept and Infliximab for the Treatment of Rheumatoid Arthritis [TA130]. https://www.nice.org.uk/guidance/ta130.

NICE, 2018. Gout: Clinical Knowledge Summary. https://cks.nice.org.uk/topics/gout.

NICE, 2018. Rheumatoid Arthritis in Adults: Management [NG100]. https://www.nice.org.uk/guidance/ng100.

Ramiro, S., Sepriano, A., Chatzidionysiou, K., et al., 2017. Safety of synthetic and biological DMARDs: a systematic literature review informing the 2016 update of the EULAR recommendations for management of rheumatoid arthritis. Ann. Rheum. Dis. 76 (6), 1101–1136.

Smolen, J.S., Landewe, R., Breedveld, F.C., et al., 2014. EULAR recommendations for the management of rheumatoid arthritis with synthetic and biological disease-modifying antirheumatic drugs: 2013 update. Ann. Rheum. Dis. 73 (3), 492–509.

van Eijk-Hustings, Y., van Tubergen, A., Bostrom, C., et al., 2012. EULAR recommendations for the role of the nurse in the management of chronic inflammatory arthritis. Ann. Rheum. Dis. 71 (1), 13–19.

USEFUL WEBSITE

Versus Arthritis. http://www.arthritiscare.org.uk.

14 ENDOCRINE SYSTEM 1
The Hypothalamus and Pituitary

CHAPTER OUTLINE

LEARNING OBJECTIVES

At the end of this chapter, the reader should be able to:

- explain the terms endocrine, paracrine and autocrine hormones
- describe the hypothalamic–pituitary axis
- describe the anatomy of the pituitary stalk and the two main pituitary lobes
- give the names, actions and some uses of the hypothalamic releasing, and inhibiting hormones
- give the names, actions and some uses of the anterior lobe hormones
- list the posterior lobe hormones and what their main actions are
- be aware of the role of the hypothalamus and the hormone leptin in appetite control

HORMONES

The endocrine or ductless glands are organs or small islands of tissue in various parts of the body. Each gland secretes a substance – or, in some cases, several substances – called *hormones*. These are released from the gland and may enter the bloodstream, circulate through the body and act on distant organs or tissues (called an 'endocrine action'); act on neighbouring cells (called a 'paracrine action'); act on the cells that released them (called an 'autocrine action'; Fig. 14.1). These describe the different forms of signalling pathways between different cell types.

Some hormones may have two or even all three types of action. Their speed of action is variable; the effects of some hormones are seen almost immediately after release (e.g. insulin), whereas others may take hours or even days to show their effects (e.g. oestrogens). After release, these hormones act upon a receptor mechanism in the organ or organs they influence, thus producing their specific actions. The actions of the various hormones differ widely, e.g. one group is concerned with metabolic processes, another with secondary sexual characteristics, etc. Sometimes, a hormone will act on another endocrine gland and stimulate it to produce a further hormone, a mechanism crucial in the control of the release of endocrine hormones such as cortisol and the sex hormones by the brain and pituitary gland.

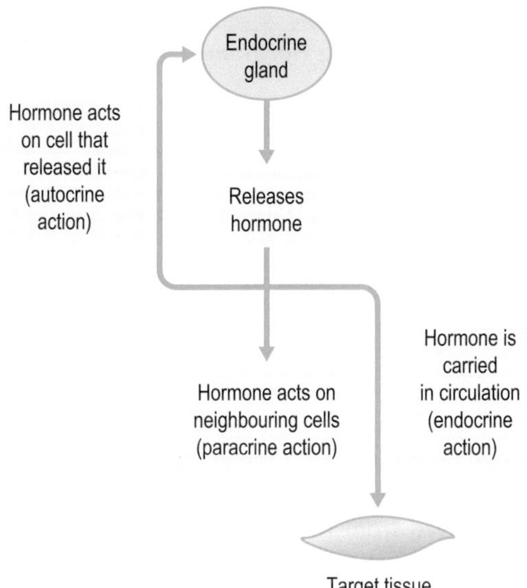

Fig. 14.1 ■ Actions of endocrine organs.

Many of these hormones have been isolated and their structure determined. This has made it possible to prepare synthetically either the hormones or analogues that are sometimes more active and more stable than the hormones themselves.

Classification of Endocrine Glands

The endocrine glands can be divided roughly into three groups:

- The pituitary gland, which secretes hormones that exercise a controlling influence over much of the rest of the endocrine system and which, in turn, is largely controlled by the hypothalamus in the brain
- Endocrine glands affecting metabolism
- Endocrine glands affecting the reproductive system.

CLASSIFICATION NOTE

The above classification is purely for the purpose of facilitating an organized division of this chapter of the book. It can be argued with much justification that since the pituitary gland controls most other glands, it affects both metabolism and reproduction, which of course it does.

This section of the chapter deals with the hypothalamic–pituitary axis, the hormones of the axis and the drugs influencing the axis.

THE HYPOTHALAMIC–PITUITARY AXIS

The pituitary is a small endocrine gland attached to the brain by a pituitary stalk and lying, almost surrounded by bone, in the base of the skull. It consists of anterior and posterior lobes. In spite of its small size, it is of great importance. It secretes a number of hormones that affect, not only various processes in the body, but also the activity of most of the other endocrine glands. It is of interest that the activity of the pituitary itself is influenced by other hormones, both released by the brain and from other glands in the body. These other hormones regulate secretion of pituitary hormones through complex and highly regulated feedback mechanisms (see later).

The release of the pituitary hormones of the anterior lobe is a complex function and for many of them, there is a specific releasing hormone, which is produced in the brain, specifically in the hypothalamus. Some of the hypothalamic hormones do not stimulate, but inhibit, release of anterior lobe hormones instead (Table 14.1). The anterior pituitary hormones in turn stimulate the release of hormones from the endocrine glands. Those hormones exert their various effects on the body, and also travel to the brain and to the pituitary gland, where they either stimulate or inhibit the release of releasing hormones and/or the pituitary gland hormones. These regulatory actions of the endocrine hormones are called feedback effects and are of great importance in understanding the pharmacological effects of several drugs, including the contraceptive pill (see Chapter 18).

The Pituitary Stalk

The pituitary is connected to the hypothalamus of the brain by a pituitary stalk called the 'infundibulum'. The pituitary stalk contains nerves that connect the hypothalamus to the posterior lobe, and blood vessels that connect the hypothalamus to the anterior lobe. The blood vessels are called the **portal system** because they carry hormones from the hypothalamus

TABLE 14.1

Anterior Lobe Hormones and their Hypothalamic Releasing Hormones

Hypothalamic Releasing or Inhibitory Hormone	Anterior Lobe Hormone
Corticotrophin-releasing hormone (CRH)	Adrenocorticotrophic hormone (ACTH; corticotrophin)
Gonadotrophin-releasing hormone (GnRH)	Luteinizing hormone (LH) Follicle-stimulating hormone (FSH)
Thyrotrophin-releasing hormone (TRH)	Thyroid-stimulating hormone (TSH; thyrotrophin)
Growth hormone-releasing hormone (GHRH; somatorelin)	Growth hormone (GH)
Growth hormone-inhibitory hormone (GHIH; somatostatin)	Growth hormone (GH)
Dopamine (DA) (inhibits release of prolactin), TRH, prolactin-releasing peptide (PRP) (stimulates release of prolactin)	Prolactin

to the pituitary. The nerves to the posterior lobe carry both electrical signals and the hormones **oxytocin** and **vasopressin** (otherwise known as antidiuretic hormone, see later), which are stored in the posterior pituitary until release into the general circulation.

CONTROL OF PITUITARY HORMONE RELEASE

There are two groups of pituitary hormones:

- anterior lobe hormones
- posterior lobe hormones.

Control of Anterior Lobe Hormone Release

The release of anterior lobe hormones is governed largely by the hypothalamic releasing hormones. The hypothalamic hormones and the anterior lobe hormones they control are shown in Table 14.1. The anterior pituitary manufactures the hormones but their release is regulated by the hormones secreted from the hypothalamus.

The hypothalamic releasing hormones (which help to stimulate the anterior pituitary hormones) and inhibitory hormones are:

- CRH – corticotrophin-releasing hormone
- GnRH – gonadotrophin-releasing hormone
- TRH – thyrotrophin-releasing hormone
- GHRH (also known as somatorelin) – growth hormone releasing hormone
- GHIH (somatostatin) – growth hormone inhibiting hormone
- Dopamine (DA).

These hormones, with the exception of dopamine, are all peptides and are important because they, or the drugs derived from them, are used both therapeutically and diagnostically.

CRH

CRH is corticotrophin-releasing hormone. It is a peptide synthesized in the hypothalamus and it causes the release of adrenocorticotrophic hormone (ACTH) from the anterior pituitary. It is used clinically mainly as a diagnostic tool to test the ability of the pituitary to release ACTH. Cortisol and the synthetic steroids such as prednisolone inhibit its release by a negative feedback mechanism and this in part explains some of the adverse effects of this class of drug, particularly when they are administered systemically. CRH is now also known to be important in the control of food intake and the problem of obesity, and drugs are being sought to modulate its action in the treatment of obesity, which is a major and growing global problem.

NURSING NOTE

Patients on long-term oral steroids such as prednisolone must be weaned off them gradually. This is because prolonged use of prednisolone completely suppresses the CRH–ACTH–cortisol system, which normally protects the patient from stress and is important in glucose metabolism. Gradual reduction in prednisolone allows cortisol levels to rise again (see also later).

GnRH

GnRH is gonadotrophin-releasing hormone. It is synthesized in the hypothalamus and travels to the anterior pituitary in the portal system of blood vessels (see earlier). GnRH causes the release of luteinizing hormone (LH) and follicle-stimulating hormone (FSH) from the anterior lobe. It is therefore the prime hormone of fertility. GnRH is released from the hypothalamus in regular pulses, and this pulsatile release has been used to induce ovulation in certain cases of infertility through the use of synthetic analogues of GnRH (see Chapter 18). The release of GnRH is subject to the negative feedback effects of the sex hormones, and this negative feedback effect is partly how the combined contraceptive pill works (see Chapter 18).

Paradoxically, if GnRH or its synthetic analogues are used continuously, there is a virtual shutdown of the LH/FSH pituitary system and infertility results. This phenomenon is used to treat certain sex hormone-dependent cancers, particularly prostate cancer and other issues where sex hormones need to be suppressed, such as endometriosis, hirsutism and precocious puberty. Continuous suppression of oestrogens in women can produce unwanted effects, particularly those normally associated with menopause, such as hot flushes, vaginal dryness, headache, decreased libido and osteoporosis. GnRH receptor antagonists are also available and are currently being used and tested for various endocrine cancers and for infertility.

TRH

TRH is thyrotrophin-releasing hormone. It is synthesized in the hypothalamus and travels to the anterior lobe, where it releases thyrotrophin (thyroid-stimulating hormone, TSH). A synthetic analogue of TRH, called 'protirelin', is used to test the integrity of the TRH–TSH system and to check for hyperthyroidism. In normal subjects, an injection of protirelin will elicit a release of TSH from the anterior lobe. In hyperthyroid patients, there is elevated thyroxine from the thyroid gland. This has a negative feedback effect on TSH release from the anterior lobe, and so an injection of protirelin will have little or no effect on TSH release. TRH has also been found to cause prolactin release, although the physiological significance of this action of TRH is still unclear.

GHIH (Somatostatin)

Somatostatin inhibits the release of growth hormone (GH) from the anterior lobe. It is thus part of the normal mechanism for the control of GH release. It is therefore potentially an important tool for the treatment of acromegaly (see later), when there is excess GH release from the pituitary or from a pituitary tumour. A long-acting synthetic analogue of somatostatin, called octreotide, has been introduced for this purpose.

Uses of Octreotide. By suppressing the release of GH in patients with acromegaly, octreotide can control the symptoms when surgery is impossible or incomplete. The main problem with the use of this drug is that it is expensive. Octreotide also suppresses the release of several hormones in the stomach and intestine, and reduces the blood flow to the gut. As a result of these actions, it can be given to control certain types of diarrhoea, including that occurring in people with HIV infection, and it is also used to reduce the bleeding from oesophageal varices (dilated veins in the lower oesophagus, which may rupture), and in the treatment of certain tumours of the intestine. Adverse effects include gastritis and gallstone formation.

CLINICAL NOTE

Octreotide is a peptide and, if given orally, will be digested before it can exert a response. Thus, its only route of administration is parenteral.

GHRH (Somatorelin)

GHRH is a very powerful hypothalamic hormone that causes the release of GH from the anterior lobe. A synthetic derivative, sermorelin, has been introduced as a diagnostic tool to test the integrity of the GH releasing system.

Dopamine

Dopamine is an important neurotransmitter, both in the brain and elsewhere in the body, and has also been discovered to be a hypothalamic hormone that is released from nerve endings into the portal blood supply to the anterior lobe, where it inhibits prolactin release. It is therefore part of the mechanism that controls lactation (see later). Dopamine is therefore potentially a useful clinical tool for suppression of lactation but cannot be administered as a drug. A dopamine analogue called 'bromocriptine' is used instead.

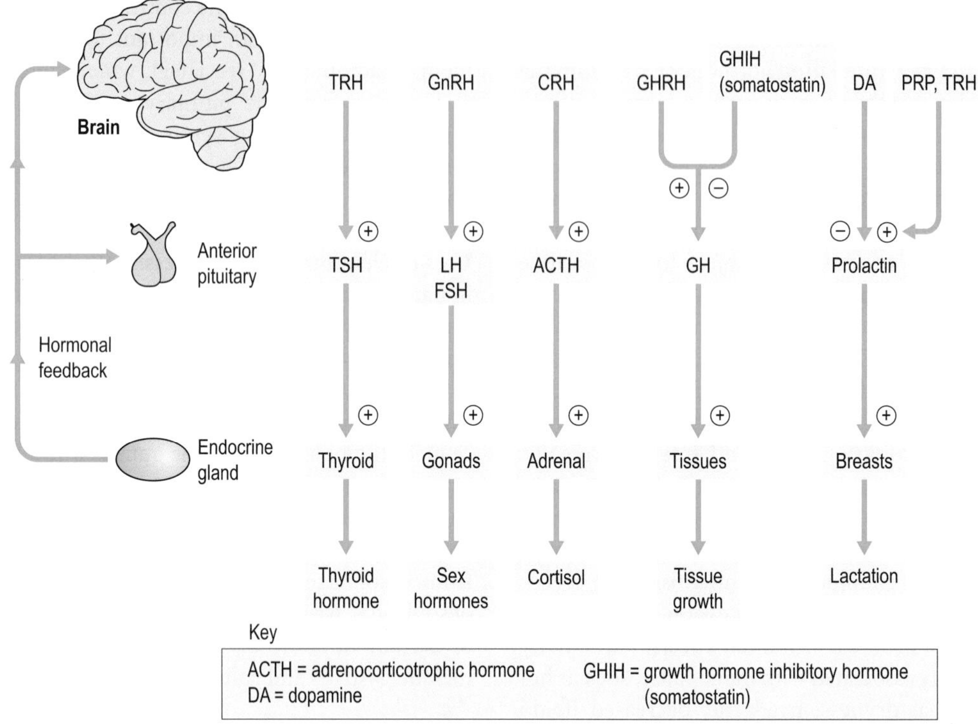

Fig. 14.2 Hormones of the hypothalamus, anterior pituitary and endocrine glands. (For abbreviations, see Table 14.1.)

Bromocriptine is an interesting drug that is extracted from ergot. It acts on the pituitary in the same way as the naturally occurring substance dopamine and inhibits the release of various hormones, particularly prolactin and GH (see later). It also stimulates dopamine receptors in the basal ganglia and thus relieves the symptoms of Parkinson's disease (see Chapter 21). Bromocriptine can be administered orally and is well absorbed. The drug is also used in the treatment of certain forms of infertility.

Prolactin-releasing peptide is a hypothalamic hormone that stimulates prolactin release. Its role in the control of prolactin release is still unclear and is being investigated.

The relationships between the hypothalamic hormones and those of the anterior pituitary are shown in Fig. 14.2.

CLINICAL NOTE

The Medicine and Healthcare Products Regulation Agency (MHRA, 2014) note that bromocriptine is associated with cardiac, pulmonary and retroperitoneal fibrosis. Prior to prescribing bromocriptine, patients should have an echocardiogram to exclude any valvulopathy and be monitored for shortness of breath or respiratory symptoms, such as a persistent cough, and for any renal symptoms.

Hormones of the Anterior Lobe

These comprise:

- adrenocorticotrophic hormone (ACTH; corticotrophin)
- luteinizing hormone (LH)
- follicle-stimulating gonadotrophins hormone (FSH)
- thyroid-stimulating hormone (TSH; thyrotrophin)
- growth hormone (GH; somatotrophin)
- prolactin.

Adrenocorticotrophic Hormone

Release of ACTH. ACTH release from the anterior lobe is under the control of hypothalamic CRH (see

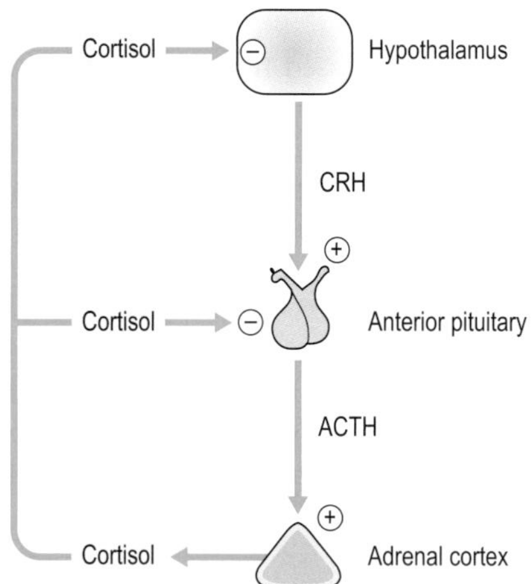

Fig. 14.3 ■ Negative feedback action of cortisol on corticotrophin-releasing hormone (CRH) and adrenocorticotrophic hormone (ACTH) release.

earlier) and of cortisol. CRH causes ACTH release. High levels of cortisol suppress ACTH release from the anterior lobe and they suppress CRH release from the hypothalamus. When cortisol levels fall, then more CRH and consequently more ACTH are released. These actions of cortisol both at the level of the brain and the anterior lobe provide a regulatory mechanism for the release of CRH, ACTH and cortisol (Fig. 14.3).

Stimulation of the Synthesis and Release of Cortisol from the Adrenal Cortex. ACTH rapidly stimulates the synthesis and release of cortisol from the adrenal cortex. It does this by increasing concentrations of adrenal cholesterol, which is the precursor for all steroid synthesis in the adrenal gland.

Trophic (Growth) Action on Adrenal Cortex Cells and Regulation of Adrenal Enzymes that Synthesize Cortisol. ACTH actually promotes the growth of the cells that produce cortisol, and also of the production of the enzymes that catalyse the synthesis of cortisol. This explains why the adrenal cortex atrophies (shrinks) in patients who receive chronic treatment with glucocorticoids such as prednisolone (see Chapter 17). In these patients, prednisolone shuts down the release of both CRH and ACTH. This is why it is important not to cease steroid treatment suddenly, but to reduce it gradually to stimulate a return to normal adrenal production.

Uses of ACTH. ACTH has been used to test the cortisol releasing system and occasionally in some autoimmune diseases such as lupus. ACTH itself is not much used anymore because it is immunogenic, i.e. it stimulates an allergic response. Instead, a synthetic compound, **tetracosactide** (also known as cosyntropin), is used, mainly for testing adrenal function.

Tetracosactide is available as a rapidly acting preparation for IM or IV use. For testing adrenal function, the medication is injected intramuscularly. Blood levels of cortisol are measured before and 30 min after injection. If the adrenals are working properly, the injection is followed by a rise in the blood levels of cortisol.

LH and FSH (Gonadotrophins)

LH and FSH are called 'gonadotrophins' because they are concerned with the growth and structural maintenance of the male and female gonads, and with the synthesis and release of the gonadal sex hormones. LH causes ovulation and promotes testosterone production in the male. FSH promotes follicular growth in the ovary and development of the spermatozoa. They are dealt with more fully in Chapter 18.

Thyroid-stimulating Hormone (Thyrotrophin)

Release of TSH. TSH is released from the anterior lobe in response to TRH from the hypothalamus (see earlier). The release of TSH is regulated by a negative feedback effect of thyroid hormone. If for any reason thyroid function is depressed, e.g. by drugs or disease, then the pituitary secretes large amounts of TSH. The positive effect of TSH on thyroid hormone release, and the negative feedback effect of thyroid hormone on TSH, are both used in a number of tests of thyroid function.

Actions of TSH. TSH controls every aspect of the production and release of thyroid hormone from the thyroid gland. The thyroid gland releases thyroid hormone, which regulates body metabolism. The actions of TSH on thyroid hormone are covered in more detail in Chapter 15.

Growth Hormone (Somatotrophin)

This hormone stimulates growth both in soft tissue and in bone. GH release from the pituitary is complicated as there are at least two substances from the brain that control its secretion (see earlier). Unfortunately, most animal somatotrophin is ineffective in humans, so human growth hormone must be used. This has now been synthesized using biotechnology and the product is called 'somatropin'. In patients with dwarfism due to hormone deficiency, treatment must be started before epiphyseal fusion (closure of the ends of the long bones) has occurred and continued until growth is complete. Somatropin is given subcutaneously weekly and the dose-adjusted as necessary. Unfortunately, GH is expensive.

Overproduction of somatotrophin by the pituitary gland will produce gigantism in children and acromegaly in adults.

Prolactin

Milk Production. Prolactin, the so called 'lactogenic' hormone, produces its maximum effect on the breast, which has already been prepared throughout pregnancy by oestrogens and progesterone (see Chapter 18). Its production by the pituitary can be suppressed by bromocriptine (see earlier), which is used when it is necessary to suppress lactation.

Inhibition of Ovarian Function. Prolactin also has a powerful inhibitory effect on ovarian function, and high blood levels of prolactin during the period of lactation are probably responsible for the delayed return of menstruation after pregnancy. Prolactin levels are also raised in both males and females during stress, and there is evidence from animal studies that this may account to some extent for the reduction in fertility due to stresses caused by, e.g. population overcrowding and hierarchical conflicts in communities.

The functions of the various anterior lobe hormones are summarized in Fig. 14.4.

Hormones of the Posterior Lobe

Two important hormones – oxytocin and vasopressin (also known as antidiuretic hormone, ADH) – can be extracted from the posterior lobe of the pituitary. These are both peptides, but they have very different functions (Fig. 14.5). The posterior pituitary does not produce hormones but it helps store and secrete the hormones which are produced by the hypothalamus.

Oxytocin

This hormone is released from the posterior lobe as part of the suckling reflex and causes milk ejection from the breast (see Fig. 14.5). Oxytocin also causes contraction of the uterus in labour and is considered in more detail in Chapter 18.

Vasopressin (Antidiuretic Hormone)

Vasopressin has two actions. In comparatively large doses, it causes vasoconstriction with a concomitant rise in blood pressure, but its more important effect from the therapeutic aspect is concerned with water balance, as it is the antidiuretic hormone.

Vasopressin Release. If the intake of water is limited, the blood becomes slightly more concentrated, which affects special receptors in the base of the brain. These stimulate the posterior pituitary to secrete more vasopressin. Vasopressin increases the reabsorption of water by the renal tubules, and thus decreases the amount of urine and conserves the body water. If the intake of water is increased, the production of vasopressin drops and the output of urine by the kidneys is increased, thus balancing the intake and output of water by the body.

Therapeutic Use of Vasopressin: Diabetes Insipidus. Occasionally, damage to the posterior pituitary or closely related structures produces a disease called 'diabetes insipidus', in which little or no vasopressin is produced. There is thus a continuously high output of urine, which in turn requires the drinking of vast quantities of water if dehydration is to be avoided. Nurses will probably encounter this condition most commonly in patients who have had hypophysectomy (surgical removal of the pituitary gland) and who therefore have no vasopressin.

The disorder can be controlled by the administration of vasopressin, which is given as an injection. It was previously used as a snuff but has now been replaced by **desmopressin**. Desmopressin is a synthetic drug structurally related to vasopressin.

Therapeutic Use of Vasopressin: Bleeding from Oesophageal Varices. The vasoconstrictor properties of vasopressin can be used in the treatment of bleeding from oesophageal varices. The vasoconstriction lowers pressure in the portal vein and allows the bleeding vein

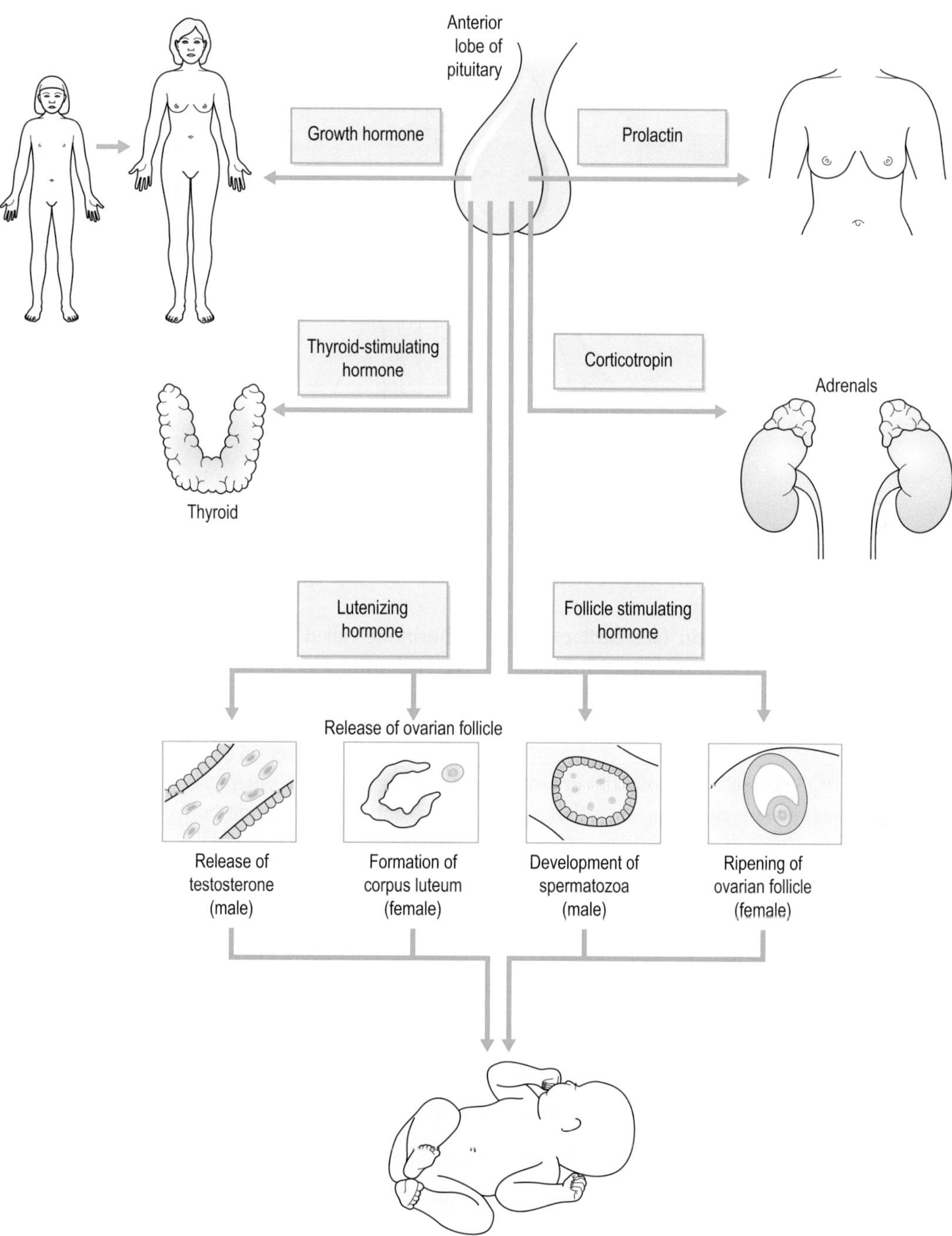

Fig. 14.4 ■ Hormones released by the anterior lobe of the pituitary gland, showing their main sites of action.

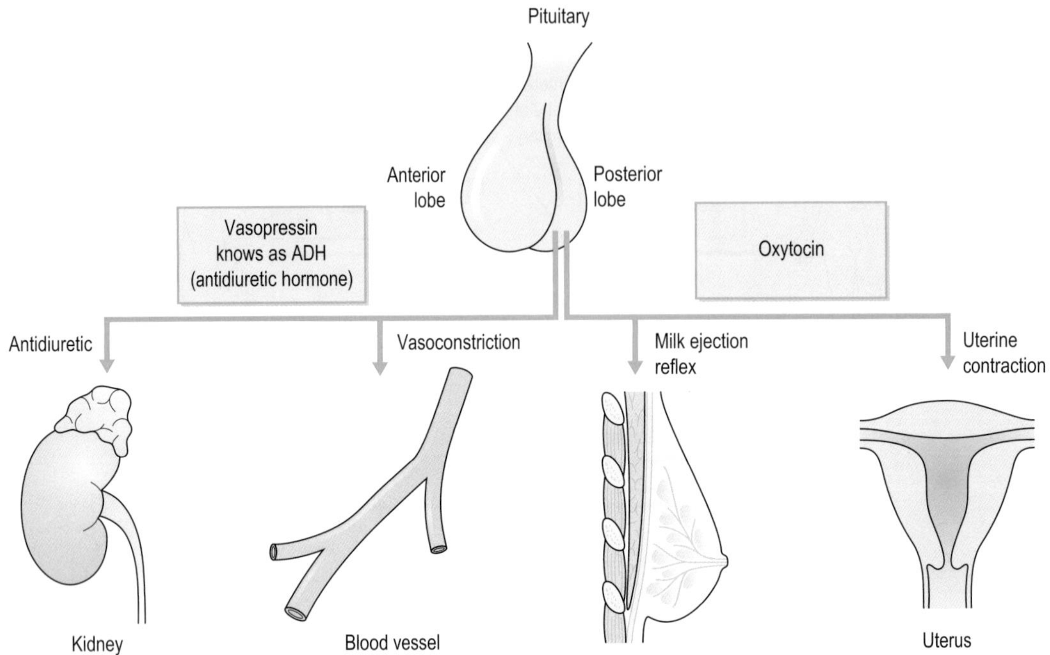

Fig. 14.5 Hormones released by the posterior pituitary gland and their sites of action.

to clot. Vasopressin or somatostatin (see earlier) can be used and are administered by intravenous infusion for the initial control of oesophageal variceal bleeding.

CLINICAL NOTE

Desmopressin can be given orally, intranasally or intramuscularly. It has a very long action such that one or two doses daily suffice to control diabetes insipidus, and it is now the preferred drug for treating this condition. Unlike vasopressin, desmopressin does not cause vasoconstriction. Treatment should aim at reducing the patient's urine output to about 2 L/day. Desmopressin can also be used to treat nocturnal enuresis in patients with normal pituitary function, by reducing night-time urine volume. However, care must be taken to prevent fluid overload. Desmopressin is administered orally or intranasally at bedtime.

THE HYPOTHALAMUS AND OBESITY

A relatively new discovery is that appetite and feeding behaviour are under the influence of a regulatory endocrine system involving the hypothalamus, fat cells and a hormone called 'leptin', released by fat cells. Fat cells secrete **leptin**, which is released into the bloodstream. In the ventromedial nucleus of the hypothalamus, there is a group of cells called 'the satiety centre', which regulate feeding behaviour. Leptin acts on these cells to inhibit the release of two neurochemicals, called 'neuropeptide Y' and 'agouti-related peptide', both of which stimulate feeding behaviour in experimental animals. Leptin was originally discovered in a mutant strain of obese mice which eat constantly and develop a condition resembling type II diabetes, which causes them to die prematurely. The mice were discovered to have no leptin and have mutations of the gene that normally produces leptin. A group of patients have been identified who also have a mutant leptin gene; these patients eat virtually constantly and become grossly obese before the age of 10. Leptin also raises body temperature slightly, directly stimulates fatty acid oxidation in liver and skeletal muscle, and appears to act directly on circulating T lymphocytes, although the significance of this is at present unknown.

Leptin, chemically, is a polypeptide containing 146 amino acids and it is anticipated that a better understanding of this hormone will lead to improved treatments for obesity.

SUMMARY

- Feedback mechanisms are exploited for drug design.
- Patients are weaned gradually off corticosteroids.
- GnRH shuts down pituitary release of LH if the pituitary is continuously exposed to it, and this is used to treat prostatic carcinoma.
- Feedback mechanisms can be exploited to test the integrity of the feedback system (e.g. using protirelin).
- Somatostatin inhibits growth hormone secretion and is therefore used to treat acromegaly.
- Bromocriptine acts like dopamine and can be used to block prolactin release, and therefore stop lactation.
- Synthetic analogues of ACTH can be used to test the integrity of the cortisol regulatory system.
- Human genetically engineered growth hormone is used to treat dwarfism, but must be started before epiphyseal closure has occurred.
- Stress raises prolactin levels and this can cause impotence in men.
- Vasopressin or synthetic analogues can be used to treat diabetes insipidus and bleeding from oesophageal varices.
- Hypothalamic feeding centres are a target for the hormone leptin, a newly discovered satiety hormone.

REFERENCES AND FURTHER READING

Alexandraki, K.I., Grossman, A.B., 2019. Management of hypopituitarism. J. Clin. Med. 8 (12), 2153.

Camilleri, M., 2019. Gastrointestinal hormones and regulation of gastric emptying. Curr. Opin. Endocrinol Diabetes Obesity 26 (1), 3–10.

Huirne, J.A.F., Lambalk, C.B., 2001. Gonadotropin-releasing-hormone-receptor antagonists. Lancet 358 (9295), 1793–1803.

Kieffer, V., Davies, K., Gibson, C., et al., 2015. Society for Endocrinology Competency Framework for Adult Endocrine Nursing, 2nd edn. Endocr. Connect 4 (1), W1–W17.

MHRA, 2014. Ergot Derived Antagonists: Risk of Fibrotic Reactions. https://www.gov.uk/drug-safety-update/ergot-derived-dopamine-agonists-risk-of-fibrotic-reactions.

Mundell, L., Lindemann, R., Douglas, J., 2017. Monitoring long term oral corticosteroids. BMJ Open Qual. 6 (2), e000209.

Perez-Lloret, S., Rascol, O., 2010. Dopamine receptor agonists for the treatment of early or advanced Parkinson's disease. CNS Drugs 24 (11), 941–968.

USEFUL WEBSITE

Colorado State University. http://www.vivo.colostate.edu/hbooks/pathphys/endocrine/hypopit/anatomy.html.

15 ENDOCRINE SYSTEM 2
Hormones and Metabolism – Thyroid and Parathyroid Disorders

CHAPTER OUTLINE

LEARNING OBJECTIVES

At the end of this chapter, the reader should be able to:

- describe the anatomical location of the thyroid gland
- explain how thyroid hormones are synthesized, stored in the thyroid and how they are released
- give the causes, consequences and treatments of hypothyroidism
- describe the symptoms and types of hyperthyroidism
- explain the surgical treatment of thyrotoxicosis
- list the drugs used to treat thyrotoxicosis
- describe the actions of parathyroid hormone
- describe the treatment of hypercalcaemia
- explain how calcium absorption is facilitated and how osteoporosis is treated

THE THYROID GLAND AND THYROID HORMONES

Introduction

The thyroid consists of two lobes connected by an isthmus and is situated in the neck, in front of the trachea (Fig. 15.1). Structurally, the thyroid gland is made up of **follicles**, which consist of a single layer of epithelial cells enclosing a lumen. The lumen is packed with a colloidal protein called 'thyroglobulin', which both forms and stores the thyroid hormones in an inactive form (Fig. 15.2). Iodine is an essential component of the two thyroid hormones: thyroxine (T4) and triiodothyronine (T3) (see later). With appropriate stimulation, notably through the action of thyroid-stimulating hormone

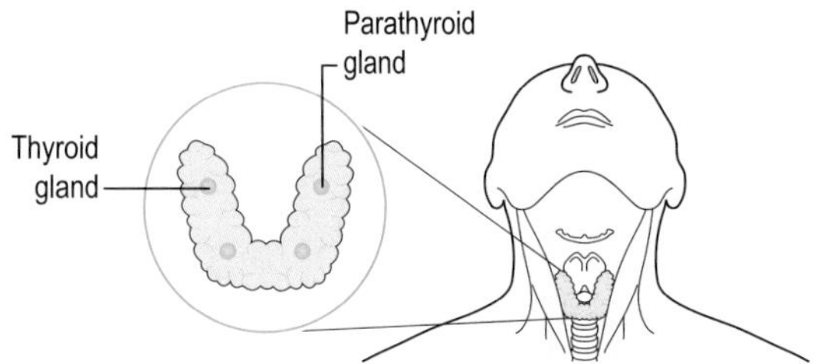

Fig. 15.1 ■ The thyroid and parathyroid glands.

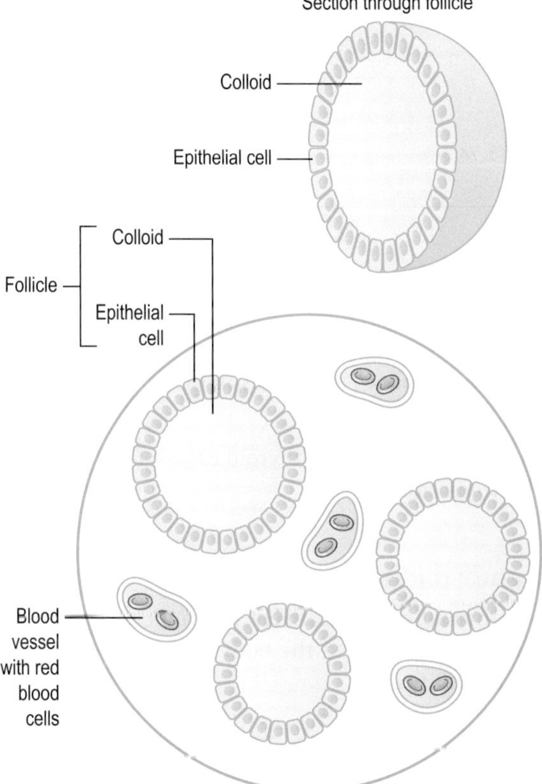

Fig. 15.2 ■ Microscopic view of thyroid gland and follicle.

(TSH; thyrotrophin), both T4 and T3 are released into the bloodstream (Fig. 15.3).

On reaching body tissues, T4 is converted to T3, which is the more active hormone. T3 exerts its effects on the cell by binding both to receptors inside the cell in a manner like that of the steroid hormones, resulting in changes in protein synthesis, and to receptors on the cell surface (see later). The effect of thyroid hormones is to increase tissue metabolism and thus to raise the basal metabolic rate. They are also important in promoting growth. In healthy people, the release of thyroid hormone is precisely adjusted to maintain the metabolic rate at a satisfactory level. When thyroid hormone levels are normal, the patient is described as *euthyroid*. When they are clinically elevated, the patient is *hyperthyroid*. When they are clinically depressed, the patient is *hypothyroid*.

Production and Release of Thyroid Hormones

Uptake of Iodide into the Thyroid

When iodine ions (known as *iodide*) enter the circulation, they are rapidly and powerfully taken up into the thyroid by an energy-dependent mechanism that can pump iodide into the thyroid against a concentration gradient of anything up to 50:1. This means that the thyroid gland can take up and concentrate even small amounts of iodide absorbed from a person's diet.

Biosynthesis of T3 and T4

Once iodide is in the thyroid, the enzyme *thyroid peroxidase* (TPO) oxidizes it to iodine, which is then incorporated into tyrosine residues on the protein *thyroglobulin*, both forming and storing T3 and T4 in inactive form as part of the protein, a complex referred to as **colloid**. The colloid is then stored in the lumen of the follicle. When circulating TSH binds to its receptor on the thyroid cell, this triggers a response, whereby droplets of the colloid are reabsorbed into the thyroid epithelial cell and by the action of other enzymes, the hormones are released from the colloid, activated and secreted from the cell into the circulation. Drugs to treat thyrotoxicosis target some of the steps in the synthesis of thyroid hormones (see later). The process is summarized in Fig. 15.3.

Plasma Binding of Thyroxine and Thyroid Function Tests

Once in the circulation, a specific thyroxine-binding protein, *thyroxine-binding globulin* (TBG), binds some of the thyroid hormones, as they are carried to their sites of action. There is a dynamic equilibrium in the circulation between the bound and free forms of thyroid hormones. This is clinically important, since it is only the free fraction of hormone that is available to the tissues, and free levels of thyroid hormones may be

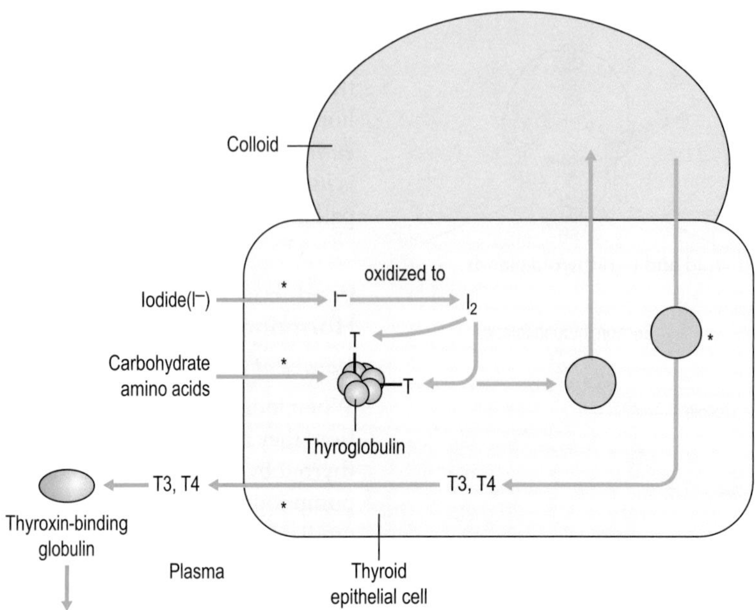

Fig. 15.3 ■ Production, storage and release of thyroid hormones. Iodide is taken up into the thyroid cell and oxidized to iodine, which is incorporated into tyrosine, on thyroglobulin. The protein is stored as colloid, until thyroid stimulating hormone (TSH) causes the cell to break down thyroglobulin and release triiodothyronine (T3) and thyroxine (T4), which are released into the circulation. *CHO*, Carbohydrate; *T*, tyrosine residue on thyroglobulin; I_2, iodine. Starred (*) reactions are promoted by TSH.

measured in patients, as well as total levels. The levels of TBG are also measured in some tests. As mentioned in Chapter 14, the ability of the pituitary to release TSH in response to hypothalamic TSH-releasing hormone (TRH) is also used to diagnose forms of thyroid disease.

Action of Thyroid Hormones

When T4 reaches its site of action, it is converted to T3, which binds to receptors on the cell surface and increases the cell's uptake of amino acids and glucose to increase metabolism. T3 is also absorbed into the cell, where it binds to intracellular receptors in the mitochondria and in the cell nucleus to generate energy, and new proteins, respectively.

ABNORMALITIES OF THYROID FUNCTION

These can be divided into:

- **hypothyroidism** (thyroid deficiency; leading to *myxoedema*)
- **hyperthyroidism** (thyroid excess; leading to *thyrotoxicosis*).

Hypothyroidism

Hypothyroidism is relatively common and means a reduced availability to the body of thyroid hormone. It can result from:

- Impairment of the TRH–TSH system of the brain and pituitary, sometimes as a consequence of pituitary tumours.
- Insufficient iodine in the diet; this leads to simple or non-toxic goitre. Iodine deficiency is the most common cause of hypothyroidism worldwide but is uncommon in high- and middle-income countries. Insufficient dietary iodine causes an increase in TSH secretion, which in turn causes thyroid growth, causing the goitre in the neck. The enlarged thyroid is nevertheless unable to produce sufficient thyroid hormone, due to the iodine deficiency. Non-toxic goitre can also occur through the eating of certain plants, such as cassava root.

- **Hashimoto's thyroiditis**, an immunological disorder, leading to the destruction of thyroid follicles. It is the most common cause of hypothyroidism in populations with sufficient iodine in the diet. The presence of antibodies directed against TPO are of particular importance in diagnosing Hashimoto's thyroiditis.
- Transient disorders of thyroid function may occur during and after pregnancy.
- Treatment with radioactive iodine, which may be used to treat hyperthyroidism (see later).

When thyroid deficiency is severe, it causes a condition called 'myxoedema'. The symptoms of myxoedema are:

- bradycardia (slowed heart rate)
- lethargy
- sensitivity to cold
- coarse, dry skin and hair
- heavy periods
- mental slowing
- weight gain
- altered sensation due to neuropathies.

Untreated, severe hypothyroidism is eventually fatal.

Provided the TRH–TSH system is intact, the levels of TSH will be **raised** in hypothyroidism, and measuring TSH aids both diagnosis and treatment of this condition.

CLINICAL NOTE

Drug metabolism is affected by a hypothyroid state and lower doses may be necessary until normal thyroid function is restored.

Congenital Hypothyroidism

The thyroid system is essential in the newborn infant for normal growth and development through the direct actions of T3 on the cells, and through the influence of TSH on growth hormone (GH) release from the anterior lobe. If severe thyroid deficiency occurs in infants from birth and is left untreated for too long, it will give rise to **congenital hypothyroidism** (sometimes referred to as *cretinism*), where development in the baby is stunted, causing small stature, intellectual disability, neurological impairment and coarsened facial features and skin. In many countries, thyroid function is tested at birth, and prompt treatment with thyroxine has almost eliminated the consequences of congenital hypothyroidism.

Treatment of Hypothyroidism

If hypothyroidism is the result of iodine deficiency, then treating the deficiency will treat the disease. In some countries, table salt is fortified with iodine in order to prevent hypothyroidism. Other forms of hypothyroidism are treated with synthetic thyroid hormones, which are available as oral tablets. Two preparations are effective in the treatment of thyroid deficiency: levothyroxine and liothyronine. Some proponents of 'natural' health remedies advocate the use of dried animal thyroid extract, which was originally the only form of treatment available for hypothyroidism. It is difficult to standardize the dose and therefore the effect of this treatment, and it is not recommended.

Levothyroxine. Levothyroxine sodium (T4; previously known as thyroxine sodium) tablets given orally are absorbed from the intestinal tract, but the full effect builds slowly over several weeks. It is the preferred form of treatment in most cases of hypothyroidism. Dosage is guided by measurement of the TSH level. The aim of treatment is to normalize the TSH. A high TSH indicates too low a dose (or poor concordance with treatment). A low TSH indicates too high a dose. When starting and changing treatment, the TSH should be measured after 6 weeks. When treatment is established, a check of the TSH annually suffices.

It is important to start treating newborn infants with hypothyroidism as soon as possible because if they are left hypothyroid for too long, the changes may be irreversible. In myxoedema it is important to start with a small dose, particularly in elderly people and people with established heart disease, as the stimulating effect on the heart may cause angina or even heart failure. Treatment of hypothyroidism is usually lifelong, although some forms of hypothyroidism, particularly that associated with pregnancy, can be transient.

NURSING NOTE

Effects of overdosage: Large doses will cause an excessive rise in metabolic rate and the symptoms of thyrotoxicosis, with loss of weight, tachycardia, nervousness and tremors. Although the dose can be monitored by the clinical response of the patient, it is preferable to measure the plasma T4 and TSH occasionally to ensure that the correct amount of hormone is being given.

Liothyronine. Liothyronine is the generic name of triiodothyronine (T3). Its actions are similar to those of thyroxine, but are much more rapid in onset, the maximum effect being seen after 3 days. Liothyronine is not as useful as thyroxine in treating myxoedema, because the control of the disease is apt to be uneven, but it is useful if a rapid effect is required. Most patients do not require liothyronine, but a few do not get adequate symptom relief with levothyroxine and do appear to benefit from the addition of a small dose of liothyronine.

Hyperthyroidism (Thyrotoxicosis)

Hyperthyroidism is relatively uncommon, compared to hypothyroidism. TSH levels will typically be **very low** or unmeasurable.

Symptoms of Hyperthyroidism

The overall effect of hyperthyroidism is a raised metabolic rate, which is manifested by:

- raised temperature and sweating
- excessive sensitivity to heat
- nervousness and tremor
- susceptibility to fatigue
- tachycardia (racing heart)
- weight loss with associated increase in appetite
- protrusion of the eyeballs in some patients
- atrial fibrillation (common).

Types of Hyperthyroidism

There are several types of hyperthyroidism, but the two most common types are:

- Graves' disease (diffuse toxic goitre; exophthalmic goitre)
- toxic nodular goitre.

Graves' Disease. This is an autoimmune disease in which the patient develops circulating antibodies that stimulate the TSH receptor on the surface of the thyroid gland cell. This results in increased thyroid hormone secretion unrelated to the normal demands of the body. Aberrant types of the TSH receptor may also be expressed. Patients with this disease may have protruding eyeballs (exophthalmos), an effect of the autoantibodies on non-thyroid tissues.

Toxic Nodular Goitre. This is due to a tumour and can develop from simple non-toxic goitres that result from dietary deficiencies of iodine. Tumours may be single or multiple. Most are not cancerous.

CLINICAL NOTE

Thyroid storm (or thyrotoxic crisis) is a term used to describe a severe acute attack of thyrotoxicosis. It may occur in people with untreated or under-treated hyperthyroidism. Triggers include trauma, infection and childbirth. It presents with hyperthermia, tachycardia, heart failure, vomiting, diarrhoea, jaundice, confusion or coma. It is rare, and potentially life-threatening.

TREATMENT OF THYROTOXICOSIS

Surgery

For otherwise healthy patients with thyrotoxicosis, a treatment course with a thionamide may produce prolonged remission. Otherwise either surgery or treatment with ^{131}I (radioactive iodine) produces satisfactory results, and the complications and failure rates are about equal for both methods of treatment. Surgery has the advantage of getting a quick result, but many patients prefer to avoid an operation, and treatment with radioactive iodine is being increasingly used.

Surgery is usually indicated for patients with nodular goitres and when the goitre produces compression of the trachea. It is usual practice, prior to surgery, to make the patient euthyroid by treatment with a drug such as carbimazole, and this may be followed by a short course of aqueous iodine (see later). This pre-treatment also makes the thyroid less vascular and easier for the surgeon to handle. The patient may also be treated with β-blockers such as propranolol prior to operating. The problems faced by a patient and the therapeutic approach used with these drugs are illustrated in Case History 15.1.

CASE HISTORY 15.1

Miss K was 22 years old when she noticed that she had a mild tremor of her hands. During the following 3 months she noticed a progressive weight loss in spite of a healthy appetite, together with palpitations, diarrhoea and an alteration in her menstrual cycle. She was upset when a relative complained to her that she was excessively irritable. She went to her GP, who suspected an overactive thyroid gland (hyperthyroidism) and sent off blood for thyroid function tests. These showed a decrease in thyroid-stimulating hormone (TSH) and a considerable and abnormal level of thyroid hormone (T4). The GP started her on carbimazole to control the overactive thyroid, and, as the effects take up to a few weeks to be noticed by the patient, propranolol was prescribed to control the symptoms. The GP referred her to the endocrinology clinic at the local hospital. Antibody tests confirmed an autoimmune thyroiditis and Miss K was warned that it was likely that the overactivity would eventually settle and that her thyroid function might swing to the other extreme and necessitate taking long-term thyroxine (T4). Had she had Graves' disease, which accounts for 75% of cases of hyperthyroidism in the UK, she might have needed surgery for thyroid enlargement or – had she been over 40 years of age – radio-iodine, which, to avoid the long-term risk of thyroid cancer, is not given to the younger patients.

Use of Drugs to Treat Thyrotoxicosis

The following drugs are used:

- thionamides
- radio-iodine (radioactive iodine; ^{131}I)
- aqueous iodine solution (Lugol's solution).

The Thionamides

These comprise:

- carbimazole (and its metabolite methimazole)
- propylthiouracil.

Mechanism of Action. These drugs inhibit thyroid hormone production, by acting as a preferred substrate for iodination by TPO (see Fig. 15.3). In addition, propylthiouracil blocks the conversion of T4 to T3 in target tissues.

Therapeutic Use. The thionamides are given orally. After administration, carbimazole is rapidly metabolized in the blood to methimazole. Carbimazole is therefore an example of a prodrug. Methimazole is available in the USA and other countries (not the UK) as an oral drug and is used instead of carbimazole. This class of drugs act quickly to block the iodination of thyroglobulin, but the beneficial effects may not be seen for anything up to 2 months. This is because circulating T3 and T4 have long half-lives, partly because they are strongly bound to plasma proteins and also because the thyroid has large stores of the hormones in the colloid. Propylthiouracil may act faster than other drugs because of its blocking action on the conversion of T4 to T3 in the target tissue. Propylthiouracil is not used as first-line treatment, except in thyroid storm or the first trimester of pregnancy, as it carries a small risk of causing severe liver injury. After thyroid function returns to normal, the thyroid may still be enlarged.

The drug is usually continued, but at a reduced dosage, for about 18 months, after which treatment may be further reduced and eventually stopped. Treatment effect is monitored by measuring free T4 and TSH. About 60% of patients will remain well, but 40% will relapse and may require either further drug treatment, surgery or radio-iodine. Long-term treatment with thionamides is avoided, where possible.

Adverse Effects. These include rashes, joint pains, enlarged lymph nodes and fever. Transient depression of the white cell count develops in around 10% of patients and, rarely, dangerous agranulocytosis may occur; therefore, severe sore throats or other infections should be reported immediately.

Carbimazole should be given with care to pregnant women as excessive dosage may suppress the fetal thyroid, causing goitre and hypothyroidism. It is also excreted in maternal milk and may have similar effects on the newborn.

Radio-iodine

Radio-iodine is a radioactive isotope of iodine. As it decays to a more stable form, it emits radiation that kills cells, particularly cells undergoing cell division. It is a rare example of a 'magic bullet', i.e. a drug that targets one particular organ or group of cells selectively. It does this because of the unique iodine-concentrating mechanism of the thyroid gland.

Administration. ^{131}I is given orally and is rapidly absorbed from the stomach and intestines. The thyroid takes it up in exactly the same way as dietary iodide is taken up, and it is incorporated into thyroglobulin. In the treatment of thyrotoxicosis, large doses are given to stop production of thyroid hormone.

Action and Use of ^{131}I. The radio-iodine emits mainly β-particles and some γ-rays. The β-particles penetrate only a few millimetres and so their cytotoxic action is confined almost entirely to the thyroid, where they have a very powerful destructive action. Since ^{131}I is incorporated into T3 and T4, some radioactivity will get into the general circulation, but, because the treatment is so powerful, the isotope quickly destroys the tissue that releases it. ^{131}I has a short half-life of about 8 days, and radioactivity has decayed away completely by about 2 months after the treatment has been administered.

Because of its powerful destruction of thyroid tissue, ^{131}I treatment will usually cause hypothyroidism, especially in patients with Graves' disease, but this is easily treated by administration of thyroxine.

Precautions with ^{131}I. Radioactive iodine should not be used to treat thyrotoxicosis during pregnancy or if the mother is breastfeeding. There are also doubts about its use in children and young women. Special care is required in the handling of and disposal of urine, etc., from these patients, as it will be radioactive. Staff who handle and administer ^{131}I must wear personal radiation dosimeters and be routinely screened for thyroid radioactivity, and patients should be nursed in isolation.

Other Uses of ^{131}I. Radioactive iodine is also used to destroy malignant cells in carcinoma of the thyroid gland.

Aqueous Iodine Solution/Saturated Potassium Iodide Solution

Aqueous iodine, also called Lugol's solution, is a solution of potassium iodide and iodine. Saturated potassium iodide solution is a similar preparation. Either may be administered orally and will temporarily inhibit thyroid hormone release. While this was used in the past to rapidly treat thyrotoxicosis, it is now only used (sometimes) as pre-treatment for around 2 weeks before thyroid surgery for Graves' disease, as this reduces the vascularity and friability of the gland. Lugol's solution has an unpleasant taste and is sometimes prescribed with milk to improve palatability.

Adverse Effects. Patients may develop adverse effects such as skin rashes, sneezing, lacrimation (watering eyes), conjunctivitis and salivary gland pain.

Other Drugs

β-Blockers reduce those symptoms of thyrotoxicosis that are due to sympathetic overactivity, including tachycardia, tremor, sweating and anxiety. In addition to their actions on the sympathetic system, they reduce the conversion of T4 to T3 in the tissues. They are useful for the rapid control of these symptoms, particularly in the preparation for operation. It must be remembered, however, that they do not cure thyrotoxicosis; so, if they are stopped, the symptoms will return. Corticosteroids reduce tissue conversion of T4 to T3 and may have a role in the treatment of severe hyperthyroidism.

NURSING NOTE

Patient education in the recognition of the side-effects associated with the use of thyroid drugs is important in monitoring the effectiveness of treatment. Nurses play an important role in helping patients understand their condition and educating them to be able to recognize and act on side-effects of medication or effectiveness of treatment.

SUMMARY

- Measurement of TSH and anti-TPO antibodies with measurement of circulating T4, and of the free fraction of T4 are important tools in diagnosis.

- TSH measurement is important in the monitoring of thyroid disease. It should be measured 6 weeks after dose changes and otherwise, annually.
- Treatment of myxoedema should be initiated with small doses of thyroxine, to minimize cardiac adverse effects.
- Congenital hypothyroidism should be tested for at birth and treated as soon as possible after diagnosis.
- Aqueous iodine tastes unpleasant and can be given in milk to improve palatability.
- Patients prescribed thionamides should be advised to report sore throats or any infections immediately.
- Drugs given to pregnant women to reduce thyroid hormone secretion can also suppress the normal fetal thyroid and make the fetus hypothyroid.
- Staff who handle ^{131}I must be monitored routinely for thyroid radioactive levels.
- Patients should be made euthyroid prior to thyroid surgery.

BONE METABOLISM, THE PARATHYROID GLANDS AND CALCIUM

Bone metabolism is of considerable medical interest and importance due to increased longevity and the problem of bone loss with ageing. Advances in our understanding of the process of bone remodelling have led to the introduction of powerful drugs that slow the rate of bone loss.

The normal process of bone remodelling is controlled by a balance between osteoblasts, which secrete new bone matrix, and osteoclasts, which break down bone matrix. This balance is affected by several chemical factors, notably:

- the turnover of calcium and phosphates
- the action of certain cytokines
- the hormones: calcitonin and parathyroid hormone
- the vitamin D family.

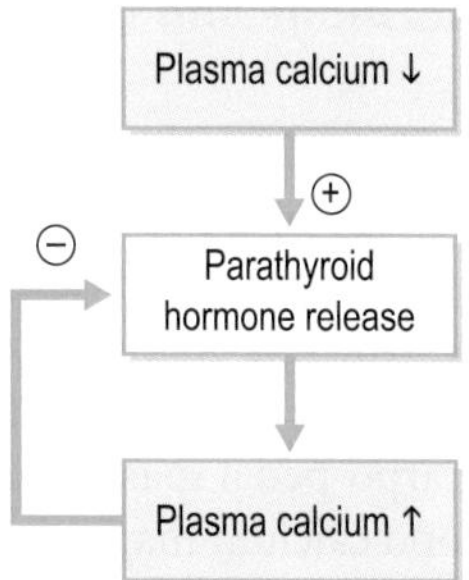

Fig. 15.4 ■ Control of parathyroid hormone (PTH) release.

THE PARATHYROID GLANDS AND PARATHYROID HORMONE

The four tiny parathyroid glands are situated in the neck in close relationship with the thyroid gland (see Fig. 15.1). They control the levels of calcium and phosphorus in the blood, and their excretion by the kidney. Parathyroid glands secrete parathyroid hormone (parathormone, PTH). A fall in the level of blood calcium concentration stimulates the parathyroids to produce more PTH, which mobilizes calcium from bone and decreases its loss through the kidney, thus returning the blood calcium level to normal. This in turn reduces the release of PTH (Fig. 15.4). Parathyroid glands may become under- or overactive, although overactivity is more common, and may be primary or secondary in cause. Primary implies an abnormality of the gland, such as a tumour; secondary means that the parathyroid glands are overstimulated due to some other cause, often chronic kidney disease.

Actions of Parathyroid Hormone

The overall effect of PTH is to increase plasma concentrations of calcium. PTH does this by:

- mobilizing calcium from bone
- increasing production of calcitriol, a member of the vitamin D_3 family, which in turn increases calcium absorption from the gastrointestinal tract
- enhancing calcium reabsorption from the kidney tubules
- increasing phosphate excretion.

Parathyroid Hormone and Calcium Deficiency

PTH deficiency results in an increase in blood phosphorus and a decrease in blood calcium levels (hypocalcaemia). Hypocalcaemia can lead to a disorder known as **tetany**, which is characterized by increased contractility of skeletal muscles with spasm of the hands and feet (carpo-pedal spasm), and of the larynx. A decrease in blood calcium may result from:

- Parathyroid underactivity: this may result from thyroid or parathyroid surgery. Autoimmune and other causes are rare. Hypomagnesaemia (low magnesium levels) may lead to parathyroid underactivity. Hypomagnesaemia is sometimes seen in chronic alcohol abuse, and occasionally in patients on long-term proton pump inhibitors, such as omeprazole.
- lack of calcium in the diet, particularly if the patient is also deficient in vitamin D
- alkalosis.

Alkalosis, although not always associated with low blood calcium, causes a decrease of ionized calcium in the blood and it is the ionized fraction that is important in preventing tetany.

Treatment of Tetany

In cases of tetany due to parathyroid deficiency, several treatments are available:

- calcium
- PTH
- vitamin D.

Calcium

Giving calcium salts may quickly relieve acute attacks of tetany due to low blood calcium. They are usually administered in the form of **calcium gluconate** or **calcium chloride**. Calcium gluconate, if given slowly intravenously, produces rapid, but short-lived relief. Calcium salts can also be given orally, not only to relieve tetany, but also to prevent chronic calcium deficiency developing, particularly in those who absorb calcium poorly, and after menopause.

Calcium Absorption. Poor calcium absorption can occur under the following conditions:

- vitamin D deficiency
- following gastrectomy or gastric bypass
- in steatorrhoea (abnormally fatty faeces)
- in elderly subjects.

Prolonged calcium deficiency, especially when combined with vitamin D deficiency may lead to decalcification of bones. Calcium and vitamin D deficiency in children leads to the condition called *rickets* where long bones are soft, painful and deformed. In adults, it causes a condition known as *osteomalacia*, where pain is more prominent and fractures are common.

CLINICAL NOTE

Calcium solutions are very irritant and if given subcutaneously or intravenously can cause tissue necrosis. In oral form, tablets can be chewable or soluble, improving adherence. In cases of extreme hypocalcaemia intravenous calcium gluconate can be given; the patient's heart rate and blood pressure should be continuously monitored.

Parathyroid Hormone

Parathyroid hormone (PTH) is rarely used in clinical practice, and only by specialists in the treatment of PTH deficiency. Careful monitoring of plasma calcium is required. It is now produced using recombinant DNA technology and allergic reactions are much less common than with earlier preparations. It is given as a once daily subcutaneous dose that can be self-administered. Hypercalcaemia is the most significant unwanted effect. In young people with unfused bone epiphyses, there is an increased risk of osteosarcoma developing. This is also true in Paget's disease, where the osteosarcoma risk is already increased. It should only be used in patients in whom adequate calcium levels cannot be achieved with the use of calcium and vitamin D. Patients should have normal vitamin D and magnesium levels before starting treatment.

Teriparatide is a recombinant or synthetic form of PTH comprising only the first 34 amino acids of the PTH molecule. This is the biologically active part of the molecule, and it has similar effects to PTH.

However, its bioavailability differs, and this leads to it having the effect of increasing bone density through the stimulation of osteoblasts. It can therefore be used as a treatment for osteoporosis (see later). It should only be used for up to 2 years and is given by once daily injection. Osteosarcoma risk may also be increased, as with PTH. It is also available in combination with denosumab (see later). An unlicensed indication is to speed the healing of bone fractures or treat non-union of fractures.

Vitamin D

Plasma calcium levels can also be raised by treatment with vitamin D, which increases the absorption of calcium from the intestine. Vitamin D may be required:

- if the patient has insufficient exposure to sunlight
- in various disorders in which resistance to the action of vitamin D occurs
- in PTH deficiency.

Vitamin D (cholecalciferol or ergocalciferol) itself can be used, or substances that have a similar action, such as dihydrotachysterol or alfacalcidol. These drugs are considered in more detail in Chapter 11.

HYPERCALCAEMIA

Hypercalcaemia may be mild, moderate or severe, depending on the level of calcium in the blood, adjusted for the level of albumin, to give the biologically active ionized calcium level (known as the *adjusted, corrected, unbound* or *free calcium level*). Mild hypercalcaemia is fairly common and is often related to primary hyperparathyroidism. Severe hypercalcaemia is dangerous and is often related to malignancy. The symptoms of hypercalcaemia are related to the calcium level and the rate of onset of the hypercalcaemia. They include:

- bone pain and fractures
- muscle weakness and neurological abnormalities
- neuropsychiatric disorders, including depression, confusion and psychosis. Fatigue is common
- gastrointestinal disturbances, particularly constipation, but also anorexia and nausea. Pancreatitis and peptic ulcers can occur, rarely
- renal colic may occur due to calcium stone formation. Diabetes insipidus may occur, leading to thirst, polyuria and dehydration
- hypertension, ECG abnormalities and cardiac arrhythmias may occur, although serious arrhythmias are rare
- hypercalcaemia is one of the causes of severe itch.

There are many causes of hypercalcaemia, of which the most common and significant include:

- Primary hyperparathyroidism, mostly caused by a solitary benign parathyroid tumour (adenoma)
- Malignancy is the second most important cause; 80% of malignancy related hypercalcaemia is caused by a direct effect of the malignancy itself and is **not** caused by bone breakdown in bone metastases
- Drugs may cause hypercalcaemia. Thiazide diuretics can cause mild hypercalcaemia. Lithium may cause more severe hypercalcaemia. Vitamin D overdose and vitamin A overuse may also lead to the condition
- Antacids taken with calcium salts and vitamin D may cause severe hypercalcaemia with renal impairment and metabolic alkalosis
- Granulomatous diseases, including sarcoidosis and tuberculosis may lead to hypercalcaemia
- End-stage renal failure may lead to hypercalcaemia due to PTH over secretion (*secondary*, and later, *tertiary* hyperparathyroidism). Hypercalcaemia is also sometimes seen in the recovery phase from acute kidney injury
- Mild hypercalcaemia is sometimes seen in thyrotoxicosis.

Treatment of Hypercalcaemia

This depends on the underlying condition and the severity of the hypercalcaemia and its associated symptoms. In mild to moderate hypercalcaemia without severe symptoms, the main approach to treatment is to identify the cause and any possible exacerbating factors and to treat them, where possible. The definitive treatment for primary hyperparathyroidism is parathyroidectomy. If surgery is not appropriate, then the drug **cinacalcet** may be used by specialists. This reduces the secretion of PTH, and also has a role in the treatment of the secondary hyperparathyroidism of end-stage renal failure. It is given by mouth. **Etelcalcetide** is a similar drug also used in secondary hyperparathyroidism, given by intravenous injection, three times a week.

Severe hypercalcaemia, especially with severe symptoms, is an emergency, requiring hospital treatment with intravenous rehydration and intravenous bisphosphonate therapy (pamidronate or zoledronate) (see later). The drug denosumab may also have a role in treating severe hypercalcaemia, not responsive to other treatments.

CALCITONIN

Calcitonin is a hormone produced in the C cells of the thyroid gland, but which is concerned with calcium balance. It inhibits the action of bone osteoclasts, which are concerned with bone resorption. Therefore, calcitonin lowers the concentration of calcium in the blood and increases its deposition in bone. In humans, its function in calcium homeostasis seems to be of limited importance. It is used therapeutically in disorders where there is a rapid breakdown of bone, such as Paget's disease, and sudden immobility due to accident or injury – for a few weeks only. It was commonly used to treat malignancy-related hypercalcaemia, but intravenous bisphosphonates have largely replaced it for this indication.

A form of calcitonin from salmon is given by subcutaneous or intramuscular injection. The dose and frequency of administration depend on the disorder being treated. Adverse effects include nausea, vomiting and flushing after the injection, and pain at the site of injection. Allergic reactions are relatively common.

OSTEOPOROSIS AND ITS TREATMENT

In this condition, the rate of bone resorption exceeds that of bone replacement, so there is a loss of bone mass, resulting in a tendency to fractures, particularly of the vertebrae, the upper end of the femur and the lower end of the radius. Osteoporosis is responsible for a great deal of morbidity and some mortality among elderly people. With increasing age, bone mass diminishes and there is a markedly rapid loss of bone in women after the menopause.

Postmenopausal women are especially prone to fractures. Other risk factors include a family history of osteoporosis, inactivity, smoking, alcohol overuse, low weight and being of Asian or Caucasian origin. Osteoporosis can also result from various endocrine disorders, malabsorption of calcium, rheumatoid arthritis and the prolonged use of corticosteroids such as prednisolone.

Prevention and control of osteoporosis are achieved using:

- the bisphosphonates
- other drugs: raloxifene, denosumab, teriparatide
- calcium and vitamin D (as considered previously)
- hormone replacement therapy (HRT).

The Bisphosphonates

These comprise:

- **disodium alendronate**
- **sodium clodronate**
- **ibandronic acid**
- **disodium pamidronate**
- **disodium risedronate**
- **zoledronic acid.**

This group of drugs are used to treat osteoporosis in men and women. They may also be used to prevent osteoporosis in patients with proven reduced bone mineralization (osteopenia), and where they are judged to be at high risk of osteoporosis, where other strategies have been ineffective. Their use has increased greatly over the past two decades, but some important adverse effects have also been identified.

Mechanism of Action

The bisphosphonates mimic the action of a body chemical called 'pyrophosphate', but they are more stable. They are absorbed onto the calcium-containing crystals in bone and slow both their rate of formation and dissolution. It should be appreciated that bone is not an inert structure, but rather is always being broken down and reformed. In Paget's disease and in malignant disease involving bone, this process accelerates, resulting in pain, and in the release of calcium into the blood with consequent hypercalcaemia. Bisphosphonates, by slowing bone 'turnover', relieve pain and control hypercalcaemia. They inhibit osteoclast activity and promote osteoblast activity in bone. They have been found to be very effective in reducing the incidence of fractures in the elderly. It should be remembered that osteoclasts are cells that resorb bone and osteoblasts form new bone.

Clinical Use

Etidronate was the first of these drugs to be developed. The doses needed were high and many patients on etidronate developed osteomalacia (softening of the bones), It has now been withdrawn by its manufacturers, following the development of **disodium alendronate**, which is 1000 times more potent than etidronate in slowing bone resorption. The drug has a very long half-life – more than 5 years – because it binds so strongly to bone. Many trials of the drug found that alendronate significantly improves bone density in the hip and the spine after 2–4 years, and most of the improvement occurs within the first year of treatment.

In the UK, alendronate has a licence for the prevention and treatment of osteoporosis, in men and women. It is given orally, as is **disodium risedronate,** which has similar indications, but can also be used to treat Paget's disease of the bone. **Disodium pamidronate** is given by intravenous infusion to treat bone pain or hypercalcaemia due to secondary malignant deposits in bone. **Sodium clodronate** has similar indications but can be given orally. **Ibandronic acid** is another intravenous (also oral) preparation with similar indications, but which can also be given as a monthly infusion to treat postmenopausal osteoporosis. **Zoledronic acid** is another intravenous drug, which can be used for all of the indications of the other drugs but has the significant advantage of only needing a *once yearly* infusion to treat osteoporosis in men and women. Some of the oral drugs are given once a week, others may be given daily.

For many of these drugs, it is recommended that they be taken with calcium and vitamin D supplements, and it is important to check the specific recommendations for each drug.

CLINICAL NOTE

All the oral bisphosphonates have potential to cause oesophageal ulceration, and perforation has been reported. It is important to ensure that the drugs do not remain in the oesophagus after taking them. Their absorption is affected significantly by food (in particular, calcium, antacids, iron and mineral supplements). Precise instructions vary between drugs, but in general, patients are advised to take the medication on an empty stomach, at least 30 min before the first food and drink of the day, or at least 2 h after eating or drinking. The medication should be taken with a full glass of water, and the patient should sit or stand upright for 30 min after taking it.

Adverse Effects

The adverse effects of the bisphosphonates vary to some extent, due to the chemical differences between them. In addition to the oesophageal ulceration risk for oral forms (patients should be warned of this), allergic reactions, skin reactions, malaise and other side-effects are common. They vary in their severity and the great increase in use of these drugs is a testament to their general tolerability.

There are some rare but serious side-effects of which all patients should be made aware:

Atypical Femoral Fractures. Low impact fractures of the femur have been reported rarely, in patients taking bisphosphonates for osteoporosis. All patients should be warned to report thigh or groin pain, and the need for treatment beyond 5 years should be considered on an individual basis.

Osteonecrosis of the Jaw. This is where an area of jawbone is not covered by gums and begins to die. It is more common with bisphosphonate treatment, and is most common with intravenous treatment, particularly zoledronate. Before bisphosphonate treatment is started, patients must have a dental check, and any treatment must be undertaken promptly, and for intravenous bisphosphonates, the dental treatment should be completed before therapy begins. Patient education (including written information) is important. Patients should be advised to have regular dental checks, maintain good oral hygiene and report any tooth or jaw problems early. Osteonecrosis can normally be treated with conservative measures.

Osteonecrosis of the External Auditory Canal. This has also been reported, very rarely. Patients should be advised to report ear pain, discharge or infection.

Other Drugs Used in Osteoporosis

Currently, the bisphosphonates are the most important drugs used to prevent and treat osteoporosis. Some other drugs are used, particularly when bisphosphonates are not tolerated.

Teriparatide has been discussed earlier. It can be given by daily injection for up to 2 years. It can also be combined with **denosumab**, a biologic drug, which can also be used to treat fractures from malignant metastases in bone. Denosumab is given by injection, every 6 months for osteoporosis, monthly for other indications. It inhibits osteoclast formation, function and survival and so decreases bone resorption. Like the bisphosphonates, denosumab treatment is associated with an increased risk of femoral fractures, osteonecrosis of jaw and external auditory canal. The same precautions and educational advice apply to its use as to bisphosphonates. It can also cause hypocalcaemia, and sometimes hypercalcaemia when it is discontinued.

Raloxifene is a type of drug known as a selective oestrogen receptor modulator (SERM). It has mainly oestrogen-like effects in bone – increasing bone density, although in breast and uterine tissue, it antagonizes the effects of oestrogen. It is used to prevent and treat osteoporosis in postmenopausal women. It is taken orally and is rather less effective than bisphosphonates. It is also used in postmenopausal women who are judged to be at high risk of breast cancer, to reduce their risk of developing this cancer.

Hormone Replacement Therapy

Hormone replacement therapy (HRT) is the regular taking by women of small doses of oestrogen, alone or with synthetic progestogens, and is discussed in Chapter 18. HRT is very effective in preventing bone loss, but when it is discontinued, bone density declines at the same rate that it does at the natural menopause. HRT was widely used for osteoporosis prevention and treatment but has fallen out of favour over the last two decades, when the magnitude of the increased risk of breast cancer with prolonged use became apparent. HRT should now normally be used for the shortest period of time possible to treat severe menopausal symptoms.

CLINICAL NOTE

Emergent data from the USA suggest that over an 18-year study period when HRT was compared with placebo, there was no difference in deaths relating to cardiovascular disease or cancer when the study and control groups compared. Furthermore, initiation between the age of 50 and 59 may have a lower impact on mortality. This suggests that HRT is safe, nonetheless it should be used for the shortest time to achieve desired effect (Pinkerton et al., 2019).

Other Strategies for Preventing Osteoporosis

Other preventative measures to reduce the risk of osteoporosis include regular weight-bearing exercise, an adequate intake of calcium and vitamin D, drinking alcohol within recommended limits at most and stopping smoking.

SUMMARY

- Dental checks and careful attention to dental hygiene are important before and during bisphosphonate treatment.
- Patients must be well-informed about the necessary precautions when taking oral bisphosphonates, and education must be given about the rare serious adverse effects.
- Patients with osteoporosis should be prescribed calcium with vitamin D and should be encouraged to take exercise and give up smoking.

REFERENCES AND FURTHER READING

de Silva, S.W., de Silva, S.D.N., de Silva, C.E., 2019. A patient with extensive cerebral calcification due to pseudohypoparathyroidism: a case report. BMC Endocr. Disord. 19 (1), 142.

NOGG, 2017. Clinical Guideline for the Prevention and Treatment of Osteoporosis. National Osteoporosis Guideline Group. https://www.sheffield.ac.uk/NOGG/mainrecommendations.html.

Pinkerton, J.V., Conner, E.A., Kaunitz, A.M., 2019. Management of menopause and the role for hormone therapy. Clin. Obstet. Gynecol. 62 (4), 677–686.

Ross, D., 2017. Patient Education: Hyperthyroidism (Overactive Thyroid) (Beyond the Basics). https://www.uptodate.com/contents/hyperthyroidism-overactive-thyroid-beyond-the-basics.

Santoro, N., Gonzales, F., Thanh-Ha, L.U.U., 2019. Practical approach to managing menopause. Contemp. Ob/Gyn. J. 64 (12), 26–30.

Tabangcora, I., 2017. Thyroid Agents. Online publication. Nurseslabs. https://nurseslabs.com/thyroid-agents.

Vestergaard, P., Rejnmark, L., Weeke, J., et al., 2002. Smoking as a risk factor for Graves' disease, toxic nodular goitre, and autoimmune hypothyroidism. Thyroid 12 (1), 69–75.

16 ENDOCRINE SYSTEM 3
Hormones and Metabolism – Diabetes

CHAPTER OUTLINE

LEARNING OBJECTIVES

At the end of this chapter, the reader should be able to:

- explain the basics of the actions, release and mechanisms of action of insulin
- state the two types of diabetes mellitus
- list the types of insulin available for treating type 1 diabetes
- describe how insulin is given by injection and be able to give the standard strength of insulin injections
- explain the basics of monitoring treatment with insulin
- recognize the signs of hypoglycaemia
- describe the use of insulin in special circumstances such as pregnancy and diabetic coma
- list the different types of oral hypoglycaemic agents
- outline the initial lifestyle and drug management of a patient with type 2 diabetes
- describe the actions of glucagon
- outline the management of patients with obesity, including aspects of diet and lifestyle

THE PANCREAS

The pancreas is a large gland lying across the upper part of the posterior abdominal wall (Fig. 16.1). It produces several digestive enzymes that drain into the duodenum. Scattered throughout the gland are small collections of tissue known as the 'islets of Langerhans'. These islets contain two important types of cell, called alpha

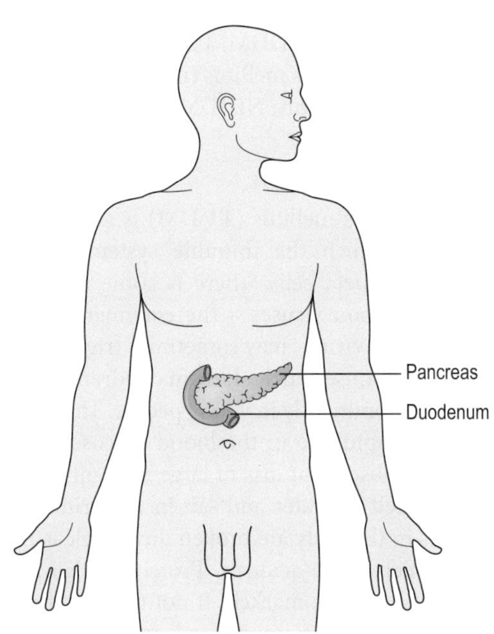

Fig. 16.1 ■ Anatomical location of the pancreas.

(α) and beta (β) cells. The alpha cells secrete glucagon and the beta cells secrete insulin. Insulin and glucagon are important components of the body's mechanism for controlling glucose metabolism. A further subset of cells found in the pancreas are known as delta (δ or D) cells and these produce the hormone somatostatin.

The Normal Control of Glucose Metabolism

Circulating concentrations of glucose are monitored and controlled by the endocrine system. When circulating glucose concentrations rise, e.g. after a meal, insulin is released from the beta cells of the pancreas into the bloodstream and causes glucose to be taken up into the tissues, where it is converted into energy stores such as liver glycogen and fat or used to generate metabolic energy. Insulin release and glucagon suppression after a meal is controlled by complex feedback mechanisms. Peptide hormones, known as incretins, are released from the gut after a meal and are an important part of these mechanisms (Fig. 16.2).

When circulating concentrations of glucose fall, then insulin release is suppressed and other hormones – glucagon, adrenaline, the adrenal glucocorticoids and thyroxine – stimulate the breakdown of fats and glycogen to glucose, which enters the circulation.

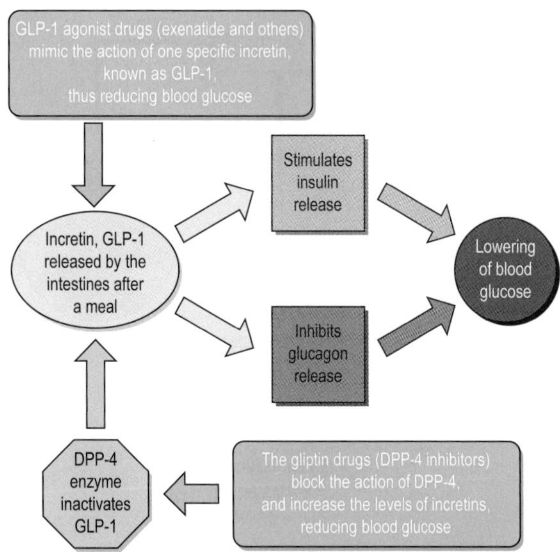

Fig. 16.2 ■ The influence of incretins on control of glucose levels. *DPP-4*, Dipeptidyl peptidase-4; *GLP-1*, glucagon-like peptide 1.

Insulin is therefore the only endocrine hormone that is *hypoglycaemic*, i.e. lowers plasma glucose. Glucagon, adrenaline, the adrenal glucocorticoids and thyroxine are *hyperglycaemic*. A hormone such as insulin that promotes the conservation of energy and tissue growth is termed *anabolic*. Hormones that promote the breakdown of tissues to provide energy are termed *catabolic*.

INSULIN

Insulin is a protein hormone whose release from the pancreatic beta cells is stimulated by glucose and other factors. It was the first hormone to be discovered and crystallized, and its discovery meant that many thousands of people, who would otherwise have died from diabetes, could be treated.

Actions of Insulin

Insulin lowers the concentration of glucose in the blood by:

- stimulating the uptake of glucose by the tissues
- converting glucose to glycogen in the liver, where it is stored
- increasing the production of fat and protein.

These actions are summarized in Fig. 16.3.

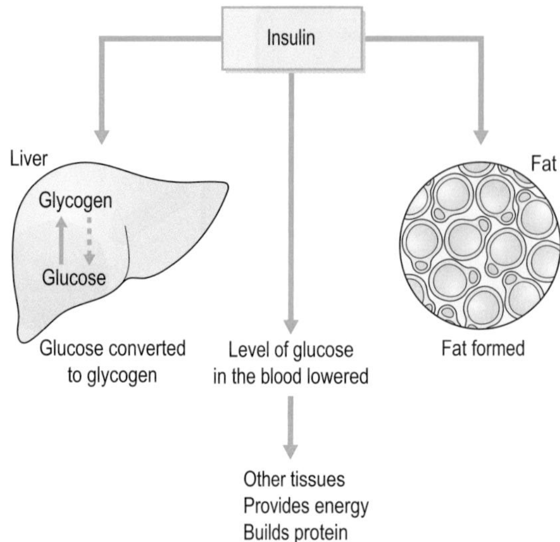

Fig. 16.3 The metabolic effects of insulin.

Release of Insulin

Insulin is released from the beta cells when the concentrations of glucose in the blood rise, e.g. after a meal. Several other substances, e.g. amino acids, carbohydrates and fatty acids, will stimulate insulin release, as will feedback hormones such as the incretins, but the most powerful trigger for insulin release is the **blood glucose level**.

Mechanism of Action of Insulin

Insulin binds to a specific insulin receptor on cell membranes and this triggers the cell's response. An important action is the transport of glucose and other sugars away from the blood and into the cell. Glucose is transported into the cell across the cell membrane by molecules called 'glucose transporters', and insulin increases the activity of the glucose transporters.

DIABETES MELLITUS

The term 'mellitus' is derived from the Latin word *mel*, meaning honey. There is a popular tale that in bygone days doctors diagnosed the disease by tasting the patient's urine, which tasted sweet because of the glucose in it.

Types of Diabetes Mellitus

Diabetes mellitus is a disease caused by lack of insulin, **and/or** lack of effect of insulin on its target tissues (known as *insulin resistance*). There are two main types:

- Type 1 diabetes mellitus (insulin-dependent diabetes mellitus; IDDM; T1 DM)
- Type 2 diabetes mellitus (non-insulin-dependent diabetes mellitus; NIDDM; T2 DM).

Type 1 Diabetes Mellitus

Type 1 diabetes mellitus (T1 DM) is an autoimmune disease in which the immune system attacks and destroys the beta cells. There is some evidence that certain common viruses – the *enteroviruses*, such as Coxsackie B4 virus – may sometimes trigger this autoimmune response, particularly in children. The disease occurs predominantly in young people. This deficiency leads to a rapid rise in the blood glucose concentration with subsequent loss of large amounts of glucose accompanied by water and salt in the urine. In addition, fats in the body are broken down, releasing ketoacids, which cause acidosis. Protein is also lost, and weight loss may be marked. If not treated, the patient will die from these unopposed anabolic effects and dehydration. They will often lapse into a coma (hyperglycaemic ketoacidosis). The only treatment for T1 DM is insulin (see later).

Type 2 Diabetes Mellitus

Type 2 diabetes mellitus (T2 DM) has historically occurred in overweight middle-aged or elderly people. A modern development in high-income countries and also in countries where income levels are rapidly increasing, is the appearance of obesity and T2 DM in young people, and even in children. This may be due to the large increase in food intake, particularly the eating of fast or processed foods containing high levels of sugars. In some societies, notably among Native Americans, the situation has become so bad that upwards of 60% of an entire community may suffer from obesity and T2 DM, partly through genetic susceptibilities and also through the ingestion of large amounts of carbohydrates and fats that are not part of a traditional diet. It is noteworthy that in high-income countries, obesity and T2 DM are particularly seen in relatively poorer members of society.

In this type of diabetes there is *insulin resistance*. This means that the tissues such as the liver, muscles and fat do not respond normally to the action of insulin. The consequence of this is that normal levels of insulin do not lead to a normal reduction in the blood glucose. The elevated glucose levels stimulate the pancreas to produce large amounts of insulin which in part counter the insulin resistance, but in time, the pancreas becomes 'exhausted' and loses the ability to produce insulin. T2 DM always begins with increased insulin production (unlike T1 DM), but over 10 years or so, insulin production declines. As a consequence, in time, almost all T2 DM patients will require treatment with insulin, a fact that has not always been understood by patients or their medical attendants. Insulin resistance is in part due to abnormally high levels of fat cells in the body, hence the association with obesity. However, insulin resistance and T2 DM can occur in people who are not overweight. The blood glucose concentration is raised with glycosuria, but ketoacidosis is less common, and the symptoms are often those of the late complications of diabetes, such as infection. The treatment of T2 DM is given later.

Later Complications of Both Type 1 and Type 2 Diabetes Mellitus

- Damage to small arteries leads to damage to the retina of the eye, declining renal function and serious interference with the circulation to the legs, often causing ulceration and sometimes requiring amputation. Large arteries are more prone to atherosclerosis and so ischaemic heart disease is common. Peripheral nerves may be damaged (peripheral neuropathy).
- Patients with diabetes are particularly prone to infection and these infections may, in turn, exacerbate the diabetes, sometimes leading to ketoacidosis and coma. Good control of the diabetes reduces the severity of the complications but does not entirely prevent them.

TREATMENT OF TYPE 1 DIABETES

Dietary Management

Patients with T1 DM require insulin to replace the deficiency. The daily amount of insulin should balance their daily carbohydrate intake, and both factors depend on their lifestyle and work habits. Younger and/or more active people will require more dietary carbohydrate and more insulin than older and/or less active people. The objective is to maintain good health as judged by their subjective feelings and their weight (which should be kept at the correct level for their age and height), and to keep their blood glucose levels near normal (Fig. 16.4).

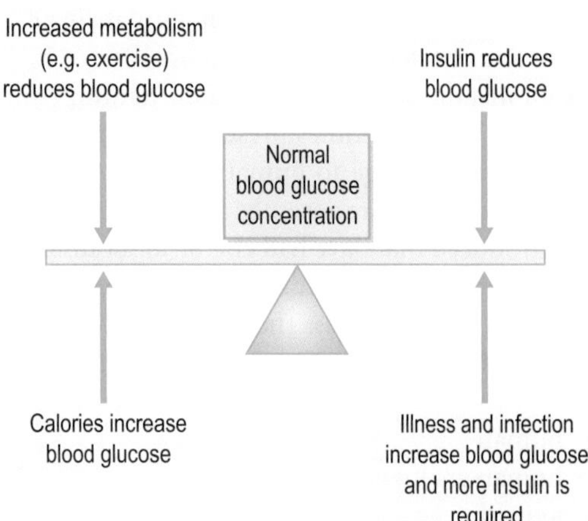

Fig. 16.4 ■ Balancing patients with diabetes.

There are many dietary schemes, and it is too lengthy a subject to discuss here in detail. Briefly, about 50% of the calories in the normal, healthy diet should be from carbohydrate in forms that are slowly absorbed, such as wholemeal bread, potatoes and other starchy vegetables, but not rapidly digestible sugars such as sweets and cakes. About 35% of the calories may come from fat and the rest from protein.

Because such patients are at high risk of cardiovascular disease, patients with diabetes should avoid foods that have a deleterious effect on plasma lipids. Hypertension, if present, should be treated, exercise encouraged and smoking avoided.

Insulin

It is important to remember that the most important unwanted effect of treatment with insulins is hypoglycaemia. Patients and their carers should know the signs of hypoglycaemia and understand how to treat it.

Sources of Insulin

Insulin is available in many preparations that vary in their onset and duration of action. Previously, insulin was extracted from the pancreas of animals and needed extensive purification. It is now possible to produce human insulin, usually by a recombinant

DNA method. The DNA code for human insulin is inserted into bacteria, which then synthesize it. Virtually all insulin now used is **human insulin**. Animal insulins are still sometimes prescribed for adults who do not wish to change to human insulins, but this is increasingly rare. More recently, human insulins have been introduced that have had chemical modifications to alter their onset or duration of action compared with the unmodified types. These are known as **human insulin analogues**. Thus, the sources of insulins are:

- human
- human analogue
- animal.

Insulins are available in forms that are:

- short-acting
- intermediate-acting
- long-acting.

Pre-mixed combinations of short-acting and intermediate-acting insulins are also available, with the proportion of short-acting insulin varying between 15% and 50%. The insulins used may be animal, human or human analogue. They are intended to provide a convenient (but less flexible) combination of onset and duration of action and should be given before meals. These are known as **biphasic insulins**.

Short-acting Insulins (Soluble Insulins)

These may be used in the long-term control of diabetes, combined with longer-acting insulin. They are given 15–30 min before meals. Soluble insulins may be used in insulin infusion pumps for subcutaneous delivery of insulin; however, the short-acting insulin analogues are more commonly used. Soluble insulins are the only type suitable for intravenous injection and are used for the treatment of diabetic coma (ketoacidosis), and to provide cover in diabetic patients undergoing surgery or suffering from other illnesses. Following subcutaneous injection, their action starts after about 30 min and continues for ~9 hours (h). After intravenous injection, their onset is immediate, but the half-life is only a few minutes.

Insulin lispro, **insulin aspart** and **insulin glulisine** are short-acting human insulin analogues, which are very rapidly mobilized from the subcutaneous injection site. They act even more quickly than soluble insulin (15 min against 30 min) and their duration of action is between 2–5 h. They are used immediately *before* a meal, to control the rise in blood sugar and mimic more closely the response of the normal pancreas. Short-acting insulin analogues are widely used in high- and medium-income countries. They are considerably more expensive than soluble insulin. There are theoretical reasons to support their use and most clinicians regard them as superior to soluble insulins; however, there is little high-quality evidence to demonstrate their superiority in terms of clinically important endpoints (such as kidney or eye disease).

The routine use of rapid acting insulins immediately *after* meals is not recommended, as glucose control has been shown to be substantially worse than when they are used before a meal.

Intermediate-acting Insulin

Isophane Insulin (NPH Insulin). This is a suspension of insulin with protamine. After injection, the blood glucose falls after approximately 1–2 h, a maximal effect at 3–12 h, and a duration of action of 11–24 h. It is given once or twice daily and may be combined with a short-acting insulin, either by the patient or as a premixed biphasic insulin.

Long-acting Insulins

Insulin Detemir. This insulin analogue is identical to insulin in amino acid sequence and composition but has been made more fat-soluble through the addition of a fatty acid molecule. This makes the insulin more slowly absorbed from the fat stores after subcutaneous injection, thereby making it more long-lasting. Also, the fatty-acid addition causes it to be bound to circulating albumin, which holds it in the bloodstream longer. It is given once or twice daily according to patient requirements. This is the preferred basal insulin for people with T1 DM.

Insulin Glargine. This is an insulin analogue that forms microcrystals under the skin. The microcrystals dissolve slowly and release insulin into the bloodstream. The onset of action is 1 h after injection, and full activity is reached within 4–5 h. This activity is maintained at a constant level for 24 h. It is given once daily.

Insulin Degludec. This is an ultra-long-acting insulin analogue with a duration of action of up to 42 h after injection. It is used to provide a very stable *basal* level of insulin activity and is given once a day.

For all of these insulins, a true steady state level is achieved after 2–4 days. The absence of peaks and troughs in activity is thought to be beneficial.

These insulin analogues have largely replaced the older long-acting insulins, insulin zinc suspension and protamine zinc insulin. Skin reactions were particularly common with the latter of these.

Administration of Insulin

Because insulin is a peptide, it is broken down by peptidase enzymes in the stomach and therefore has to be given by injection. One regimen is to give short-acting insulin 15–30 min before the three main meals and intermediate-acting or long-acting insulin at night; alternatively, both short- and intermediate-acting insulin can be given before breakfast and the evening meal. In some patients, provided the dose is small, a single injection of intermediate-acting insulin is adequate. The type of insulin, dosage and frequency of administration are modified in the light of the patient's response, until optimum control is obtained. People with T1 DM are very sensitive to the effects of insulin and starting doses should be small and increased in small increments. Typically, someone with T1 DM requires between 0.5–1 unit of insulin/kg weight each day. Insulin is increasingly used to treat T2 DM when pancreatic function declines. Here, because of insulin resistance, the doses of insulin need to be much higher than in T1 DM, and basal long-acting insulins are often used.

Strength of Insulin Preparations

All insulins are now of standard strength: 100 units in 1 mL. They should only ever be administered using U100 syringes, that are marked in units of insulin.

Storage

Insulin should be stored in the refrigerator (not the freezing compartment), but the bottle in current use can safely be kept at room temperature.

CLINICAL NOTE

Insulin prescribing is high risk, and is a focus of quality and safety in health care (Bain et al., 2019). It is regarded as a 'Never Event' to give the wrong insulin dose due the use of syringes or other delivery devices that are not specifically made for insulin administration. Similarly, administration of the wrong dose due to misreading a prescription is a 'Never Event'. Insulin doses should never be abbreviated. 'Units' or 'International Units' should always be written in full on the prescription and the prescriber should be contacted if this is not the case. Check carefully the strength of insulin in vials and pen cartridges before administration, against the prescription.

Injection of Insulin

If at all possible, patients receiving insulin are instructed how to inject themselves and this instruction is often given by a nurse.

The best sites for subcutaneous injection of insulin are the front of the thighs, the abdomen and the outer side of the upper arm. A different site should be used each time, but it must be remembered that the rate of absorption of insulin into the circulation varies with different parts of the body. Therefore, it is better to use the same area, but not exactly the same site, at the same time of day.

CLINICAL NOTE

If a patient is able to, they should be encouraged to continue injecting their insulin within the tertiary hospital setting. The patient should be provided with an individual sharps container, supplies for continuing to check their blood glucose level and a self-administration assessment so that they do not reduce their skills.

Other points of note about injecting insulin are:

- A microfine IV needle and syringe or a 25 gauge 3⁄8 inch needle should be used. The skin should be pinched up and the needle introduced at an angle of 90 degrees.
- No alcohol should be used for skin cleaning as it hardens the skin, and the injection site should not be massaged after injection.

- Special syringes and insulin pens are available for those with poor eyesight or other disabilities.

Other Injection Apparatus

Insulin Pens. These are devices that contain a cartridge of insulin in a ready to use form with a pre-selectable dose. A wide range of insulins are available in cartridges and they are convenient and easy to use.

Insulin Pumps. These give a continuous subcutaneous infusion of insulin for those with T1 DM. The patient wears the pump and the rate of infusion is modified according to the patient's needs, thus producing a very fine control of the diabetes. They are increasingly being used, particularly in patients whose diabetes is difficult to control. Active younger people particularly benefit from their use, especially when combined with new continuous blood glucose monitoring devices. The latest generation of pumps incorporate these glucose monitors and automatically adjust insulin delivery according to glucose levels.

While needle technology has improved, there have been attempts to introduce inhaled insulin as an alternative to administration by injection. To date, however, these new inhaled preparations have not found favour, partly because of the inconvenience of the inhalation devices.

CLINICAL NOTES

- Patients should be taught to monitor their response to treatment by regularly measuring glucose levels in the blood.
- Insulin passports should be filled in with the latest insulin dosage and a record of a glucose level recorded regularly.

Glucose Concentrations

In normal subjects, the blood glucose concentration varies from 3 to 7 mmol/L. The object of treatment is to keep the blood glucose as near as possible to these levels. In patients receiving insulin, this is best achieved by measuring the blood glucose using a drop of blood from a finger-prick applied to a test strip and read using a meter. Alternatively, a continuous glucose monitoring device may be worn. Patients with T1 DM should check their blood glucose before meals as a minimum. If they are unwell, then much more frequent monitoring is required (see later). The blood glucose concentration should be kept as close to physiological levels as possible, while avoiding hypoglycaemic attacks.

The proportion of haemoglobin in the red cells that is glycosylated (i.e. combined with glucose) (**HbA_{1c}**) provides an indicator of the blood glucose concentration over the previous 3 months and is a very useful indicator of real-life diabetic control in patients with T1 and T2 DM. The target level of HbA_{1c} should be set in consultation with the patient, but T1 DM guidelines recommend 48 mmol/mol (6.5%) or lower. With T2 DM, particularly in older people, this level may not be safely achievable without the risk of dangerous hypoglycaemia.

Urine testing for glucose has no role in the modern management of diabetes and is a poor method of screening for diabetes. It should only be used if no other monitoring method is available. If diabetes is seriously out of control, the urine will show the presence of ketones, which may indicate that ketoacidosis is developing. This requires immediate treatment (see later). Unwell diabetes patients should have their urine dipstick tested for ketones.

Hypoglycaemia

Overdosage with insulin causes an undue decrease in the blood sugar (hypoglycaemia; 'hypo'). This leads to faintness, dizziness, tremor, sweating and abnormal behaviour, which may be mistaken for drunkenness. If no treatment is given, convulsions, coma and death may occur. It can quickly be relieved by giving sugar or glucose: 4 teaspoonfuls or lumps of sugar in half a glass of fruit juice followed by two biscuits is effective. Glucose solution can also be given by slow intravenous infusion into a large vein using a large-gauge needle, but care must be taken, as glucose is an irritant in higher concentrations if extravasation occurs.

Glucagon by injection is also effective and is useful if the patient is too drowsy to swallow. Glucagon (see later) may be administered through most routes by injection, e.g. IM or SC, and can also be given by IV injection or infusion. It is often prescribed on an 'if necessary' basis for inpatients being treated with insulin.

About one-quarter of patients with long-term diabetes may not be aware that they are becoming hypoglycaemic. Alcohol and β-blockers may aggravate this condition.

Driving a Car. A patient may lose control of a vehicle as a result of hypoglycaemia. Special care is therefore necessary, and patients who are being treated with insulin are required by many licencing authorities to check their blood sugar before setting out and at 2-hourly intervals during a long journey. Sugar should always be available in the car.

CLINICAL NOTE

Hypoglycaemia is a common complication for people living with diabetes (Khunti et al., 2016). Clinicians should support people with diabetes by educating them on the signs and symptoms of hypoglycaemia, advise on what to do if symptoms occur and to avoid hypoglycaemia by eating and exercising at regular intervals (Johnson-Rabbett and Seaquist, 2019).

Insulin in Special Circumstances

Details of the methods used under the following circumstances vary, but the general principles are the same.

Pregnancy

During pregnancy, the metabolic rate rises, and this increases the demand for insulin. In fact, the condition may first manifest itself during pregnancy. It is necessary to control the diabetes as well as possible during pregnancy, usually giving insulin two or three times daily. Poor control increases the incidence of fetal abnormality and perinatal problems. After delivery of the placenta, insulin requirements fall, and dosage adjustment will be necessary.

Intercurrent Illness

A patient's insulin requirement will rise because of an increased metabolic rate through stress, such as the presence of an intercurrent illness, and this situation is a potent cause of diabetic ketoacidosis and coma; therefore, it is important not to reduce insulin dosage. It may be necessary to change the regimen to 1–6 units/h of soluble insulin given by intravenous infusion, together with fluid and glucose as determined by blood glucose estimations.

It is extremely important that patients with T1 DM (and to a lesser degree those with T2 DM on insulin) and their family members understand that they need to continue their insulin when they are ill, even if they are not eating, and that they may need to increase their insulin dose. Frequent blood glucose monitoring is essential and medical attention should be sought if glucose levels are rising.

Major Surgery

It is preferable that patients with diabetes who require surgery are first on the morning operating list. The morning dose of insulin is not given, but at least an hour before surgery, an infusion of glucose with a suitable dose of potassium is started. Soluble insulin is commenced at the same time. The precise dose will depend on factors such as the patient's weight. All doses and concentrations of solutes required prior to surgery need to be calculated and prescribed by the anaesthetist. The rate of insulin infusion is subsequently adjusted depending on the blood glucose levels.

Diabetic Ketoacidosis and Coma

Patients with diabetes who are not treated, or who develop some infection during treatment, may rapidly develop diabetic ketoacidosis (DKA) and coma. They not only have a very high blood glucose level, but are also producing large quantities of ketone bodies, which can be detected in the urine and, being acids, lead to an acidosis. The excessive diuresis produced by the glucose in the urine leads to severe depletion of sodium, potassium and water. Such patients are seriously ill and need urgent treatment with insulin, rehydration and correction of electrolyte imbalances. The symptoms of DKA include rapid weight loss, nausea or vomiting, abdominal pain, fast and deep breathing, sleepiness, a sweet smell to the breath, a sweet or metallic taste in the mouth or a different odour to urine or sweat.

Soluble insulin should be given intravenously by an infusion pump in this condition. The rate is adjusted to produce a fall in the blood glucose concentration of about 5 mmol/h. The aim is to reduce the level to about 11 mmol/L and maintain it until oral feeding and subcutaneous injection of insulin can be introduced. At the same time, water and electrolyte imbalance are corrected by giving an infusion of normal saline containing a suitable level of potassium chloride. Insulin treatment will shift potassium from the plasma into the cells, hence the need for the additional potassium to maintain safe plasma levels. Restoration of electrolyte and water balance is usually sufficient, and the kidneys will correct the acidosis by excreting acid urine. Occasionally, however, the acidosis is so severe that it is necessary to infuse sodium hydrogen carbonate until the degree of acidosis is improved. Frequent examination of the urine for sugar and ketones, of the blood sugar hourly, and of the electrolytes is important in controlling treatment. Subsequent doses of insulin are determined by the blood glucose concentration.

The possibility of infection as a cause of DKA should not be forgotten, and if this is found, it should be treated by the appropriate antibiotic. Deep vein thrombosis is a common complication and prophylactic subcutaneous heparin may be prescribed.

MANAGEMENT OF PATIENTS WITH TYPE 2 DIABETES MELLITUS

Aims of Treatment

The main objective in treating T2 DM is to prevent the development of the late complications of the condition. These are myocardial infarction, vascular disease, renal failure, retinopathy and neuropathy. This is best achieved by controlling plasma glucose, lipids and blood pressure (if raised), and by avoiding risk factors such as smoking and obesity. Some 75% of T2 DM patients will be overweight and all should be offered guidance on weight loss. The 'diabetic diet' is essentially a normal healthy diet with no added sugar. Sucrose (white and brown sugar), honey and glucose should be largely avoided, and most carbohydrates should be complex and minimally processed in the form of whole grains. Green vegetables should form a large part of the diet and dietary fibre intake should be increased. The intake of saturated animal fat should be low. When the appropriate weight has been reached, the diet should be adjusted to maintain it at that level. Regular exercise, tailored to the abilities of the patient, is also beneficial by increasing insulin sensitivity. Patient education is very important, and structured education programmes exist in many countries to assist newly diagnosed patients. There is increasing evidence that bariatric surgery has a role in the management of severely obese diabetic patients.

This regimen is intended to keep the HbA_{1c} at 48 mmol/mol (6.5%) in patients not taking a drug associated with hypoglycaemia. Ideally, the plasma total cholesterol should be 4 mmol/L or less. Blood pressure control is also very important in reducing diabetic complications and several guidelines currently (NICE, 2020) suggest a target of 140/80 or less for patients without complications and 130/80 or less for patients with microvascular complications (eye or renal disease). Angiotensin-converting enzyme (ACE) inhibitors or angiotensin receptor antagonists (see Chapter 6) are the preferred hypotensive drugs in this setting as they also decrease renal damage. In elderly patients, the requirements may be relaxed a little. It is recognized that personalized targets for blood pressure and HbA_{1c} should be agreed for many patients and that individualized care plans developed in collaboration with the patient may improve concordance and outcomes. While patients with T2 DM have often been prescribed blood glucose monitors, these are of little value for most patients and should not be routinely prescribed unless there is evidence suggesting hypoglycaemia or the patient is on insulin therapy or a sulphonylurea (see later).

It is important to regularly – usually once or twice a year – assess renal function, lipids and urinary microalbumin levels and check for peripheral neuropathy, peripheral artery disease and foot health and diabetic retinopathy. Nurses have an important role in managing these routine reviews.

Older guidelines suggested a period of lifestyle changes as described previously before starting medication. It is now recognized that most T2 DM patients will benefit from early treatment with metformin, as this drug reduces insulin resistance in all patients and does not cause hypoglycaemia. If metformin is not tolerated (even in MR form) or contraindicated, then another oral antidiabetic drug may be offered.

HbA_{1c} should be measured no more frequently than every 3 months, but if target levels are not achieved, then treatment should be intensified, but with a target HbA_{1c} of 53 mmol/mol (7%), as more intensive drug treatment increases the risk of hypoglycaemic attacks.

Treatment is intensified by a gradual stepwise introduction of other antidiabetic drugs. There are several different classes of drugs for the treatment of T2 DM, which are discussed individually later. At each step, a drug from a different class should be introduced and the dose increased to moderate (rather than maximum) levels, and the effect assessed. Various combinations of drugs are recommended, and local and national guidelines should be consulted. However, if available, the recommended (NICE, 2020) order of introduction, by class, is:

- a gliptin (dipeptidylpeptidase-4 inhibitor; DPP-4i)
- a thiazolidinedione (pioglitazone in the UK)
- a sulphonylurea or meglitinide
- a flozin (sodium-glucose cotransporter-2 inhibitor; SGLT-2i).

If patients are not controlled on three drugs, then changing to metformin, a sulphonylurea and a glucagon-like peptide-1 (GLP-1) mimetic may be appropriate in some cases. However, for many patients, insulin therapy is more appropriate, often combined with metformin and sometimes with other drugs. For some patients it is appropriate to suggest insulin therapy if their diabetes is not well controlled on metformin plus one other drug.

CLINICAL NOTE

Medicines adherence in people living with type 2 diabetes is a major public health issue. A systematic review of 21 studies, six of which were conducted in the UK, cited diabetes medicines' non-adherence as the most common cause of hospital admission related to adverse drug events (Al Hamid et al., 2014). At review points, clinicians should explore with the patient how effectively they are taking their medicines and triangulate this with glycaemic control. People with depressive symptoms and diabetes (Gonzalez et al., 2008) may be more susceptible than most to non-adherence and motivation to adhere to medication regimens should be explored.

Oral Antidiabetic Agents

Oral antidiabetic drugs include:

- metformin
- gliptins
- thiazolidinediones
- sulphonylureas
- meglitinides
- SGLT2i
- GLP-1 agonists
- acarbose.

Metformin

Metformin belongs to a group of drugs called 'biguanides'. It was discovered 90 years ago and has fallen in and out of favour down the years. It was only introduced in the USA in 1995. It is firmly back in favour, as it is one of the few drugs which combats insulin resistance directly and does not lead to weight gain, unlike many other antidiabetic drugs (and even insulin, when given for T2 DM).

Mechanism of Action. Metformin's mechanism of action is not fully understood but is thought to include:

- reduced glucose production and release from the liver
- reduced glucose absorption from the gut
- stimulation of glucose uptake into muscle and other tissues.

Other Effects.

- Metformin does not cause hypoglycaemia
- Metformin does not cause weight gain, possibly because it does not stimulate appetite.

Clinical Use. Metformin is a first-line treatment for T2 DM and can be used in combination with other antidiabetic drugs (including insulin) in a stepwise fashion, as previously described. Metformin is also occasionally used combined with insulin in patients with T1 DM. Metformin is sometimes used to reduce the symptoms associated with polycystic ovarian syndrome, a gynaecological condition that is associated with insulin resistance. There is interest in other possible clinical uses of metformin, including cancer treatment, non-alcoholic fatty liver disease and even as a drug to reduce the effects of natural ageing.

Metformin treatment is gradually increased over a period of a few weeks to minimize gastrointestinal side-effects. If tolerated, a dose of 2 g/day should be aimed for in many patients. If gastrointestinal side-effects are troublesome, modified-release preparations of metformin should be tried, as they are often better tolerated.

In some countries, metformin is available as a fixed dose combination pill with either a sulphonylurea, pioglitazone, a gliptin or repaglinide.

Adverse Effects and Contraindications.

- Transient gastrointestinal disturbances (the most common)
- Long-term use may interfere with vitamin B_{12} absorption.
- Very rarely, metformin may cause lactic acidosis, which is often fatal. The principal risk factor for lactic acidosis is reduced renal function (which often occurs as a diabetic complication). It is important to include renal function in diabetic checks and the drug should be discontinued if the eGFR falls below 30 mL/min per 1.73 m^2.

CLINICAL NOTE

Metformin is commonly associated with adverse drug reactions (Pirmohamed et al., 2004) and hospitalization, and is one of the drugs listed as those in the 'Sick Day Rules' (SPSP, 2020). If a patient has an illness that may put them at risk of dehydration and acute kidney injury it may be prudent to withhold metformin until health is restored. During medicines' review and routine checks clinicians may need to remind people with type 2 diabetes of sick day rules thus preventing unnecessary hospital admission.

Gliptins (DPP-4i)

Although relatively new drugs, these have become an important addition to the treatments available for T2 DM. They are a preferred drug for initial intensification of treatment in addition to metformin.

There are many gliptins on the market worldwide, all distinguished by the appearance of *gliptin* in the generic name. They are generally similar to each other. The gliptins available in the UK are:

- sitagliptin
- alogliptin
- linagliptin
- saxagliptin
- vildagliptin.

Mechanism of Action. They work by inhibiting the action of an enzyme called 'dipeptidylpeptidase-4' (hence DPP-4i). This in turn increases the levels of the incretin hormones released by the intestines after meals. This has the effect of increasing insulin secretion and lowering glucagon secretion.

Other Effects.

- They do not cause hypoglycaemia when used alone or with metformin, but may increase the hypoglycaemic effects of sulphonylureas
- They do not cause weight gain, which is a considerable advantage.

Clinical Use. They are generally used in combination with metformin, but may be used in combination with other antidiabetics, including insulin.

Adverse Effects and Contraindications. The gliptins are generally well-tolerated even in more fragile patients. Side-effects and cautions are similar in this group, with some specific differences that should be checked before prescribing, due to the large numbers of gliptins available on the market. There have been reports of liver dysfunction with vildagliptin and liver function testing is required during its use.

- Pancreatitis is the most important, although rare, adverse effect. All patients should be advised to urgently report severe abdominal pain and immediately discontinue use.
- Hypersensitivity reactions can include serious skin reactions and also pulmonary fibrosis.
- Joint and muscle pain is relatively common as are gastrointestinal symptoms and flu-like symptoms.
- There is a suggestion of increased risk of heart failure with at least some gliptins and it may be less appropriate to prescribe them in patients with established heart failure.

- Drug interactions are not generally significant, except with saxagliptin, which interacts with drugs that inhibit cytochrome P3A4/5 enzymes, such as ketoconazole and clarithromycin. The saxagliptin dose should be reduced.

The Thiazolidinediones (Glitazones)

These drugs were introduced in the late 1990s and were the first novel antidiabetic agents to be introduced for many years. Although initially popular, the first of the class (troglitazone) had to be withdrawn due to severe liver toxicity. While the newer glitazones do not seem to have this problem, hepatic monitoring is advised. They are not as widely used as they were and concerns about adverse effects may continue to limit their use. The only drug in the class available in the UK is **pioglitazone**. In some markets others are available, of which the most important is **rosiglitazone**.

Mechanism of Action. They reduce insulin resistance by increasing the dependence of peripheral tissues on circulating glucose for metabolism, rather than other energy sources, such as circulating fatty acids. This has the effect of reducing blood glucose concentrations.

Other Effects.

- Pioglitazone reduces the incidence of micro- and macrovascular cardiovascular events and atheromatous plaque progression. This is probably also true for rosiglitazone, contrary to earlier research, which raised concerns about increased cardiovascular risk.

Clinical Use. Pioglitazone may be used alone but is more commonly used in combination with metformin. It may also be combined with a sulphonylurea or insulin.

Adverse Effects and Contraindications.

- Liver function should be checked before treatment and periodically thereafter.
- Fluid retention often occurs and may precipitate heart failure. This seems to occur more frequently when combined with insulin. Cardiovascular disease increases the risk. Careful monitoring for signs of heart failure is required.
- There is a small increased risk of bladder cancer. These drugs should not be used if there is a past history of bladder cancer or if there are substantial risk factors for bladder cancer. Patients should be counselled to report haematuria or other urinary symptoms.
- Bone density may be reduced, and fractures are more common, particularly in women.

CLINICAL NOTE

Patients prescribed glitazones should be advised to contact their prescriber or nurse specialist if they develop signs such as dark urine, yellowish tinge to the skin, abdominal pain or light-coloured bowel motions. This may be indicative of abnormal liver function and will require medical review.

Drug Interactions. Pioglitazone induces an enzyme that is partly responsible for its metabolism in the liver. The same enzyme metabolizes a number of other drugs, including calcium channel blockers, erythromycin, ciclosporin, statins and glucocorticoids such as prednisolone. It may therefore reduce the plasma levels of these drugs and thus reduce their effectiveness.

The Sulphonylureas

For many years, these were the main antidiabetic drugs. One of the earliest of them was chlorpropamide, now not available in most countries. It has a very long duration of action and hypoglycaemia was a substantial risk, particularly in the elderly. For similar reasons, **tolbutamide** and **glibenclamide** are rarely used now, although the hypoglycaemic risk is less with them. The second- and third-generation drugs still risk hypoglycaemia, but their shorter durations of action make this less likely. The sulphonylureas are used less than they were, but remain important and inexpensive drugs.

In the UK, the commonly used sulphonylureas are:

- gliclazide
- glimepiride
- glipizide.

Other second- and third-generation sulphonylureas are available in some countries.

Mechanism of Action. They mainly lower blood glucose levels by increasing insulin production by the pancreas. There may be other mechanisms of action too.

Clinical Use. Usually in combination with metformin. Sulphonylureas are all given orally and differ largely in their duration of action. Gliclazide is the one most used. Its effects last up to 24 h and it rarely causes hypoglycaemic episodes. At most strengths, it need only be taken once a day. It takes about 5 h to achieve a peak response. This means that it can be taken before breakfast and gives good cover for lunch and supper.

Adverse Effects.

- Hypoglycaemia is the most important adverse effect. Patients should be provided with blood glucose monitoring strips and told to check their blood sugar if they feel unwell. They should be warned of the symptoms of 'hypos'. This is particularly important with car drivers.
- Weight gain is an issue with these drugs and can make it difficult to achieve diabetic control.
- blood dyscrasias (abnormalities)
- fluid retention
- hypoglycaemia
- skin rashes.

The Meglitinides

The meglitinides, **nateglinide** and **repaglinide** (and **mitiglinide** in some countries), were introduced in the late 1990s and have the theoretical advantage of stimulating insulin production postprandially, meaning that they deal with the rise in circulating glucose that occurs immediately after a meal. They have a rapid onset and short duration of action and should be taken immediately before a meal. This flexibility in use may be beneficial in some patients, but in general they appear to offer few advantages over sulphonylureas in clinical use. They may not be combined with other antidiabetic drugs, apart from metformin, which limits their usefulness.

Adverse Effects.

- weight gain
- nausea and other gut upsets are common
- hypoglycaemia can occur
- skin rashes
- acute coronary syndrome risk may be increased.

SGL2 Inhibitors (the Flozins)

The sodium-glucose cotransporter 2 inhibitors (SGL2i or flozins) are a new class of antidiabetic drug. Those available in the UK are:

- canagliflozin
- dapagliflozin
- empagliflozin.

Mechanism of Action. By inhibiting the enzyme SGL2 in the kidney, they inhibit reabsorption of glucose from the urine. They thus promote glycosuria and lower blood glucose.

Clinical Use. They are used most commonly in combination with metformin, but also as monotherapy or in combination with other antidiabetics, including insulin. Their use tends to lead to weight loss, which is beneficial.

Adverse Effects.

- The induced glycosuria increases the risk of urine infections and vaginal and penile candidiasis.
- *Fournier's gangrene*, a rare but potentially disfiguring or life-threatening infection of the genitalia or perineum, has been reported. Patients should be counselled to seek urgent attention if they develop pain, redness or swelling in these areas.
- Serious, life-threatening, DKA has occurred, sometimes with near normal blood glucose levels. Patients should be warned of the symptoms of DKA, and if DKA is suspected, urine should be tested for ketones, even if blood sugar is near normal.

GLP-1 Agonists (Incretin Mimetics)

The glucagon-like peptide-1 receptor agonists (GLP-1 agonists) or incretin mimetics are the latest addition to the range of new antidiabetic drugs available, mostly introduced in the 2010s.

The ones currently available are:

- exenatide
- liraglutide
- lixisenatide
- dulaglutide
- semaglutide.

Mechanism of Action. Like the gliptins, these drugs use the incretin mechanisms. While the gliptins increase levels of natural incretins, the GLP-1 agonists mimic the action of one of the incretins, GLP-1, by acting as a long-acting agonist for its receptor. These drugs thus have many of the effects of the gliptins but are considerably more potent. They stimulate postprandial insulin release and reduce glucagon release. They also have subtle effects in reducing fat deposition in the liver and slowing gastric emptying. They reduce appetite and tend to promote weight loss, which is a considerable benefit.

Clinical Use. These drugs are peptides and so have to be given by SC injection, which limits their patient acceptability (and also increases their cost, as special injection devices must be used). Most are given once or twice a day, but semaglutide is given as a once weekly injection, and exenatide is available in a once weekly modified-release form. They may be used as monotherapy, but this is unusual, and they are mostly used in conjunction with other antidiabetic drugs or insulin. A pre-mixed presentation of lixisenatide and insulin glargine is available. Particular care needs to be taken in selecting the correct dose strength of this mixture.

Adverse Effects.

- Life-threatening episodes of DKA have occurred in patients treated with these drugs in combination with insulin, particularly if the insulin dose has been reduced. Insulin dose reduction must be done slowly with careful blood monitoring, and patients must be made aware of the risk factors and symptoms of DKA.
- Gastrointestinal upsets are common.
- Urticaria and angioedema have been reported.
- Acute pancreatitis has been reported, rarely. It may be severe or fatal. Patients must be warned to seek urgent help if they develop acute abdominal pain.

Acarbose

Mechanism of Action. Acarbose is an inhibitor of the enzyme intestinal α-glucosidase. This enzyme is part of the gastrointestinal mechanism for converting carbohydrate to glucose.

Clinical Use. Taken orally before meals, this agent inhibits the digestion of complex carbohydrates such as sucrose and starches, thus preventing their absorption, but it does not interfere with glucose absorption. The postprandial rise in the blood sugar is reduced. However, the unabsorbed carbohydrates in the bowel may cause flatulence and diarrhoea. Acarbose has a smaller effect than other antidiabetic drugs and is not commonly used. It may have a role where other antidiabetics are not tolerated.

Insulin

Insulin may be used in combination with other agents if the patient's own pancreatic reserve is exhausted. Unlike T1 DM, the daily doses are much higher, and the monitoring requirements are less stringent, as hypoglycaemia is less likely. Twice, or even once daily dosage with a basal insulin may be all that is required. Unfortunately, weight gain is a common unwanted effect of insulin treatment in T2 DM.

The practical problems associated with the management of NIDDM are illustrated in Case History 16.1

GLUCAGON

Glucagon is a polypeptide hormone secreted by the alpha cells of the pancreatic islets of Langerhans.

Release of Glucagon

Glucagon is released in response to high plasma levels of amino acids, especially arginine, e.g. after a high-protein meal. It is also released in response to circulating adrenaline and increased sympathetic or parasympathetic activity. Release of glucagon is inhibited by another hormone, somatostatin, which is released from other cells in the pancreatic islets, called

CASE HISTORY 16.1

Mr. T had a strong family history of type 2 diabetes, but over time he became obese due to a typical Western diet and a sedentary job. He had noticed progressive tiredness, nocturia and an increasing thirst, unfortunately quenched mainly by high-sugar fizzy drinks. His diabetes went undiagnosed for 2 years, until he visited his GP about another matter and mentioned his symptoms. Blood tests taken then showed a high level of glucose and the diagnosis was confirmed with two raised HbA_{1c} levels. He was referred to a structured diabetes education programme, which he found very helpful. He managed to lose some weight and increased his exercise levels. At diagnosis, he was started on metformin and the dose was increased to 2 g/day. Initially this led to satisfactory diabetic control. He was regularly reviewed in a nurse-led diabetic clinic at his GPs. Kidney function, HbA_{1c} and urine microalbumin were checked twice a year and his blood pressure was checked. He required treatment for hypertension with the ACEI drug, ramipril. He had yearly retinal photography. With time, his diabetic control worsened, partly due to weight gain and he developed background diabetic retinopathy. He was started on sitagliptin, which improved his control. In time, he may require more intensive treatment, and in due course is likely to require insulin therapy.

'D cells'. In contrast to insulin, however, plasma concentrations of glucagon do not fluctuate, but remain fairly steady throughout the day.

Actions of Glucagon

Glucagon:

- stimulates glycogen breakdown to glucose in the liver
- inhibits glycogen synthesis
- inhibits glucose oxidation
- causes lipolysis in fat
- increases breakdown of muscle
- increases release of insulin.

The overall result is to increase blood glucose. Glucagon's actions oppose those of insulin. It also limits its own actions by stimulating insulin release.

Clinical Use

Glucagon is used to raise blood sugar in patients who are hypoglycaemic, e.g. after an overdose of insulin. It can be administered IM, SC or IV. Nausea and vomiting is a common consequence of glucagon use.

THE NURSE AND THE PATIENT WITH DIABETES AT HOME

The management of patients with diabetes is a team activity involving the patient, the doctor, the nurse, the dietician and the pharmacist. Increasingly, people with diabetes are stabilized and controlled in the community. Specialist nurses supervise treatment in hospital clinics and in primary care. Most diabetes monitoring is now nurse-led, and it is common for the education required for insulin initiation to be delivered by nurses in the community, particularly for T2 DM. Education is key for all people living with diabetes and many countries have structured education programmes, generally nurse- and dietician-led.

APPETITE SUPPRESSION AND OBESITY

Obesity is a serious health hazard and is increasingly common throughout the world. In 2018, 28% of the population of the UK were clinically obese (i.e. they have a body mass index (BMI) of over 30). It is strongly associated with heart disease, hypertension, NIDDM and arthritis of weight-bearing joints.

The essential cause is an imbalance between calorie (food) intake and energy expenditure (exercise). Normally, various mechanisms within the body keep these in balance, but even a small disturbance in this balance can lead to increasing deposition of fat. This is particularly liable to occur with a sedentary occupation and the consumption of energy-rich foods, which are, unfortunately, features of a modern lifestyle. Genetic factors can also play a part in maintaining the balance between calorie intake and energy expenditure, and obesity often runs in families.

Management

The definitive treatment of obesity is to decrease calorie intake and increase energy expenditure. In spite of extensive literature on all types of diet, it remains essential to eat less. The actual composition is less important than its calorie content, and a normal, mixed diet, low in fat and sugar, is adequate. The diet should be combined with a programme of exercise related to the age and health of the patient, to increase energy expenditure.

An average woman, not engaged in an active occupation, in their early 30s, needs about 2000 calories a day to maintain a stable weight. A similar man requires about 2500 calories a day. Calorie requirements are greater in younger and more active people and less in older and sedentary people. A daily reduction of 500–600 calories a day on these levels will lead to weight loss of between 0.5 and 1 kg a week, which is a safe and sustainable level of weight loss. The aim should be to reduce the weight to the healthy BMI. The formula for BMI is: 'kg/m^2', i.e. Weight (kg)/(Height (m))^2. The normal range is between 20 and 25.

Drugs Used to Treat Obesity

The history of drugs introduced to treat obesity has been very disappointing, with many drugs introduced only to be withdrawn when dangerous adverse effects became apparent. In general, drugs are a poor choice, as they do not promote the long-term healthy eating habits that enable weight loss to be maintained. Sustaining and then maintaining weight loss is extremely difficult with any diet, and there is increasing interest in the use of bariatric surgery to produce and maintain weight loss in morbidly obese people. Although such surgery may seem extreme (and is very expensive), it may be lifesaving and highly cost-effective in preventing morbidity. Patients who have had some forms of bariatric surgery may not absorb certain vitamins adequately and will require vitamin supplements.

Drugs should never be the sole element of treatment of obesity but may have a role as part of a treatment plan, particularly in initiating weight loss or overcoming 'plateaus' in weight loss.

The only drug currently licenced in the UK for the treatment of obesity is **orlistat**.

Orlistat

Orlistat inhibits the action of lipase in the intestine, thus reducing fat absorption. It causes steatorrhoea: oily, smelly, hard to flush stools. This limits its acceptability, and patients should be warned of this. It can help in weight loss, and its adverse effects encourage a low-fat diet, which is also beneficial. It may impair the absorption of fat-soluble vitamins, particularly vitamin D, and supplementation may be advisable. Orlistat might affect the absorption of other drugs. It may be wise to separate administration. This is particularly important with antiepileptics, antiretrovirals and drugs that have a narrow therapeutic index.

CLINICAL NOTE

For optimum benefit, orlistat should be taken with three main meals a day and, if a meal is missed, the dose or orlistat should also be missed. Treatment can cause flatulence, which can often be reduced by lowering fat content in food ingested. In a recent systematic review, dietary modifications, exercise regimens and orlistat treatment achieved a similar effect on weight loss in people with heart failure, suggesting lifestyle modifications are as important as drug treatment when caring for people with obesity (McDowell et al., 2018).

Centrally Acting Appetite Suppressants

Centrally acting appetite suppressants, including stimulants and serotonergic drugs (such as dexfenfluramine, fenfluramine, sibutramine, and rimonabant), have been used in the past, but in UK practice have been withdrawn or are not recommended due to serious safety concerns or their potential for addiction.

Drugs to Promote Satiety

Bulk forming agents such as **sterculia** and **methylcellulose** have been used to promote the feeling of satiety and control appetite. While they are probably safe, there is little evidence to suggest that they are effective.

CLINICAL NOTE

Devices for the administration of insulin are changing all of the time; you will see many different types of administration devices, insulin vials and insulin cartridges. Before administration, regularly check the dosage, the concentration of insulin and how it is administered to the patient. There have been incidents of patient overdosing or underdosing due to faulty devices, incorrectly loaded insulin administration devices or incorrect concentration calculations.

SUMMARY

- Children should be encouraged to limit the intake of fast foods that are rich in carbohydrates and fats, particularly highly processed foods.
- Good dietary management is critical in diabetes.
- Slowly absorbed carbohydrates such as potatoes and wholemeal bread are preferable to sweets and cakes.
- In IDDM, insulin analogues may be useful if given immediately before a meal for controlling the rise in blood sugar.
- Intermediate-acting insulin may be combined with soluble insulin.
- The sites of injection with insulin should be varied and the site should not be massaged after injection.
- Spirits for cleaning injection sites cause skin hardening.
- Special syringes are available for patients who are disabled or who have poor eyesight.
- Many patients find insulin pens more convenient.
- Patients need to know how to monitor their own glucose levels and how to restore glucose after overdosage with insulin.
- Patients new to insulin must be warned to check glucose levels before driving and at regular intervals during a long car journey, if driving.
- Metformin is the cornerstone of T2 DM treatment and should be introduced at diagnosis in most cases.
- Other antidiabetic drugs are introduced in a stepwise process.
- The gliptins are increasingly used as the first treatment intensification, combined with metformin.
- Patient education in diabetes is a critically important responsibility of the health team.
- Obesity is a growing problem in the UK and health workers should play a large part in educating patients about balancing calorie intake and exercise.

REFERENCES AND FURTHER READING

Al Hamid, A., Ghaleb, M., Aljadhey, H., Aslanpour, Z., 2014. A systematic review of hospitalization resulting from medicine-related problems in adult patients. Br. J. Clin. Pharmacol. 78 (2), 202–217.

Bain, A., Silcock, J., Kavanagh, S., et al., 2019. Improving the quality of insulin prescribing for people with diabetes being discharged from hospital. BMJ Open Qual. 8 (3), e000655.

Capaldi, B., 2007. Optimising glycaemic control for patients starting insulin therapy. Nurs. Stand. 21 (44), 49–57.

Gonzalez, J.S., Safren, S.A., Delahanty, L.M., et al., 2008. Symptoms of depression prospectively predict poorer self-care in patients with Type 2 diabetes. Diabet. Med. 25 (9), 1102–1107.

Johnson-Rabbett, B., Seaquist, E.R., 2019. Hypoglycemia in diabetes: the dark side of diabetes treatment. A patient-centered review. J. Diabet. 11 (9), 711–718.

Khunti, K., Alsifri, S., Aronson, R., et al., 2016. Rates and predictors of hypoglycaemia in 27,585 people from 24 countries with insulin–treated type 1 and type 2 diabetes: the global HAT study. Diabetes Obes. Metab. 18, 907–915.

Levich, B., 2011. Diabetes management: optimizing roles for nurses in insulin initiation. J. Multidiscip Healthc. 4, 15–24.

Marín-Peñalver, J.J., Martín-Timón, I., Sevillano-Collantes, C., Del Cañizo-Gómez, F.J., 2016. Update on the treatment of type 2 diabetes mellitus. World J. Diabetes 7 (17), 354–395.

McDowell, K., Petrie, M.C., Raihan, N.A., Logue, J., 2018. Effects of intentional weight loss in patients with obesity and heart failure: a systematic review. Obes. Rev. 19 (9), 1189–1204.

NICE, 2020. Type 2 Diabetes in Adults: Management [NG28]. https://www.nice.org.uk/guidance/ng28/chapter/recommendations.

Pirmohamed, M., James, S., Meakin, S., et al., 2004. Adverse drug reactions as cause of admission to hospital: prospective analysis of 18 820 patients. BMJ 329, 15.

RCN, 2020. Diabetes: Education, Prevention and the Role of the Nursing Team. https://www.rcn.org.uk/clinical-topics/diabetes/education-prevention-and-the-role-of-the-nurse.

SPSP, 2020. Medicines Sick Day Rules Card. Scottish Patient Safety Programme. https://ihub.scot/improvement-programmes/scottish-patient-safety-programme-spsp/spsp-medicines-collaborative/high-risk-situations-involving-medicines/medicines-sick-day-rules-card.

WHO, 2016. Global Report on Diabetes. World Health Organization. https://apps.who.int/iris/bitstream/handle/10665/204871/9789241565257_eng.pdf.

USEFUL WEBSITES

Diabetes UK. https://www.diabetes.org.uk.

National Institute for Health and Care Excellence (NICE). https://www.nice.org.uk.

17 ENDOCRINE SYSTEM 4
Hormones and Metabolism – The Adrenal Glands

CHAPTER OUTLINE

LEARNING OBJECTIVES

At the end of this chapter, the reader should be able to:

- list the different classes of adrenocortical hormones
- give examples of synthetic glucocorticoids and mineralocorticoids
- describe the physiological actions of cortisol
- describe the survival response to stress and the role played by cortisol
- explain the consequences and dangers associated with prolonged use of glucocorticoids and explain the consequences of aldosterone excess
- discuss the dangers associated with the sudden cessation of long-term glucocorticoid therapy
- list the important uses of the glucocorticoids, including replacement therapy in Addison's disease

THE ADRENAL GLANDS

The two adrenal glands are situated at the upper pole of the kidneys. They consist of an outer layer or *cortex* and a central portion or *medulla* (Fig. 17.1). These two parts of the adrenal gland produce hormones of very different composition and function and they will therefore be considered separately.

THE CORTEX

A number of hormones are produced by the adrenal cortex that all belong to the class of chemical substances known as 'steroids'. Three main groups may be identified:

- mineralocorticoid hormones
- adrenal sex hormones
- glucocorticoid hormones (also called 'corticosteroids' or simply 'steroids').

Mineralocorticoid hormones are concerned with salt (sodium) and water control; the most important is **aldosterone**. Aldosterone increases reabsorption of sodium by the kidney, thus raising the amount of sodium in the body, which in turn causes water retention. It also increases excretion of potassium by the kidney. The main trigger to the release of aldosterone is the renin mechanism (see Chapter 6 and Fig. 6.1) and its main function is to ensure that the volume of fluid in the circulation and tissue spaces is kept constant. This has an important effect on the control of blood pressure.

Excess of aldosterone gives rise to hypertension and sometimes oedema. Very rarely, aldosterone-producing tumours arise in the adrenal gland,

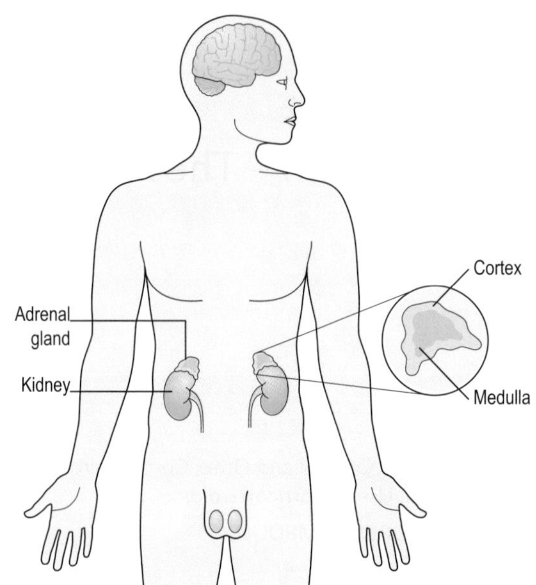

Fig. 17.1 ■ Anatomical location and structure of the adrenal gland.

causing *Conn's syndrome*, which is characterized by hypertension and low plasma potassium levels with muscle weakness. Many of the synthetic glucocorticoids, such as prednisolone and dexamethasone, which are widely used to treat inflammatory conditions will, in higher doses, activate aldosterone receptors, and cause oedema. Aldosterone is not available for clinical use as a drug; however, the synthetic corticosteroid **fludrocortisone** has mineralocorticoid activity and can be used to replace its effects.

Adrenal sex hormones are only secreted in small amounts and are of comparatively little importance as sex hormones when compared with the role of the gonadal sex hormones in the regulation of sexual reproduction. Both male and female sex hormones are secreted in both men and women. Excessive secretion of testosterone from adrenal tumours, leads to *virilism* in women, which is the development of male secondary sex characteristics, such as beard growth and voice deepening. In men, oestrogen secreting adrenal tumours can cause *feminization*, often first presenting as breast development (*gynaecomastia*).

Glucocorticoid hormones are concerned with metabolism of carbohydrate, fat and protein and will also modify the response of the body to injury. The chief glucocorticoid released from the adrenal is **cortisol**. Another, minor corticosteroid, is **cortisone**, which has similar effects.

GLUCOCORTICOID HORMONES

Control of Cortisol Release

Cortisol release is controlled by ACTH (adrenocorticotrophic hormone, corticotrophin), which is produced by the anterior pituitary. The release of ACTH is in turn stimulated by corticotrophin-releasing hormone (CRH), a hypothalamic releasing hormone. The mechanism is such that when the amount of cortisol in the blood increases it 'switches off' the release of corticotrophin by the pituitary and the release of CRH in the hypothalamus. This is a negative feedback action that prevents large changes in the blood cortisol concentration (see Chapter 14 and Fig. 14.3). Failure of the anterior pituitary gland or its hypothalamic control leads to *secondary* adrenocortical insufficiency and is one of the causes of Addison's disease, discussed later.

Cortisol secretion varies during the day, following a diurnal pattern where the level peaks in the early morning (around 8 a.m.) and reaches its lowest level at about midnight–4 a.m., or 3–5 h after the onset of sleep. Cortisol secretion is increased in response to stress, and even the stress of a difficult venepuncture can sometimes lead to a falsely elevated level.

Classification

There are a number of synthetic compounds with similar actions to those of cortisol. The members of the whole group are commonly called the 'corticosteroids', 'glucocorticoids' or simply the 'steroids':

- betamethasone
- beclomethasone dipropionate
- fluticasone propionate
- fluticasone furoate
- budesonide
- mometasone
- dexamethasone

- methylprednisolone
- prednisolone
- prednisone
- triamcinolone.

Hydrocortisone is a synthetic form of cortisone.

The synthetic corticosteroids vary in their potency and bioavailability and this determines their clinical uses. These differences in potency are of particular importance for the clinical uses of corticosteroids in skin diseases and are discussed further in the chapter on dermatological drugs (see Chapter 24).

Most of these steroids are available in many forms and delivery systems. These include tablets, injections, depot injections, ointments, creams, foams, metered-dose inhaled mists and powders, and drops.

Effects of Cortisol and Other Corticosteroids

These can be considered as:

- physiological effects
- adverse effects.

Physiological Effects of Cortisol

Cortisol is the major naturally occurring glucocorticoid hormone in humans. In the blood, cortisol is carried mostly bound to a specific protein, corticosteroid-binding globulin (CBG). CBG also binds progesterone. Only the free, unbound fraction of cortisol is available to act in tissues; CBG thus acts as a buffer, preventing excess amounts of cortisol from gaining access to cells. Cortisol:

- raises blood glucose
- promotes survival responses to stress.

The synthetic glucocorticoids also have these metabolic effects, and are generally more potent than cortisol.

Effects on Blood Glucose. Cortisol has both *anabolic* and *catabolic* actions. In the liver, it stimulates the production of several key enzymes involved in gluconeogenesis, i.e. production of newly synthesized glucose. This is an *anabolic* action. In fat and muscle, however, cortisol stimulates the breakdown of these tissues to mobilize energy. This is a *catabolic* action that also results in an increase in glucose synthesis.

Survival Response to Stress. Cortisol plays a critical role in the body's response to stress, both physical and psychological. Stress initially leads to cortisol release, together with release of catecholamines (adrenaline and noradrenaline) from the adrenal medulla (see later), and the release of noradrenaline from sympathetic nerve terminals. The mobilization of energy stores is used in the 'fight or flight' reaction to stress. If the stress is prolonged then cortisol production declines, but in chronic low-grade stress, whether physical or psychological, cortisol is still elevated and can lead to effects that are similar to overuse of synthetic corticosteroids:

- muscle wasting
- suppression of the immune system and atrophy of its tissues involved with immune responses
- hyperglycaemia
- gastric ulceration
- vascular damage
- reduced sensitivity to insulin.

These effects are not nearly as marked as when synthetic corticosteroids are used in high doses, as discussed later. However, they help explain some of the negative physical effects of prolonged physical or psychological stress.

Adverse Effects of the Synthetic Glucocorticoids. Synthetic corticosteroids are important, often life-saving, drugs. It is sometimes necessary to use them in high doses for long periods of time. Sometimes they are also inappropriately overused. Prolonged use of high doses of the glucocorticoids can result in:

- suppression and atrophy of the adrenal cortex
- effects on carbohydrate metabolism
- effects on electrolytes – oedema
- suppression of inflammatory responses
- suppression of immunity
- gastric ulceration
- suppression of stress responses

- growth retardation in children
- skin thinning, acne and striae (stretch marks)
- bone thinning and osteoporosis
- muscle weakness and wasting
- psychological effects (euphoria)
- reduced response to stress
- 'moon face'
- diabetes
- hirsutism
- raised blood pressure
- masked infection.

Adrenal Cortical Suppression. Prolonged treatment with steroid hormones causes failure of cortisol production and eventual atrophy of the adrenal cortex. If this treatment is stopped suddenly or if the requirement is increased by stress or infection, the adrenal cortex cannot produce adequate amounts of cortisol and a shock-like state develops . It may take the adrenal cortex up to 2 years to recover after prolonged steroid treatment. **Long courses of steroids should never be stopped suddenly, and the dose should be increased in stress or infection.** This is of great importance and is discussed further, later.

Effects on Carbohydrate Metabolism. Glucocorticoids stimulate the production of glucose and decrease sensitivity to insulin. This may be sufficient to make the patient transiently diabetic during treatment, or they may unmask a previously unrecognized tendency to type 2 diabetes.

Effects on Electrolytes. Glucocorticoids cause retention of sodium and water and loss of potassium via the kidneys, although they are not as powerful as aldosterone. They do this in part by activating aldosterone receptors in the kidney. The retention of sodium and water may lead to oedema and hypertension in some patients.

Effects on Inflammation. Glucocorticoids reduce all inflammatory processes and also the generalized reactions of inflammation such as pyrexia (raised temperature) and malaise. The reduction of inflammation is a key clinical use of these drugs. However, it may also be dangerous, because inflammation is the body's method of dealing with infections. If inflammatory reactions are reduced, then infections may spread widely without the seriousness of the position being apparent to the practitioner or the patient (see also Masked Infection, later).

Effects on the Stomach. Glucocorticoids may provoke gastric ulcers through an increased gastric acidity and other mechanisms. If perforation of the ulcer occurs, the damping effects of glucocorticoids on inflammation may mask the symptoms of the perforation, with disastrous results. While enteric-coated steroid tablets were developed, in the hope that this might protect the stomach, there is no good evidence that enteric coatings reduce the risk of ulceration.

Effects on Immunity. The immune reaction is suppressed, and patients become more vulnerable to infections. This is partly due to damping down the antigen–antibody response and possibly also to the reduced production of antibodies. For the same reasons, allergic reactions of various types are inhibited. Glucocorticoids also cause atrophy of tissues of the immune system and they inhibit mitosis, and therefore suppress production of cells of the immune system.

Effects on Bone. Glucocorticoids reduce bone production and prolonged treatment can cause osteoporosis. Avascular necrosis of bone, producing severe pain and usually affecting the hips, is a rare adverse effect. Occasional bone densitometry scans are advisable in patients on long-term steroids.

Psychological Effects. Glucocorticoids usually produce a feeling of well-being (euphoria). Occasionally depression can occur. High doses of steroids can (rarely) provoke psychotic reactions, such as mania, particularly in older people. Children sometimes show behavioural problems when given short courses of corticosteroids, which are often given to treat asthma attacks.

Responses to Stress. As noted previously, stress causes an increased secretion of cortisol. In patients on high doses of glucocorticoids this stress response is suppressed. Failure of this response can lead to a shock-like state if the patient is subsequently stressed, particularly if glucocorticoids are stopped suddenly (see later). Stress in this context includes infections, as discussed later. Stress (including infections and surgery) may require an increase in steroid dose.

Masked Infection. Any infectious disease may spread rapidly and yet produce minimal signs in patients receiving chronic glucocorticoid treatment. Such a situation requires prompt treatment with appropriate medicines for the type of infection, together with an increase in the dose of glucocorticoid. For example, chickenpox, which is usually a mild disease, may become life-threatening in patients taking glucocorticoids if they have no immunity from a previous attack. Such patients should avoid contact with chickenpox or herpes zoster. A similar risk applies to patients with measles.

Miscellaneous Effects. In large doses, glucocorticoids will produce a clinical picture similar to that of Cushing's disease. The patient will develop a round 'moon-like' face, hair on the face and body, a tendency to acne and purple striae on the trunk (Fig. 17.2). Occasionally, muscle weakness and wasting occur, and the skin becomes thin and very susceptible to bruising. There is redistribution of body fat that can result in the so-called 'buffalo hump'. Patients may develop raised blood pressure. Patients receiving chronic treatment with glucocorticoids may also develop cataracts or glaucoma.

The various adverse effects are summarized in Fig. 17.2. However, it must be stressed that many of these adverse effects are only seen if glucocorticoids are given in high doses systemically for prolonged periods.

Just what constitutes 'high' and 'prolonged' is not absolutely clear and will vary from person to person. However, long-term use of corticosteroid doses equivalent to less than 5 mg of prednisolone a day seems to be associated with relatively few unwanted effects and to be reasonably safe, but will still require slow discontinuation over weeks or even months. Use of high doses of steroids for more than 14 days can lead to some suppression of the adrenal cortex and so the steroid dose should be reduced and stopped slowly. How slowly depends on how long the course has been. For example, in most cases, a 5-day course of prednisolone at 40 mg/day can be stopped without reducing first. However, if the course was 5–14 days in duration, it would be wise to taper the daily dose to zero over a week. If the course was more than 14 days, then a longer tapering of the dose would be required.

Sometimes, it can be difficult to judge how much adrenal cortex suppression has taken place after long-term steroid treatment. Various tests are available that measure how well the adrenal cortex and its control systems respond to stimulation. A commonly used test in the UK is the **Synacthen test**. Synacthen is a brand name for the drug **tetracosactide acetate**. It is a synthetic peptide that has a structure identical to the biologically active part of ACTH. If the adrenal cortex

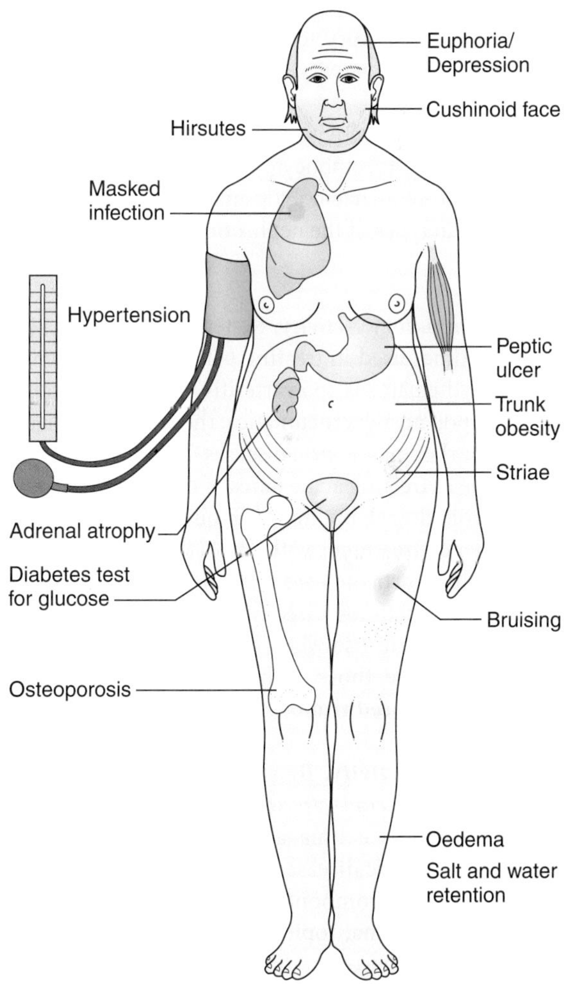

Fig. 17.2 ■ Side-effects of the steroids.

is able to respond to stimulation, then an injection of Synacthen will provoke cortisol production that can be measured in a blood test.

Clinical Use of Corticosteroids

The therapeutic uses of corticosteroids may be considered under two headings:

- Suppression of some disease processes
- Replacement of steroid hormones, which, for some reason, are deficient.

Suppression of Disease Processes

These include:

- antiinflammatory activity
- anti-allergic activity and suppression of immunity
- anti-tumour activity
- idiopathic thrombocytopenic purpura
- certain acute haemolytic anaemias
- certain types of the nephrotic syndrome.

Antiinflammatory Activity. Systemic glucocorticoids are sometimes used in treating patients with systemic lupus erythematosus, polyarteritis nodosa, temporal arteritis, polymyalgia rheumatica, rheumatoid arthritis and other rheumatological diseases. They are of particular value in treating acute flares of the diseases (using high steroid doses), but may be required for long-term maintenance treatment with low doses. In these disorders, glucocorticoids are administered orally or by injection (sometimes directly into inflamed joints). The best drugs to use when antiinflammatory effects are required are those with little sodium-retaining action, such as **prednisolone**.

Anti-allergic Activity. By suppressing allergic reactions, glucocorticoids are useful in the treatment of such disorders as asthma, allergic rhinitis (hay fever) and eczema. These diseases have both an allergic and an inflammatory component, and steroids are helpful for both. In asthma, topically active glucocorticoids (e.g. beclomethasone dipropionate, budesonide, mometasone or fluticasone) are normally used by the inhaled route to reduce systemic exposure and thus reduce the side-effect profile (see Chapter 9). The same drugs may be used as nasal sprays to treat allergic rhinitis. In more severe asthma attacks, oral prednisolone may be given in relatively high doses for short courses. In patients with status asthmaticus, cortisol (hydrocortisone) is given intravenously and repeated every 6 h; such treatment may be life-saving. In eczema and many other inflammatory skin conditions, topical steroids in ointments, creams and foams are used. Prolonged use of potent topical steroids may lead to skin thinning. Steroid preparations may also be used as ear, eye or nose drops. Use of topical steroids is discussed further in the chapters on respiratory, skin and ENT disorders (Chapters 9, 24, 25).

Suppression of Immunity. Glucocorticoids are also used to suppress the immune and inflammatory responses to prevent organ rejection after transplantation.

Anti-tumour Activity. Glucocorticoids have some anti-lymphocyte activities and are therefore sometimes used in combination with cytotoxic drugs to treat lymphomas and some leukaemias. Large doses of prednisolone, for example, are given over 1 or 2 weeks. Dexamethasone is given in the palliative treatment of either primary or secondary brain tumours, where it is probably effective by reducing oedema possibly due to vasoconstrictor activity.

Miscellaneous Uses. Glucocorticoids produce an improvement in idiopathic thrombocytopenic purpura, in certain acute haemolytic anaemias and in certain types of nephrotic syndrome. In these disorders, large systemic doses are usually required. These conditions are a consequence of immune overactivity and dysfunction and steroids may be of use in other similar conditions.

Ideally, oral steroids should be given with food at breakfast. At this time, natural steroid production is at a maximum, and so the exogenous glucocorticoids cause the least suppression of adrenal function. In children, long-term treatment with systemic glucocorticoids retards growth, which may be minimized by giving the hormone on alternate days. Evening dosage with glucocorticoids should be avoided, as this may keep the patient awake at night.

Replacement Therapy

Glucocorticoid hormones are also used to replace the normal secretions of the adrenal glands when the adrenals have been destroyed by disease (**Addison's disease**) or surgically removed. Failure of ACTH production by the pituitary gland also leads to loss of adrenal function. When this occurs, the kidneys are no longer able to retain sodium, which is excreted in the urine, and the body thus becomes depleted of sodium. This in turn leads to collapse, with vomiting and low blood pressure. This is referred to as an Addisonian crisis.

The aim of treatment in this disorder is to replace the missing hormones. In an acute Addisonian crisis with a collapsed and severely ill patient, cortisol (hydrocortisone) is given intravenously and repeated as required. Saline and glucose are also infused and any concurrent infection is treated vigorously.

For maintenance treatment, it is important to use a glucocorticoid with sodium-retaining properties. Cortisol (hydrocortisone) morning and night is satisfactory and may be combined with fludrocortisone to further reduce salt loss. A rough check of adequate replacement can be achieved by measuring the blood pressure supine and erect. If inadequate, there will be a large postural fall in blood pressure. Other indications are the weight and general well-being of the patient.

In a patient with Addison's disease, or with adrenal suppression due to long-term steroid treatment, then stress or infection requires an increase in steroid dose. If this is not done, then an Addisonian crisis may occur.

NURSING NOTE

1. Patients receiving long-term treatment with glucocorticoids will require double their usual dose if they develop a moderate illness, and treble their usual dose for a severe illness. They must be taught to recognize stress situations.
2. Before any operation, the surgeon and anaesthetist must be informed if the patient is receiving glucocorticoids due to risk of adrenal suppression. Patients must also inform their doctor and dentist if they are receiving glucocorticoids.
3. If doses in excess of 15 mg daily are prescribed, patients may also require a drug to reduce the risk of gastric ulceration, e.g. omeprazole or ranitidine.
4. If treatment with glucocorticoids lasts more than 14 days, withdrawal must be gradual, as adrenal suppression may have occurred. Patients must be taught not to suddenly stop taking glucocorticoids.
5. All patients receiving long-term treatment with glucocorticoids should carry a card detailing their treatment.
6. Careful monitoring of adverse effects (see Fig. 17.2) is important.
7. Nurses should wear gloves to apply topical glucocorticoids and wash hands afterwards, as these drugs are easily absorbed through the skin.
8. If topical corticosteroids are applied to broken skin, greater systemic absorption will occur.

THE ADRENAL MEDULLA

The adrenal medulla produces both adrenaline and noradrenaline, which are released into the circulation. The properties of these substances are discussed in more detail in Chapter 8. Tumours of the medulla occur rarely (e.g. phaeochromocytoma) and may produce both these substances in excessive amounts.

SUMMARY

- The adrenal glands are situated at the upper pole of the kidneys.
- High doses of glucocorticoids have aldosterone-like effects.
- Prolonged use of glucocorticoids will reduce the body's ability to respond to stress.
- Do not allow patients to stop taking glucocorticoids suddenly. This will leave them defenceless against stress. The dosage should be gradually reduced.
- Low daily doses of glucocorticoids are used to treat many immune mediated disorders.
- Prescribing glucocorticoids for patients with peptic ulcers is dangerous.
- Patients on long-term glucocorticoid treatment should have bone densitometry scans periodically.

- Patients on long-term glucocorticoid treatment should avoid contact with herpes zoster, measles and chickenpox.
- Prednisolone is often the glucocorticoid of choice because it has relatively little salt-retaining activity.
- Glucocorticoids are best taken in the morning with breakfast. Evening doses may cause insomnia.

REFERENCES AND FURTHER READING

Bidder, T.M., 2019. Effective management of adult patients with asthma. Nurs. Stand. 34 (8), 43–50.

Cheng, O.T., Souzdalnitski, D., Vrooman, B., Cheng, J., 2012. Evidence-based knee injections for the management of arthritis. Pain Med. 13 (6), 740–753.

Chua, A., Cramer, C., Moudgil, A., et al., 2019. Kidney transplant practice patterns and outcome benchmarks over 30 years: the 2018 report of the NAPRTCS. Pediatr. Transplant. 23 (8), e13597.

Liu, D., Ahmat, A., Ward, L., et al., 2013. A practical guide to the monitoring and management of the complications of systemic corticosteroid therapy. Allergy Asthma Clin. Immunol. 9 (1), 30.

Onselen, J.V., 2019. Enabling self-management of eczema in primary care. Pract. Nurs. 30, S9–S13.

Pinkerton, E., Good, P., Kindl, K., et al., 2019. Quality use of medicines: oral corticosteroids in advanced cancer. Palliat. Med. 33 (10), 1325–1326.

Siegel, A., Kreider, K., 2019. Physiologic steroid tapering. J. Nurse Pract. 15 (6), 463–464.

USEFUL WEBSITES

BNF. https://bnf.nice.org.uk/treatment-summary/corticosteroids-inflammatory-disorders.html.

Medic8. http://www.medic8.com/healthguide/articles/adrenaldisorders.html.

NICE. https://cks.nice.org.uk/topics/corticosteroids-oral.

Patient. http://www.patient.co.uk/showdoc/30002010.

Versus Arthritis. https://www.versusarthritis.org.

18 ENDOCRINE SYSTEM 5
Hormones and Reproduction

CHAPTER OUTLINE

LEARNING OBJECTIVES

At the end of this chapter, the reader should be able to:

- describe the main phases of the menstrual cycle and the roles of the various hormones
- list the therapeutic uses of the oestrogens and the different types of oral contraceptive pill, and give a few examples of each
- explain the mechanisms of action and administration of the different types of oral contraceptives
- describe the beneficial and reported adverse effects, and the controversies surrounding the use of oral contraceptives
- describe the symptoms of menopause, the types of preparations used for hormone replacement therapy (HRT), and how they are used
- discuss the obstetric use and risks associated with the use of prostaglandins, ergometrine and oxytocin
- list the drugs used for pregnancy termination and describe the treatments for menorrhagia and dysmenorrhoea
- describe the premenstrual syndrome (PMS) and its symptoms

THE FEMALE SEX HORMONES

It is important to understand the hormonal background of the normal menstrual cycle and of pregnancy before considering how the individual hormones and this system can be regulated pharmacologically.

The Menstrual Cycle

The primary purpose of the menstrual cycle is to grow an ovarian follicle and its enclosed ovum to a point when the ovum is released from the follicle and is ready to be fertilized, while at the same time preparing the female reproductive tract for the entry of the male sperm, and for the implantation of the fertilized egg into the inner wall or endometrium. The critical event is the explosive rupture of the follicle at mid-cycle and the release of the ovum into the fallopian tubes, where the egg will be fertilized by sperm if they are present. The fertilized egg will travel down to the uterus, dividing as it goes, where it will implant itself in the endometrium of the uterus. If the ovum is not fertilized and implantation does not occur, progesterone secretion stops and this may be one of the triggers for menstruation. The entire process is superbly orchestrated by the combined and synchronized actions of hormones from the brain, the anterior pituitary and from the ovary itself.

Hormonal Control of the Menstrual Cycle

This is facilitated by:

- a hypothalamic hormone: gonadotrophin-releasing hormone (GnRH)
- anterior pituitary gonadotrophins: follicle-stimulating hormone (FSH) and luteinizing hormone (LH)
- ovarian sex hormones: oestradiol-17β and progesterone.

The menstrual cycle and ovulation are made possible through the operation of feedback systems involving the hypothalamus, anterior pituitary and the sex hormones oestradiol-17β and progesterone, which are released by the ovarian follicle and corpus luteum, respectively. The feedback systems are similar in principle to those that govern the secretion of thyroid hormone and cortisol, in that hormones act on the pituitary and the hypothalamus to suppress the release of hormones that cause sex hormone release from the gonads. They differ from systems that control, e.g. thyroxine release, in that there are also positive feedback effects at the level of the pituitary and the hypothalamus in operation to cause more release of sex hormones at critical times of the menstrual cycle. The menstrual cycle has three main components: the **proliferative** phase, the **luteal** phase and **menstruation**.

Proliferative Phase of the Cycle

In primates, including humans, the hypothalamus synthesizes, and once every 60–90 min releases, into the pituitary portal system, a peptide called *gonadotrophin-releasing hormone or GnRH* (see also Chapter 14). This intermittent release of GnRH is called a 'pulsatile' release. GnRH acts on anterior pituitary cells called 'gonadotrophs', causing them to release FSH into the general circulation. In the ovary, FSH promotes the growth of the follicles. Each follicle contains an ovum and, for some reason, one follicle (and sometimes two follicles) develops faster than the others and it becomes the Graafian follicle, while the other follicles degenerate. The Graafian follicle synthesizes the powerful oestrogenic hormone oestradiol, which is released into the general circulation. Another two oestrogenic hormones released into the circulation are 'oestrone' and 'oestriol'.

As the Graafian follicle matures, it releases more and more oestradiol-17β into the circulation. Oestradiol travels throughout the body, where it prepares the reproductive tract for the coming ovulation:

- In the uterus it causes the regeneration of the endometrium or inner lining of the uterus.
- In the anterior pituitary, though a negative feedback effect, it prevents GnRH from causing a release of LH from gonadotroph cells, thus preventing LH from reaching the follicle before the follicle is ready to be ruptured.
- Oestradiol works to prepare the gonadotrophs of the anterior pituitary so that they become more sensitive to hypothalamic GnRH.
- Another important job of oestradiol is to cause a large increase in the concentration of progesterone receptors in the endometrium, anterior pituitary and hypothalamus. This is done to prepare these tissues for the rise in progesterone secretion that will occur after ovulation. This period before ovulation is called the 'follicular' or 'proliferative' phase of the cycle.

Ovulation

Ovulation, the successful releasing of an egg from the ovary, occurs about halfway (day 14) through the normal 28-day menstrual cycle due to a mid-cycle explosive discharge of LH from the anterior pituitary. However, the length of the menstrual cycle is variable between women and normal cycles can vary from 21 days to 40 days. Ovulation can also vary between 10 and 16 days prior to the women's period, depending on her cycle length. Following ovulation, the egg is viable for only 24 hours.

The LH surge occurs because oestradiol has made the anterior pituitary gonadotrophs exquisitely sensitive to hypothalamic GnRH. In addition, for some unknown reason, the powerful negative feedback effect of oestradiol on LH release is overcome. This LH surge causes the rapid swelling and rupture of the follicle, and the egg is released. The ruptured follicle now becomes the *corpus luteum* (Latin for 'yellow body').

Knowledge of these events during the menstrual cycle has made it possible to advise on how to optimize the chances of becoming pregnant (conception) as well as provision of contraception.

The Luteal Phase

The part of the cycle following ovulation is called the 'luteal' phase. The corpus luteum produces the hormone progesterone, which has a number of critical actions:

- Progesterone causes further thickening of the endometrium through the build-up of glands and laying down of glycogen; this is called a 'secretory endometrium'.
- Progesterone exerts a negative feedback effect on the anterior pituitary, suppressing the release of LH.
- Progesterone, perhaps by an action on the hypothalamus, causes an increase in body temperature of about 0.5°C, its so-called thermogenic effect.
- Progesterone is responsible for some water and salt retention and is mildly anabolic.
- Progesterone ensures that any incoming sperm will find a hostile environment by making the cervical mucus more viscid and less alkaline.

The endometrium now passes into what is called its 'secretory' phase. If implantation of the fertilized ovum does not occur, the corpus luteum regresses and the superficial part of the endometrium breaks down and is discharged as the menstrual flow (Fig. 18.1).

Conception

It is not always easy for couples to conceive, and the information available about the menstrual cycle enables healthcare professionals to give advice. Theoretically, the couples should have intercourse anywhere from 4–5 days before ovulation to 24 h afterwards, with the best chances of conception if intercourse is within the time window of 24 h before or after ovulation. The figures arrived at here are based mainly on the fact that spermatozoa live up to 7 days in the fallopian tubes after sex and the egg is viable for 24 h after ovulation. The most fertile days for a woman with a 28-day cycle are days 12–18, with ovulation occurring typically on day 14. However, it is clinically appropriate to advise

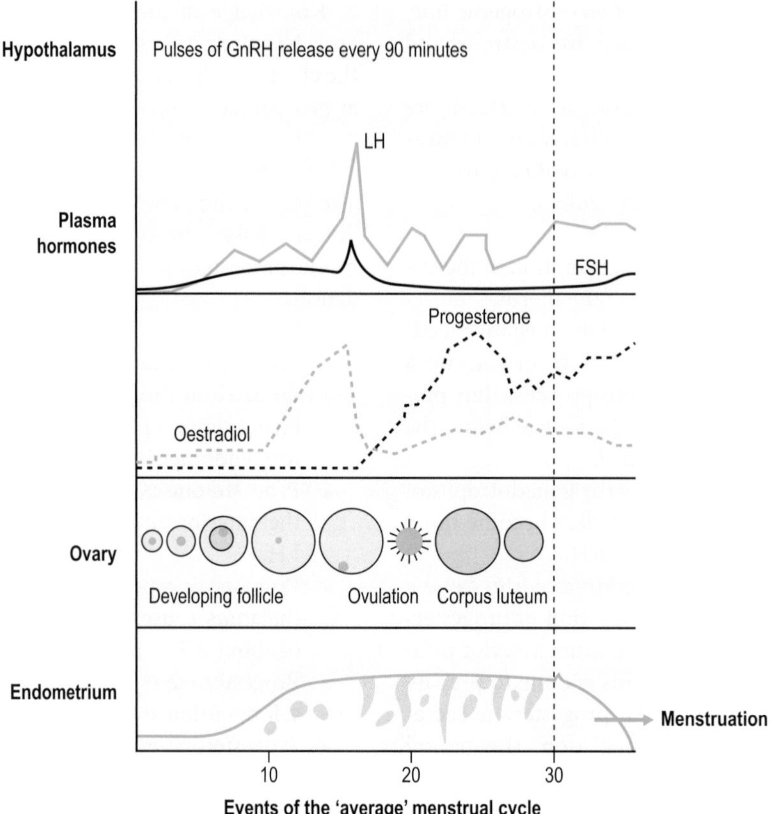

Fig. 18.1 ■ Events of the 'average' menstrual cycle. *FSH*, Follicle-stimulating hormone, *GnRH*, gonadotropin-releasing hormon; *LH*, luteinizing hormone. (Reproduced with permission from: Greenstein B. 1994. Endocrinology at a glance. Blackwell Sciences, Cambridge MA; 49.)

patients on regular sexual intercourse every 2–3 days to help optimize the chances of a successful pregnancy. This also aids in helping reduce stress for couples associated with working out the ovulation period per cycle. Signposting couples to useful resources such as those produced by the Family Planning Association (e.g. leaflets on *Planning a pregnancy*) can help aid the preconception advice given.

Pregnancy

If a fertilized ovum is implanted in the uterus, the corpus luteum does not immediately regress, but continues to produce its hormones. This function is eventually taken over by the placenta. Throughout pregnancy, large quantities of progesterone and oestrogens are produced by the placenta, and can be recovered from the urine. The human placenta produces a gonadotrophic hormone called *human chorionic gonadotrophin (HCG)* during the early months of pregnancy and its presence in the urine forms the basis of various tests for pregnancy. The placenta also produces large amounts of the oestrogenic hormone oestriol, and levels of oestriol are used to monitor the growth of the fetus. The most important clinical monitoring aid for fetal development, however, is through the use of ultrasound.

Just before parturition, the production of progesterone ceases and this may be involved with the start of labour.

The knowledge of the various negative feedback mechanisms governing LH and FSH release has provided the rationale for the design of the oral contraceptives (see later).

THE MALE SEX HORMONES

The hypothalamus of the postpubertal male puts out regular pulsatile doses of GnRH and in response, the anterior pituitary puts out FSH and LH. FSH promotes the development of the spermatozoa and LH promotes the production of testosterone by the interstitial Leydig cells of the testis. Testosterone exerts androgenic and anabolic effects (see later), and also has a negative feedback effect on LH secretion from the anterior pituitary, thus regulating its own production in the testis.

Clinical Use of GnRH Analogues

GnRH is a peptide hormone, which when administered to the pituitary in a pulsatile fashion, ensures normal anterior pituitary function and continued fertility. If GnRH for some reason is not produced, infertility results. If, on the other hand, the pituitary receives a *continuous* exposure to GnRH, it actually shuts down gonadotrophin production by the anterior pituitary cells. These phenomena have been exploited either to restore fertility or to prevent sex hormone production by the gonads. GnRH has been prepared synthetically and more stable and powerful analogues introduced.

Synthetic GnRH and GnRH Analogues

These comprise:

- **gonadorelin**, which is synthetic GnRH
- **buserelin**
- **goserelin**
- **leuprorelin**
- **nafarelin**, which is about 200 times more powerful than GnRH.

The last four drugs are synthetic analogues of gonadorelin. An analogue of a hormone is a synthetic compound with a (usually) slightly modified chemical structure, but similar biological actions. The analogues mentioned here all act on the GnRH receptors on anterior pituitary cells and are therefore also called *agonists*.

Therapeutic Uses

Gonadorelin. Gonadorelin is used to induce ovulation in some cases of infertility. It is given as a pulsed injection every 90 min using a miniaturized pump.

GnRH Analogues (e.g. Zoladex). These are usually given as subcutaneous, long-acting implants. They initially increase the release of gonadotrophins, followed by a falling off of gonadotrophin secretion due to pituitary desensitization. This results in decreased activity of the male and female gonads and reduced secretion of the sex hormones. GnRH analogues are used for the treatment of severe cases of endometriosis, carcinoma of the prostate as well as hormone receptor positive breast cancer. The aim is to shut down the production of the sex hormones, which aggravates these conditions. They are also used before surgery in women, together with iron supplements, to treat anaemia due to uterine fibroids.

GnRH analogues may be used off-label and prescribed by a specialist for severe premenstrual syndrome and perimenopausal depression when other therapies have failed. Patients prescribed GnRH analogues for this purpose will also be experiencing temporary/reversible menopause and therefore should be considered for prescription of hormone replacement therapy (HRT) and will likely undergo monitoring of bone density annually due to risk of osteoporosis (RCOG, 2016).

CLINICAL NOTE

When these GnRH analogues were first introduced and implanted into men with carcinoma of the prostate, the initial stimulus to gonadotrophin release caused a sometimes-fatal acceleration of the carcinoma due to increased testosterone production. To counteract this, patients are also treated with a drug such as **cyproterone acetate** (see later), which blocks the action of androgens on their receptors.

Clinical Use of Gonadotrophins and Antagonists

These comprise:

- FSH
- human chorionic gonadotrophin (HCG)
- human menopausal gonadotrophin (HMG)
- clomifene
- danazol.

These hormones and synthetic compounds are used therapeutically and are now considered in detail (Fig. 18.2).

FSH and LH

FSH is available as **urofollitropin** and as **follitropin alpha**. It is extracted from the urine of postmenopausal women. In the female, it causes ripening of the ovarian follicles and the production of oestrogen, and in the male it is necessary for the production of spermatozoa. It is given by injection. Pituitary LH is not used, but its actions are available as HCG. It is extracted from the urine of pregnant women. In the female it produces the corpus luteum and in the male it stimulates the interstitial cells of the testis to produce androgens. It is given by injection.

In **female infertility**, FSH and HCG are given by injection to induce normal ovarian function. FSH is given first to produce an ovarian follicle, followed by HCG to induce ovulation, or they may be given together as HMG. They will only be successful if infertility is due to lack of normally secreted gonadotrophins and not if there is primary ovarian failure.

Clomifene and Cyclofenil

Clomifene is a synthetic compound that blocks the action of oestradiol on its receptors (see more later). This releases the anterior pituitary from oestradiol's negative feedback effects, and large amounts of LH and FSH are released. Clomifene stimulates increased secretion of gonadotrophins and is used in the treatment of **infertility due to failure of ovulation**. It is given daily for 5 days, early in the menstrual cycle. It may be so successful that it results in twins, but multiple pregnancies can be avoided by careful dosing. Adverse effects include flushing, headaches, nausea, weight gain and visual disturbances.

CLINICAL NOTE

Women who are being offered ovulation induction with gonadotrophins should be informed about

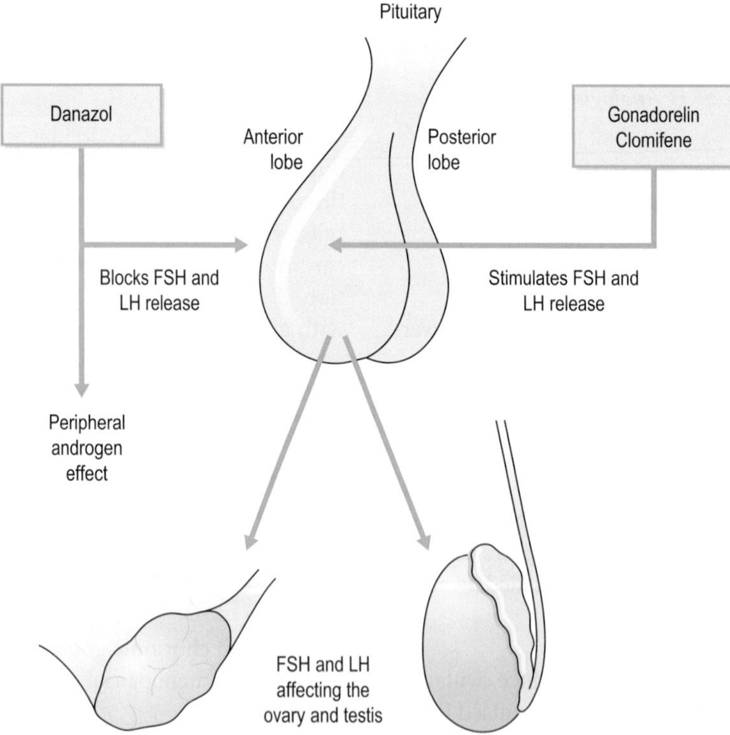

Fig. 18.2 ■ Medicines modifying the release of follicle-stimulating hormone (FSH) and luteinizing hormone (LH) and thus modifying gonadal activity.

the possibility of multiple pregnancy and ovarian hyperstimulation and they should undergo ovarian ultrasound monitoring to assess this (NICE, 2013).

Danazol

Danazol inhibits GnRH and gonadotrophin release and is used to treat endometriosis, and various benign breast disorders: e.g. **cyclical breast pain** that does not respond to conservative measures. This is due to swelling and tenderness of the breasts, which occurs during the second half of the menstrual cycle and is associated with the corpus luteum. If the symptoms are severe, danazol is effective in prevention, but its adverse effects are troublesome. The adverse effects reflect the fact that these compounds are androgen derivatives and cause abnormal hair growth, acne, fluid retention, weight gain and nausea. Patients should also be counselled about danazol causing deepening of the voice and enlargement of the clitoris. If used for treatment in women, they should concurrently be using effective non-hormonal contraception, as it can lead to developmental problems in the fetus.

CLINICAL NOTE

Patients may ask about gamolenic acid, which is extracted from evening primrose oil; anecdotally it may be felt to decrease the sensitivity of the breasts to hormones. However, NICE currently does not recommend the use of evening primrose oil for cyclical breast pain due to limited evidence of its benefits when compared with placebo (NICE, 2016).

SUMMARY

- GnRH analogues are used to treat endometriosis and prostatic carcinoma.
- When GnRH is started in patients with prostate carcinoma, they should take an androgen receptor blocker as well.
- FSH and HCG (or if given combined as HMG) will be successful in treating infertility only if infertility is caused by a lack of normally secreted gonadotrophins.
- Clomifene is used to treat infertility due to failure of ovulation and can cause multiple births and ovarian hyperstimulation.
- Danazol is used to treat cyclical breast pain, although danazol has unpleasant side-effects.

THE OESTROGENS

As mentioned previously, **oestradiol** is the main female sex hormone and the most potent. **Oestrone** is also a female sex hormone, but is shorter-acting. **Oestriol** is produced in large amounts during pregnancy, but its function is obscure.

Therapeutic Use of Oestrogens

The oestrogens comprise **natural oestrogens** and **synthetic oestrogens** (Table 18.1). Oestradiol-17β is the principal oestrogen secreted by the ovary, but there are a number of oestrogens that are used therapeutically. Oestrogens are used for:

- combined contraceptive methods (oral, transdermal, vaginal rings)
- HRT (oral and topical which includes topical gels and transdermal patches)
- atrophic vaginitis (as a topical vaginal cream).

ORAL CONTRACEPTION

There are two main types of oral contraceptive pill:

- the combined oral contraceptive pill
- the progestogen-only pill.

Combined Oral Contraceptive Pill

The combined oral contraceptive pill (COCP) is very widely used and is the most effective method of

TABLE 18.1
Oestrogens

Natural Oestrogens	Synthetic Oestrogens
Oestradiol-17β	Ethinylestradiol
Oestrone	Mestranol
Oestriol	Dienestrol[a]

[a]Used topically in the vagina.

preventing conception. It is a combination of an oestrogen and a progestogen, and acts in several ways. The oestrogen used is ethinylestradiol or mestranol. The content of oestrogen is 20–50 micrograms (μg). The progestogen used includes: desogestrel, gestodene, drospirenone, levonorgestrel or norethisterone, norgestimate and dienogest. The COCP can be used for contraception in women until the age of 50 years old, as long as there are no contraindications as outlined by the UK Medical Eligibility Criteria (UKMEC; see later).

Mechanism of Action

- The oestrogen inhibits the release of FSH by a negative feedback effect, thus inhibiting follicular development.
- The progestogen inhibits the release of LH, so that ovulation cannot occur. Together, the two chemicals render the endometrium hostile to implantation.
- Both drugs may upset the coordinated contractions of the fallopian tubes, uterus and cervix.

Usually, the composition of the COCP is unaltered throughout the full monthly course; these are known as 'monophasic'. There are a few preparations in which pills of varying composition of the two hormones are given sequentially, these are termed 'multiphasic'. Of the many preparations now available, the most effective and widely used are those in which both an oestrogen and a progestogen are given throughout the course, with a failure rate of less than 0.5 per 100 women-years. Table 18.2 shows the oestrogen and progestogen content of some of the preparations in use.

Using the Combined Oral Contraceptive Pill

- It is usual to start with the lowest-dose formulation because the risk of thrombosis (see later) is related to the oestrogen content. Preparations containing 20–35 μg of ethinylestradiol are usually prescribed.
- Correct use of the COCP is over 99% effective if used perfectly, but with typical use, 9% become pregnant in their first year of use.
- The COCP is usually started on the first day of the menstrual cycle (first day of bleeding) and

TABLE 18.2
Oral Contraceptives

		PROGESTOGEN ONLY[a]	
Generic name		Proprietary name	Dose (micrograms)
Desogestrel		Cerazette	75
Etynodiol		Femulen	500
Levonorgestrel		Norgeston	30
Norethisterone		Noriday	350
		COMBINED PREPARATIONS	
Preparation		Oestrogen (μg)	Progestogen (μg)
Ethinylestradiol 1 norethisterone			
BiNovum		35	500
Brevinor		35	500
Loestrin 20		20	1000
Norimin		35	1000
Ovysmen		35	500
Ethinylestradiol 1 levonorgestrel			
Microgynon 30		30	150
Ovranette		30	150
Ethinylestradiol 1 desogestrel			
Mercilon		20	150
Marvelon		30	150
Ethinylestradiol 1 gestodene			
Femodene		30	75
Ethinylestradiol 1 norgestimate			
Cilest		35	250
Triphasic preparations			
Ethinylestradiol 1 norethisterone			
Trinovum	(7 days)	35	500
	(7 days)	35	750
	(7 days)	35	100
Ethinylestradiol 1 levonorgestrel			
TriRegol	(6 days)	30	50
	(5 days)	40	75
	(10 days)	30	125
Logynon	(6 days)	30	50
	(5 days)	40	75
	(10 days)	30	125
	(7 days) inactive pill		

TABLE 18.2—cont'd

		Combined preparations	
Ethinylestradiol 1 gestodene			
Triadene	(6 days)	30	50
	(5 days)	40	70
	(10 days)	30	100

[a]Microval was discontinued by Wyeth in 2005.

continued for 21 days, then stopped for 7 days, during which bleeding occurs. The regimen is then repeated. However, following the 2019 updated guidelines by the FSRH (2016), they suggest there is no health benefit from the 7-day hormone free interval. Women can safely take fewer (or no) hormone free intervals, which would avoid bleeds, as well as can help control some other symptoms such as abdominal cramps. If the hormone free interval is taken, shortening it to 4 days could potentially reduce pregnancy risks.

- If the COCP is started within the first 5 days of the cycle, there is no additional need for contraception. If it is started at any other point then barrier contraception should be advised for the next 7 days.
- The COCP must be taken regularly and missed pill rules applied specific to the pill as per patient drug information.
- If a low-dose combination pill fails to control the cycle after 3 months, alternatives such as triphasic preparations should be tried.
- In the past, following childbirth, a progesterone only pill was preferred if the woman was breastfeeding, due to concerns regarding its effect on milk production. However, if not otherwise contraindicated, the COCP can be used first-line, even if breastfeeding, as it is felt that, by the time it is initiated in breastfeeding women (usually from 6 weeks postpartum) milk supply is already well established. If women do report concerns about a drop in milk supply, then it would be sensible to offer an alternative form of contraception.

THE UK MEDICAL ELIGIBILITY CRITERIA

The UKMEC offers guidance to providers of contraception regarding who can use contraceptive methods safely (FSRH, 2016). The World Health Organization has developed guidelines (WHO, 2015) for the provision of contraception to people with a range of medical conditions. It is primarily aimed at developing countries, where the risks associated with pregnancy are high.

The UKMEC splits each of the categories of contraceptives (COCP, progesterone only pill, intrauterine contraception and emergency contraception) into four categories (FSRH, 2016):

- Category 1: No restriction on the use of the method
- Category 2: Condition where the advantages of the method outweighs the risks
- Category 3: Theoretical or proven risks outweigh the advantages of using the method. Therefore, consideration of specialist intervention should be sought. This is because the method of contraceptive use is not usually recommended unless other more appropriate methods are not available or not acceptable.
- Category 4: Condition represents an unacceptable health risk and the considered contraceptive method should not be used.

The recommendations from the UKMEC are the same for all COCPs, irrespective of their progestogen content. The oestrogen transdermal patch and vaginal rings are relatively new contraceptives and there is still limited information that is available on safety profile; however, the limited evidence available place them in the same category as COCPs in the UKMEC tables.

Beneficial Effects of the Combined Contraceptive Pill

There is a reduced risk or incidence of:

- intermenstrual bleeding
- irregular periods
- iron deficiency anaemia
- premenstrual tension

- acne improvement
- benign breast disease
- uterine fibroids
- functional ovarian cysts
- thyroid disease
- unwanted pregnancy
- reduced risk of ovarian, endometrial and colorectal cancer.

Some authorities (Baird and Glasier, 1993) regard the COCP as safe for most women during their reproductive years. Women who smoke or suffer from obesity or hypertension do have a slightly higher risk of adverse effects (see more later).

Reported Adverse Effects and Unanswered Questions about the Combined Pill

- Thrombosis
- Migraine
- Dizziness, flushing, nausea, irritability and mood disturbance
- Gastrointestinal upsets
- Acne and skin pigmentation
- Gallstones
- Cardiovascular problems
- Weight gain
- Cancer.

Thrombosis. Taking the oral contraceptive carries a slightly increased risk of venous and cerebral thrombosis. In addition, there is a slightly increased risk of cerebral arterial disease. The overall mortality is about 2 per 100,000. Older women who smoke heavily are especially at risk from thromboembolic complications. Heavy smokers aged 40–44 years have an excess mortality of 54 per 100,000 women, and they should therefore use some other form of contraception. Thrombosis is believed to be due to the oestrogen in the COCP. For this reason, the oestrogen content of these preparations is kept as low as possible.

The associated arterial disease is due to the progestogen fraction of the COCP, which alters the blood lipids. The progestogens desogestrel and gestodene are less likely to cause changes in plasma lipids and, therefore, might be expected to reduce the risk of vascular disease (e.g. coronary thrombosis and strokes). However, evidence has emerged that they may actually increase the incidence of venous thrombosis in the legs and, thus, the risk of pulmonary embolism.

The incidence of venous thrombosis is approximately:

- 5 per 100,000 women per year – no contraceptive
- 15 per 100,000 women per year – with older progestogens
- 25 per 100,000 women per year – with desogestrel or gestodene (third-generation pill)
- 60 per 100,000 women per year – in pregnancy.

In view of this very small risk of thrombosis with the third-generation COCP, which is considerably less than that of pregnancy, they can be prescribed after a discussion with the patient. This is usually when other COCPs with a lower thrombosis risk have not been well tolerated.

Migraine. Women using the COCP who develop migraine with aura are at increased risk of strokes than women using the COCP without migraine.

Breast Cancer. Current evidence supports a slight increase in risk of breast cancer among women taking the COCP and this increases with duration of use. After 10 years of stopping the COCP, the woman is not thought to be at an increased risk.

Cancer of the Cervix. There is some evidence that cancer of the cervix is increased slightly in women taking the COCP for more than 5 years. It should therefore be encouraged that women take part in the cervical screening programmes.

Cardiovascular Problems. There is a very small increased risk of myocardial infarction and ischaemic strokes with use of the COCP. Women can develop hypertension when taking the COCP, which may resolve on stopping it. It is recommended to have an annual pill check, which includes a blood pressure assessment as well as a BMI check and assessment of other drug interactions, as well as any adverse effects.

Nausea. It is probably related to the oestrogen dosage and can usually be relieved by changing to a preparation with less oestrogen.

Weight Gain. There is no clear evidence that the COCP causes weight gain.

Mood Changes. Some women may experience negative mood changes but the evidence is not entirely clear or consistent on this. If present, an alternative COCP can be tried. If there are other features of premenstrual syndrome present then the continuous use of the COCP may be of benefit.

CLINICAL NOTE

In the UK, women aged 25–49 years are advised to have cervical smears every 3 years. Those aged 50–64 years are invited every 5 years.

Cancer of the Ovary and Uterus. The use of oral contraceptives reduces the risk of endometrial, ovarian and colorectal cancer.

At 10 years after discontinuation of the COCP there appear to be no long-term ill-effects.

CLINICAL NOTE

It is important to point out that many different COCPs are available, and it is usually possible to find one that best suits the woman requiring this form of contraception.

Drugs that Interfere with the Actions of Oral Contraceptives

Certain drugs when taken with oral contraceptives will increase the rate of breakdown of the oestrogen they contain and thus decrease their efficiency, and can lead to an unwanted pregnancy. Drugs that induce hepatic enzyme activity such as phenobarbital, carbamazepine, phenytoin, isoniazid and griseofulvin have also been suggested to interfere with the actions of contraceptives. Women requiring such treatments should be advised to use alternative forms of contraception, e.g. long-acting reversible contraception such as intrauterine devices or parenteral medroxyprogesterone acetate (contraceptive injection). This should then be continued for the duration of the treatment and for 4 weeks after stopping the treatment.

Antibacterials that do not induce liver enzymes do not require additional contraceptive precautions unless diarrhoea or vomiting occurs.

CLINICAL NOTE

Nurses working in family planning clinics and health centres have an important role in teaching women about taking oral contraceptives and allaying their anxieties.

If concerned, women should be advised to seek advice from specially trained nurses or their doctor. Stopping the Pill may result in an unplanned pregnancy. Women should be encouraged to express any dissatisfaction they may have so that they do not suddenly stop the Pill, with unfortunate consequences.

Nurses should ensure that the patient is well educated about other medications that may interfere with the contraceptive pill, e.g. antibiotics. Alternate contraception should be used if there is a fear that the contraception pill is interfered with.

Contraindications to the Use of the Combined Oral Contraceptive Pill

Contraindications include:

- Thromboembolic disease, past or present
- Carcinoma of the breast or uterus
- Focal migraine
- Hypertension (UKMEC3 – if blood pressure is more than 140/90 mmHg)
- Severe liver disease or recent viral hepatitis, previous cholestatic jaundice of pregnancy
- Pregnancy
- Porphyria
- Pemphigoid gestationis.

Progestogen-only Pill, Implants and Injections

It is possible to give preparations that only contain a progestogen (POP); however, although they impair fertility, they prevent ovulation in only about half the menstrual cycles, so are less efficient as contraceptives. If used correctly, the combined pill provides the most effective contraceptive available and failure rarely occurs.

This method, which inhibits ovulation and changes the character of the cervical mucus, is less 'safe' than the combined pill, but has virtually no risk of thrombotic disease (see earlier) and may be preferred in older women or those at risk of thrombosis. The POP is started on day 1 and taken at the same time each day throughout the cycle with no break. If started within the first 5 days of the menstrual cycle it provides immediate protection, otherwise additional contraceptives, e.g. barrier methods should be used for the first 2 days until it becomes effective.

Progestogens can also be given as depot injections, e.g. Depo Provera, which is the main injectable contraceptive in the UK and is given every 12 weeks. There is a disadvantage of possible delay in return of fertility. There is also an increased risk of osteoporosis.

Implants are flexible plastic rods that are inserted into the upper arm (implants) under a local anaesthetic and are effective for about 3 years. If the implant is not inserted within the first 5 days of the cycle, an additional 7 days of, e.g. barrier methods are recommended. If side-effects occur, the implants can be easily removed.

The main adverse effects of the POP are:

- Amenorrhoea, which is common in women taking this form of the pill. This is usually a welcomed effect in many women.
- Spotting – slight blood loss – may occur through much of the cycle.
- Breast-tenderness, weight gain and acne. These often subside within a few months of using the POP.

INTRAUTERINE SYSTEM

This releases a progestogen, levonorgestrel, directly into the uterine cavity. The mechanism of action is to prevent endometrial proliferation within the uterus and to thicken the cervical mucus to prevent pregnancy. There are now different IUS available on the market including the commonly used Mirena as well as the newer, smaller and lower dose of levonorgestrel called Jaydess. Both are used as contraceptives but Mirena is also indicated in idiopathic menorrhagia as well as for endometrial protection for HRT. The Jaydess may be more useful for women who prefer a regular bleed and may be more advantageous to use in young nulliparous women due to its smaller dimensions, thus theoretically allowing easier insertion (FSRH, 2014).

Emergency Contraception

The risk of pregnancy after unprotected sexual intercourse is about 1:20. It is possible to reduce the risk of pregnancy by using emergency contraception as a 'morning after' pill (oral hormonal method, which includes levonorgestrel or ulipristal acetate) or insertion of an intrauterine copper device. They should be offered soon after unprotected sex to increase their effectiveness.

The copper coil is the most effective emergency contraception and can be inserted up to 5 days after unprotected sex or up to 5 days after the earliest likely calculated ovulation. This can then also be used for ongoing contraception.

Levonorgestrel is effective up to 72 h after unprotected intercourse. The dosage of levonorgestrel is variable according to patient's body weight. Those over 70 kg should be considered for the higher dose (unlicensed). Ulipristal acetate can be given up to 120 h after unprotected sex. Following hormonal emergency contraception, women should be offered ongoing contraception either in the form of long-acting reversible contraception (e.g. IUS/IUD, implants, contraceptive injections) or suitable oral hormonal contraception. Following levonorgestrel, hormonal contraception can be started immediately; however, after ulipristal acetate, women should wait 5 days prior to starting hormonal contraception as ulipristal may reduce the effectiveness of the hormonal contraception. However, it is pertinent to advise the patient to abstain/use the barrier method in the interim until the hormonal contraceptive becomes effective.

SUMMARY

- The UKMEC is a guide to assess who can use different methods of contraception safely depending on their medical conditions and should be assessed when initiating or reviewing contraceptive methods in patients.
- The combined pill is the most effective oral contraceptive if taken correctly.
- Always start with the lowest-dose formulation of the combined pill.
- If a dose of the COCP is missed, other precautions, e.g. barrier method should be used additionally for 7 days.
- After childbirth, start the COCP after 3 weeks postpartum if not breastfeeding and no other venous thromboembolic risk factors.
- If breastfeeding, initiation of COCP should be 6 weeks onward (UKMEC 2). Less than 6 weeks postpartum breastfeeding women are UKMEC Category 4.

- Patients about to start on the COCP should first be fully briefed on possible adverse effects and especially about thrombosis.
- There may be a case for avoiding oral contraceptives that contain desogestrel or gestodene in patients who are overweight, immobile or who have a history of thrombosis.
- Women should be encouraged to have cervical smears and take part in screening if available.
- There is evidence that taking oral contraceptives reduces the risk of endometrial and ovarian cancer.
- Oral contraceptives reduce the efficacy of antihypertensive treatment, and their potency may be reduced by drugs such as some broad-spectrum antibiotics that reduce the absorption of oestrogens. Drugs such as phenobarbital, carbamazepine, isoniazid, griseofulvin, phenytoin and rifampicin (the most troublesome in this respect) enhance the breakdown of oestrogens by the liver.
- The occurrence of breakthrough bleeding may give a warning that an oral contraceptive is ineffective and it may be necessary to use a pill that contains more oestrogen.
- The progestogen-only pill is not as efficient as the combined pill, but carries virtually no risk of thrombotic disease.
- Progestogen-only contraceptives can also be given as depot injections, implants and intrauterine systems (IUS).
- Amenorrhoea (the absence or stopping of menstrual periods) is common with the progestogen-only pill and women should be taught the early signs and symptoms of pregnancy to avoid anxiety.
- Migraine, epilepsy and depression may be worsened if oral contraceptives are used.

HORMONE REPLACEMENT THERAPY

The menopause commences with a woman's last menstrual period and she is considered to be postmenopausal 1 year after her last menstrual period. Menopause is a retrospective diagnosis and can be clinically challenging, often due to the use of various contraceptive methods by women, which can often cause women to become amenorrhoeic (e.g. through the use of progesterone pill or an intrauterine device) . In the UK, the average age of menopause is 51 years old but menopause usually occurs from 45–55 years old. Women are advised to take contraceptive precautions for at least 1 year after menstruation ceases if they are aged over 50 years (or at least 2 years if aged under 50). However, you may have symptoms several months to years before you reach menopause and this is called the 'peri-menopause'. Premature menopause is defined as menopause occurring before 40 years of age and this is important to manage to help reduce the risk of heart disease and osteoporosis.

The menopause may be associated with a number of disorders. Women can have varying distressing symptoms during the menopause and it is important to individualize treatment for women based on their individual needs.

There has been controversy on the use of HRT stemming from the Women's Health Initiative study. This was one of the largest studies of women on HRT. A stem of the trial was halted early, as it was found that oestrogen with synthetic progesterone combination was associated with increased risk of breast cancer, heart disease and stroke. It did find some benefits, including lower rates of colorectal cancer as well as fewer hip fractures. The MHRA (2019) have issued a warning stating that the risk of breast cancer falls after stopping HRT but some risk can persist for more than 10 years after stopping HRT. The British Menopause Society suggests that healthy women younger than 60 years should not be concerned about the safety profile of HRT. They have stated that combined HRT use is associated with an extra five breast cancers per 1000 women after 7.5 years of use over the age of 50, with no increase in mortality

Menopausal Symptoms

Menopausal symptoms are due to oestrogen deficiency, which occurs due to the ovaries no longer producing oestrogen and as a result they stop releasing eggs. These symptoms can be physical, psychological and sexual, including:

- Physical symptoms: joint pains, fatigue, palpitations, hot flushes/night sweats (vasomotor), increased fracture risk due to osteoporosis
- Psychological: insomnia, mood disturbance
- Sexual: reduced libido, vaginal dryness – itching, soreness and recurrent urinary tract infections as well as dyspareunia (difficult or painful sex).

Osteoporosis. Osteoporosis, an imbalance of bone resorption and bone formation resulting in low mass bone density, which subsequently increases risk of fracture, is a serious problem in postmenopausal women. Oestrogen treatment is possibly the most effective way of preventing this in premature menopause. In addition, HRT appears to give some protection against coronary artery disease, stroke and, possibly, Alzheimer's disease. The treatment of osteoporosis is dealt with more fully in Chapter 15.

Hot Flushes. Their cause is unknown, but may be due to the rise in circulating LH. They respond to treatment with oestrogen, which brings LH levels back down again.

Aim of Hormone Replacement Therapy

The aim of HRT is to replace the sex hormones lost due to cessation of ovarian function at menopause, and the approach favoured is to restore, approximately, the chemical pattern of hormones present in blood during the menstrual cycle.

Preparations

HRT preparations comprise:

- oestrogen–progestogen combinations
- oestrogen patches/gels
- conjugated oestrogens
- tibolone.

Oestrogen–Progestogen Combinations

Most patients receiving HRT will have an intact uterus. The unopposed action of oestrogens stimulates the endometrium and may ultimately cause a carcinoma of the uterus. To prevent this happening, the **oestrogen is combined with a progestogen** to mimic the normal menstrual cycle, with regular shedding of the endometrium. A monthly course consists of an oestrogen given daily and a progestogen for the last 10–14 days of the cycle. Withdrawal bleeding may occur. A convenient preparation is *Prempak-C*, in which an oestrogen is given throughout the cycle and a progestogen (norgestrel) for the last 12 days. It is presented in a specially designed pack for ease of recognition. Other similar preparations are available.

Oestrogens

Oestrogens can also be given as a **patch** or **gel** applied to the skin. The patch available in the UK contains oestradiol, which diffuses through the skin and is effective for 3–4 days, after which the patch is replaced. Cyclical progestogen treatment causing monthly bleeding is still required. If the patient has had a hysterectomy, the progestogen is not needed and replacement can be with an oestrogen alone, e.g. **conjugated oestrogens** (Premarin). It is felt that transdermal preparations are the safest forms of HRT (oestrogen patch/gel), which can be combined with progestogens (in women who have an intact uterus), e.g. Mirena IUS or micronized progesterone (Utrogestan).

Oestrogens can also be applied topically into the vagina. They are used in atrophic vaginitis, which occurs in postmenopausal women due to oestrogen deficiency. Ovestin cream is applied daily for 3–4 weeks and then reduced. There is some controversy over the use of topical oestrogen in women with a history of oestrogen-dependent breast cancer. The American College of Obstetricians and Gynaecologists (ACOG, 2016) recommend that the data does not support an increased risk of cancer recurrence among women undergoing treatment for breast cancer or those with a personal history who use vaginal oestrogen to relieve urogenital symptoms. However, it is sensible to use non-hormonal approaches as first-line choices for managing the urogenital symptoms. If they are unsuccessful, then with the oncologist's involvement to help balance risks and benefits, a low-dose vaginal oestrogen can be considered.

Tibolone is a synthetic androgenic hormone that helps control postmenopausal symptoms. The drug is not available in USA or Canada but is approved in many countries worldwide, including the UK, although it is less commonly used. Tibolone has androgenic side-effects such as hirsutism and acne. Due to its androgenic effects, it can positively improve sexual function. In addition to its androgenic effects, it also has oestrogenic and progestogenic effects. There remains some uncertainty about its effects on breast cancer and cardiovascular disease.

Raloxifene has effects similar to oestrogens on blood and lipids, but blocks oestrogen action on the breast and uterus. It reduces osteoporosis and its use is not associated with menstrual bleeding. It is no longer recommended as treatment for primary prevention of osteoporotic fragility fractures in postmenopausal women (NICE, 2008b); instead it is indicated for women for secondary prevention of osteoporotic fragility fractures who are unable to tolerate bisphosphonates. It has been shown to reduce the risk of breast cancer but increases the risk of thrombosis. It does not control the vasomotor symptoms.

Factors to Consider When Prescribing Hormone Replacement Therapy

Symptoms to be Treated

On balance, HRT is indicated in postmenopausal women if they have symptoms (e.g. vaginitis, flushing) or are at special risk of osteoporosis or cardiovascular disease, e.g. women with premature menopause. Before starting treatment, counselling about the risks of HRT is pertinent and ideally should include written information or the women should be signposted to resources such as menopause matters website. Women should also be encouraged to take part in regular screening and be made 'breast aware' (being able to spot changes). Some vaginal bleeding can be common after HRT initiation for up to 3–6 months. However, if it persists beyond this, then sinister underlying causes need to be excluded and HRT discontinued interim.

Duration of Treatment

Duration of treatment depends on the therapeutic objectives. To relieve menopausal symptoms, 5 years is usually adequate. To prevent arterial disease, stroke and osteoporosis, lifelong treatment might be desirable, but 10 years is perhaps more practical because of the slightly increased risk of breast cancer, which is related to the duration of treatment. HRT prescription should be assessed annually (with discussion about risks) and be individualized to the woman.

Risks

Many practitioners consider that most women should use HRT, provided there are no contraindications. However, possible problems, which must be weighed against the benefits, are:

- There may be a slightly increased risk of carcinoma of the breast, particularly in older women and those taking hormones for more than 5 years.
- There is a slight risk of venous thrombosis.

Adverse Effects of Hormone Replacement Therapy

Adverse effects include nausea, weight gain, headache and fluid retention. Breast swelling may occur early in treatment, but usually subsides within 3 months.

SUMMARY

- If a woman has had a hysterectomy, a progestogen is not needed for HRT, preparation containing only oestrogens may be used.
- Women with an intact uterus do need co-prescription of licensed HRT progesterone, e.g. Mirena IUS or micronized progesterone.
- Transdermal oestrogens (patches/gel) are the safest available HRT preparations.
- Before starting HRT treatment, counselling of risks should take place.
- Women should be made breast aware and encouraged to attend screening.
- HRT treatment is usually adequate to relieve menopausal symptoms.
- Lifelong treatment may be desirable to prevent stroke, arterial disease and osteoporosis, although 10 years may be more practical because of the slightly increased risk of breast cancer.

DRUGS THAT AFFECT UTERINE SMOOTH MUSCLE

These comprise:

- Prostaglandins
- Ergometrine
- Oxytocin
- Syntometrine.

The Prostaglandins

These substances are formed by most cells of the body and are released from the cell membranes as a result of a range of stimuli. They usually produce their effects locally rather than at distant sites in the body, and many of them are removed from the circulation when they pass through the lung.

Prostaglandins and Pathology

Prostaglandins have been implicated in a number of pathological processes:

Inflammation. Prostaglandins of the E series are the mediators of some of the changes (swelling, redness and pain) seen in acute inflammation. This is important, since drugs such as aspirin and other nonsteroidal antiinflammatory drugs (NSAIDs), which block the production of prostaglandins, reduce the symptoms and signs of inflammation.

Thrombosis. Two types of prostaglandins or chemically-related compounds appear to be involved in thrombosis. Thromboxanes stimulate clumping of platelets and constriction of blood vessels, and thus encourage thrombosis, whereas prostacyclin (PGI2) has the reverse effect. Through use of low doses of aspirin, the balance between the availability of PGI2 and thromboxane goes in favour of PGI2 leading to a reduced risk of myocardial infarction and stroke (see Chapter 7 for more details).

Effects on Uterine Muscle. Prostaglandins cause contraction of the uterine muscle and are concerned with both menstruation and childbirth. Prostaglandins are also responsible for much of the pain associated with dysmenorrhea and this is why NSAIDs are effective in this condition. Prostaglandin E_2 can be used to induce labour or terminate pregnancy by causing the uterus to contract (see later).

Effects on the Stomach. Prostaglandins increase mucus secretion by the cells lining the stomach and thus protect the mucosa against ulcer formation.

Therapeutic Uses of Prostaglandins

Vaginal prostaglandin E2 is the preferred method of induction of labour. **Dinoprostone** (prostaglandin E_2) can be given by vaginal tablets, gel or controlled-release pessary to induce labour. The patients should be informed about the associated risks of uterine hyperstimulation. Continuous electronic fetal heart rate and uterine contraction monitoring should be available on induction of labour. Women should also be informed that induced labour is likely to be more painful than spontaneous labour and therefore discussion of various analgesics may be even more pertinent. If there is uterine hyperstimulation following induction, then NICE (2008a) suggests consideration of tocolysis (which inhibits uterine contractions, see later).

Misoprostol and mifepristone are only offered for induction of labour to women who have intrauterine fetal death (see later).

SAFETY POINT

Dinoprostone increases the effects of oxytocin and these drugs should never be given together. The bladder should be emptied before insertion and the patient should lie down for 15 minutes after insertion.

Gemeprost (a prostaglandin E_1 analogue) pessaries are inserted into the vagina to soften the cervix and thus facilitate abortion during the first 2 months of pregnancy. Adverse effects include nausea, vomiting, diarrhoea, headache and fever.

Ergometrine

Ergometrine (see also the ergot alkaloids, Chapter 21) is rapidly absorbed either from the intestinal tract or from the site of injection. This is the chemical that was responsible for the spontaneous abortions suffered by those who ate contaminated rye. Its chief action is to cause contractions of the uterus. With small doses, these contractions are rhythmic, but with larger doses they become very powerful and more or less continuous. They are brought about by a direct action of ergometrine on the uterine smooth muscle. The uterus is especially sensitive to ergometrine at the time of childbirth. It has little effect on other smooth muscles throughout the body.

Therapeutic Use of Ergometrine

Ergometrine is given after childbirth to cause the uterus to contract and thus prevent bleeding. It should not be given before delivery, even if the uterus is sluggish, as it may produce such powerful contractions that the uterus is ruptured, or risks hypoxia to the fetus. Increased contractions of the uterus are seen within 5 min of intramuscular injection.

Oxytocin

Oxytocin (see also Chapter 14) is a hormone released from the posterior pituitary gland. It causes contraction of the smooth muscle of the uterus. This effect is not marked until the later stages of pregnancy and at parturition, when extremely small amounts of oxytocin will cause powerful uterine contractions.

Therapeutic Use of Oxytocin

Oxytocin is used to induce labour. For this purpose, it is usual to use synthetic oxytocin (**Syntocinon**), as the naturally prepared oxytocin contains a small amount of vasopressin. Oxytocin is given by intravenous infusion in saline and the rate of infusion is regulated according to the response of the patient. There is a risk of rupture of the uterus with oxytocin and it should only be used to induce labour under expert supervision. Oxytocin is also used after delivery of the placenta to cause uterine contraction, but its effects are not as prolonged as those of ergometrine. For this reason, it is sometimes combined with ergometrine as **Syntometrine** (see later). Whole posterior pituitary extract should not be used, because of its vasopressor effects.

Adverse Effects of Oxytocin

In addition to producing powerful uterine contractions, oxytocin can cause a rise in blood pressure and water retention. It should not usually be combined with prostaglandins to induce labour.

Syntometrine

Syntometrine is a mixture of ergometrine and oxytocin. It is given intramuscularly and combines the rapid action of oxytocin on the uterus with the prolonged contraction caused by ergometrine. It is commonly used after the expulsion of the placenta to prevent bleeding.

Termination of Pregnancy

The termination of pregnancy is ethically and morally challenging and there may be restrictive abortion laws in many countries. The Abortion Act 1967 legalized abortions in the UK, by registered medical practitioners. Later in 1990, the time frame for carrying out abortions was lowered from 28 weeks to 24 weeks through the Human Fertilization and Embryology Act 1990.

In the UK, abortions can be carried out in a licensed clinic or in an NHS hospital. The method for conducting abortions is dependent upon the gestation of pregnancy. In the first trimester (up to 12 weeks of pregnancy), drugs can be used for termination of pregnancy, referred to as a medical abortion. After 12 weeks, surgical dilatation is conducted with evacuation of uterine contents; a **gemeprost** pessary may be given to help soften the cervix.

Most terminations of pregnancy are carried out in the first trimester. Drugs used to terminate pregnancy in the first trimester are:

- **mifepristone**
- misoprostol (a synthetic **prostaglandin**).

Mifepristone blocks the action of progesterone at its receptors in the uterus. It also helps to ripen the cervix. Misoprostol has potent effects on stimulating the uterus causing contractions, which results in the expulsion of tissue.

There is a risk of infection after termination; however, NICE (2019) no longer recommends routine antibiotic prophylaxis to women having a medical abortion but prophylactic antibiotics are recommended in women having a surgical abortion.

Women who are rhesus D negative and who have an abortion after 10 weeks' gestation should also be offered anti-D prophylaxis.

Tocolytic Agents (Drugs Inhibiting Uterine Contractions)

Tocolytic agents help relax the myometrium to postpone premature labour. They may help provide time to administer corticosteroids to help maturation of fetal lungs or help implement other measures to improve perinatal health, such as transfer to a neonatal intensive care facility.

Atosiban, an oxytocin receptor antagonist, as well as **nifedipine**, a calcium channel blocker, can have fewer side-effects in comparison to β_2 receptors agonists. Stimulation of β_2 receptors in uterine muscles will diminish uterine activity. The β_2 agonists **salbutamol** and **terbutaline** are sometimes used in the management of premature labour between 22 and 37 weeks of pregnancy and are usually given by intravenous infusion for this purpose. There is a real risk of fluid overload.

Menorrhagia

Heavy bleeding during a period is very common and may sometimes be serious enough to require a

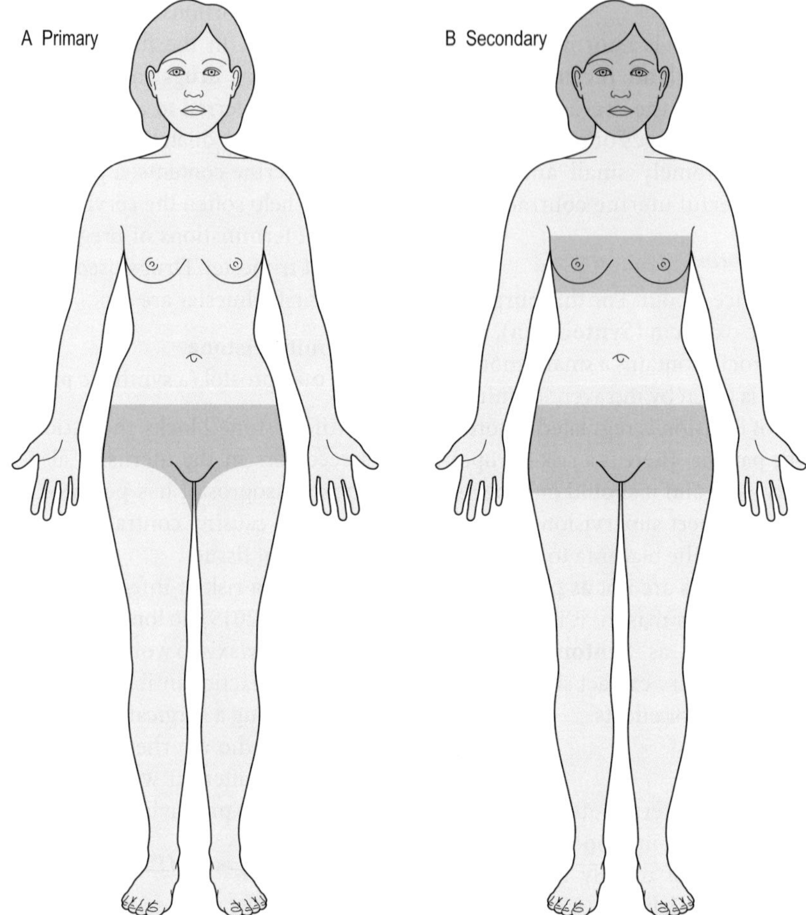

Fig. 18.3 ■ (A) Primary and (B) secondary sites of discomfort in primary and secondary dysmenorrhoea.

hysterectomy. The majority of patients have no underlying pelvic disease, known as abnormal uterine bleeding (formerly known as dysfunctional uterine bleeding).

Treatment options:

- A **levonorgestrel intrauterine system** (LNG-IUS) is first-line treatment for menorrhagia in women without identified pathology (or fibroids less than 3 cm).
- **Combined hormonal pill** or a cyclical oral **progestogen.**
- **Mefenamic acid**, a weak NSAID, is widely used, with some success, to control pain and reduce bleeding.
- **Tranexamic acid**, which inhibits the breakdown of fibrin, is more effective. It is given orally when bleeding has started and continued for 3–4 days. Adverse effects include nausea, vomiting and blurred vision. It is contraindicated in thromboembolic disease.
- If the pharmacological treatments are unsuccessful and fibroids are identified, then surgical treatments can be offered including uterine artery embolization, myomectomy, hysterectomy or endometrial ablation.

Dysmenorrhoea

Dysmenorrhoea means painful periods. It can be subdivided into primary or secondary causes (Fig. 18.3).

Primary Dysmenorrhoea

Primary dysmenorrhoea is common in young women and does not have any underlying pelvic pathology. Usual symptoms are low backache and colicky pain in the pelvic area. This is due to the cyclical release of prostaglandins in the uterus, leading to contraction of the uterine muscle and constriction of the arteries supplying the muscle, with consequent ischaemia. Other symptoms include nausea, vomiting, diarrhoea and faintness. NSAIDs, e.g. **ibuprofen** or **mefenamic acid**, should give relief by inhibiting prostaglandin synthesis. Ideally, they should be taken after menstrual bleeding has commenced, to avoid the ingestion of drugs by a possibly pregnant woman. If this fails, oral contraceptives (oestrogen/progestogen) are frequently effective.

Secondary Dysmenorrhoea

Secondary dysmenorrhoea affects women in their late 20s and 30s, causing a dragging pain, often preceded by headaches. As its name implies, this occurs in response to some pathological condition (fibroids, endometriosis) and treatment is by removal of the cause.

Premenstrual Syndrome

The cyclical appearance of a cluster of symptoms in the second half of the menstrual cycle which terminate abruptly with the onset of menstruation is known as the 'premenstrual tension syndrome' (PMS). Although PMS is very common, only about 5% of women experience symptoms severe enough to disrupt their lives. There can be a variety of symptoms, both emotional and physical (Table 18.3). A small number of women suffer from premenstrual dysphoric disorder, which is an intense form of PMS.

TABLE 18.3

Symptoms of Premenstrual Tension (PMS)

Emotional Symptoms	Physical Symptoms
Depression	Headache
Tension	Breast swelling and discomfort
Crying	Bloating
Aggression	
Failure to concentrate	

The range of these symptoms suggests that there is more than one cause; in-keeping with this theory, women respond differently to prescribed treatments. However, its relationship with the menstrual cycle indicates that PMS is probably related to the hormonal and metabolic changes that occur. A diary of symptoms can help with the diagnosis as well as monitoring of treatments. The cause of PMS remains unknown and is likely multifactorial.

A selection of possible aetiological factors and treatments is given below:

- *Brain neurotransmitters.* Attention is now directed to the relationship between ovarian hormones and neurotransmitters in the brain. It is thought that progesterone or, more probably, one of its metabolites interacts with the GABA or 5-hydroxytryptamine (5-HT; serotonin) systems and a disorder of these interactions is responsible for PMS. Serotonin appears to play the most important role in the aetiology of PMS; therefore serotonin reuptake inhibitors (SSRIs) are the most effective for the disorder.
- *Changes in water and salt balance.* Although feelings of bloating and swelling are frequent symptoms, there is some controversy over whether fluid retention actually occurs.
- *Elevated prolactin levels.* Prolactin is released from the anterior pituitary and stimulates lactation. When a woman is not lactating, a hormone inhibitor suppresses prolactin secretion. Some women with PMS have raised prolactin levels. Bromocriptine, which inhibits prolactin release, has been found useful for some symptoms, especially breast discomfort, but adverse effects may be troublesome.
- *Diminished progesterone levels.* These have been suggested as an aetiological agent, but injection of progesterone or of a synthetic substitute has not been shown to be beneficial.
- *Changes in prostaglandin E_1 levels.* This appears important in hormone balance and it has been suggested that PMS is a manifestation of deficiency. Gamolenic acid (evening primrose oil) is converted into prostaglandin E_1 and, given

as *Efamast*, some women find this effective but lacks good evidence base. Conversely, prostaglandin synthesis inhibition by mefenamic acid can improve headaches, aches and pains.
- *Diet.* Various dietary modifications have been tried. A balanced diet should be encouraged for mild symptoms along with other lifestyle measures.

In summary, there is no overall regimen to control PMS. In patients with mild symptoms, it is probably best to employ lifestyle changes including exercise, balanced diet and stress management. There is limited evidence that complementary therapies are effective. With more severe symptoms medical treatment can be trialled. This includes non-hormonal therapy and hormonal therapies.

Non-hormonal Therapy for PMS

Antidepressants such as SSRIs, e.g. sertraline, are the first choice of treatments for severe PMS if lifestyle changes have failed to control the symptoms.

Hormonal Therapy for PMS

Oral contraceptive if not contraindicated is the first-line hormonal treatment (in particular those containing drospirenone) and taking it continuously rather than cyclical may be more beneficial for the patient. Other options include using transdermal oestrogen (gel/patches with opposing progesterone if the patient has an intact uterus), however the patient may also require additional contraception. Danazol may be considered by a specialist, in patients who have breast tenderness. GnRH analogues (see earlier) may be required, e.g. goserelin (which can also help confirm the diagnosis), if other therapies have failed but will require monitoring for osteoporosis and patients may also be commenced on HRT, as the treatment causes a temporary menopause.

Surgical Treatment for PMS

As a last resort, surgical treatment may be offered if other therapies have failed. This can include a total hysterectomy and oophorectomy. However, as this will result in menopause, HRT may need to be considered for the patient.

SUMMARY

- Dinoprostone and oxytocin should never be given together.
- Ergometrine should never be given before delivery.
- Oxytocin is not effective until the later stages of pregnancy, and is extremely potent at onset of labour.
- There is a risk of rupture of the uterus with oxytocin and it should be used with care.
- Oxytocin can cause a rise in blood pressure and water retention, particularly if it is used in the form of a pituitary extract, which could well contain vasopressin.
- Oxytocin should not usually be combined with prostaglandins to induce labour.
- Syntometrine is commonly used after delivery of the baby to prevent bleeding.
- Tocolytic agents help to postpone premature labour.
- LNG-IUS is first-line treatment for menorrhagia without pathology (or in women with fibroids less than 3 cm).
- Dysmenorrhea can be primary or secondary; the latter is associated with pathology (e.g. fibroids, endometriosis).
- PMS is very common and likely has a multifactorial aetiology, with serotonin playing an important role. Treatment is through lifestyle advice, hormonal or non-hormonal methods.

MALE SEX HORMONES

Testosterone

The interstitial cells of the testis produce the male hormone testosterone. It is responsible for the secondary male sex characteristics, including distribution of hair, deepening of the voice, and enlargement of the penis and seminal vesicles. Testosterone can be isolated from the testis, but is usually prepared synthetically. Its synthesis and release from the testis is controlled by LH (see Chapter 14 and Fig. 14.4). The actions of testosterone that virilize are called 'androgenic actions'.

Therapeutic Use

Testosterone or synthetic analogues are used in the treatment of testicular hormone deficiency and carcinoma of the breast.

Testicular Hormone Deficiency. **Testosterone** is used in the treatment of testicular hormone deficiency. This may be of unknown origin or due to injury or disease of the testis, or it may be secondary to lack of gonadotrophic hormone following pituitary gland disease. Treatment with androgen is pointless for impotence and impaired spermatogenesis, unless there is associated hypogonadism. If this is detected, then treatment should be under specialist supervision. Esters of testosterone (e.g. *Sustanon*) can be given intramuscularly every 3 weeks and are released slowly from the injection site. They are the preferred method of replacement. Testosterone is also available in topical applications (e.g. *Testogel*), which may be more desirable for patients rather than injections.

Carcinoma of the Breast. Testosterone is effective in about 30% of premenopausal patients with advanced carcinoma of the breast for relieving symptoms and causing temporary regression of secondary deposits. It does, however, have virilizing effects. When given to women, testosterone causes the growth of facial hair, deepening of the voice and acne.

Androgen Antagonists

Cyproterone acetate and **flutamide** block the action of testosterone at its receptor. They are used in various endocrine disorders where there is overproduction of this male hormone, causing hirsutism in the female (when it may be combined with an oestrogen) and hypersexuality in males. These drugs are also used in treating carcinoma of the prostate.

Finasteride blocks the enzyme 5α-reductase that converts testosterone into a powerful androgenic metabolite called '5α-reductase' in the prostate gland, thus causing the prostate to decrease in size. This drug is used to treat benign enlargement of the prostate.

Carcinoma of the Prostate. The structural and functional integrity of the prostate depends on continued stimulation by testosterone and this also applies to carcinomatous tissue in the prostate. When widespread deposits have developed, strategies that interfere with hormone stimulation of these secondaries can control the disease. This can be achieved by giving an oestrogen (usually diethylstilbestrol), but adverse effects (feminization and fluid retention) can be troublesome. Alternatively, a gonadorelin analogue may be used. This initially causes increased testosterone activity, which can be controlled by cyproterone but, after about 2 weeks, LH release is inhibited, resulting in a fall in testosterone levels and a regression of the tumour.

Anabolic Hormones

The structure of these male sex hormones has been modified so that they have little masculinizing effect but they have considerable anabolic action and are capable of building up protein in bone and other tissues. They were used to treat osteoporosis in women but are no longer advocated for this. They are used to treat some aplastic anaemias. Anabolic steroids also produce an increase in muscle bulk and have been used by athletes to improve their performance, which is dishonest and undesirable and also carries the possibility of adverse effects.

Male Erectile Dysfunction (Impotence)

Impotence is a common disorder. Its incidence increases with age and it may have a considerable effect on the well-being of the individual. The cause can be psychological, physical or a combination of both.

Erection depends on the relaxation of the corpus cavernosum (penile smooth muscle), with subsequent engorgement with blood following psychological or tactile stimulation. The autonomic nervous system is involved in the control of this activity with nitric oxide being the important neurotransmitter mediating the vascular relaxation.

Drugs can be used in two ways with respect to erectile dysfunction:

- Drugs may interfere with sexual performance
- Drugs can also improve performance.

Drugs that Interfere with Male Sexual Performance

Among those implicated are various centrally acting drugs (alcohol, tricyclic antidepressants, neuroleptics), antihypertensives (particularly thiazides and beta blockers) and cimetidine (due to its oestrogen-like action).

Drugs that Help Induce an Erection

An effective method is the intracavernosal injection of **papaverine** or **prostaglandin E_1** (e.g. alprostadil), which relaxes the vascular smooth muscle in the penis and produces a satisfactory erection. After preliminary training, the drug can be self-administered. The erection should not be allowed to continue for more than 4 hours. Alternatively, a small pellet of prostaglandin E_1 can be inserted into the urethra and enough is absorbed to achieve an erection in a proportion of patients. However, the use of such drugs can be associated with local pain and are not as convenient for patients as the use of orally active drugs.

Sildenafil (***Viagra***) is an orally active phosphodiesterase-5 inhibitor, which causes relaxation of the corpus cavernosum in the blood vessels of the penis, leading to vasodilatation and an enhanced erection when taken an hour or two before intercourse. It is effective in the majority of men with impotence, whatever the cause. Other orally active phosphodiesterase-5 inhibitors include tardenafil and vardenafil.

Adverse effects are rarely serious and include headache, flushing and occasional disturbances of colour vision. It should not, however, be combined with nitrate-containing preparations such as glyceryl trinitrate (including patients using GTN spray as required) or patients taking nicorandil.

When drugs are not effective, various mechanical or surgical treatments are available for the management of erectile dysfunction. These measures can be used alongside psychosexual counselling.

REFERENCES AND FURTHER READING

ACOG, 2016. The use of vaginal estrogen in women with a history of estrogen-dependent breast cancer. In: Committee Opinion No 659. American College of Obstetricians and Gynecologists.

Baird, D.T., Glasier, A.F., 1993. Hormonal contraception. N. Engl. J. Med. 328 (21), 1543–1549.

Chalouhi, S., 2017. Menopause: a complex and controversial journey. Post. Reprod. Health 23 (3), 128–131.

French, K., 2017. The Role of Nurses in the Provision of Contraception in Primary Care. Nursing in Practice. https://www.nursinginpractice.com/professional/the-role-of-nurses-in-the-provision-of-contraception-in-primary-care.

FSRH, 2014. New Product Review: Jaydess Levonorgestrel Intrauterine System (LNG IUS). Faculty of Sexual & Reproductive Healthcare, RCOG. https://www.fsrh.org/standards-and-guidance/documents/cec-ceu-newproductreview-jaydess-apr-14.

FSRH, 2016. UK Medical Eligibility Criteria for Contraceptive Use (UKMEC). Faculty of Sexual & Reproductive Healthcare, RCOG. https://www.fsrh.org/standards-and-guidance/documents/ukmec-2016.

Gersh, F.L., Lavie, C.J., 2020. Menopause and hormone replacement therapy in the 21st century. Heart 106 (7), 479–481.

Gourdin, T., 2020. Recent progress in treating advanced prostate cancer. Curr. Opin. Oncol. 32 (3), 210–215.

Kelsey, S., 2017. Methods of contraception: the nurse's role in providing care and advice. Nurs. Stand. 32 (13), 52–63.

Matheson, L., Nayoan, J., Rivas, C., et al., 2020. A qualitative exploration of prostate cancer survivors experiencing psychological distress: loss of self, function, connection, and control. Oncol. Nurs. Forum 47 (3), 318–330.

MHRA, 2019. Hormone Replacement Therapy (HRT): Further Information on the Known Increased Risk of Breast Cancer with HRT and its Persistence after Stopping. https://www.gov.uk/drug-safety-update/hormone-replacement-therapy-hrt-further-information-on-the-known-increased-risk-of-breast-cancer-with-hrt-and-its-persistence-after-stopping.

Mitidieri, E., Cirino, G., d'Emmanuele di Villa Bianca, R., Sorrentino, R., 2020. Pharmacology and perspectives in erectile dysfunction in man. Pharmacol. Ther. 208, 107493.

NICE, 2008a. Inducing Labour [CG70]: Recommended Methods for Induction of Labour. https://www.nice.org.uk/guidance/cg70.

NICE, 2008b. Raloxifene for the Primary Prevention of Osteoporotic Fragility Fractures in Postmenopausal Women [TA160]. https://www.nice.org.uk/guidance/ta160.

NICE, 2013. Fertility Problems: Assessment and Treatment [CG156]. https://www.nice.org.uk/guidance/cg156.
NICE, 2016. Breast Pain – Cyclical. https://cks.nice.org.uk/breast-pain-cyclical.
NICE, 2019. Abortion Care [NG140]. https://www.nice.org.uk/guidance/ng140.
RCOG, 2016. Management of Premenstrual Syndrome. Green-top Guideline No. 48. https://www.rcog.org.uk/globalassets/documents/guidelines/gt48managementpremensturalsyndrome.pdf.
WHO, 2015. In: Medical Eligibility Criteria for Contraceptive Use, fifth ed. https://www.who.int/reproductivehealth/publications/family_planning/Ex-Summ-MEC-5/en/.

USEFUL WEBSITES

British Menopause Society (BMS). https://thebms.org.uk/.
Patient. http://www.patient.co.uk.
SexWise, Planning a Pregnancy. https://www.sexwise.fpa.org.uk/planning-pregnancy.

19 NERVOUS SYSTEM 1
General Anaesthesia and Local Anaesthetics

CHAPTER OUTLINE

LEARNING OBJECTIVES

At the end of this chapter, the reader should be able to:

- outline preoperative assessment procedures taken before general anaesthesia and surgery
- give an account of the role that drugs have in the preoperative preparation of the patient for general anaesthesia and surgery
- describe the main elements of general anaesthesia and have an understanding of the groups of drugs involved
- explain how muscle relaxants work and how their effects may be reversed using drugs
- describe the ways in which local anaesthetics may be used and of some of the differences between the various drugs

HISTORY

Three important drugs, capable of producing general anaesthesia when inhaled in sufficient quantity, were introduced to medicine within a time span of 5 years in the mid-19th century. These inhalational anaesthetic agents are:

- ether
- nitrous oxide
- chloroform.

In 1842, William E. Clark of Rochester, New York, used **ether** to provide general anaesthesia for the extraction of a tooth. **Nitrous oxide** was first used as a general anaesthetic in 1844 by Horace Wells, a dentist from Hartford, CT. He had first persuaded a travelling lecturer in chemistry to give him nitrous oxide while a fellow dentist took out one of his teeth; he then used it successfully on his own patients. James Y. Simpson of Edinburgh introduced the use of **chloroform** in 1847 for general surgery and obstetrics and he administered it to Queen Victoria in 1853 at the birth of Prince Leopold. Chloroform remained popular for over 100 years but is no longer used as a general anaesthetic. Ether remains in use in some lower income countries due to its high therapeutic index and low price. Nitrous oxide remains in daily use worldwide. Despite the sophistication of modern anaesthetic practice, the precise mode of action of most general anaesthetics is poorly understood. This is probably a reflection of the fact that the phenomenon of consciousness and its relationship to brain function remains largely mysterious.

PREOPERATIVE ASSESSMENT OF THE PATIENT

The patient's medical history must be thoroughly assessed, and existing medicine use and drug allergies and any pre-existing medical conditions (e.g. diabetes mellitus, heart, liver or respiratory disease, or problems with blood coagulation) identified before elective surgery. Previous anaesthetic problems should be enquired after (particularly suxamethonium apnoea – see later). Examination should include:

- measurement of blood pressure and heart rate
- check of veins for ease of cannulation
- examination of the lungs, including chest X-rays if indicated
- ECG if indicated
- identification of heart murmurs
- check for loose teeth and crowns that may be damaged during intubation, and false teeth or bridges, which should be removed
- check for impaired mobility of the temporomandibular joints (TMJ; connects the lower jaw to the skull) and for rheumatoid arthritis (RA)-associated mobility problems of the neck
- Blood tests may be required, particularly in older patients. Kidney and liver function are often checked, as is a check on the haemoglobin level. Checks for haemoglobinopathies, such as sickle cell disease, may be necessary.

PREMEDICATION

Premedication is the administration of drugs to patients 1–2 hours before anaesthesia and surgery. The objectives of premedication are:

- to relieve anxiety
- to reduce the production of saliva
- to reduce the volume, and increase the pH, of the gastric contents.

The use of premedication has declined considerably as newer anaesthetics and techniques have been introduced and it is common practice not to administer any drugs to patients for the above purposes before anaesthesia and surgery. If drugs are used, they are generally given orally and rarely by intramuscular (IM) or intravenous (IV) injection. Intramuscular premedication, in particular, is not tolerated well by children. Some drugs may still sometimes be necessary before surgery, e.g. steroids and antibiotics.

Drugs used for premedication include:

- Drugs to reduce anxiety (anxiolytic drugs)
- Muscarinic receptor antagonists to reduce secretions
- Drugs to reduce gastric acidity.

Relief from Anxiety

Most patients are anxious before anaesthesia and surgery. Many feel a general sense of nervousness or apprehension. Others have more specific concerns such as fears of:

- injections
- pain after surgery
- waking up in the middle of the operation
- dying and not waking up at all
- the embarrassment of nakedness
- talking aloud while asleep (and perhaps giving away personal secrets)
- the loss of control over themselves and their environment
- having the wrong operation
- what the surgeon may find something wrong with them.

CLINICAL NOTE

Comprehensive preoperative information is important, this is of particular importance when dealing with parents of children undergoing surgery. In children, a systematic review of eight studies reported a reduction in anxiety with the use of clown therapy (Zhang et al., 2017). This intervention involves the introduction of a clown actor to prepare the child for surgery in a way that the child will find engaging, non-threatening and understandable. Transferring these principles to the adult population, information conveyed should be straightforward, clear, simple and accurate. Taking a patient-centred approach and addressing any specific concerns that the patient has will reduce anxiety. Teach-back techniques to check understanding may also ensure that the patient has made an informed choice for the procedure.

Anxiolytic Drugs

Several of the benzodiazepine group of drugs may be used to help reduce anxiety before anaesthesia and surgery. **Temazepam** is the most commonly used. It is well absorbed and effective given orally (there is no injectable preparation). **Midazolam** is only available as an injection solution, but this can be used orally. It is, however, more effective if given intranasally or sublingually, and is sometimes given by these unusual routes in children. The injection solution is extremely bitter tasting. It has a shorter duration of action than temazepam. Other drugs in this group that can be used are **diazepam** and **lorazepam. Alimemazine** (trimeprazine, a phenothiazine) is still sometimes be used for oral premedication in children. It can cause marked pallor and tachycardia. **Dexmedetomidine** and **clonidine hydrochloride** are α_2-adrenergic agonists with sedative properties. Dexmedetomidine is used for sedation in intensive care units, and clonidine hydrochloride is occasionally used for sedation when other methods prove ineffective.

Opioids

Morphine and other opioid analgesics (see Chapter 20), although good anxiolytics, are only used for premedication for patients who are in pain before surgery.

CLINICAL NOTE

Anxiolytics act on receptors in the central nervous system. These drugs work on gamma-aminobutyric acid (GABA), a natural neurotransmitter, which slows down the body's central nervous system to promote relaxation and induce sleep. Anxiolytics stimulate the inhibitory action of these receptors, reducing anxiety and inducing sleep. While their drug action is not entirely understood, it is thought that stimulation results in an increase in chloride ions and reduces excitation of GABA receptors. Preoperative medication is infrequently given due to the need for early postoperative mobilization, which can be delayed if patients are given preoperative medication.

Reducing the Production of Saliva

Excessive salivation can present problems in safe airway management, particularly during the induction of anaesthesia. It is a more common problem in children than in adults. Premedication with drugs that reduce these oral secretions is occasionally used, especially in preparation for an awake fibreoptic intubation, before certain complex examinations of the upper airway in children, and before the use of ketamine. Muscarinic receptor antagonists (anticholinergic drugs) are used for this purpose.

Glycopyrronium (glycopyrrolate) is most commonly used. It may be given intravenously minutes before the induction of anaesthesia, to reduce secretions immediately.

Hyoscine reduces secretions effectively and has mild sedative and amnesic effects that can sometimes be useful. Unlike atropine, it can cause bradycardia, and postoperative confusion and restlessness may be a problem, particularly in the elderly.

Atropine is now rarely used for premedication, although it was the first of this type of drug to be introduced. Tachycardia and CNS stimulation may be problematic when it is used.

Reducing the Volume and Acidity of Gastric Contents

A reduction in the volume, and a decrease in the acidity, of gastric contents reduces some of the risks of vomiting, regurgitation and of subsequent inhalation of gastric contents during general anaesthesia. In most cases, the most effective way of doing this is to ensure the patient is 'nil by mouth' for 2–3 h before surgery (historically, the fasting time was much longer, and local policies vary). Drugs are commonly used to achieve these effects in surgical emergencies when there is no time for fasting, and during labour when women face the possibility of elective or emergency surgery under general anaesthesia. They may also be used in other patients known to have significant gastro-oesophageal reflux.

Metoclopramide hastens gastric emptying. It is given on the morning of, or a few hours before, delivery in obstetric patients or general anaesthesia. It may be given orally or intravenously. **Sodium citrate** raises the pH of gastric contents by neutralizing acid in the stomach. It is given orally about 30 min before general anaesthesia.

Ranitidine also raises the pH of gastric secretions. It is an H_2-receptor antagonist that reduces gastric acid production and so increases the pH of gastric contents. It is usually given on the night before, and the morning of, delivery in obstetric patients or general anaesthesia. It can be given orally or intravenously.

Intravenous Induction Agents

These drugs are given intravenously to induce unconsciousness. In most cases, anaesthesia is maintained using an inhalational **anaesthetic mixture of oxygen (with or without nitrous oxide)** and a volatile anaesthetic agent. Increasingly, anaesthesia may be maintained using intravenous agents on their own (**total intravenous anaesthesia, TIVA**).

Propofol

Propofol is the most widely used agent in adults and children. It has powerful sedative and amnesic effects. Recovery from its effect is more rapid and complete than from any other intravenous induction agent. Thus the 'hangover effect' of anaesthesia is greatly reduced. It is therefore particularly suited to use in day surgery units and for short procedures. It is very rapidly metabolized (in a few minutes) and can be used as a continuous low-dose intravenous infusion along with remifentanil (see later) to provide prolonged periods of anaesthesia or to sedate patients for hours or days in intensive care units. Injection of propofol is followed by a short period of apnoea and a drop in blood pressure.

CLINICAL NOTE

Pain on injection is the most common side-effect, with one study reporting the side-effect in three out of five patients receiving the drug. Pre-treatment of the vein with lidocaine or using the antecubital vein appears to be the most effective interventions (Jalota et al., 2011).

Etomidate

Etomidate is metabolized rapidly and recovery is fast, with little hangover effect. It has little effect on blood pressure and for this reason, is sometimes chosen for use in patients with cardiac problems. Uncontrolled muscle movements are an unwanted effect that can be minimized by pre-treatment with a benzodiazepine drug.

Thiopental

Thiopental is a barbiturate that was first used in 1934. Its use has declined markedly as safer agents have become available and more affordable. Unconsciousness occurs about 20 seconds after injection and continues for several minutes. The termination of its action occurs as the drug is redistributed away from the brain into other tissues, particularly muscle and fat. It is metabolized very slowly (several hours) and so cannot be used as a continuous intravenous infusion, as it would then accumulate and lead to prolonged sleepiness or unconsciousness when discontinued, unlike propofol. The hangover effect is a problem with its use. Patients often report the subjective sensation of the smell of rotten onions or garlic as thiopental is injected.

Loss of muscle tone and therefore of normal airway control occurs immediately after injection, as does a short period of respiratory depression and sometimes apnoea. Thiopental normally causes a small drop in blood pressure. A marked fall in blood pressure may occur if the injection is given too rapidly, the dose is too large, or if the patient is elderly, has significant cardiac disease or is hypovolaemic. Accidental injection into an artery or outside of the vein is dangerous as ischaemia and tissue damage can follow. Overdose is often fatal, and the drug is much used in veterinary euthanasia.

Ketamine

Ketamine is unique among the induction agents. It is mainly used for paediatric anaesthesia. It is also extensively used in veterinary anaesthesia. Some of its effects are noted here:

- It can be given intramuscularly as well as intravenously.
- It has potent analgesic activity and produces a state known as dissociative analgesia in which the patient looks dreamily awake and may move around but is, in fact, unaware of his or her surroundings and is free of any pain.
- Muscle tone is maintained and therefore the patient retains the ability to maintain his or her own airway despite being unconscious. Respiration is generally not depressed. It is thus of particular value when access to the head and neck is not possible, as occurs in children receiving radiotherapy, some civilian transport disasters and in casualties in the field of battle.
- It may cause a rise in blood pressure.
- During recovery, nightmares and hallucinations are common, except in children. These effects are so unpleasant in adults that the drug is rarely used in them except in the unusual circumstances referred to above. Pre-treatment with benzodiazepines may reduce these problems. Its dissociative and hallucinatory effects have led to it becoming a 'street' drug of abuse.

NURSING NOTE

After ketamine has been used, let the patient wake up peacefully, preferably in a quiet room with subdued lighting, and do not prod or shout at the patient to wake him or her up more quickly. This will reduce the incidence and severity of emergence phenomena – nightmares and unpleasant hallucinations.

MAINTENANCE OF ANAESTHESIA

After induction of anaesthesia, it is maintained using a combination of drugs, whose effects combine to complement each other and to facilitate surgery. These comprise:

- inhalational anaesthetics
- short-acting opioids
- muscle relaxants – and the drugs that reverse their effects.

Inhalational Anaesthetics

Nitrous oxide is sometimes called 'laughing gas', as it causes some patients to laugh during the induction of anaesthesia if it is used on its own. It is a faintly smelling gas that is compressed and stored as a liquid in cylinders (coloured blue in the UK). It is only a weak anaesthetic and it needs to be combined with other inhalational agents or intravenous drugs. It must always be used in combination with oxygen. However, unlike the other inhalational anaesthetics, it has a strong analgesic effect in concentrations less than those required to produce unconsciousness. This analgesic effect is used when nitrous oxide is used as a carrier gas for the volatile anaesthetic agents, as it enables these to be used in lower concentrations than would otherwise be needed to produce anaesthesia. However, the use of nitrous oxide as a carrier gas is falling from favour and it is no longer recommended for most general anaesthetic purposes.

Entonox takes advantage of the analgesic properties of nitrous oxide. It is a 50:50 mixture of nitrous oxide and oxygen, stored as a compressed gas in cylinders (coloured blue and white in the UK). It is used for self-administered pain relief in labour, and by ambulance crews and others who treat pain outside hospital. It is also useful for rapid but potentially painful procedures, such as when very painful dressings are applied. Nitrous oxide should not be used if there is a possibility that the patient has a pneumothorax, as it may worsen this condition.

Volatile Anaesthetic Agents

Sevoflurane, **desflurane** and **isoflurane** are potent halogenated hydrocarbons and have similar structures and effects. They are referred to as volatile anaesthetic agents as they are liquids at room temperature, and it is the vapour from the liquid that is inhaled as the anaesthetic. They require a carrier gas, always containing oxygen and sometimes containing nitrous oxide, to deliver them, and vaporizers capable of delivering accurate concentrations in the range of 0.25%–8.0%. Unlike nitrous oxide, they have no analgesic properties in sub-anaesthetic concentrations. **Sevoflurane** is very rapid acting and recovery is also rapid. It is particularly suitable for inducing anaesthesia in children, as it has a weak and not unpleasant smell and can be used to induce anaesthesia on its own in a few breaths using a mask, without any need for injections. **Desflurane** is even more rapid in action, but it is somewhat irritant and so is not used as an induction agent. A clear role for it has not been established in UK practice. **Isoflurane** use has declined, although it remains a useful and safe drug that is considerably less expensive than the others. Induction takes a little longer than the newer agents, and it may cause a drop in blood pressure and cardiac output in some cases. It is the recommended drug for obstetric anaesthesia in the UK but is only licensed for veterinary anaesthesia in some countries. All the agents in this class may trigger malignant hyperpyrexia (see later).

The first of this class of anaesthetic was **halothane.** It was introduced in 1956 and rapidly replaced the use of ether. It is more extensively metabolized than any of the other drugs in this class, and this may explain its very rare but serious side-effect of liver damage, often fatal. Repeated exposure to halothane increases the risk of this happening. It is no longer used in high and middle-income countries but is still available in some low-income countries. It was replaced by **enflurane,** which is metabolized to a far smaller degree, but this has itself been largely replaced by the agents discussed earlier. It is available in middle and low-income countries and is much preferable to halothane.

Ether is an historically important drug that is no longer used except in a few parts of the world where resources and skills are limited. It is cheap, potent and fairly safe and can be used with simple and portable equipment using room air instead of cylinder oxygen. Induction of, and recovery from, anaesthesia is very slow, and it has a pungent and unpleasant smell. It is inflammable and also explosive, and this represents a major hazard.

CLINICAL NOTE

It is important that any patients receiving a general anaesthetic should have their cardiac status, vital signs and urine output monitored throughout. As mentioned previously, some anaesthetics can cause myocardial depression and can also have a depressant effect on the hypothalamus causing hypo- or hyperthermia.

Future Developments

All of the volatile anaesthetic agents in use are potent greenhouse gases, which may contribute to Global Warming. Increasing awareness of this has led to refinements in anaesthetic practice that have reduced the amounts released into the atmosphere. It has also driven renewed interest in TIVA, which uses no inhalational agents. The noble gas **xenon** is a potent inhalational anaesthetic agent with many advantages, including no greenhouse effect and no risk of malignant hyperpyrexia. Its use remains under investigation. Its greatest disadvantage appears to be its cost, as it has to be extracted from air, where it is present in tiny amounts.

CLINICAL NOTE

Clinicians should make a point of knowing when an inflammable inhalational anaesthetic such as ether is going to be used, as may happen in less-developed countries, and ensure that qualified electricians have checked for properly earthed equipment.

Short-acting Opioid Analgesics

Long-acting opioids such as morphine are described in Chapter 20. In patients whose lungs are ventilated during anaesthesia, potent and short-acting opioids are commonly used and safe. They have three valuable actions that contribute to anaesthesia:

- profound analgesia
- sedation and, in large doses, anaesthesia
- intense respiratory depression (a useful effect).

They have little effect on blood pressure and cardiac output and in large doses, they reduce the need for inhalational anaesthetic agents to a minimum. Where available, **remifentanil** is increasingly used, as unlike any other μ-opioid agonist, it is rapidly metabolized by non-specific tissue and plasma esterases and thus its elimination is unaffected by renal or hepatic function. The action of remifentanil is so short that it can only be administered as a continuous infusion. Once an infusion is discontinued, the effects of remifentanil are gone within 3–6 min. If postoperative analgesia is required it should be given as, or before, the infusion is stopped, using other longer-acting opioids such as morphine. Because of its potency, short action and lack of cardiovascular side-effects, it is useful in cardiac surgery, and is much used in TIVA. It does not have a place in the management of postoperative pain. A curious unwanted effect is increased postoperative sensitivity to painful stimuli (hyperalgesia).

Fentanyl is still widely used. Others in this class include **alfentanil**. The main differences between all of them are their doses and duration of action (Table 19.1).

As with the longer-acting opioids, their action may be reversed at the end of anaesthesia using **naloxone** (see Chapter 20). This may be necessary to correct any respiratory depression but will also reverse any analgesia and may leave the patient in pain.

TABLE 19.1
Short-acting Opioids

Opioid	Approximate duration
Alfentanil	10 min
Fentanyl	30 min
Remifentanil	A few minutes

CLINICAL NOTE

Patients respiratory rates should be monitored to detect adverse events such as respiratory depression. A systematic review of 12 papers noted that there was increased risk of respiratory depression in people with pre-existing cardiac or respiratory disease or people with obstructive sleep apnoea (Gupta et al., 2018).

Muscle Relaxants

The introduction of muscle relaxants into anaesthetic practice in the 1940s has been claimed as the greatest single advance in anaesthesia made in the 20th century.

Curare was the first such drug to be used and is an alkaloid extracted from the bark, leaves and vines of the tropical plant *Chondrodendron tomentosum*, found around the upper reaches of the Amazon River. Crude preparations of this plant have long been used by South American Indians to poison the tips of their arrows and blow darts. Since the 1940s many new relaxants have been produced, and those in current use, and some of the differences between them, are listed in Table 19.2.

TABLE 19.2
Muscle Relaxants

Drug	Type of Blocker	Duration of Action (min)	Reversal of Action	Other Points
Vecuronium	Competitive	20–30	Sugammadex or Neostigmine (with atropine or glycopyrronium)	Very commonly used, has a specific reversing agent
Rocuronium	Competitive	20–30	Sugammadex or Neostigmine (with atropine or glycopyrronium)	Fastest onset of action of all competitive blockers, has a specific reversing agent
Atracurium	Competitive	20–30	Neostigmine (with atropine or glycopyrronium)	Remains widely in use around the world
Cisatracurium	Competitive	20–30	Neostigmine (with atropine or glycopyrronium)	Causes less histamine release than atracurium
Mivacurium	Competitive	10–15	Neostigmine (with atropine or glycopyrronium)	Often causes marked histamine release, leading to cutaneous flushing and tachycardia
Gallamine, Pancuronium	Competitive	45–60	Neostigmine (with atropine or glycopyrronium)	Older, rarely used drugs. Should not be used in renal failure as renal secretion is significant
Suxamethonium	Depolarizing	2–5	Cannot be reversed with drugs	Causes postoperative muscle pain and tenderness. Prolonged action in 1 in 2800 patients

Most anaesthetics involve the use of muscle relaxants. There are three main indications for their use:

- To facilitate intubation of the trachea with an endotracheal tube at the beginning of anaesthesia.
- To relax muscles sufficiently to make surgery possible. This applies particularly to abdominal surgery, for which relaxed muscles are necessary for easy access to, and closure of, the abdomen.
- To permit artificial ventilation. There are many situations in anaesthesia in which it is better to ventilate lungs mechanically rather than let patients breath spontaneously, and these include chest surgery, anaesthesia in patients with severe cardiorespiratory disease and lengthy surgery of any kind.

THE NEUROMUSCULAR JUNCTION

Muscle relaxants act at the neuromuscular junction (or motor endplate) by blocking the transmission of nerve impulses from the nerve to skeletal muscle (Fig. 19.1). When a nerve supplying a voluntary muscle is stimulated, acetylcholine is liberated from vesicles in the nerve ending and acts on special receptor sites on the muscle to produce changes that are known as depolarization. This is followed by contraction of the muscle fibre. The acetylcholine is then rapidly broken down by the enzyme cholinesterase and repolarization of the muscle occurs. The muscle is now ready to be stimulated again. Should depolarization persist (see depolarizing muscle relaxants, later), then the muscle remains unresponsive to further stimulation.

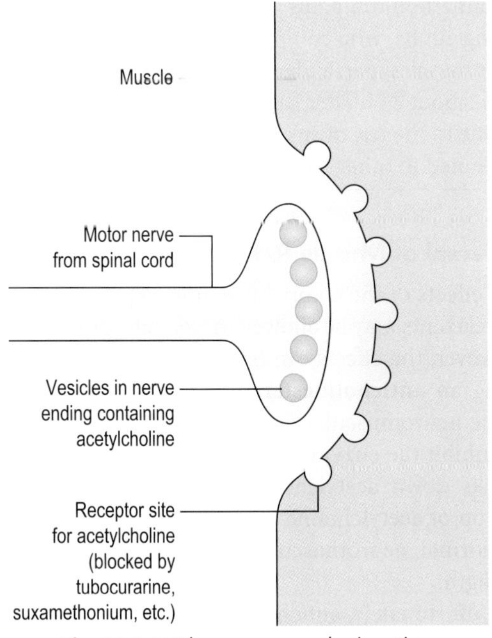

Fig. 19.1 ■ The neuromuscular junction.

Competitive Muscle Relaxants

Two types of blockade of the neuromuscular junction are produced by muscle relaxants. Most muscle relaxants are competitive or non-depolarizing blockers. These drugs occupy the receptor site for acetylcholine and so render ineffective the acetylcholine released following nerve stimulation. There are two groups of competitive muscle relaxants: the 'aminosteroid group', which includes rocuronium, vecuronium and pancuronium; and the 'benzylisoquinolinium group', which includes atracurium, cisatracurium, gallamine and mivacurium.

Of all of these drugs, rocuronium and vecuronium are probably the most important in current anaesthetic practice.

Rocuronium has the fastest onset of action of all non-depolarizing relaxants, particularly if given in a high dose, and is increasingly used as an alternative to suxamethonium when rapid intubation of the trachea is indicated at induction of anaesthesia. It is excreted unchanged in the urine and is therefore not suitable for use in patients with poor or no renal function. In an emergency, its action (and that of vecuronium) can be reversed by the use of sugammadex.

Vecuronium also has a medium duration of action of 30–60 min. It is not associated with histamine release and has no effect on cardiac function or blood pressure. A small amount is excreted renally but, nevertheless, it can safely be used in patients with renal failure. It is still commonly used and has the advantage of being simply reversible with the use of sugammadex.

Atracurium, is still fairly commonly used. Atracurium has a medium duration of action of 30–60 min. It is associated with some histamine release, which can cause skin flushing and a slight tachycardia, and a drop in blood pressure. It breaks down under the influence of body temperature and pH, and thus its elimination is independent of renal or hepatic function.

Cisatracurium is a single isomer of atracurium and causes less histamine release than atracurium (atracurium is a mixture of 10 isomers), but it is otherwise very similar to atracurium.

Mivacurium has a short duration of action of 15–30 min. It causes considerable histamine release, with consequent marked skin flushing, tachycardia and hypotension.

Gallamine and **Pancuronium** are older drugs with a longer duration of action of 60–90 min. They are excreted predominantly by the kidney and should therefore not be used in patients with renal failure. Pancuronium is sometimes used for long procedures and in the management of patients on ventilators in the intensive care unit. Gallamine has a vagolytic effect that leads to a significant tachycardia.

CLINICAL NOTE

Muscle relaxants have no analgesic or amnesic properties and, when given for a prolonged period of time, e.g. in critical care, a benzodiazepine and, where indicated, an analgesic should be given.

Depolarizing Muscle Relaxants

Suxamethonium is the only representative of this group in current use. It is useful because of its rapid onset of action, but in UK practice, is gradually being superseded by the use of rocuronium. It occupies the nicotinic receptor sites for acetylcholine on skeletal muscle and initially stimulates the muscle into contracting, visible as the 'twitching' or fasciculation that occurs almost immediately after it is injected. It then produces a state of persistent depolarization of the muscle cell membrane, during which no further stimulation of the muscle fibre is possible. There are several special points to note about suxamethonium:

- It has a quick onset of action of about 60 seconds; therefore, it is used in patients who may have full stomachs in whom rapid tracheal intubation is indicated.
- It has a short duration of action of 5–10 min.
- It is normally rapidly broken down by the enzyme plasma cholinesterase. About 1 in 3000 of the population have a familial and genetically determined variant of this enzyme, which breaks down suxamethonium more slowly and leads to a prolonged period of paralysis of up to 2–3 h. This is referred to as 'suxamethonium apnoea'.
- A common side-effect of the drug is muscle pain and tenderness, particularly in the chest and abdomen. It can be severe and occurs about 24 h after the medicine has been given. It is likened to the pain and tenderness experienced after severe, unaccustomed exercise and is usually seen in young fit adults. It is rare in children.
- A marked bradycardia is sometimes seen following a second injection of suxamethonium in adults and following the first injection in children. It is easily treated with atropine or glycopyrronium.
- In certain situations, such as following major burns or trauma or in acute peripheral neuropathies, it can cause a dangerous rise in serum potassium with consequent life-threatening cardiac arrhythmias.
- There are no drugs that can be used to reverse its actions.

CLINICAL NOTE

'Suxamethonium pains': look out for patients, usually young adults, who complain of pain and tenderness in their muscles, particularly of their chest and abdomen, about 24 h after surgery. These symptoms may be due to the use of suxamethonium but are often attributed to other factors. They can be very severe.

Reversal of Muscle Relaxants

The effects of the competitive, non-depolarizing muscle relaxants may be allowed to wear off spontaneously. However, the effects can be reversed more quickly by using an **anticholinesterase**. Anticholinesterases act at the neuromuscular junction, where they temporarily inhibit the enzyme cholinesterase, which normally breaks down acetylcholine, and allows the concentration of acetylcholine to rise and so help the return of normal neuromuscular transmission and muscle strength.

Unfortunately, anticholinesterases also have effects at sites other than the neuromuscular junction, where acetylcholine also acts as a neurotransmitter, namely at peripheral parasympathetic nerve endings. The most important side-effects of these drugs are:

- a bradycardia, which can be severe and therefore dangerous
- an increase in salivation and in tracheobronchial secretions
- an increase in peristaltic activity in the gut that causes colic and diarrhoea and can disrupt bowel anastomoses following surgery.

Of interest, these symptoms are also the symptoms of poisoning with nerve weapons, including Sarin and VX, which are themselves highly potent anticholinesterases.

Fortunately, these unwanted effects of anticholinesterases can be prevented by the administration of one of the muscarinic receptor antagonist group of drugs (see later), which must be given at the same time as, or before, the anticholinesterase. Thus, a common mixture used to reverse the effects of competitive muscle relaxants at the end of anaesthesia is that of the anticholinesterase drug, neostigmine, and the muscarinic receptor antagonist, **glycopyrronium** (see later).

Neostigmine has a maximal effect after 5–7 min, although an initial effect may be seen after 2 min. Its action lasts about 30 min. As noted earlier, it must be preceded by, or given at the same time as, a muscarinic receptor antagonist, usually glycopyrronium.

Edrophonium is another anticholinesterase drug that is also effective in reversing the effects of muscle relaxants, although it is not commonly used for this purpose. It possibly has a quicker onset of action and a slightly shorter duration of action than neostigmine. It may also be used in the assessment and management of patients with myasthenia gravis.

Sugammadex is not an anticholinesterase, but is the first specific antidote to the skeletal muscle relaxants rocuronium and vecuronium. It strongly binds to these drugs and has none of the unwanted effects of the anticholinesterases. This easy and side-effect-free reversal of muscle relaxation has contributed to the increased use of rocuronium and vecuronium.

Anticholinergic Drugs (Muscarinic Receptor Antagonists)

Not to be confused with anticholinesterases (see earlier), these drugs temporarily block the effects of acetylcholine, particularly at postganglionic parasympathetic nerve endings, and have three uses during anaesthesia:

- to increase the pulse rate
- to reduce tracheobronchial and salivary secretions
- to prevent the increase in peristaltic activity that occurs after the administration of neostigmine or edrophonium.

Atropine was the earliest of these drugs, although it is not so widely used as glycopyrronium during anaesthesia. It can be given orally as part of premedication. It has a slight central stimulant effect.

Glycopyrronium (glycopyrrolate) is widely used during general anaesthesia. Its onset of action is slower, and its duration of action is longer, than atropine. Its effect on reducing secretions is more potent than that of atropine. In the doses generally used, it causes less tachycardia than atropine. It is not used for premedication before anaesthesia, as it is not absorbed from the gastrointestinal tract. It does not cross the blood–brain barrier and so does not cause any CNS stimulation.

MALIGNANT HYPERPYREXIA

Susceptibility to this extremely rare disorder is familial and genetically determined. Malignant hyperpyrexia may be triggered by exposure to suxamethonium (but not to any of the non-depolarizing muscle relaxants) and to any of the halogenated hydrocarbon inhalational anaesthetics – halothane, enflurane, isoflurane, sevoflurane or desflurane – but not to nitrous oxide or, curiously, almost any other drug.

Malignant hyperpyrexia starts with excessive metabolic activity in muscle cells, which leads to muscle rigidity, a high temperature and widespread severe metabolic disturbances. It used to have a high mortality. It is important to be aware of the possibility of this condition in postoperative patients.

Dantrolene, if given promptly and combined with aggressive treatment of the metabolic problems, markedly reduces mortality from this disorder. It is a skeletal muscle relaxant that acts at an intracellular level (but not by blocking the neuromuscular junction) and reduces the excessive metabolic activity seen in muscle cells during malignant hyperpyrexia. Every operating department should stock sufficient amounts of the drug to treat at least one patient. It may take 20 min to prepare for use and is expensive.

LOCAL ANAESTHETICS

Local anaesthesia for surgery was first used in 1884 when Carl Koller, in Vienna, used cocaine for ophthalmic surgery. The use of cocaine for nerve blocks was first described by William S. Halstead in 1885; unfortunately, Halstead later became addicted to cocaine after he had experimented on himself with too many nerve blocks.

Local anaesthetics produce a reversible inhibition of conduction along nerves and, in sufficient concentration, produce a complete sensory and motor blockade. However, the fine, unmyelinated, nerve fibres that conduct pain sensation are more easily blocked by local anaesthetics than the thicker, heavily myelinated, motor fibres that supply muscle, and so it is possible to provide good analgesia without loss of too much motor function. This is best illustrated by observing the effects of an epidural during labour, in which there is good pain relief and yet the patient is still able to move their legs.

There are several routes by which local anaesthetics can be given:

- Direct application to mucous membranes
- Direct application to the skin
- Intradermal injection
- Local infiltration of subcutaneous tissues, muscles, other soft tissues or periosteum
- Infiltration around local nerves
- Extradural injection (an 'extradural', 'epidural' or 'caudal')
- Subarachnoid injection (a 'spinal')
- Intravenous injection – intravenous regional anaesthesia (Bier's block).

Intravenous regional analgesia, otherwise known as a Bier's block, in an arm is established as follows. The arm is elevated for a few minutes to encourage the drainage of as much blood as possible. Further exsanguination may be achieved by applying an Esmarch bandage around the arm. A previously applied padded double cuff orthopaedic tourniquet is inflated to well above arterial blood pressure and maintained at that pressure for the duration of the block. Then, 40 mL of 0.5% prilocaine is injected into a previously inserted cannula in a vein in the dorsum of the hand. The prilocaine now spreads throughout all the vessels in the arm below the tourniquet and after a few minutes, this will produce complete analgesia of the arm below the cuff. The tourniquet is not released for at least 20 min to prevent toxic doses of prilocaine reaching the heart or brain. Bier's block remains useful, but complications due to cuff deflation and subsequent prilocaine cardiotoxicity have reduced its popularity. Careful attention to, and maintenance of, the equipment used with properly trained personnel following clear local guidelines are key to its safe use. Lipid emulsion (***Intralipid***) should always be available in case of accidental prilocaine toxicity.

Lidocaine is the most commonly used local anaesthetic. It has a rapid onset of action and a duration of action of 1–2 h. By mixing it with adrenaline (epinephrine), its duration of action can be usefully prolonged. It is available in various concentrations and preparations, including an aerosol spray for use on mucous membranes such as in the mouth, pharynx or trachea.

Lidocaine also depresses myocardial excitability and is sometimes used to suppress ventricular arrhythmias such as may follow myocardial infarction or cardiac arrest. For this purpose, it is given as a bolus intravenous injection or as a continuous, low-dose infusion. It will, however, as with all local anaesthetics, cause myocardial depression in overdose.

Prilocaine is similar to lidocaine, but has a slightly longer action than lidocaine. It is less toxic than lidocaine and is therefore the preferred drug for intravenous regional anaesthesia. It is commonly used, mixed with felypressin, for dental blocks. In doses twice the recommended maximum, it causes cyanosis due to the formation of methaemoglobin.

***EMLA* cream (eutectic mixture of local anaesthetics)** is a unique preparation. If powders of lidocaine and prilocaine are mixed together, then a *eutectic* mixture is created – that is, the mixture changes consistency from a powder to a paste. Substances are then added to this paste to make a cream containing 2.5% lidocaine and 2.5% prilocaine suitable for application to the skin. Absorption through the skin is slow, but application for at least 45 min produces adequate analgesia, and *EMLA* cream is now used extensively to allow pain-free venepuncture, particularly in children, and for other minor procedures.

Bupivacaine has a slow onset of action, sometimes taking up to 30 min for its maximum effect. It has about twice the duration of action of lidocaine and its effects may last 2–4 h. It is particularly popular and suitable for continuous epidural analgesia in labour and for postoperative pain relief. It is more toxic on the heart than other local anaesthetics and must therefore never be used for intravenous regional anaesthesia.

Levobupivacaine is a more recent drug. It is an isomer of bupivacaine that is probably less cardiotoxic.

Ropivacaine is similar to bupivacaine in structure and effect. It has a marginally shorter duration of action, and is less cardiotoxic than bupivacaine. More interestingly, it is associated with less motor blockade for the same degree of sensory blockade. Thus, an epidural or spinal anaesthesia produced using ropivacaine leaves the patients with greater power in – and more use of – their legs than they would have had if bupivacaine had been used to provide the analgesia.

Tetracaine has a slow onset and long duration of action. It is too toxic to be used by injection or to be used on highly vascular mucous membranes, where its rapid absorption may quickly lead to toxic effects. It is mostly used for conjunctival anaesthesia in the eye. It may also be used to provide skin anaesthesia for venepuncture (see later). It is a good vasodilator.

Tetracaine gel (*Ametop*) is a preparation, like *EMLA* cream, that is designed to enable pain-free venepuncture. It contains tetracaine only. It may have a quicker onset of action than *EMLA* cream and it may cause more vasodilatation and so make venepuncture easier. It should be removed after 60 min as it can cause marked skin irritation if left on too long.

Oxybuprocaine is only used as a local anaesthetic in the eye. It causes less initial stinging sensation, and has a shorter duration of action than amethocaine.

Cocaine, the first of the local anaesthetics, is a very different drug from all other local anaesthetics. It is an alkaloid obtained from the leaves of a tree, *Erythroxylon coca*, found in Bolivia, Brazil, Peru and other South American countries. For centuries it has been chewed by the peoples of these countries to produce euphoria and to increase their capacity for physical work.

Cocaine is absorbed well by mucous membranes and is used to provide surface analgesia for eye surgery and throat and nose surgery, where its intense vasoconstrictor effect is also a useful feature. It is available as a paste, and as a solution of various concentrations, for these purposes. It is too toxic to be used by injection.

Cocaine has widespread sympathomimetic actions, causing mydriasis (dilatation of the pupil), marked vasoconstriction, hypertension, tachycardia and ventricular arrhythmias. In overdose, sudden death due to ventricular fibrillation occurs. Headache, nausea, vomiting and abdominal pain are common. It causes excitement, restlessness, euphoria and confusion and, with increasing dosage, CNS depression, coma and convulsions. It is a drug of addiction and a controlled drug. In most countries it has fallen out of use because of the abuse problems. However, no single drug combines its useful features for ENT and eye surgery.

There are many other local anaesthetics, both old and new. **Procaine** is an old drug that is now rarely used. **Mepivacaine** and **articaine** are used in dentistry. **Benzocaine** is used as a constituent of proprietary drug mixtures, particularly those used for sore throats, mouth ulcers and musculoskeletal conditions.

CLINICAL NOTE

When using local anaesthetic, assessment of vital signs and movement and sensation of affected limbs. Epidural anaesthesia in particular can cause hypotension and to avoid this, patients should be well hydrated prior to local anaesthetic induction. Some patients may report itching and this may be a sign that the patient is allergic to the analgesic agent. In such cases, the infusion should be stopped, patient monitored and alternative local anaesthetic or analgesia sought.

Vasoconstrictors and Local Anaesthetics

Most local anaesthetics are also vasodilators, which, by increasing local blood flow, hasten the removal of the drug from the site of action. If adrenaline (epinephrine) is mixed with the drug, then the vasoconstriction it produces will delay the removal of the drug and so prolong its duration of action.

Adrenaline (epinephrine) must never be used with prilocaine when used for intravenous regional anaesthesia, because of the obvious danger that, if the cuff were to deflate unexpectedly, then large doses of adrenaline (epinephrine) could reach the heart. Neither should vasoconstrictors be used with local anaesthetics for blocks around the base of the penis or for 'ring' blocks of the fingers or toes; they may severely interrupt the blood supply and cause permanent ischaemic damage to the penis or digit. They should be used with great caution on the ear and nose, for similar reasons. And particular care should always be taken when injecting local anaesthetics mixed with adrenaline (epinephrine) not to inject the drug intravenously by accident.

Felypressin (**Octapressin**) is a safer alternative to adrenaline (epinephrine). It is an analogue of vasopressin and is a powerful vasoconstrictor but has none of the potentially serious effects that adrenaline (epinephrine) has on the heart. It is generally only used, mixed with local anaesthetics, for dental blocks.

CLINICAL NOTE

Do not forget that the patient will be conscious during procedures carried out under local anaesthesia. Conversation between staff should be at a minimum, but the patient should be reassured throughout. A second nurse or assistant should be in attendance to not only reassure the patient but observe the patient for any side-effects to pain, medication or other needs.

Toxicity of Local Anaesthetics

All local anaesthetics have dangerous side-effects at doses only a little above those that may be used for some of the more extensive regional blocks. Care must therefore be taken in calculating the total dose used when establishing any block. The development of toxicity is dependent not only on the total dose of local anaesthetic given, but also on such factors as:

- the concentration used
- the route by which the drug is given
- the vascularity of the tissues being injected
- the age and weight of the patient
- the time period over which the local anaesthetic is administered.

The most common cause of life-threatening systemic toxicity is the accidental injection of a local anaesthetic into a vein.

CLINICAL NOTE

- A 1% solution equals 1 g in 100 mL or 10 mg in 1 mL.
- Only by knowing this can the amount of drug given be calculated.

Signs of Toxicity

Early signs of toxicity are tingling of the tongue and lips, tinnitus, tremor, light-headedness and drowsiness; they progress to unconsciousness and convulsions, and then cardiac and respiratory depression. Convulsions may also be the presenting feature of toxicity, and cardiac arrest may be the first sign of toxicity due to bupivacaine.

Treatment of Toxicity

As well as cardiac monitoring and supportive treatment, infusion of a lipid emulsion (***Intralipid***), more commonly used for Total Parenteral Nutrition, has been shown to reduce cardiac toxicity in accidental local anaesthetic overdose, presumably because the lipid soluble drugs dissolve into the lipid droplets.

SUMMARY

- Patients should be given a thorough examination, including review of medical history and pre-existing medication, some days before general anaesthesia and surgery.
- Premedication is not as much used as before, but certain drugs such as steroids and antibiotics may still be required.
- Patients may have many diverse fears before surgery and should be listened to carefully and be reassured.
- Opioids should only be used as premedication before surgery for patients who are in pain and not as anxiolytics.
- Children who have had ketamine should be allowed to wake up peacefully in a quiet, darkened room, as this will reduce the possibility of nightmares.
- In children, oral administration is the preferred route.
- Reducing the acidity of gastric contents with an H_2 antagonist before surgery will reduce the

chances of regurgitation and subsequent inhalation of vomit, e.g. during labour under general anaesthesia.

- Propofol is useful for induction of anaesthesia and for TIVA.
- Entonox is useful in labour as an analgesic.
- Nurses who work under more primitive conditions should be aware of the dangers associated with the use of inflammable general anaesthetic gases.
- Short-acting opioid anaesthetics are useful in anaesthesia of ventilated patients.
- Muscle relaxants are a very important part of general anaesthesia.
- Some muscle relaxants such as mivacurium will cause histamine release.
- Sugammadex will reverse the effects of rocuronium and vecuronium.
- No drugs will reverse the actions of suxamethonium.
- Anticholinesterases have very many effects, since they act at every site where acetylcholine is released as a neurotransmitter.
- Atropine is a long-acting drug and may not be suitable for short procedures.
- The volatile anaesthetic agents and suxamethonium may trigger malignant hyperpyrexia in some patients.
- Bupivacaine should never be used for intravenous regional anaesthesia.
- Tetracaine is too toxic to be used by injection or on highly vascular mucous membranes.
- Adrenaline (epinephrine), if injected with a local anaesthetic, will cause local vasoconstriction; this will delay removal of the drug from its site of action and thus prolong its duration of action.
- Local anaesthetics combined with adrenaline (epinephrine) should not be injected into peripheries such as digits, ear lobes, the tip of the nose or the penis.
- Felypressin is a safer alternative to adrenaline (epinephrine).
- It is very dangerous to inject a local anaesthetic accidentally into a vein, and care should be taken to check that the needle is not in a vein by withdrawing the plunger briefly before injecting; if blood is drawn up into the syringe, remove the needle immediately.
- Epinephrine should not be confused with ephedrine; the two names are very similar.

REFERENCES AND FURTHER READING

Caplin, M., 2015. Utilizing teach-back to reinforce patient education. Orthop. Nurs. 34 (6), 365–368.

Gupta, K., Nagappa, M., Prasad, A., et al., 2018. Risk factors for opioid-induced respiratory depression in surgical patients: a systematic review and meta-analyses. BMJ Open 8 (12), E024086.

Hounsome, J., 2017. A systematic review of information format and timing before scheduled adult surgery for peri-operative anxiety. Anaesthesia 72 (10), 1265–1272.

Jalota, L., Kalira, V., George, E., et al., 2011. Prevention of pain on injection of propofol: systematic review and meta-analysis. BMJ 342, d1110.

Sheenm, M.J., Fang, L., Shung, T., 2014. Anesthetic premedication: new horizons of an old practice. Acta. Anaesthesiol. Taiwan 52 (3), 134–142.

Zhang, Y., Yang, Y., Lau, W.Y., et al., 2017. Effectiveness of pre-operative clown intervention on psychological distress: a systematic review and meta-analysis. J. Paediatr. Child Health 53 (3), 237–245.

USEFUL WEBSITES

Association for Perioperative Practice. https://www.afpp.org.uk/home.

Anaesthetic and Recovery Nurses Association. https://www.barna.co.uk.

Patient. General Anaesthesia. http://www.patient.co.uk/showdoc/40024458.

Resuscitation Council (UK). https://www.resus.org.uk/library/2015-resuscitation-guidelines/hospital-resuscitation.

20 NERVOUS SYSTEM 2
Opioid Analgesics

CHAPTER OUTLINE

LEARNING OBJECTIVES

At the end of this chapter, the reader should be able to:

- outline the gating theory of pain
- describe what opium is, the important opioid drugs, their therapeutic uses and adverse effects
- describe the symptoms of morphine and heroin overdosage and emergency treatment
- describe what is meant by an opioid agonist, partial agonist and antagonist, and give examples of each
- discuss the concept of 'total pain'
- discuss the need for individualized pain control programmes
- explain the need to determine the cause of pain in patients with terminal disease
- describe the treatments for opioid non-responsive pain

Analgesics are drugs that relieve pain. They are of great importance in patient care, as pain is a common and distressing feature of many conditions. It must be remembered, however, that pain has its uses, both as a warning of the presence of disease and also, by its nature, it may help in localization and diagnosis of the underlying cause. It is debatable whether chronic pain has any physiological role, except as an unwelcome and constant reminder of ongoing tissue damage.

THE PERCEPTION OF PAIN

The most important principle underlying pain perception is that the brain perceives pain. No matter how bad the damage to the body is, if nerve connections carrying pain signals to the brain are interrupted, e.g. through damage to the spinal cord, the patient will feel no pain.

Mechanism of Pain Perception

The Gating Theory of Pain

The mechanism of pain perception is summarized in Fig. 20.1. The central nervous system (CNS) is constantly receiving nerve impulses arising in the body from the skin and internal organs. Under certain circumstances the brain interprets these as pain. There are a number of theories to explain how this occurs and the most popular today is the 'gate' (input control) theory. This states that high-intensity stimulation activates a network of fine nerves at the periphery that terminate centrally in the posterior horn of the spinal cord. From here, nerve impulses are relayed via the spinothalamic tract to the thalamus in the brain, where they are felt as pain. There is then a further relay system to the cerebral cortex, where discrimination and interpretation occur.

The passage of nerve impulses through the relay 'gate' in the posterior horn is modified by:

- Ascending impulses from the periphery to the brain
- Descending impulses from the brain to the periphery.

Ascending Impulses from the Periphery to the Brain

Low-intensity ascending nerve impulses unrelated to pain dampen the transmission of pain impulses. This explains why methods such as transcutaneous stimulation or counter-irritation applied to a painful area can relieve pain by 'closing the gate'. An example is the application of creams containing skin irritants to painful joints or muscles (e.g. *Deep Heat* cream, which contains capsicum extracted from hot chillies). Heat therapy, e.g. through the use of lamps and heated pads, is also used to treat pain.

High-intensity impulses from an area of tissue damage (as may occur after surgery) overcome the low-intensity ascending nerve impulses and facilitate transmission through the 'gate' and thus increase painful sensations. This may be reduced by blocking impulses from the area of damage by **local anaesthesia** or by giving an **analgesic** just before an operation (as discussed in Chapter 19).

Descending Impulses from the Brain to the Periphery

Nerve fibres arising in the brain and descending in the spinal cord terminate in the posterior horn and damp down transmission through the gate, and thus decrease the sensation of pain.

DRUGS THAT RELIEVE PAIN

Sites of Action

Drugs that relieve pain may act at various sites along the pain pathways:

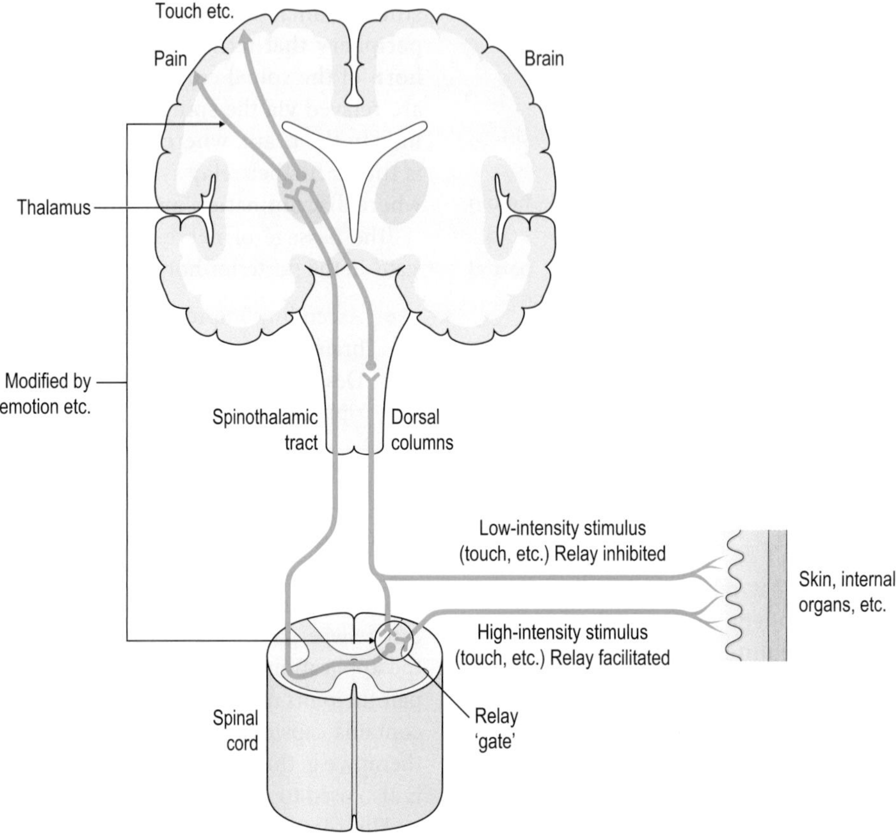

Fig. 20.1 ■ Pathways involved in perception of pain.

TABLE 20.1
Opioid Analgesics

Type	Name
Natural	Morphine; codeine
Synthetic	Diamorphine; methadone; pethidine; dihydrocodeine; fentanyl

- They may act on the brain and spinal cord and reduce the appreciation of pain. This is the major site of action of opioid analgesics.
- They may suppress conduction in nerves carrying impulses from the painful area. This is where local anaesthetics act.
- They may reduce inflammation and other causes of pain in the painful area. This is the site of action, e.g. of the non-steroidal antiinflammatory drugs (NSAIDs; see Chapter 13).

Analgesics can be broadly classified for practical purposes as:

- Opioid analgesics (Table 20.1)
- Non-opioid analgesics.

Non-opioid analgesics and local anaesthetics are dealt with in Chapter 19.

ANALGESICS FOR THE TREATMENT OF ACUTE PAIN

Acute pain is frequently generated by surgery, but may occur as a result of trauma, or as part of a medical illness such as myocardial infarction or some form of colic.

Attitudes to Acute Pain Relief

Patients needing opioids for the treatment of acute pain were too easily labelled as addicts and yet dependence and respiratory depression are rarely associated with the treatment of acute pain with opioids. The unimaginative approach of the 'give as necessary' 4-hourly prescription, which is not regularly given, and which does not allow for the opportunity to titrate the dose and frequency against the needs of the patient, can lead to the emergence of extreme pain. The patient then becomes tense, sweaty and exhausted, and needs a large dose of opioid for adequate relief of pain.

The Pain Relief Programme

A programme for pain relief needs to take some important factors into account:

- Patients vary considerably in their sensitivity to pain and response to analgesics, so the programme should be individualized.
- The pain relief programme for an individual patient will depend on the severity, nature and cause of the pain. It may include a wide range of analgesics and, in addition, local anaesthetics and drugs that are specific for certain types of pain (e.g. colchicine for treating patients with gout; see Chapter 13).

The World Health Organization (WHO) analgesic ladder is commonly used to help in the management of acute and chronic pain. It is impossible to specify regimens for all types of pain, but certain general rules should be followed:

- The programmes must be flexible and aim to keep the patient free of pain.
- Many programmes have a continuous background of analgesia with facilities for a top-up (perhaps with a more powerful analgesic) if the pain breaks through.
- A combination of drugs and treatments should always be considered. This can be very successful. Thus, paracetamol may be combined with an NSAID (see Chapter 13) and an opioid – and a local anaesthetic technique may be used as well.
- Anxiety markedly exacerbates the perception of pain. Explanation and reassurance are powerful tools with which to reduce anxiety and therefore the perception and distress of pain. Patients undergoing surgery must be given a full description of postoperative pain problems and the steps that will be taken for their relief. Consideration needs to be given to treatment of anxiety and depression, which can be present in many chronic conditions and can result in increased perception of pain.

Combination of pharmacological and non-pharmacological therapies may need to be implemented in successful management of chronic pain. Non-pharmacological management can include exercise (e.g. through physiotherapy), TENS (transcutaneous electrical nerve stimulation), acupuncture and psychological interventions (e.g. cognitive behavioral therapy). It is recommended that in hospitals there should be specialized teams of doctors and nurses dedicated to help in management of complex chronic pain issues.

Patient-controlled Analgesia

Pain in postoperative and some terminally ill patients can be effectively controlled by the self-administration of analgesia via a syringe pump set up to deliver a preset dose of the drug when a delivery button is pressed by the patient (Fig. 20.2). A number of patient-controlled analgesia (PCA) devices are commercially available, all designed so that dose, rate and frequency of administration can be controlled and pre-set. A number of drugs have been used successfully in this way, including morphine and pethidine.

Trials have demonstrated high levels of acceptance of PCA among patients in hospital and the community, where small, portable PCA machines have been

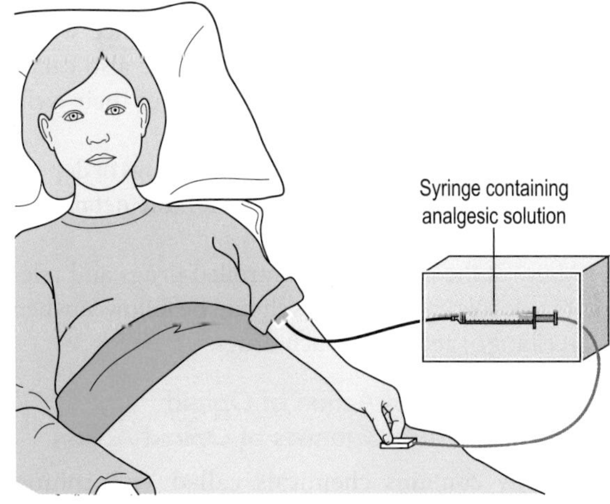

Fig. 20.2 ■ Principles of patient-controlled analgesia (PCA).

used. Part of the success of PCA is related to the feeling of control it gives patients and the confidence that they will not have to wait for the nurse to give an injection to relieve pain. Nursing time is saved as, once the device is set up, it obviates the need to prepare and administer routine injections. However, nurses still have a responsibility for monitoring the adequacy of analgesia and the appearance of side-effects such as nausea or respiratory depression. This is best done by using written protocols that should define the monitoring and actions necessary to maintain adequate analgesia, and to manage properly the side-effects of the drugs.

Patients must be taught how to use the device before they need it. For surgical patients this should be before their operation, as a heavily sedated postoperative patient will not be receptive to lengthy explanations. Patients going home with PCA machines should have the opportunity to become familiar with their use before they are discharged.

Principles of PCA (see Fig. 20.2).

- A patient can self-administer a bolus of analgesic on demand
- The machine is programmed to allow self-dosage only at pre-set intervals between 'lock-out' times
- Continuous low-level dosage can be programmed
- The syringe is securely locked into a case
- The programming panel is securely locked and the key kept secure.

OPIOID ANALGESICS

The term 'opioid' is applied to any substance which has an opium-like action. The opioids are also called *narcotics* or *narcotic analgesics*, because of their well-known drowsiness effects.

Nearly all the opioids are potentially drugs of dependence and this subject is discussed in more detail later in this chapter (see Chapter 23).

Many of the opioids are controlled drugs and relevant protocols and guidelines should be followed when prescribing or managing such drugs.

The Mechanism of Action of Opioid Analgesics and Antagonists of Opioid Action

The body contains chemicals called 'endorphins' and 'enkephalins'. These are the body's own type of opioid. Two of these, β **endorphin** and **metenkephalin**, act on special opioid receptors in the nervous system, particularly in the midbrain and posterior horn of the spinal cord. When these receptors are stimulated, transmission of nerve impulses related to pain are inhibited and the appreciation of pain is suppressed. It seems likely that β endorphin and metenkephalin are part of a system in the brain that controls pain appreciation and may be involved in such phenomena as acupuncture. Opioid drugs also react with these receptors and thus relieve pain. There are several types of opioid receptor in the nervous system, but the most important for pain control by opioids are called **mu (μ) receptors** and are responsible for the analgesia, euphoria and respiratory depression seen with most opioid analgesics. Although the most important actions of the opioids occur in the CNS, there is now some evidence that they may also react with receptors on the peripheral nerves, which augments their analgesic action. Endorphins, incidentally, are released during physical exercise and may be responsible for the feeling of well-being that participation in sports so often engenders.

Opioids and Related Drugs

Some opioids, e.g. **morphine** and **diamorphine** (heroin), are full agonists. Some, such as buprenorphine, are partial agonists. **Naloxone** is a drug that is a pure competitive antagonist at opioid receptors (Fig. 20.3).

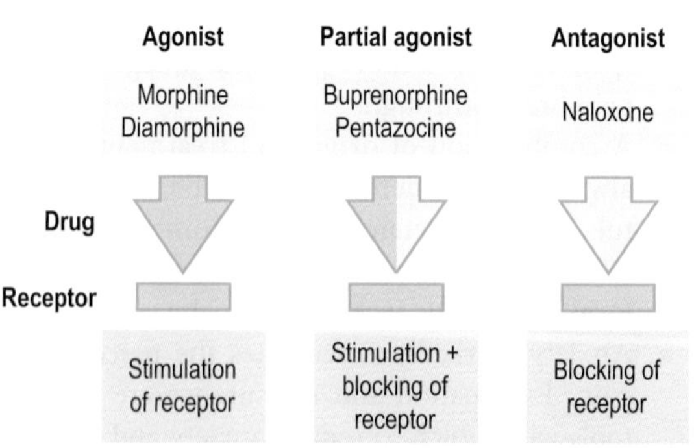

Fig. 20.3 Mode of action of opioid agonists, antagonists and partial agonists.

Agonists. Examples are:

- Morphine
- Diamorphine
- Methadone
- Pethidine (meperidine)
- Oxycodone
- Fentanyl
- Codeine
- Dihydrocodeine.

Partial Agonists. Examples are:

- Buprenorphine
- Meptazinol
- Tramadol.

Antagonists. Examples are:

- Naloxone
- Naltrexone.

Opium: The Source of Morphine

Opium is obtained from the unripe seed capsule of the poppy *Papaver somniferum*. Opium has been used for thousands of years in the Orient, and was smoked in opium dens. The drug produces euphoria and the user slips into a deep sleep, called the 'yen', which is often characterized by vivid dreams. The poppy is now grown in the UK as well (at secret locations) for commercial development of morphine. Crude opium is a brownish gum-like material and contains a number of substances, the most important being **morphine**, **codeine** and **papaverine**. Morphine is the most powerful of these alkaloids and the actions of morphine and opium are similar and may be considered together.

OPIOID AGONISTS

Morphine

Administration of morphine can be through various routes:

- Oral
- Intramuscular injection
- Intravenous injection
- Infusion via a syringe pump.

Oral

Morphine can be given orally as an immediate-release tablet every 4 h. For long-term control of pain there are slow-release tablets, which are only needed twice or once daily, or as an aqueous solution.

When given orally as a single dose, morphine's effect is greatly reduced because the liver breaks down about 75% of the dose through first pass metabolism before the drug reaches the circulation. With repeated oral dosage, however, it is very effective. This may happen because the metabolite morphine-6-glucuronide (see later) is slowly excreted and with repeated doses accumulates sufficiently to help produce satisfactory analgesia.

Injection

The modes of injection are:

- Subcutaneous
- Intravenous
- Continuous subcutaneous infusion.

When given by injection, morphine produces analgesia rapidly. The analgesic effect of morphine usually lasts about 4 h after injection, but depends to some extent on the severity of the pain, the sensitivity of the patient to the drug, and on the dose. The dosage in severe pain or in acute left ventricular failure depends on many circumstances, including the age, weight and general health of the patient.

Morphine can also be given slowly intravenously. The analgesic effect starts within 20 min of subcutaneous injection and 10 min of intravenous injection, and peaks after about 1 h. PCA is a useful system which relies on a pump system and is controlled by the patient to help administer strong analgesia to respond to their required needs. This is particularly useful after operations and they do have a safety lockout period to prevent overdosing of the medication (see earlier).

Morphine in small doses can also be given by continuous subcutaneous infusion. This allows the dose to be modified as required and can be very useful in severe and fluctuating pain. However, this method needs careful titration of the dose in relation to the therapeutic effect and fixed dose regimens are not very successful. Administering morphine via continuous subcutaneous infusion can be done via a syringe pump, which is particularly useful for managing patients with palliative care needs.

Metabolism and Excretion

After absorption, morphine is combined in the liver to form several substances, one of which (morphine-6-glucuronide) has powerful analgesic properties of its own. The kidney excretes these substances. Repeated doses of morphine will induce a state of tolerance to the drug, so that increasing doses may be required to produce an effect.

Central Nervous System Actions

The most important actions of morphine are on the CNS. The effects may be divided into **depressant** and **stimulant**. Morphine also causes the development of **tolerance** and **dependence** to its central actions. Drug dependence is discussed more fully in Chapter 23.

CNS Depressant Effects.

- Morphine depresses the appreciation of pain by the brain and thus acts as a powerful analgesic.
- It relieves all types of pain.
- If the pain is felt at all, it seems to have lost its unpleasant nature.
- Morphine depresses the emotional component of pain, namely anticipation and fear of pain. It is euphoric and allays anxiety.
- It depresses respiration in large doses. However, patients are often left in pain through erroneous fears about respiratory depression.
- It depresses the cough centre and thus damps down the cough reflex.
- It is a mild hypnotic and may produce drowsiness and sleep.

CNS Stimulant Effects.

- Morphine stimulates the chemoreceptor trigger zone (CTZ; see Chapter 10 and Fig. 10.3) in the brainstem causing nausea and vomiting in about 30% of patients, particularly if they are mobile.
- The pupils of the eye are constricted.
- Morphine stimulates the vagus nerve. This action is particularly liable to be troublesome when morphine is used for the pain associated with coronary thrombosis, as it may cause undue slowing of the pulse and lowering of the blood pressure.

Peripheral Actions (Outside the CNS)

Constipation.

- Morphine decreases the peristaltic activity of the bowel and at the same time, increases the tone of gastrointestinal smooth muscle, leading to constipation.

Increase in Biliary Pressure.

- Morphine causes spasm of the sphincters, including the sphincter of Oddi at the lower end of the bile duct, and thus produces a rise in pressure in the biliary system.

Urinary Retention.

- Morphine interferes with bladder function, which may cause urinary retention, particularly after an operation.

Histamine Release.

- Morphine can lead to the degranulation of mast cells leading to the release of histamine which can cause 'pseudo-allergic responses' such as hives and occasionally bronchoconstriction.

Tolerance to Morphine

Tolerance may be defined as the phenomenon whereby successively more of a drug is needed to produce the same effect. Tolerance develops only to the CNS actions of morphine, and long-term diamorphine (heroin) addicts take doses (as much as 50 times the doses normally used to obtain the therapeutic effect of pain relief) that would normally kill the naive user. However, the same addicts still develop chronic constipation (a peripheral effect of morphine) from a much smaller dose that would not satisfy their craving. There are several theories to explain tolerance, but the actual mechanism of tolerance is unknown. The understanding of tolerance is important because if a patient has become tolerant to the drug then abrupt withdrawal of it will cause withdrawal symptoms. Thus the patient will likely need support with a slow step-wise weaning of the drug.

Common Uses of Morphine

- **Pain control**
- **Cough**
- **Dyspnoea.**

Pain Control. Morphine is very useful for pain control in:

- surgical emergencies
- the postoperative period
- following injury
- after a coronary thrombosis
- controlling severe pain in terminal cancer on a regular basis (see later)
- acute failure of the left ventricle with pulmonary oedema.

Morphine is still one of the best analgesics for temporary severe pain. Morphine is useful after a coronary thrombosis. Its mode of action under these circumstances is not clear, though it probably acts by its widespread sedative effect on the CNS and by dilating veins and relieving congestion in the pulmonary circulation of the lungs.

Signs of Overdosage

A patient who has received an overdose of morphine is drowsy or unconscious. The skin is cyanosed and sweating. Respiration is depressed and the pupils are pinpoint. The treatment for overdosage is immediate endotracheal intubation to aid respiration and administration of an opioid antagonist (see later).

NURSING NOTE

Patients who have been given morphine should be monitored appropriately using local guidelines for both pain and conscious status.

Diamorphine (Heroin)

Diamorphine is obtained by chemical modification of morphine. When given by injection it enters the nervous system more rapidly than morphine, so its action starts a little sooner. Thereafter, it is quickly converted to morphine in the body. When given orally, diamorphine is all converted to morphine in the liver before it enters the systemic circulation; therefore their actions are similar except that the effects of diamorphine are seen a little earlier after injection. It is more soluble than morphine and this is useful when large doses are required by injection.

Although diamorphine is more popular than morphine among addicts, it is difficult to see a scientific reason for this and it may be for social or mythological reasons.

Adverse Effects of Morphine and Diamorphine

Some of these adverse effects comprise:

- Pseudo-allergic symptoms
- Bradycardia
- Confusion
- Constipation
- Dependence
- Dry mouth
- Hallucinations and nightmares
- Hypersensitivity
- Hypotension

TABLE 20.2

Adverse Effects of Morphine, Diamorphine and Other Powerful Opioids (Based on the Guy's, St Thomas' and Lewisham Formulary)

Adverse Effect	Approximate Frequency (%)	Dose- related	Tolerance	Comments
Constipation	100	No	No	Prophylactic laxative (e.g. Senokot) required
Nausea	30	Yes	Yes (5–7 days)	Prophylactic antiemetic if needed
Sedation	30	Yes	Yes (3–4 days)	Usually mild Wears off in 48 h
Confusion, nightmares, hallucinations (particularly at night)	1	No	No	Try reducing dose, then consider haloperidol 2 mg at night

- Nausea
- Respiratory depression
- Sedation
- Urinary retention.

Some features of these adverse effects are summarized in Table 20.2.

Hypersensitivity. Certain patients are very sensitive to powerful opioids and a normal dose may produce signs of overdose. The most important of this group are patients whose respiratory centre is under stress, i.e. those with chronic obstructive pulmonary disease (COPD) and in patients having an asthmatic attack. Patients with liver damage or impaired renal function suffer an exaggerated and prolonged response. Finally, the elderly and paediatric patients are especially sensitive and they should only be given a small dose until their sensitivity to the drug is known.

Dependence. This can develop rapidly when opioids are used in a social context, but they very rarely present a problem when used therapeutically, either in an acute painful situation or in the treatment of patients in the palliative care setting. However, their use in chronic, painful but non-fatal, disorders should be avoided.

Pseudo-allergic Responses. Morphine is chemically a base and can cause the degranulation of mast cells leading to symptoms that are similar to an allergic reaction.

Pregnancy. Morphine will also cross the placental barrier and affect the fetus, a point of importance in midwifery.

Drug Interactions. Opioids increase the effect of other central depressants, as do monoamine oxidase inhibitors (MAOIs), which are particularly dangerous with pethidine (see later).

Methadone

Methadone is a synthetic analgesic. Its analgesic action is as powerful as that of morphine, but it has little of morphine's euphoric and sedative effect. Like morphine, it also has a depressing effect on the cough centre, but the effect on the respiratory centre is not so marked. However, methadone can cause dependence, especially if given by injection. It is rapidly and well absorbed after oral administration or subcutaneous injection and is less liable to produce vomiting than morphine. Its action is longer-lasting than that of morphine and this can make repeated dosage difficult. Methadone should not be given more than twice daily to avoid accumulation.

Therapeutic Uses

Pain. Methadone may be used as a substitute for morphine in the treatment of severe pain.

Cough. In small doses methadone may be useful as an antitussive to relieve cough in terminally ill patients.

Heroin Withdrawal. Methadone is used orally as a substitute for morphine or diamorphine in the treatment of drug dependence (in UK this is the only licensed therapeutic indication). The drug prevents the severe symptoms associated with the withdrawal from heroin. It is rarely required more frequently than every 12 h in the management of opioid withdrawal.

NURSING NOTE

Patients treated with oral tablets or liquid forms of methadone for treatment of heroin dependence have been known to crush the tablets and use the liquid to inject them intravenously, producing the euphoric effects. Nurses who work with patients dependent on opioids should be aware of the problems associated with methadone and its uses, as well as withdrawal symptoms.

Pethidine (Meperidine)

Pethidine is a synthetic substance that is chemically related to atropine. It is well absorbed after oral or subcutaneous administration. It is less powerful than morphine, and has less effect in therapeutic doses on the cough or respiratory centre. It causes some spasm of the muscle of the bile ducts, but does not lead to constipation. Pethidine does not cause constriction of the pupils and is therefore used in head injuries where observation of the pupil size may be important. However, pethidine can cause dependence.

Therapeutic Uses

Pethidine is used in the treatment of moderately severe pain, particularly those arising from the viscera. It can be administered orally or by intramuscular injection. For many years it was given to relieve pain in the later stages of labour, as it is short-acting, thus avoiding prolonged depression of the infant's respiration immediately after birth. There is now good evidence that, although it produces sedation, it is an ineffective analgesic in these circumstances and it is increasingly being replaced by epidural analgesia. Its action lasts 2–3 h.

Oxycodone

Oxycodone is an opiate helpful in the treatment of severe pain, which is available for oral, subcutaneous and intravenous administration. It is a helpful alternative when morphine may not be suitable or tolerated, e.g. it may be suitable in patients with mild to moderate renal impairment. When switching opioids, it is important to use an analgesic conversion table (e.g. in the BNF) to calculate the equivalent dose. This helps provide adequate analgesic cover for the patient.

Fentanyl

This is one of a group of opioids that are very powerful and short-acting. They are used largely in the intraoperative period to help anaesthetic induction. Their use requires care, as severe respiratory depression is a risk. Fentanyl can also be used as a patch, applied to dry, non-hairy skin, which allows slow absorption for up to 72 h in the relief of severe pain and in patients with severe renal impairment. Owing to its complex distribution in the body, the action of fentanyl in these circumstances may continue for 24 h after removal of the patch.

NURSING NOTE

Fever can increase absorption from fentanyl patches and result in symptoms of overdose. The application of a fentanyl patch should be documented with the date and time of administration. The site should be checked regularly to ensure that the correct dose is absorbed and the patient is receiving the correct dose of pain relief. Often pain relief is not achieved due to poor compliance or the patch not being secure or becoming dislodged.

Codeine and Dihydrocodeine

Codeine is obtained from opium. It is given orally. It is a mild analgesic, having only about one-seventh of the power of morphine. Its most useful action is its depressing effect on the cough centre, although it is not as powerful as morphine in this respect. Codeine is often found in OTC remedies for cough and colds, and like morphine, also decreases peristalsis of the intestine and therefore can cause constipation.

Therapeutic Uses

Codeine is primarily used as an analgesic. It can also be combined with aspirin or paracetamol as a mild analgesic, although there is some variation in its analgesic efficacy, due to differences among patients in the metabolism of codeine. Another one of its uses is in cough mixtures because of its ability to inhibit the cough centre. These cough mixtures usually also contain syrup, whose demulcent action is useful in relieving coughs arising from the pharynx. **Do not give to diabetics.**

NURSING NOTE

Increasing the dose of codeine or dihydrocodeine above those recommended will not enhance the analgesic effect. Dihydrocodeine and probably codeine given alone are ineffective in postoperative dental pain.

Dihydrocodeine is similar to codeine and is used as a mild analgesic. It causes constipation and occasionally dizziness, low blood pressure and nausea. It is administered by intramuscular injection or as tablets. Both of these drugs are highly addictive and stricter controls over these drugs (previously available OTC in pharmacies) are now in place.

OPIOID PARTIAL AGONISTS

Opioid partial agonists differ from opioid agonists such as morphine in some of their effects. They are powerful analgesics, but are less addictive, less likely to depress respiration and are less euphoric.

Buprenorphine

This analgesic, although only a partial agonist, is as powerful as morphine. It can be given by injection or sublingually, but is not effective orally, as it is broken down in the liver in a large first pass action. Its analgesic action lasts longer than that of morphine (6–8 h) and it is less likely to depress respiration. The risk of dependence is low, but it can occur.

Buprenorphine shows a 'ceiling effect', so that increasing the dose above the usual range will not improve its efficacy. Although it competes with powerful opioids such as morphine for receptor sites in the brain, in the therapeutic dose range buprenorphine only slightly reduces the analgesic action of other opioids when they are combined. In higher doses, the antagonistic action of buprenorphine will become apparent if combined with opioid agonists.

Therapeutic Use

Buprenorphine is used to treat moderate and severe pain. It can be given by injection for postoperative pain, but it is slow to take effect. It is also given sublingually every 6–8 h for various forms of chronic pain. It is used in opioid detoxification as well (see Chapter 23).

Adverse Effects

Buprenorphine sometimes causes troublesome vomiting, which requires the drug to be stopped. Respiratory depression, although not so marked as with morphine, is only partly reversed by naloxone.

Meptazinol

This drug is similar in some respects to buprenorphine. When given by injection it has a short action (2–3 h) and is used in obstetrics, where its rapid elimination by both mother and fetus is an advantage. It is also useful for breakthrough pain in the postoperative period. There is a large first pass effect, so that only about 10% of the oral dose reaches the circulation, and it is used only for moderate pain by this route.

Tramadol

This is a weak opioid and, in addition, reduces pain appreciation by interfering with pain pathways through the spinal 'gate'. It can be given orally or systemically and is about as powerful as pethidine, its action lasting for about 6 h. The main use of tramadol is in the treatment of moderately severe pain, e.g. postoperatively, although it can be used orally for the treatment of chronic pain. Respiratory depression is not usually marked and its addiction potential is low. Adverse effects include nausea and vomiting, dizziness, constipation and a dry mouth.

OPIOID ANTAGONISTS

Several substances antagonize the actions of morphine and other opioids. Generally, they resemble morphine in their chemical structure and thus compete with it for the μ-opiod receptor sites that morphine acts on. Having occupied receptor sites, however, they produce little or no stimulation, so that the actions of morphine are reversed. Morphine antagonists are used to treat **overdosage** by opioids. The most widely used are naloxone and naltrexone.

Naloxone

Naloxone is a pure antagonist, having no stimulating actions. It reverses the effects of both natural and synthetic opioids, but with buprenorphine, a larger dose of naloxone may be required. It has no analgesic action. The drug can be administered intravenously, intranasally and intramuscularly, and it is very rapidly effective. It can also be used to terminate the action of opioid drugs in the postoperative period. Its action is relatively short (about 1 h), and if used to reverse the effects of longer-acting opioids, repeated doses might be needed. However, as it will antagonize the analgesia, it is important that the patient is not in significant pain following administration, which should also be addressed.

NURSING NOTE

If a patient is given naloxone they should be monitored carefully following administration as, due to the short action of the medication, the effects of the opioids may rapidly return.

Naltrexone

Naltrexone is an orally active opioid antagonist used in special clinics in the treatment of opioid withdrawal (see Chapter 23).

SUMMARY

- Repeated oral doses of immediate-release morphine tablets are needed to build up effective pain relief.

- With continuous subcutaneous infusions of morphine, fixed dose regimens are not generally satisfactory to control pain.
- Morphine and heroin can cause respiratory depression.
- Emergency treatment for morphine overdosage is endotracheal intubation to aid respiration and an opioid antagonist, e.g. naloxone or naltrexone.
- Morphine can cause vomiting.
- Morphine slows the pulse and lowers blood pressure.
- Opioids constipate the patient.
- Morphine can cause a 'pseudo-allergic' reaction.
- There is a danger of causing tolerance and drug dependence with chronic use of opioids.
- Opioids suppress cough.

ANALGESICS FOR TERMINAL DISEASE

Pain is often a prominent feature of terminal disease, particularly cancer. Although the use of drugs is only part of the management of the dying, the correct use of analgesics can play a very important part in the care of these patients.

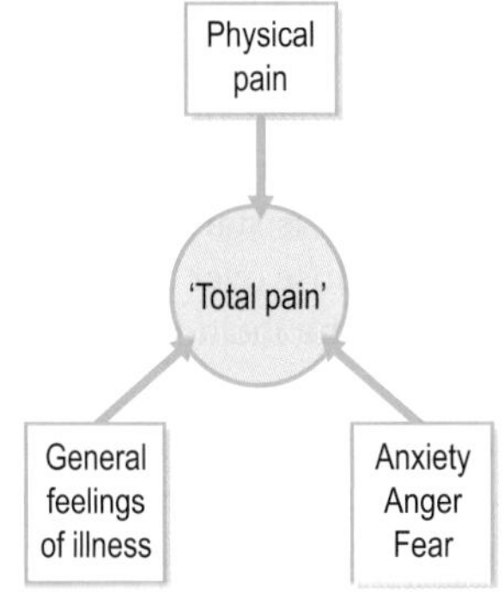

Fig. 20.4 ■ Factors that go to make up the concept of 'total pain' or anguish in the terminally ill.

Determination of the Cause of Pain

It must be realized that, in this type of patient, pain can arise in many ways and the cause should be determined, as it may have a specific remedy. It may be:

- related directly to the spread of the cancer
- the result of therapeutic measures such as surgery or wound procedures
- due to secondary deposits, particularly in bone
- due to some unrelated cause
- due to a combination of these factors.

Concept of Total Pain

Whatever the cause of the pain, unresolved fear or anxiety may make it worse. A vicious cycle of pain and distress is thus engendered, relieved only by resolution of the anxiety, as well as the alleviation of physical pain. The concept of 'total pain' introduced by Cicely Saunders to incorporate physical, social and emotional factors is crucial if the patient's problems are to be fully addressed (Fig. 20.4).

Adjusting the Dose of Analgesic to Keep the Patient Pain-Free

The nurse has a fundamental role in the assessment of the patient's pain. Nursing interventions may include regular administration of analgesia and also active listening to the patient's worries and anxieties. Evaluation of the response to such interventions is important in the ongoing care of that individual. Pain cannot be treated in isolation, but must be regarded as one facet of the patient's physical and mental state. The nurse is critically important in the titration of the drug against the pain (Fig. 20.5).

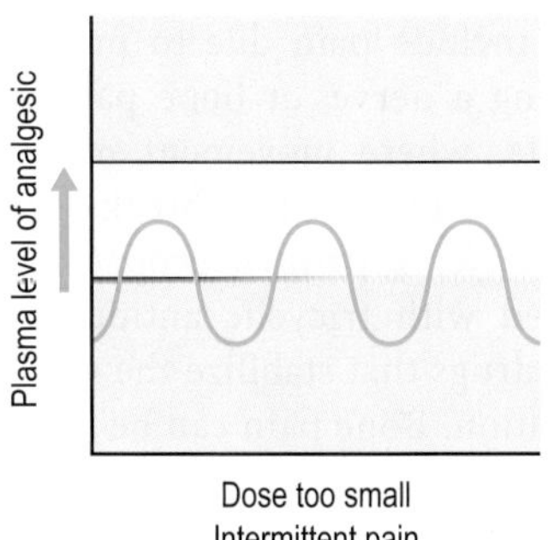

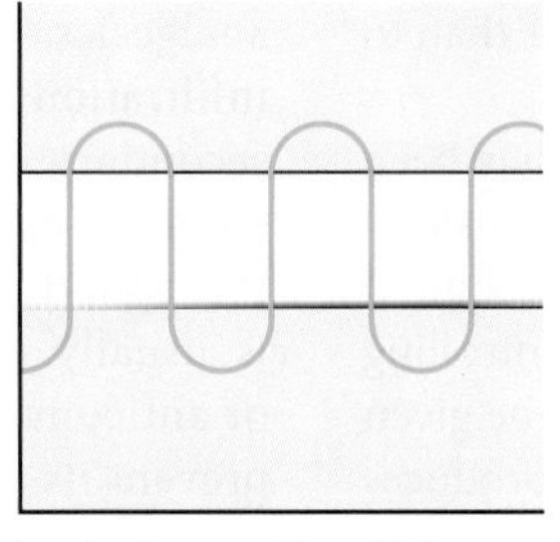

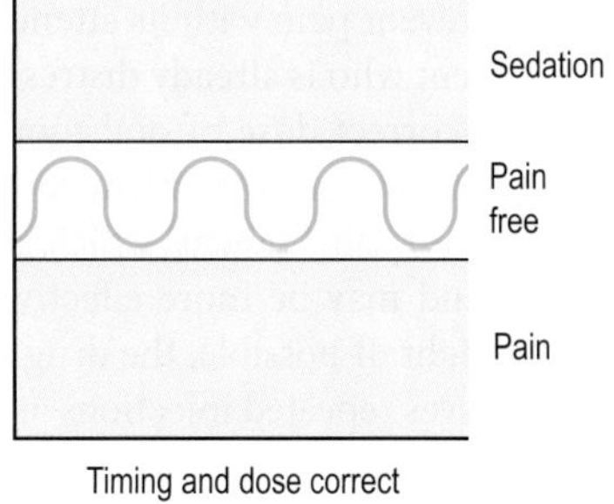

Fig. 20.5 ■ Adjusting the dose to keep the patient free from pain.

Mild Pain

For mild pain, weak analgesics such as paracetamol may be adequate. Co-codamol (paracetamol and codeine) is useful and, if given regularly can be more effective if simple analgesia (e.g. paracetamol or ibuprofen) alone is not sufficient. For pain arising from secondary deposits in bone, antiinflammatory analgesics such as naproxen (see Chapter 13) are sometimes very effective, alone or combined with opioids.

Moderate-to-Severe Pain

Moderate-to-severe pain should be treated by giving opioid analgesics regularly, titrated against the patient's pain.

The most effective drugs are morphine and diamorphine. As diamorphine is largely converted to morphine in the body, their actions and efficacy are essentially the same. However, diamorphine is more soluble than morphine and is thus better for injection if a small volume is required.

The opioid should be prescribed regularly and given regularly. For the average patient, morphine orally as an elixir in chloroform water has been used in the past but is seldom given now. (The shelf-life of morphine in chloroform is 3 months unopened or 1 month if in use.) Immediate-release tablets are usually satisfactory. Lower doses are required in elderly patients, very ill patients and sometimes in those with impaired liver or renal function. Higher doses will be necessary for those patients who are already on, or have recently been on, opioids. The frequency of administration is commonly fixed at every 4 h, but this, like the dose, needs to be kept under regular review.

At first, the patient may need additional doses as required when the pain breaks through. This should be noted and incorporated in the regular 4-hourly schedule. The object is to keep the patient pain-free. It is easier to prevent pain with its attendant fear than to relieve a patient who is already distressed.

Once the correct dose of oral morphine has been established, it may be convenient to change to slow-release (SR) morphine tablets, which are only required twice daily and may be more effective in controlling the pain at night. If possible, the drug should be given orally. This saves repeated injections and also produces a smoother and more prolonged analgesic effect. Dosage schedules should be regularly reviewed and titrated against the patient's pain and well-being.

Side-effects

Side-effects may develop with the use of opioids. They should be anticipated and treated as necessary. Constipation may be a particular problem and a stool softener (docusate) combined with a bowel stimulant (*Senokot*) is very effective.

With this regimen, tolerance to the analgesic action of the drug does not usually develop. A need to increase the dose of the drug usually indicates advance of the disease. The risk of dependence is not relevant in the terminally ill patient.

Other Routes of Administration

Sometimes it is necessary to give opioids by injection intravenously or subcutaneously, when the dose should be reduced (refer to BNF for dose conversion tables). In very severe pain or when vomiting makes oral administration impossible, opioids can be given by subcutaneous infusion. Diamorphine is used in this situation because of its solubility. The procedure is as follows:

- A single 4-h dose is given subcutaneously before the syringe pump is set up.
- The 24-h requirement of the analgesic is calculated and dissolved in water.
- The syringe pump is started at a rate adjusted to give the correct dose over 24 h.
- Antiemetics can be included in the syringe such as cyclizine.
- Careful monitoring of the therapeutic effect and degree of sedation are necessary, and adjustment of the dose made as required.

Opioid Non-responsive Pain

Certain types of pain respond poorly to opioid analgesics. These include pain due to pressure or infiltration affecting a nerve, or bone pain due to secondary deposits, where movement may cause an acute exacerbation of pain that breaks through the opioid control. Nerve pain (neuropathic pain) is usually managed with tricyclic antidepressants or anticonvulsant drugs that stabilize the nerve and prevent its stimulation. Bone pain can be helped by radiotherapy (if this is possible), NSAIDs, bisphosphonates and by preventing movements that cause pain.

Treatments for Opioid Non-responsive Pain

- **Entonox** (50% oxygen + 50% nitrous oxide) by inhalation can be used to cover painful procedures.
- **Lidocaine** medicated plasters may help in patients suffering with localized pain.

Other Methods

The use of analgesics is not the only way to relieve pain in terminal cancer. Radiotherapy is very effective, particularly in treating secondary deposits in bone. In recent years, various types of nerve block either at the level of the peripheral nerve or in the spinal cord have been developed, which can relieve pain without any systemic effects. These blocks may be temporary or permanent.

Analgesics in Non-painful Terminal Disease

Many patients with malignant disease or dying from other diseases such as renal failure do not have pain, but they may experience considerable malaise and anxiety. The use of opioids in these circumstances is more controversial. Some people consider that opioids should be used only for pain relief. In these patients, opioids may also be useful for controlling cough and relieving the sensation of dyspnoea.

Analgesics and Chronic Non-terminal Pain

For some types of chronic pain the cause is obvious (e.g. arthritis; see Chapter 13); in others, it is obscure. Psychological factors play some part in most types of pain, but may play a major part in the more obscure varieties. This means that there are many types of treatment, depending on the cause and severity of the pain, and it is only possible here to make some general statements:

- Before starting treatment it is very important to listen to patients and to assess their perception of the pain, and how it affects their daily life.
- Management with the appropriate drugs will be enhanced by considerable supportive therapy, and various techniques for dealing with pain by psychotherapeutic methods are available.
- Alternative methods of pain relief, i.e. nerve block and TENS, which probably act by closing the relay gate in the spinal cord, may prove helpful in some patients.
- Do not forget that depression often presents as obscure chronic pain. In this case, antidepressants are effective.
- It is important to avoid drugs with a high risk of dependence. Even so-called 'low-risk' analgesics are not entirely safe, e.g. buprenorphine dependence does occur. In prescribing analgesics the patient should be assessed carefully and prescriptions should not be repeated endlessly. The NSAIDs (see Chapter 13) are free from the risk of dependence, but are not free of adverse effects.

Gabapentin and Pregabalin (Gabapentinoids)

Gabapentin is a non-opioid drug that can reduce the nociceptive processes involved in the central sensitization of pain. It is licensed for neuropathic pain treatment as well as an anticonvulsant. Pregabalin is a related drug. Gabapentinoids are subject to misuse and therefore should be used with caution following a history of previous drug abuse.

TERMINAL CARE SERVICES AND THE PAIN CONTROL TEAM

Hospice Care

The object of hospice care is to help maintain an acceptable quality of life while enabling a patient to die peacefully, with special reference to the person's values, preferences and outlook on life. This may be achieved through a team approach in various settings.

The hospice movement has expanded considerably over the last 25 years and there are now many units offering hospice facilities or home palliative care. Referral may be through the GP or arranged on hospital discharge.

The Hospital Support Team

A more recent development is the hospital support team. The team is usually multidisciplinary, sometimes working in conjunction with the radiotherapy or oncology departments. The hospital support team provides skills in symptom control and pain relief and can offer emotional support to patients and carers, while fulfilling an educational role within the hospital.

Pain Control Teams

Pain control teams have been developed to cope with the problem of those in chronic pain. Although many of these patients have terminal cancer, there are other types of chronic pain, such as postherpetic neuralgia, various long-term pains following injury such as amputation, and pain for which there is no obvious cause, but where psychological factors may play a part.

The team usually comprises one or two doctors who are interested in the subject (e.g. anaesthetists), nursing staff (often a sister who is specially trained) and a psychiatrist. They deal with patients who have been referred to them in hospital; they may run an outpatient service and may also undertake home visiting.

Many types of chronic pain are made worse by depression, fear and anxiety and here the psychiatrist can help through explanation, reassurance and the judicious use of drugs such as antidepressants. As in so many areas of treatment, the control of pain is becoming a team activity.

Note: Please refer to Summary of Product Characteristics of the drugs mentioned in this chapter for further description as the above information may not summarize all essential details.

REFERENCES AND FURTHER READING

Chandler, A., Preece, J., Lister, S., 2002. Using heat therapy for pain management. Nurs. Stand. 17 (9), 40–42.

Cowan, D., 2007. Pandemonium over painkillers still exists. Br. J. Community Nurs. 12, 166–169.

Fishbain, D.A., 2008. Pharmacotherapeutic management of breakthrough pain in patients with chronic persistent pain. Am. J. Manag. Care 14 (5 Suppl. 1), S123–S1288.

Francis, L., Fitzpatrick, J.J., 2013. Postoperative pain: nurses knowledge and patients experiences. Pain Manag. Nurs. 14, 351–357.

Griffith, R., 2006. Controlled drugs and the principle of double effect. Br. J. Community Nurs. 11, 352–357.

Griffith, R., 2006. The role of nurse prescribers and the management of controlled drugs. Nurse Prescribing 4 (4), 155–160.

Grossman, S.A., Dunbar, E.M., Nesbit, S.A., 2006. Cancer pain management in the 21st century. Oncology 20, 1333–1339.

Idvall, E., Ehrenberg, A., 2002. Nursing documentation of postoperative pain management. J. Clin. Nurs. 11 (6), 734–742.

Mackintosh, C., 2007. Assessment and management of patients with post-operative pain. Nurs. Stand. 22 (5), 49–55.

Morrison, L.J., Morrison, R.S., 2006. Palliative care and pain management. Med. Clin. North Am. 90, 983–1004.

Pickrell, L., Duggan, C., Dhillon, S., 2001. From hospital admission to discharge; an exploratory study to evaluate seamless care. Pharm. J. 267, 650–653.

Stenner, K., Courtenay, M., 2013. A qualitative study on the impact of legislation on prescribing of controlled drugs by nurses. Nurse Prescribing 5 (6).

USEFUL WEBSITES

Care Quality Commission. https://www.cqc.org.uk/sites/default/files/The_safer_management_of_controlled_drugs_Annual_update_2019.pdf.

NICE. Controlled drugs: safe use and management [NG46]. https://www.nice.org.uk/guidance/ng46.

21 DRUGS USED IN NEUROLOGICAL DISEASES
Migraine, Epilepsy and Parkinson's Disease

CHAPTER OUTLINE

LEARNING OBJECTIVES

At the end of this chapter, the reader should be able to:

- describe the treatment of acute migraine
- describe preventative treatments for migraine
- recognize risk factors for medication overuse headache
- summarize the ILAE 2017 classification of epilepsies
- give an account of the different age-related causes of epilepsy and list the main approaches to the treatment of epilepsy with drugs
- provide examples of epilepsy drugs, their adverse effects, contraindications and monitoring requirements
- describe the use of drugs to treat status epilepticus
- explain how to treat febrile convulsions and about reassuring parents
- give an account of antiepileptic drugs, pregnancy and eclampsia
- discuss the epileptic patient's special needs and problems, e.g. driving
- give the two main approaches to the treatment of Parkinson's disease with drugs and be able to give examples
- give an account of the problems associated with the use of levodopa and other drugs

MIGRAINE

Introduction

Migraine is characterized by recurrent attacks of moderate to very severe headache, often unilateral and pulsating, which may be associated with vomiting and preceded by visual (or other neurological) disturbances (the aura). Its often-familial attacks may be precipitated by trigger factors, such as certain foods, alcohol, stress, and hormonal influences, such as premenstrual tension or the taking of the oral contraceptive pill. Avoidance of trigger factors is important, if possible, especially in children and adolescents. The causes of migraine are not well understood, and older theories that implicated changes in the cerebral circulation as the underlying cause have been discarded, although changes in blood flow may contribute to the condition. It appears that chemical compounds and hormones, such as serotonin and oestrogen, play a role in pain sensitivity for migraine sufferers. Some of these substances also cause cerebral vasodilatation, and it is striking that drugs such as 5-HT receptor agonists, that lead to vasoconstriction, also help halt a migraine attack. It is clear, however, that there is more to migraine than just cerebral vasodilatation. Migraines are common and can be very disabling, especially if frequently recurrent.

Treatment of Acute Attacks

Treatment is by analgesic drugs or 5-HT receptor stimulating drugs.

Analgesic Drugs

The headache often responds to simple analgesics such as aspirin or paracetamol or a non-steroidal antiinflammatory drug (NSAID), especially if started early in the attack. There is research evidence that suggests that a single dose of three regular aspirin tablets (~1000 mg, as regular tablets vary slightly between countries) is nearly as effective as the 5-HT receptor agonists in relieving migraine in many people, especially if combined with a small dose of metoclopramide (see Chapter 10) to prevent vomiting and increase the rate of gastric emptying and thus hasten absorption. Metoclopramide should be used with caution in young adults, especially women, as it may provoke frightening acute dystonic reactions affecting the face and eye muscles. Aspirin should not be used in children and young teenagers. In addition to the use of these drugs, it often helps to lie down in a quiet, darkened room. If these measures fail, as they do in about 20% of people, then a 5-HT receptor agonist can be tried.

5-HT Receptor Agonists (Triptans)

- Sumatriptan
- Naratriptan
- Zolmitriptan
- Rizatriptan
- Almotriptan
- Frovatriptan
- Eletriptan.

Not all of these drugs are available in all markets. They vary widely in price, with sumatriptan generally being the least expensive. In general, there is little difference between them in effectiveness, but for some patients, one triptan will work when another does not, so it is worth trying an alternative if treatment has not been successful. They vary in their onset of action and duration, when given orally. Oro-dispersible and nasal spray formulations are generally more rapid acting and are helpful if vomiting is marked. Subcutaneous injection is available for some of these drugs, using an autoinjector. This type of delivery is the most rapid and generally the most effective. Triptans should be taken at the start of the headache, even if mild, but not at the start of the preceding aura, if any. The initial dose can be repeated after an hour, if ineffective, but no further doses should be taken for that attack.

These drugs stimulate 5-HT receptors and lead to cerebral (and more general) vasoconstriction, but probably act to treat migraine pain in other ways as well. They should not be given to people with known coronary artery disease or cerebrovascular disease and they are not generally licensed for use in the elderly. The initial treatment should be with the lowest dose. They may be combined with an NSAID, if needed. The nasal delivery route is recommended for young people (12–17 years). Nasal and injectable forms of some triptans are also used to treat attacks of 'cluster headache', which is another severe headache syndrome with some similarities to migraine. Regular use of triptans can lead to 'medication overuse headache'.

Ergotamine is a fungal derived drug that causes vasoconstriction through a variety of actions. It was, for many years, the only non-analgesic treatment available for migraine. Its usefulness is limited by the severity of its vasoconstrictor effects, which may lead to gangrene. It should **not** be used to treat migraines but has a limited role in the treatment of cluster headaches, under expert supervision.

Opiates such as codeine have often been used to treat migraines, but they are less effective than the treatments described and run the risk of abuse and medication overuse headache. They should **not** be used to treat migraines.

Treatment to Prevent Migraine

Before starting preventative treatment, medication overuse headache must be excluded.

The aim of preventive treatment is to reduce the frequency, severity and duration of migraine attacks. Preventative treatment should be considered if:

- Migraine attacks are having a significant impact on quality of life and ability to work. These would normally be frequent attacks (more than once a week on average) or prolonged and severe attacks despite acute treatment.
- Acute treatments are contraindicated or ineffective.
- The person is at risk of medication overuse headache because they are frequently using acute drugs.

Preventative drugs need to be taken every day. No one drug is dramatically better than the others and all are limited to some extent by side-effects. For many patients, a β-blocker or amitriptyline are a sensible first choice. Lifestyle change to avoid triggers is still required, and realistic expectations should be encouraged. A good response is generally felt to be a 30%–50% reduction in frequency and/or severity of attacks.

- **Propranolol** 80–160 mg/day is more effective than other β-blockers, but is contraindicated in asthma.
- **Amitriptyline** 25–75 mg taken at night can be effective. This dose is much lower than the dose used to treat depression, and patients should be reassured that they are not being 'secretly' treated for depression.
- **Topiramate** (see later) 50–100 mg/day works well in some cases, but it has many common adverse effects, some serious, and pregnancy must be avoided during use.
- **Pizotifen** has fallen from favour, as weight gain is a troublesome unwanted effect in some patients.

Drugs such as **methysergide** and **sodium valproate** should no longer be used in migraine prophylaxis, except in exceptional circumstances, as the risks associated with their use outweigh the possible benefits in most cases.

Non-drug preventative treatments that have at least some supportive evidence include relaxation therapies, mindfulness, acupuncture and various types of cranial electrical stimulation.

CLINICAL NOTE

Migraine can have a financial, personal and professional impact (Buse et al., 2019). Drug treatment offers some support in modifying impact and, in addition, modification of lifestyle factors is thought to improve migraine symptoms. Regular exercise, adequate sleep, stress management and regular mealtimes are all thought to improve migraine symptoms (Marmura, 2018).

Medication Overuse Headache

'Medication overuse headache' is far more common than was earlier thought. It is a paradoxical, but important cause of chronic daily headache. Regular use of analgesics of any kind, or triptans, can lead to this condition. The International Classification of Headache Disorders defines it as a headache occurring on 15 days or more in a month in a patient with a headache disorder such as migraine or tension headache. The patient must have overused headache medication for at least 3 months. Medication overuse is defined as more than 10 days/month for triptans and opioids and 15 days/month for simple analgesics, including aspirin and paracetamol. It is important to exclude other causes of chronic headache, but medication overuse will often be the underlying cause. A headache diary, in which the patient records the presence and severity of headache, and the use of any medication, is very helpful in diagnosing headache disorders, particularly medication overuse headache.

The treatment is to withdraw the headache medication. This is more easily said than done, and considerable powers of persuasion may be needed, along with much support. Opioids should be withdrawn slowly; other drugs can be stopped abruptly. Unfortunately, the headaches often get worse before they get better, and it can take several weeks before they improve. Withdrawing acute treatment will not make any underlying headache disorder go away. However, this underlying disorder may be amenable to preventative treatment, as discussed earlier.

EPILEPSY

Introduction

The word **epilepsy** is derived from Late Latin *epilepsia*, from the Greek *epilambanein*, which means to seize or attack. Hippocrates wrote about epilepsy in about 400 BCE, calling it the 'sacred disease', since people experiencing seizures were assumed to be possessed by or communicating with the gods. These days, although much more is known about epilepsy, it is still not fully understood.

Epilepsy affects at least 350,000 people in the UK. About 30,000 people develop epilepsy every year and epilepsy affects about 1 in 20 people at some time during their lives. Many studies have found a slightly higher incidence among men.

Causes of Seizures

Some causes of seizures are listed here:

Neonatal Onset

- Congenital brain malformation
- Asphyxia or hypoxia or intracranial trauma during delivery
- Infection
- Intracranial haemorrhage
- Electrolyte or metabolic disturbances.

Childhood and Adolescence

- Brain tumours or trauma
- Cerebral degenerative disease or cerebral palsy
- Congenital brain malformation
- Febrile convulsions (see later)
- Chemical toxicity, e.g. lead, drugs
- Hereditary, e.g. tuberous sclerosis
- Hydrocephalus
- Idiopathic
- Infection
- Rare childhood epilepsy syndromes (Lennox–Gastaut and Dravet syndromes)
- Other diseases, e.g. renal disease.

Adult

- Birth trauma
- Brain trauma or tumours
- Cerebral degenerative disease
- Cerebral vascular disease, e.g. infarction
- Congenital disease
- Drug toxicity, drug abuse and withdrawal, including alcohol
- Idiopathic
- Metabolic disturbances.

Clearly, there is overlap among the various age groups and in many cases, the underlying cause is not identified.

Drugs that May Cause Seizures

- **Anaesthetics**, e.g. enflurane, halothane, ketamine
- **Antibiotics**, e.g. amphotericin, cephalosporins, chloroquine, cycloserine, fluconazole, isoniazid, penicillins
- **Antidepressants and antipsychotic drugs**, e.g. baclofen, cocaine, lithium, tricyclics
- **Cardiovascular drugs**, e.g. intravenous lidocaine, procaine
- **Endocrine drugs**, e.g. desmopressin, insulin, oxytocin, prednisolone
- **Radiographic contrast media**, e.g. certain meglumine derivatives, metrizamide
- **Stimulant drugs**, e.g. aminophylline, caffeine, theophylline.

This list is far from comprehensive but should alert the reader to the fact that many drugs are capable of producing seizures in some patients.

Classification of Epilepsy

Historical Classifications (Often Still Encountered)

For decades, the most common way of describing seizures was *grand mal* and *petit mal*.

More recently, the terms *partial* and *generalized* seizures are used. This divides seizures into partial (seizures starting in one area or side of the brain) and generalized (seizures starting in both sides of the brain at the same time).

Partial seizures are then defined by whether a person is aware or conscious during the seizure.

- *Simple partial seizures*: Person is aware of what happens.
- *Complex partial seizures*: Person has some impaired awareness during the seizure.

2017 ILAE Classification

Epilepsy is complex and accurate classification helps to guide treatment and predict the likely outcome. In 2017, the International League Against Epilepsy (ILAE) revised its classification of epilepsies. It is based on three main features:

- Where seizures begin in the brain
- Level of awareness during an attack
- Other features of the seizures.

The basic version of the ILAE 2017 classification is summarized here:

Where Seizures Begin

- **Focal seizures:** Previously called 'partial seizures', these start in an area on one side of the brain.
- **Generalized seizures:** Previously called 'primary generalized', these involve both sides of the brain at the onset.
- **Unknown onset:** If the onset of a seizure is not known, the seizure falls into the unknown onset category.
- **Focal to bilateral seizure:** A seizure that starts in one side or part of the brain and spreads to both sides was called a secondary generalized seizure. Now the term 'generalized' refers only to how the seizure starts. The new term for secondary generalized seizure is 'focal to bilateral seizure'.

Awareness

Whether a person is aware during a seizure is of practical importance because it is one of the main factors affecting a person's safety during a seizure.

- **Focal aware:** If awareness remains intact, the seizure would be called a 'focal aware seizure'. This replaces the term 'simple partial'.
- **Focal impaired awareness:** If awareness is impaired, the seizure would be called 'focal impaired awareness'. This replaces the term 'complex partial seizure'.
- **Awareness unknown:** Sometimes it is not possible to know if a person is aware or not, particularly if they only have seizures at night or in their sleep.
- **Generalized seizures:** These always affect a person's awareness or consciousness in some way.

Other Features of Focal Seizures

Seizure behaviours are separated into groups that involve movement:

- **Focal motor seizure:** This means that some type of movement occurs during the event. These can be twitching, jerking or stiffening movements of a body part or automatisms (automatic movements such as licking lips, rubbing hands, walking or running).
- **Focal non-motor seizure:** This type of seizure has other symptoms, such as changes in sensation, emotions, thinking or experiences.
- **Auras:** The term 'aura', which describes symptoms a person may feel in the beginning of a seizure, is not in the ILAE classification. It is still often used and is useful as it may provide patients with a warning that they are having a seizure.

Other Features of Generalized Onset Seizures

Seizures that start in both sides of the brain, called 'generalized onset', can be motor or non-motor.

- **Generalized motor seizure:** In the generalized tonic-clonic seizure there is stiffening (tonic) and jerking (clonic). This used to be called 'grand mal'. Other forms of generalized motor seizures may happen.
- **Generalized non-motor seizure:** These are *absence* seizures and used to be called 'petit mal'. These seizures involve brief changes in awareness, staring and some may have automatic or repeated movements like lip-smacking.

Myoclonic Seizures

Myoclonic jerks are a feature of several different types of epilepsy and epilepsy syndromes and can occur in people who do not have epilepsy, often when they are falling asleep. They are single or repeated involuntary contractions of muscle groups. Several antiepileptic drugs can help myoclonic seizures, but some may worsen them.

CLINICAL NOTE

Patients with epilepsy should be warned against driving vehicles, swimming and working under conditions where a seizure could produce disaster. Patient education with regards to epilepsy is important so triggers can be identified and managed. Epilepsy UK provides excellent advice for people living with epilepsy.

General Approach to the Treatment of Epilepsy

Currently used drugs aim to control epilepsy through one of three main mechanisms:

- **enhancement** of the activity of the **inhibitory** brain neurotransmitter gamma-aminobutyric acid (GABA)
- **inhibition** of the activity of the **excitatory** brain neurotransmitter glutamate
- Reducing the activity of sodium and/or calcium channels in the nerve cell membrane.

Some drugs, such as gabapentin, are effective, but the mechanism is still not well understood.

The Aims of Treatment

- The maintenance of as normal a lifestyle as possible for the patient
- Prevention of occurrence of seizures through maintenance of adequate blood levels of antiepileptic drugs
- The use of single drug therapy using careful grading of drug dosage
- Choice of drugs and dosage frequency to optimize patient compliance
- Regular monitoring for drug toxicity
- Regular monitoring of patient status regarding drug interactions.

Although there are now a number of drugs that are useful in controlling epilepsy, it is usually best to start treatment with one drug (called 'monotherapy') and use multiple drug regimens only in resistant cases. The initial dose should be low, and it should be increased until control of the seizures is achieved, or adverse effects develop.

Drugs Used in the Treatment of Epilepsy

The most important drugs used to treat epilepsy are discussed here, with some indication of their main uses. Table 21.1, summarizes the first-line treatments for different types of epilepsy.

Carbamazepine

Carbamazepine is a drug that is chemically related to the tricyclic antidepressants. It is believed to act by reducing sodium channel function in the nerve membrane and keeping the conducting nerve in an inactive state.

Therapeutic Use. Carbamazepine is widely used in the control of generalized and focal seizures. It is also used to relieve the pain of trigeminal neuralgia and in the treatment of bipolar affective disorder. It is given orally. Its rate of breakdown in the body increases with prolonged use, because, like phenytoin, it induces the liver enzymes that break it down. There is a slow-release or 'retard' formulation of carbamazepine that may be used at higher dosages, and also a suppository for when the oral route is not feasible.

Adverse Effects. Up to one-third of patients who take carbamazepine experience adverse effects, but only about 5% of patients have to discontinue treatment because of adverse effects. The most common adverse effects include rashes, dizziness and drowsiness, blurring of vision, depression of the leucocytes of the blood and, occasionally, jaundice and excessive salivary secretion. At higher doses, carbamazepine can have an antidiuretic effect and cause dyskinesia, photosensitivity and arrhythmias. It should be used with caution in cases of renal failure and the dose should be reduced in patients with liver disease.

Drug Interactions. These occur with warfarin and macrolide antibiotics such as erythromycin.

TABLE 21.1

Initial and Add-on Drug Treatment for the Different Types of Epilepsy

Epilepsy Type	Initial Treatment	Add-on Treatment (any one additional drug)	Notes
Generalized motor seizures	Sodium valproate or lamotrigine	Clobazam, lamotrigine, levetiracetam, sodium valproate, topiramate	Valproate should not be used in premenopausal women Carbamazepine and oxcarbazepine are alternative monotherapy treatments
Generalized non-motor seizures	Ethosuximide or sodium valproate or lamotrigine	A combination of any two of the first-line drugs	Valproate should not be used in premenopausal women Other drugs may be used in tertiary specialist centres
Focal and focal to bilateral seizures	Carbamazepine or lamotrigine	Carbamazepine, clobazam, gabapentin, lamotrigine, levetiracetam, oxcarbazepine, sodium valproate, topiramate	Oxcarbazepine, sodium valproate and levetiracetam are alternative initial monotherapy treatments Do not use carbamazepine and oxcarbazepine together Valproate should not be used in premenopausal women
Myoclonic seizures	Sodium valproate, levetiracetam, topiramate	A combination of any two of the first-line drugs	Valproate should not be used in premenopausal women

Oxcarbazepine

Oxcarbazepine is a pro-drug that is converted in the body to an active metabolite. It has a similar mode of action to carbamazepine but is less likely to cause the blood dyscrasias carbamazepine can cause. It does not induce liver enzymes to the same degree as carbamazepine. Its indications for use and side-effect profile are otherwise generally similar to carbamazepine.

Eslicarbazepine acetate is a very similar drug to oxcarbazepine, with similar indications and side-effects. It should not be used in patients with second or third-degree atrioventricular block on the ECG.

Sodium Valproate and Valproic Acid

Sodium valproate has been available for many years, being introduced in the early 1970s. Valproic acid was introduced in the 1990s and is generally similar. Both are often referred to as 'valproate', but should never be prescribed as such.

Sodium valproate has several central nervous system (CNS) actions. It maintains levels of GABA after the neurotransmitter has been released, by inhibiting enzymes that break it down. It also increases the breakdown of the excitatory neurotransmitter glutamate. Sodium valproate also has a weak blocking action on sodium channels in the nerve cell membrane.

Therapeutic Use. Sodium valproate is well absorbed after oral administration and has a half-life in the circulation of about 15 h. It is effective against both focal and generalized seizures. It is especially useful for treating infants, since it has relatively low toxicity and few sedative effects. Valproate is a mood stabilizer that can help keep people with bipolar affective disorder well. However, its teratogenicity seriously limits its usefulness in psychiatric practice.

Adverse Effects. **These are very teratogenic drugs,** leading to spina bifida and other serious problems. They should not be prescribed to women of reproductive age unless no other treatment is suitable. Sodium valproate fairly commonly causes a fall in the platelet count. Occasionally this is severe, and the patient should be warned to report any bruising or bleeding. It is advisable to carry out a platelet count before major surgery. Very rarely it causes serious liver damage, particularly in those with pre-existing liver disease or in children with congenital or accidental brain damage. Drowsiness, thinning of the hair (usually reversible) and weight gain are not uncommon.

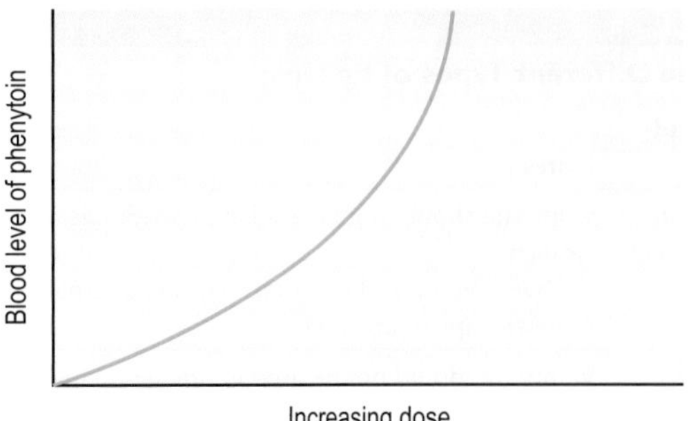

Fig. 21.1 ■ Relationship between dosage and blood level of phenytoin.

SAFETY POINT

If a woman of reproductive age is prescribed valproate, they must receive highly effective contraception and a discussion about this must be documented regularly.

Phenytoin

Phenytoin reduces the activity of sodium channels in nerve membranes. This reduces the excitability of nerve cells and prevents the abnormal electrical discharge from spreading in the brain. Phenytoin is falling out of favour and is no longer a first choice for any indication where alternatives are available. Many patients are still taking it and if it is effective, it should not be stopped. It is particularly used in the treatment of generalized motor seizures.

Therapeutic Use. Phenytoin is well absorbed by mouth and does not produce drowsiness. Its effectiveness as an anticonvulsant and the incidence of side-effects depend largely on the plasma level of the drug. Finding the correct dose may be difficult for several reasons:

- Patients vary considerably in the rate at which they break down phenytoin, so there is a wide variation of dose requirements between patients.
- The relationship between dose and plasma level is not linear; this means that a small increase in the dose may cause a considerable rise in the plasma level (Fig. 21.1).
- Because phenytoin is slowly broken down, once the daily dosage is adequate, it takes about a week for the plasma level to become steady. Therefore, the dose should not be altered at less than fortnightly (2-weekly) intervals.
- When establishing a patient on phenytoin, it is useful to measure blood phenytoin levels. Monitoring of blood phenytoin levels should **not** be routinely performed, unless to assess adherence or suspected toxicity or after adjustment of phenytoin dose. The target concentration is 10–20 mg/L.

Adverse Effects. In phenytoin toxicity there is sedation, slurred speech, ataxia and nystagmus (rapid, involuntary eye movements).

Other side-effects are fairly common and include greasy skin and hirsutism, gum hypertrophy, lymph node enlargement, rashes – some of which may be severe. Macrocytic anaemia due to folic acid deficiency can occur and, rarely, other blood disorders including dangerous agranulocytosis (failure of white cell production).

Drug Interactions.

- Phenytoin is largely bound to plasma proteins in the blood and can be displaced from these proteins by other drugs such as sodium valproate (see later), and by aspirin. This will increase the concentration of free phenytoin in the blood and therefore effectively increase the dose. Increasing the unbound fraction of phenytoin in the blood also increases the amount of phenytoin that can be metabolized in the liver, and all this results in highly unpredictable levels of phenytoin in the circulation.
- Phenytoin induces liver enzymes that metabolize other drugs such as hydrocortisone, oral contraceptives, theophylline, tricyclic antidepressants and thyroxine. This will decrease the efficacy of those drugs.

SAFETY POINT

Patients must be warned to urgently report symptoms of blood and bone marrow dysfunction, particularly fever, rash, mouth ulcers, bruising or bleeding.

Fosphenytoin

Fosphenytoin is a pro-drug that is converted into phenytoin by the liver. It is given by injection when phenytoin cannot be given by mouth, e.g. during status epilepticus, or seizures associated with head injuries or surgery. It causes less irritation at the injection site than does phenytoin. Its adverse effects and contraindications are as for phenytoin.

Lamotrigine

Lamotrigine inhibits the release in the brain of the excitatory neurotransmitters glutamate and aspartate, thus preventing seizures.

Therapeutic Use. Lamotrigine is effective in focal and generalized seizures and has been shown to be as effective as carbamazepine and better tolerated. If combined with other antiepileptic drugs, dose adjustment is necessary. Higher doses may be required with phenytoin or carbamazepine and lower doses with sodium valproate. An advantage of lamotrigine is that it is well-tolerated and causes little impairment of cognition.

Adverse Effects. Lamotrigine may cause ataxia, headaches, nausea and rashes, which may be dangerous, and which occur particularly in children. It should not be used in patients with hepatic or renal impairment.

Levetiracetam and Brivaracetam

Levetiracetam is used for monotherapy or adjunctive therapy of focal and focal to bilateral seizures. It is also used as an adjunct in treatment of generalized seizures and myoclonic seizures. Brivaracetam is a related drug that is currently only used for focal and focal to bilateral seizures. All the drugs in the 'racetam' class are thought to act on glutamate receptors in the brain.

Side-effects include skin rashes, nausea, dizziness, headaches, drowsiness, ataxia and occasionally anorexia. It can trigger mood disorders and rarely, psychosis. It is contraindicated or should be used with caution in cases of liver or renal disease, and in patients who are pregnant or breastfeeding. The structurally related drug **piracetam** is prescribed for myoclonic jerks of non-epileptic origin (*myoclonus*). The evidence for its effectiveness in treating these involuntary muscle contractions is not strong. There is some evidence that piracetam may act to improve memory and cognitive performance.

Tiagabine

Tiagabine was introduced in 1998, and is based on the structure of GABA. Like gabapentin, it was designed to pass easily across the blood–brain barrier. It prolongs the action of GABA by blocking its reuptake in CNS synapses.

Therapeutic Use. Tiagabine is used as an adjunctive treatment of focal seizures and focal to bilateral seizures. It is also used outside of its licence by some physicians to treat anxiety. It may worsen myoclonic and generalized motor and non-motor seizures.

Adverse Effects. These include diarrhoea, dizziness, confusion, headache, depression and, occasionally, psychotic episodes.

Topiramate

Topiramate has multiple actions in the brain, and many side-effects that limit its usefulness. It potentiates GABA activity in the brain and also has carbonic anhydrase inhibitory activity.

Therapeutic Use. It is a second-line treatment but can be used as monotherapy or adjunctive therapy for generalized motor seizures and focal and focal to bilateral seizures. It is used as an adjunct in the treatment of Lennox–Gastaut syndrome. It may be effective in migraine prophylaxis, if tolerated.

Adverse Effects. Topiramate has an unusually large number of side-effects, some common and some serious. Confusion and incoordination are common but can improve. Many other neurological disorders can occur. It may impair heat regulation, especially in children, leading to heat stroke with vigorous exercise. Rarely but seriously, it can provoke serious eye inflammation and acute onset myopia with secondary acute glaucoma. It is teratogenic and effective contraception should be used.

Vigabatrin

Vigabatrin inhibits the breakdown of GABA in the brain, thus enhancing its effect.

Therapeutic Use. Vigabatrin is used as an adjunct to other drugs in the treatment of focal and focal to generalized seizures. Adverse effects limit its usefulness. It may worsen generalized seizures, particularly non-motor ones, and it may worsen myoclonic symptoms.

Adverse Effects. Sedation may occur and, occasionally, gastric upsets and headaches. Behavioural problems such as irritation, aggression, hallucination and memory problems occur in about 15% of patients. Encephalopathic symptoms, including stupor and confusion have occurred rarely. Around 33% of patients develop visual field defects, which may be permanent. Visual fields should be tested before starting treatment and at 6-monthly intervals. Slow withdrawal of the drug may be necessary if field defects occur.

Zonisamide

Zonisamide is a sulphonamide anticonvulsant used to treat refractory partial seizures with or without secondary generalizations. Its mechanism of action is unknown at present but may involve acting on both sodium and calcium channels on neurones in the cerebral cortex. It also shows weak inhibition of carbonic anhydrase.

Therapeutic Use. It is used as adjunctive therapy of focal and focal to bilateral seizures. It may also be used as monotherapy. It can also be used as an adjunctive treatment for the motor symptoms of Parkinson's disease. It should be used with caution in the elderly and children, and where there is renal or hepatic impairment.

Adverse Effects. Neuropsychiatric symptoms of many sorts are common and can be severe. Dangerous weight loss has occurred, especially in children. Blood and bone marrow disorders, some severe, have occurred. Body heat regulation may be disordered. Metabolic disorders and glaucoma have been reported, rarely. It has been shown to be toxic in studies on pregnant animals, and effective contraception should be used while taking it. It should not be used in patients who are breastfeeding or who are allergic to sulphonamides.

SAFETY POINT

Fatal heatstroke has occurred in children taking zonisamide or topiramate, and parents should be warned of the risks of children overheating during exercise, and the need for adequate hydration.

Gabapentin

Gabapentin was originally designed as an analogue of GABA that would pass easily across the blood–brain barrier. However, it was discovered that gabapentin does not act as a GABA analogue, but instead appears to inhibit certain specific voltage-dependent calcium channels in CNS neurons.

Therapeutic Use. Gabapentin can be used to control focal and generalized seizures but is not generally more effective than other drugs. It is more useful in the control of neuropathic pain.

It is rapidly excreted unchanged, mainly through the kidneys, so three-times-daily dosage may be necessary. It should be used with caution in renal failure.

Adverse Effects. These include sleepiness, ataxia and fatigue. There is an association with suicidal ideation, although it is not known if this is causal or due to the conditions (such as chronic pain) that it is prescribed for. It has become a drug of abuse for its euphoric effects and there are controls on its prescribing in some countries.

Pregabalin

Pregabalin is similar to gabapentin in its mechanism of action, although it appears to be more potent.

Therapeutic Use. Pregabalin is used as adjunct therapy in the treatment of focal and focal to bilateral seizures. It is more commonly used to treat neuropathic pain, such as painful diabetic peripheral neuropathy, and to treat generalized anxiety disorder. It is contraindicated with breastfeeding and used with caution in pregnant patients or patients with kidney disease.

Adverse Effects. Minor gastrointestinal and neurological adverse effects are relatively common, but overall the drug is quite well-tolerated. More significant neuropsychiatric disturbances are uncommon, and ascites, liver and kidney disorders and pancreatitis occur rarely. It has become a drug of dependence and abuse and there are controls on its prescribing in some countries.

Ethosuximide

Ethosuximide is a structural derivative of barbiturates such as phenobarbital. It blocks all subtypes of T-type calcium channels in nerve cells, and this probably underlies its therapeutic and adverse effects.

Therapeutic Use. Ethosuximide is used to treat generalized non-motor seizures of the absence type. It is also used to treat myoclonic seizures

Adverse Effects. Ethosuximide may aggravate tonic–clonic types of generalized motor seizures and may, if necessary, be combined with a drug that controls this type of attack.

It is generally well-tolerated, with minor adverse effects including sleepiness, gastric upsets and headaches. More serious neuropsychiatric reactions have occurred rarely, and serious blood and bone marrow disorders have been reported. Occasional skin rashes, sometimes severe, have occurred.

SAFETY POINT

Patients must be warned to urgently report symptoms of blood and bone marrow dysfunction, particularly fever, rash, mouth ulcers, bruising or bleeding.

Lacosamide

Lacosamide is an amino acid derived drug that appears to work through the modulation of sodium channels in nerve cells.

Therapeutic Use. It is presently a second-line drug used as monotherapy or as an adjunct in the treatment of focal and focal to bilateral seizures. It is used in some countries as a treatment for neuropathic pain.

Adverse Effects. It is generally well-tolerated. Various forms of dizziness and vertigo are the most common reasons for discontinuing it. While neuropsychiatric disorders can occur, as with many antiepileptic drugs, the incidence of severe psychiatric disorders seems to be low. It should not be used in patients with first- or second-degree heart block on the ECG.

Benzodiazepines

The benzodiazepine drugs have a limited role in the management of epilepsy. Diazepam is the most well-known of this group of drugs. They may produce their antiepileptic effects by enhancing the inhibitory effect of GABA. They are effective in all forms of epilepsy, but cause sedation. There is also a troublesome withdrawal syndrome associated with the benzodiazepines, which can worsen epileptic seizures if these drugs are stopped. They are most useful in treating status epilepticus. Benzodiazepines are drugs of dependence and abuse.

Clobazam is a benzodiazepine that is used as an adjunct to other drugs in the treatment of epilepsy that is difficult to control. It is helpful in myoclonic seizures. It is also used by specialists in conjunction with the cannabis extract **cannabidiol** to treat some rare childhood epilepsy syndromes.

Phenobarbital

Phenobarbital is the oldest drug in use for the treatment of epilepsy. It is very dangerous in overdose and has neurotoxic side-effects. It is a drug of dependence and abuse and should not be withdrawn suddenly, as this may provoke potentially fatal seizures. It has many drug interactions.

It should not be started as epilepsy treatment. Even in low-income countries, where its low cost is an advantage, other safer drugs are now available at low cost. If a patient is on phenobarbital and stable, then they may continue taking it.

Primidone

Primidone is in many ways similar to phenobarbital and was an early antiepileptic drug. Its mechanism of action is still not understood, despite nearly 70 years of use. It is effective against all forms of epilepsy except absence attacks, but newer drugs are more effective and much safer. It has fallen out of general use, but some patients with long established and well-controlled epilepsy may still be taking it. It is still used in low-income countries. Drowsiness, ataxia, visual disturbances, nystagmus, headache and dizziness are common adverse effects. Low folic acid levels are associated with its use. This may lead to blood disorders.

Other Drugs

Other drugs are available for the treatment of epilepsy, generally as adjuncts to other drugs in difficult to control epilepsy and in the rare severe childhood epilepsies such as Lennox–Gastaut and Dravet syndromes. They are relatively rarely used and should only be started by experts in these conditions. These include **perampanel, rufinamide, cannabidiol and stiripentol. Felbamate** has a similar role but is only available in a few countries due to the risk of aplastic anaemia associated with its use.

Outcome of Treatment

A single drug controls about 80% of patients with generalized motor seizures. If monotherapy with one first-line drug is not successful, monotherapy with an alternative should be tried. Occasionally it is necessary to use combinations of drugs. When the patient has been free of seizures for 3–5 years, drug treatment may be slowly withdrawn. Many subjects will have no further seizures, but about 40% (rather less in children) will relapse.

SAFETY POINT

It is important that anticonvulsants are not discontinued suddenly, as this may precipitate seizures.

Drugs must be given as time critical and not missed. If a patient is nil by mouth or unable to eat or drink, an alternative route should be used so a dose is not missed, to avoid seizures.

Antiepileptic Hypersensitivity Syndrome

Carbamazepine, **lacosamide**, **lamotrigine**, **oxcarbazepine**, **phenobarbital**, **phenytoin**, **primidone** and **rufinamide** can trigger a rare, but potentially fatal reaction known as the *antiepileptic hypersensitivity syndrome*. **Eslicarbazepine**, **stiripentol** and **zonisamide** have not been reported as causing it, but there is a theoretical risk.

The symptoms usually start between 1 and 8 weeks of first taking the drug. Fever, rash and lymph node enlargement are most common. There may be liver dysfunction, blood, kidney and lung abnormalities, vasculitis and multi-organ failure. If this syndrome occurs, immediate withdrawal of the drug is required, **under expert supervision**, and it must not be prescribed again for that patient.

Generic Versus Branded Prescribing

While it is generally desirable to prescribe drugs by their generic names, rather than as a particular manufacturer's brand, the formulations of generic drugs vary slightly and in some cases of epilepsy, this may affect the pharmacokinetics of the drug sufficiently to lead to a loss of control of seizures in patients stabilized on one particular brand of drug. For some drugs this seems to be more of an issue than for others. In the UK, where generic prescribing of drugs is the rule, the Committee on Human Medicines and the MHRA have issued guidance as to which antiepileptic drugs should be prescribed by brand name and not switched to generic drugs. Three categories were established:

1. Prescribe by brand and do not change – carbamazepine, phenobarbital, phenytoin, primidone
2. Generally safe to prescribe generically and change brands, but for some patients who have had trouble obtaining seizure control and those for whom a breakthrough seizure would have major implications, it may be better to not change brands – clobazam, clonazepam, eslicarbazepine, lamotrigine, oxcarbazepine, perampanel, rufinamide, topiramate, valproate, zonisamide
3. Therapeutic equivalence can be assumed, and drugs prescribed generically – brivaracetam, ethosuximide, gabapentin, lacosamide, levetiracetam, pregabalin, tiagabine, vigabatrin.

Even where it is possible to prescribe generically, patient factors should be considered, as adherence to treatment is essential in epilepsy. If generic prescribing might lead to confusion or anxiety, then brand prescribing may be more appropriate. This may be particularly important if patients have learning disability, autism or mental health problems.

Driving

In the UK, a person must tell the licensing authority if they have had a seizure. They may not drive without permission from the licensing authority. The minimum period where driving is not allowed depends on whether the seizure was 'provoked' or 'unprovoked', whether it occurred while awake or asleep and the type of licence (much longer seizure-free periods, while off all antiepileptic medication in the case of bus, coach and lorry licences). The minimum period without driving varies between 6 months and 10 years. Consult guidance from your local driving licensing authority for detailed information. It is important to document that you have discussed driving with a newly diagnosed or suspected epileptic. If you learn that a patient you know to have active epilepsy is driving, you may need to inform licensing authorities as a matter of public safety.

Status Epilepticus

In status epilepticus the patient has a series of seizures, rapidly following each other. These patients require careful nursing so that they do not injure themselves. They should be nursed in the lateral semi-prone position, and the airway established; oxygen should be given by mask. Set a timer going to ensure the duration of the seizures is known. The patient should not be left unattended until the seizures have ceased. It is important to check for hypoglycaemia and correct if necessary. Medication is required to end the seizures if they last longer than 5 minutes.

The drugs commonly used are:

- benzodiazepines – lorazepam, diazepam or midazolam
- phenytoin or fosphenytoin
- phenobarbital or thiopental.

Initially **lorazepam** should be given by slow intravenous injection. **Diazepam** emulsion is an alternative, but is more irritant. In the community or in young children, rectal diazepam, administered using rectal tubes, is rapidly effective and useful particularly if intravenous injection is difficult. **Midazolam** oromucosal solution given into the buccal cavity is an alternative. Benzodiazepines should control seizures within 10 min; if the seizures persist, the dose may be repeated.

If seizures recur or persist after 25 min, then treatment with intravenous **phenytoin**, **fosphenytoin** or **phenobarbital** should be given. Intensive monitoring of vital signs and ECG is required. Phenytoin and fosphenytoin may be given intravenously. Phenytoin needs a slow injection and often causes injection site reactions, so fosphenytoin is preferred, if available.

If seizures persist or recur after 45 min, anaesthesia with thiopental, midazolam or propofol is needed. This requires full intensive care unit support.

Paraldehyde

Paraldehyde, an oily liquid with a pungent smell, has been used for many years. It is a CNS depressant that can control status epilepticus. It is given rectally, diluted in saline, or by deep intramuscular injection; however, as it is an irritant, care must be taken to avoid the sciatic nerve. Paraldehyde must be injected using a glass syringe as it dissolves plastics. It is not the preferred treatment for status epilepticus, but because it is a relatively safe drug, it can be used when facilities for close monitoring and respiratory support (if needed) are not available.

NURSING NOTE

The renewal of seizures or the emergence of toxicity after a period of good control may be due to poor adherence with medication or to an interaction with a newly prescribed medicine (Honavar et al., 2019). Studies have suggested that the use of electronic text reminders in adolescents may improve adherence to antiepileptic medicines (Yoo et al., 2020), and when people present to the emergency department with epilepsy symptoms, clinicians should explore with the patient how frequently they take their epilepsy medicines, if they ever miss a dose, and explore reasons for dose omission.

Febrile Convulsions

About 3% of infants and young children have a fit when feverish (pyrexial). Of these children, only 1% will ultimately develop true epilepsy. They tend to occur when the body temperature rises rapidly.

The immediate treatment is to lay the child semi-prone, and most convulsions stop within a few minutes. If the seizure persists, rectal diazepam as for status epilepticus (see earlier) is the safest and easiest treatment. Hospital admission may be necessary to exclude serious infection.

Prevention

The parents should be taught to reduce fever by removing excess clothing, keeping the environment cool, supplying cool drinks and giving paracetamol paediatric elixir. If attacks recur with fever, then it may be an option to give rectal diazepam when the child develops a fever. Anticonvulsant prophylactic medication, given continuously, is very rarely required.

There is a 30% chance that febrile convulsions will recur if the child has a fever, but attacks become rare after 4 years of age. It is very rare for a child to come to any harm from febrile convulsions.

CLINICAL NOTE

Although febrile convulsions are nearly always benign, nurses must remember that they may signify a serious illness (e.g. meningitis) and they are very frightening for parents. Any unusual features call for a rapid assessment by an expert.

Antiepileptics and Pregnancy

There is evidence that antiepileptic drugs given during pregnancy are associated with an increased incidence of fetal malformation, and some, such as valproate, should never normally be given in pregnancy. If possible, a single antiepileptic should be used, and the dosage controlled by repeated measurement of blood levels. Most fetal abnormalities arise during the first trimester of pregnancy and women who are taking antiepileptic drugs should be advised of the risk before becoming pregnant.

No antiepileptic drug is entirely safe in pregnancy, and women planning pregnancy should be referred to an expert to plan their treatment. In some cases, it may be appropriate to withdraw the drug before conception. In other cases, this may be too risky to the mother and the risks and benefits need to be discussed. With an unplanned pregnancy, the first trimester will often have nearly passed before the woman realizes she is pregnant. In this case, she should be encouraged to continue her medication while she is referred to an expert in epilepsy in pregnancy. If she is taking valproate, then this should be an urgent referral for expert guidance. She should be reassured that at least 90% of babies born to women taking antiepileptic drugs have no abnormalities. Folic acid supplementation before and during pregnancy reduces the risk of neural tube defects.

Many antiepileptic drugs induce liver enzymes and thus increase the rate of breakdown of oral contraceptives, so the patient's method of contraception may need to be reviewed.

Eclampsia

The control of seizures is important in the treatment of eclampsia. In the UK, this has usually been attempted by using phenytoin or diazepam. It has been shown that intravenous **magnesium sulphate** is probably more effective. Its mode of action in these circumstances is not clear, but it may relieve cerebral ischaemia by vasodilatation or minimize cerebral damage. It is given by intravenous infusion.

Prognosis in Epilepsy

The prognosis with epilepsy is variable in that 70%–80% of patients who develop epilepsy will at some stage become free of seizures with treatment. Treatment may be stopped in patients who have been free of seizures for 3–5 years. Approximately 50% of patients in this category who stop taking drugs will remain seizure-free.

The remaining 20%–30% of patients who continue to have seizures despite treatment may develop chronic active epilepsy. The prognosis for these patients is usually poorer and they often suffer from additional psychological or neurological problems.

The overall mortality rates for patients with epilepsy are about three to five times those of the general population, especially in patients with severe epilepsy and in younger sufferers. The most common causes of death include status epilepticus, accidents, suicide and tumours.

SUMMARY

- In epilepsy, it is common to use monotherapy, and multiple drug regimens only in resistant cases
- Patients with epilepsy should be warned against driving vehicles, swimming and working under conditions where a seizure could produce disaster
- Measures of plasma phenytoin concentrations can be helpful when doses are changed, but do not require regular checks
- Sodium valproate or lamotrigine are first-line treatments for generalized motor seizures (tonic-clonic). Carbamazepine and oxcarbazepine are alternatives
- Ethosuximide or sodium valproate are first-line treatments for generalized non-motor seizures (absences). Lamotrigine is a suitable alternative
- Carbamazepine and lamotrigine are first-line treatments for focal seizures. Levetiracetam or sodium valproate are suitable alternatives

- Sodium valproate, levetiracetam and topiramate are first-line treatments for myoclonic seizures
- The benzodiazepine lorazepam is useful in the treatment of status epilepticus
- It is important that anticonvulsants are not discontinued too suddenly, as this may precipitate seizures
- A patient may be allowed to drive a car after being free from primary seizures for 1 year, but not a heavy goods or public service vehicle
- For febrile convulsions, parents should be taught to reduce fever by removing excess clothing, keeping the environment cool, supplying cool drinks and giving paracetamol paediatric elixir
- Carbamazepine and sodium valproate may cause neural tube defects and phenytoin may cause a variety of abnormalities. At present, there does not appear to be an entirely safe antiepileptic drug to use during pregnancy. To minimize the risk, women should receive supplementary folic acid before (if possible) and throughout pregnancy.

PARKINSON'S DISEASE

Introduction

Parkinson's disease is a progressive degenerative disease of the brain. It occurs mainly in the elderly, although it can first manifest itself during the 40s or 50s. The onset is often gradual and insidious. It is a relatively common neurological disorder, and in the UK affects 1%–2% of elderly people.

Chief Symptoms

- Inhibition of voluntary movements (hypokinesias), which is caused partly by inertia of the motor system and partly by muscle rigidity (see later). Inertia means that movement is difficult to initiate and difficult to stop.
- Tremor at rest, often involving the 'pill-rolling' action between thumb and forefinger, is lessened during voluntary movement.
- Muscle rigidity, when muscles are stiff and difficult to move, using passive limb manipulation.

Other Clinical Features

The patient's face may be expressionless. Walking is difficult to initiate, and the patient may walk with rapid, small steps (called 'festination') or with small, shuffling steps. The patient will freeze when trying to change direction when walking and, as the disease progresses, the patient may fall down due to the gradual loss of postural reflexes. The resting tremor of the hands is noticeably worsened by stress. The patient's handwriting often becomes much smaller because of the difficulty performing fine motor movements. The patient sweats excessively and suffers from a greasy skin (seborrhoea). The digestive system is adversely affected. Swallowing becomes difficult and the patient may drool. Constipation occurs virtually invariably and often prior to motor symptoms occurring. The patient becomes depressed and may complain of difficulty with thinking (dysphrenia; cognitive impairment). In the later stages, the patient may suffer from dementia.

Causes of Parkinson's Disease and Parkinsonism

- Degenerative changes of unknown cause in nerve cells in the basal ganglia of the brain
- Drug-induced brain damage
- Cerebral ischaemia
- Viral encephalitis.

Note that the term *parkinsonism* is used to describe the symptoms of Parkinson's disease, which result from drugs or infections. The term *Parkinson's disease* is used, normally, to describe the idiopathic disease that results from the progressive degeneration of parts of the brain involved in motor coordination.

Neurotransmitters in Parkinson's Disease and Parkinsonism

Fine movements are controlled via the *extrapyramidal nerve pathways*, which have their controlling centre in the brain. There is normally a fine balance between the activity of the two neurotransmitters **dopamine** and **acetylcholine (ACh)** in two structures in the basal ganglia of the brain, the *dorsal striatum* and the *substantia nigra* and the nerve connections between them, the *nigrostriatal pathways*. These have nerve connections to the sensory cortex, motor cortex and other structures and thus to the spinal cord and finally to the voluntary muscles. Dopamine is inhibitory and ACh is excitatory. The dopaminergic nerves are found in the substantia nigra and ACh nerves are in the dorsal

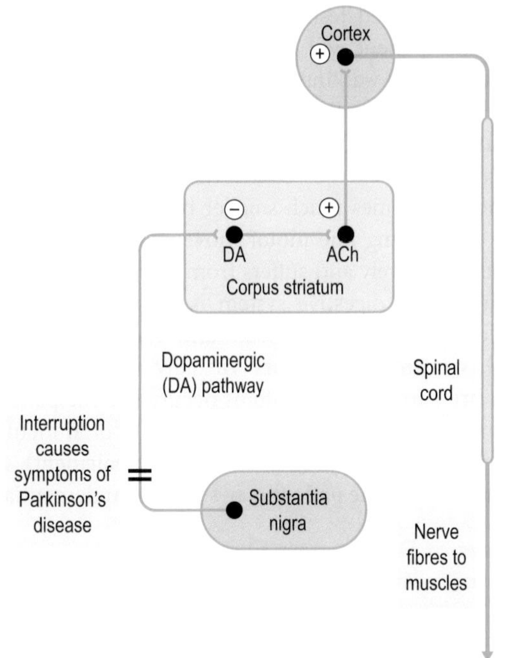

Fig. 21.2 ■ Extrapyramidal system simplified to show the role of the nigrostriatal dopaminergic pathway in the control of fine movement. +, Excitatory; −, inhibitory; *ACh*, acetylcholine; *DA*, dopamine.

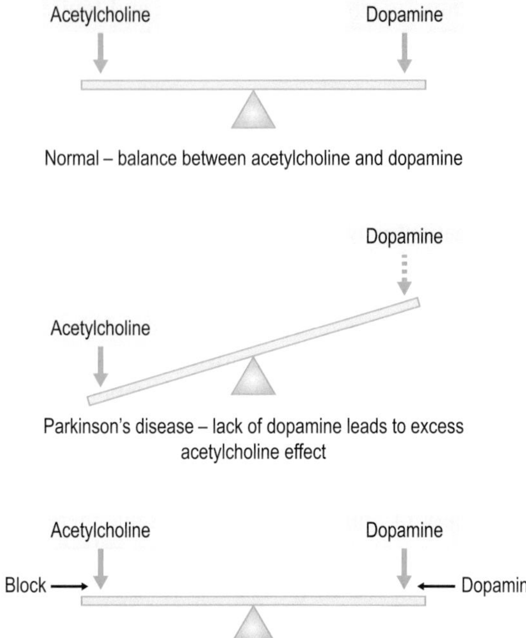

Fig. 21.3 ■ The use of drugs in Parkinson's disease.

striatum. If for any reason the inhibitory dopaminergic influence is reduced significantly, the ACh nerves become relatively overactive, resulting in the muscle tremor and rigidity of Parkinson's disease. The system is shown diagrammatically in Fig. 21.2.

It can be seen, therefore, that relief of symptoms can be achieved by reducing cholinergic activity or by increasing the amount of dopamine (Fig. 21.3).

Drug-induced Parkinsonism

Certain drugs can cause symptoms of Parkinson's disease, some temporarily and others permanently. The most famous example is that of the case of a group of Californian heroin addicts who, in 1982, developed a very severe form of Parkinson's disease. The cause was the presence in their drugs of a chemical called MPTP, which was a contaminant of the heroin substitute they were using. The MPTP was converted in their bodies to the active substance MPP, which was selectively taken up into the dopaminergic neurones of the nigrostriatal system and destroyed them. Strangely, the drug attacked only the dopaminergic neurones of the nigrostriatal system and nowhere else.

More commonly patients treated with neuroleptic drugs, particularly the older ones, such as chlorpromazine and haloperidol, can develop parkinsonism. This may be reversed if the drug is stopped, and other medications can help alleviate the symptoms if treatment is continued. Sometimes the parkinsonism continues even if the causative drug is stopped.

Drugs Used in the Treatment of Parkinson's Disease

Two main chemical approaches are used:

- to enhance dopaminergic activity
- to reduce cholinergic activity.

Drugs that enhance dopaminergic activity have largely replaced the use of drugs that reduce cholinergic activity, in the treatment of Parkinson's disease. Anticholinergic drugs still have a role in the treatment of parkinsonism, particularly if it is drug-induced.

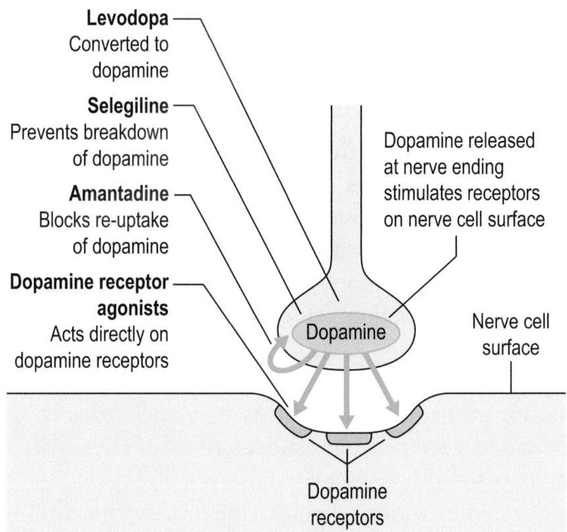

Fig. 21.4 ■ Site of action of dopaminergic drugs used in Parkinson's disease.

Drugs that Enhance Dopaminergic Activity

Drugs that increase dopamine activity (Fig. 21.4) can be subclassified as:

- drugs that replace dopamine
- drugs that act as dopamine agonists (stimulate) at dopamine receptors on nerves in the dorsal striatum normally supplied by dopaminergic nerves from the substantia nigra
- drugs that stimulate the release of dopamine from dopaminergic nerve terminals in the dorsal striatum
- drugs that block the breakdown of dopamine after it has been released from surviving dopaminergic nerve terminals in the dorsal striatum. There are at present two main types:
  - monoamine oxidase inhibitors (MAOIs)
  - drugs that block the enzyme COMT (catechol O-methyltransferase).

Drugs that Replace Dopamine: Levodopa

It is not possible to restore the deficiency in the brain by giving dopamine, as this substance will not enter the brain because it cannot cross the blood–brain barrier. Therefore, **levodopa** is used. This precursor of dopamine passes freely into the brain, where it is converted to dopamine. The dopamine then acts on dopamine receptors wherever they are found in the brain, including those in the dorsal striatum. The drug will therefore have many central actions, resulting in sometimes-troublesome adverse effects (see later). Levodopa is particularly useful in reducing rigidity but has less effect on tremor.

Levodopa and a DOPA decarboxylase inhibitor. Levodopa is broken down by an enzyme called DOPA decarboxylase, which is found particularly in the gut wall and liver. If this enzyme is inhibited by a drug which can be administered in combination with levodopa, the effects of levodopa are enhanced and prolonged and a much smaller dose of levodopa is required. This reduces the incidence of some side-effects. Two preparations that are widely used are:

- levodopa + carbidopa (**co-careldopa**; *Sinemet*)
- levodopa + benserazide (**co-beneldopa**; *Madopar*).

Therapeutic Use. Adverse effects are very troublesome when levodopa is used alone, so treatment is usually started with small doses of either co-careldopa or co-beneldopa. These doses are gradually increased until a satisfactory control of symptoms is obtained, without an unacceptable incidence of adverse reactions to the drug. The intervals between the taking of doses can be critical in determining the severity of adverse effects and will have to be chosen according to the reactions of individual patients to the drug.

The drug's efficacy falls with duration of use. The patient may show slow improvement for the first 6–18 months, and this may be maintained for 1–2 years, but thereafter the medicine loses efficacy. Patients may suffer from the 'on–off' effect. During the 'on' period, the patient walks normally, but during the 'off' period, the patient reverts to the impaired gait of Parkinson's disease. The duration of benefit of the drug often becomes shortened after prolonged use and the frequency of dosing needs to be increased, with a concomitant increase in adverse effects. This is called the 'end-of-dose' effect of levodopa.

Adverse Effects. These comprise nausea and vomiting, a postural fall in blood pressure, restlessness and involuntary facial movements, and constipation. Nausea and vomiting are very common but can be minimized by giving the drug in divided doses with meals. An antiemetic such as domperidone may be given for short periods of time. Metoclopramide and prochlorperazine may worsen Parkinson's symptoms and should not be used. Some postural fall in blood pressure is common, but rarely causes symptoms. Blood pressure should be measured before and during treatment. A few patients become restless and, at higher dose levels, involuntary movements, usually affecting the face, may occur. Constipation requires a good fluid and fibre intake.

Drug Interactions. Levodopa/decarboxylase inhibitor combinations should not be combined with MAOIs. Concomitant use of halothane, cyclopropane or trichlorethylene carries an increased risk of cardiac arrhythmias and the medicine should be stopped 8 hours before anaesthesia.

Drugs that Act as Dopamine Receptor Agonists

Non-ergot derived dopamine receptor agonists:

- Ropinirole
- Pramipexole
- Rotigotine
- Apomorphine.

Ergot-derived dopamine receptor agonists:

- Bromocriptine
- Cabergoline
- Lisuride
- Pergolide.

This group of drugs stimulates dopamine receptors in the cells of the basal ganglia. They are prescribed when treatment with levodopa is ineffective or requires supplementation, but adverse effects can limit their use. There are at least five types of dopamine receptors (called D_1 to D_5), and the more potent agonists act on both D_1 and D_2 and D_3 receptor types.

Non-ergot derived dopamine receptor agonists are the first-line choice for this class of drug and may be the initial treatment in younger patients and those whose motor symptoms are not currently causing a substantial reduction in quality of life. **Ropinirole, pramipexole** or **rotigotine** may all be tried. Ropinirole acts on D_2 receptors and pramipexole acts on D_2 and D_3 receptors. Rotigotine acts on all five currently known dopamine receptors, but particularly D_3. It has the advantage of being available as a drug delivery patch.

Ergot-based dopamine receptor agonists are less safe (see the Safety Point warnings) and are not recommended as first-line treatment. They are less expensive however, and so may be the only option in some health systems. **Bromocriptine** and **cabergoline** are almost identical. Both drugs can cause nausea and postural hypotension, and dosage requires careful adjustment. **Lisuride**, which has a short duration of action, acts mainly on D_2 receptors. **Pergolide**, which has the longest duration of action, acts on both D_1 and D_2 receptors.

SAFETY POINT

All dopamine receptor agonists are associated with increased sleepiness, and sudden onset of sleep. All patients should be warned of this possibility and to use extreme caution when driving or using machinery. If they do suffer from sudden onset of sleep, then they must refrain from driving or operating machinery. The elderly population may be particularly susceptible to adverse events and should be monitored closely for any signs (Latt et al., 2019)

SAFETY POINT

Treatment with any of the dopamine-receptor agonists is associated with impulse control disorders, including pathological gambling, binge eating and hypersexuality (Collins, 2019). Patients and their carers should be informed about the risk of impulse control disorders. The drug may need to be withdrawn or the dose reduced.

Apomorphine is a powerful dopamine receptor stimulant in the CTZ of the brain and has been used as an emetic. It is also sometimes prescribed to control the 'off' period associated with prolonged use of levodopa (see earlier). Treatment is difficult and requires close supervision and considerable patient education. Ideally, it should be initiated in hospital, and domperidone started 3 days before apomorphine to control vomiting. Apomorphine is given by multiple subcutaneous injections or by continuous subcutaneous infusion. A few patients develop postural hypotension, but the most common problem is nausea, which may be difficult to control. Domperidone should not be used long term, as there is a risk of serious cardiac arrhythmias associated with this medication.

SAFETY POINT

The Committee for the Safety of Medicines has advised that all ergot-based dopamine receptor agonists should not be used until the patient has been screened for erythrocyte sedimentation rates and for urea and electrolytes, and chest X-rays and lung function tests may be advisable. This is because this class of drugs has been associated with pericardial, pulmonary and retroperitoneal fibrotic reactions (Gupta et al., 2019).

Drugs that May Stimulate the Release of Dopamine from Dopaminergic Nerve Terminals in the Dorsal Striatum: Amantadine

Amantadine was originally introduced as an antiviral drug for the treatment of influenza. It is believed to work by increasing dopamine release from the nerve terminals and also perhaps by blocking the reuptake of dopamine into the nerve terminal, thereby maintaining concentrations of endogenously released dopamine. The efficacy of this type of drug will decrease with progressive loss of dopaminergic nerves.

Therapeutic Use. Amantadine may be used as an adjunct to other treatments if they are ineffective on their own. It is not commonly used.

Adverse Effects. These include livedo reticularis (skin discoloration), blurred vision, peripheral oedema, dizziness and gastrointestinal disturbances.

Contraindications. The drug is contraindicated in epilepsy, renal disease, pregnancy, breastfeeding and when there is a history of gastric ulceration.

Drugs that Block the Breakdown of Dopamine

These consist of MAOIs, such as selegiline and rasagiline, and COMT inhibitors, such as entacapone, tolcapone and opicapone.

Selegiline and **rasagiline** inhibit the breakdown of levodopa in the brain by selectively blocking the enzyme MAO type B. They are used in combination with levodopa with or without a decarboxylase inhibitor and this allows a smaller dose of levodopa to be used and prolongs its action. Adverse effects include confusion and nausea. Hypertension has been reported with both drugs and there are several important drug interactions, which should be checked for when prescribing. Unselective MAO inhibitors were used to treat depression, although rarely today. Eating foods rich in tyramine (e.g. strong cheeses) have led to severe or fatal hypertensive crises when combined with unselective MAO inhibitors. The risk is less with selective inhibitors, but is noted as a possible risk with selegiline, but not rasagiline.

Entacapone, tolcapone and **opicapone** are drugs that can be used only if levodopa is given as well, since they act by blocking the action of the enzyme COMT, which breaks down levodopa before it crosses the blood–brain barrier and gets into the brain. They are useful when 'end-of-dose' fluctuations in motor activity occur with levodopa (see earlier). Adverse effects include gastrointestinal disturbances, discoloured urine, dyskinesias, dizziness, dry mouth and, rarely, hepatitis. Contraindications include pregnancy and breastfeeding, liver disease and phaeochromocytoma (adrenaline-secreting tumours).

Drugs that Reduce Cholinergic Activity (Antimuscarinic Drugs)

Drugs that reduce cholinergic activity are called 'antimuscarinic' drugs or 'muscarinic receptor antagonists':

- benzatropine mesylate
- biperiden hydrochloride (in some countries only)
- orphenadrine hydrochloride
- procyclidine hydrochloride
- trihexyphenidyl hydrochloride.

Mechanism of Action. These drugs antagonize the action of the excitatory neurotransmitter ACh at its muscarinic receptors in the dorsal striatum, thus allowing dopamine to exert its inhibitory effect (see Fig. 21.2). Since ACh is such a widely used neurotransmitter, both in the brain and elsewhere in the body, these drugs will produce many unwanted adverse effects.

Therapeutic Use of Muscarinic Receptor Antagonists. These drugs reduce tremor, but have less effect on rigidity, which is generally more troublesome for the patient than is the tremor. They were used in mild cases, but they have troublesome adverse effects and have been largely replaced. They are not first-line therapy but may be used as adjunct therapy with dopamine agonists. They have a role in reducing the symptoms of drug induced parkinsonism, but not (antipsychotic) drug induced *tardive dyskinesia*, which can be very troublesome.

Trihexyphenidyl is given orally and the dose is gradually increased until a satisfactory response is obtained or the limit of tolerance is reached. **Orphenadrine** has the advantage of having a mood-lifting effect, as well as relieving the symptoms of parkinsonism. This is useful as these patients are often depressed. **Benzatropine** is in many ways similar to trihexyphenidyl. It is particularly useful for the excessive salivation often found in parkinsonism and for muscular rigidity. It is liable to cause drowsiness and is best given as a single dose at bedtime.

Adverse Effects. These include nausea, constipation, giddiness and falls, dry mouth, urinary retention and glaucoma; in overdose, confusion and hallucinations may also occur. The elderly are particularly sensitive to these effects. There is an association between the use of antimuscarinic drugs and an increased risk of developing dementia. It is not known if this is a causal association, but this has nonetheless contributed to a marked fall in the use of these drugs.

The Treatment of Parkinson's Disease

Levodopa in the form of co-careldopa or co-beneldopa is the first-line treatment for patients whose motor symptoms significantly impact their quality of life. For those patients whose symptoms are less troublesome, a dopamine receptor agonist may be offered, or a MAOI. These drugs are less effective than levodopa, but the response fluctuations, end of dose effects and dyskinesias are less problematic. Unfortunately, sleepiness (including sudden falling asleep) and impulse control disorders are more common with these drugs.

About three-quarters of patients with Parkinson's disease respond to drugs. Rigidity is usually most amenable to treatment and tremor less so. Unfortunately, in more than half the patients being treated by levodopa, its efficacy decreases with time, so that increasingly frequent dosage is required to maintain its effect and prevent the 'on–off' phenomenon, during which there are periods of weakness and loss of movement. These fluctuations can be reduced by frequent dosage or by using a controlled-release preparation. Adjunctive medication is often required as levodopa becomes less effective. A non-ergot dopamine agonist is the preferred additional drug. If this fails, a COMT or MAOI can be added to the regimen.

Family Needs in Parkinson's Disease

It is highly likely that when a patient develops Parkinson's disease, a progressively greater burden will be placed on a partner, who may be infirm through age (Theed et al., 2017). It is the responsibility of all healthcare professionals who are involved to be concerned not only about the patient but also about whether the family is coping with the problem. Specialist nurses and organizations such as the Parkinson's Disease Society and European Parkinson's Disease Society play critical and highly effective roles in this respect and the family should be put in touch with concerned groups.

Surgical Treatments in Parkinson's Disease

Neural Transplantation

Great interest was generated in the 1970s when it was discovered that fetal brain tissue could be successfully transplanted into the adult brain and function normally. On this basis, several attempts have been made to transplant human fetal tissue containing dopaminergic neurones into the brains of patients with Parkinson's disease. The results have been variable, despite the proven ability of fetal grafts to be integrated into the patient's brain. The use of human fetal tissue has raised many problems and issues, including ethical ones. Scientists are now experimenting with stem cells and animal nerve cells that produce dopamine.

Pallidotomy (Pallidectomy)

Pallidotomy is the introduction of electrodes into the brain to destroy a particular part of the brain in an area called 'the globus pallidus', which contains cells that are involved in the generation of unwanted movements. It fell out of favour when levodopa was introduced but now it is being used again because modern imaging techniques now make it possible to pinpoint with greater accuracy the cells to be destroyed.

Pallidotomy is indicated mainly for patients who develop dyskinesia due to their drugs. There are risks with this procedure, including the possibility of stroke, partial loss of vision or speech, confusion and swallowing difficulties.

Deep Brain Stimulation

This procedure is based on that of the cardiac pacemaker. It involves placing electrodes into specific brain areas, specifically the globus pallidus or the thalamus. As with pallidotomy, the aim is to stop uncontrollable movements. The electrodes are connected to a pacemaker-like device that the patient can switch on or off, depending on the symptoms.

REFERENCES AND FURTHER READING

Buse, D.C., Fanning, K.M., Reed, M.L., et al., 2019. Life with migraine: effects on relationships, career, and finances from the chronic migraine epidemiology and outcomes (CaMEO) study. Headache J. Head Face Pain 59 (8), 1286–1299.

Collins, T.R., 2019. Impulse control behaviors affect one fifth of patients with Parkinson's disease, study finds. Neurol. Today 19 (15), 30–31.

Gupta, H.V., Lyons, K.E., Pahwa, R., 2019. Old drugs, new delivery systems in Parkinson's disease. Drugs Aging 36 (9), 807–821.

Honavar, A.G., Anuranjana, A., Markose, A.P., et al., 2019. Profile of patients presenting with seizures as emergencies and immediate noncompliance to antiepileptic medications. J. Family Med. Prim. Care 8 (12), 3977–3982.

Kovosi, S., Freeman, M., 2011. Administering medications for Parkinson disease on time. Nursing 41(3), 66.

Latt, M.D., Lewis, S., Zekry, O., Fung, V.S.C., 2019. Factors to consider in the selection of dopamine agonists for older persons with Parkinson's disease. Drugs Aging 36 (3), 189–202.

Marmura, M.J., 2018. Triggers, protectors, and predictors in episodic migraine. Curr. Pain Headache Rep. 22 (12), 1.

Pooja, M.R., Ailani, J., 2017. Diagnosis and treatment of migraine. J. Clin. Outcomes Manag. 24 (11), 516–526.

Theed, R., Eccles, F., Simpson, J., 2017. Experiences of caring for a family member with Parkinson's disease: a meta-synthesis. Aging Ment. Health 21 (10), 1007–1016.

Yoo, S., Lim, K., Baek, H., et al., 2020. Developing a mobile epilepsy management application integrated with an electronic health record for effective seizure management. Int. J. Med. Inform. 134, 104051.

USEFUL WEBSITES

Epilepsy Action. https://www.epilepsy.org.uk.

Institute for Safe Medication Practices (ISMP). https://www.ismp.org/guidelines/timely-administration-scheduled-medications-acute.

National Institute for Health and Care Excellence (NICE). https://www.nice.org.uk/guidance.

Parkinson's UK. https://www.parkinsons.org.uk.

Royal College of Nursing. Parkinson's disease. https://www.rcn.org.uk/clinical-topics/neuroscience-nursing/parkinsons-disease.

22 DRUGS USED IN PSYCHIATRIC DISORDERS

Antipsychotics, Antidepressants, Anxiolytics, Hypnotics and Anti-dementia drugs

CHAPTER OUTLINE

LEARNING OBJECTIVES

At the end of this chapter, the reader should be able to:

- identify some brain neurotransmitter receptors known to be important targets for drug action in psychiatry
- discuss the special implications of administering drugs to patients with mental health problems
- give an account of classification of antipsychotic drugs into first and second generation antipsychotics, provide examples and discuss their use and adverse effects
- talk about the nature of schizophrenia and its management
- discuss acute confusional state, its causes, diagnosis, treatment and patient care
- give an account of the classification of anxiety disorders, anxiolytic drugs and treatment of anxiety disorders
- describe insomnia and talk about its treatment with different hypnotic drugs
- learn about depression, its causes and brain neurotransmitters involved
- give an account of treatment of depression with drugs (including details of SSRIs, MAOIs, tricyclics and other antidepressants) and ECT
- understand mania/bipolar disorder and learn about its management including use of lithium
- give an account of dementia and the drugs used to treat Alzheimer's disease
- know what is meant by ADHD and its treatment with various drugs

INTRODUCTION

Mental illness is one of the major causes of ill health. Many drugs have been produced in the hope that they would have some therapeutic effect. Certain mental illnesses, particularly depression and schizophrenia, are linked with chemical abnormalities in the brain. The nature of some of these abnormalities is known, but there are considerable gaps in our knowledge. Nevertheless, the knowledge gleaned so far from medical research has resulted in the introduction of drugs that are designed to target brain mechanisms that may alleviate some of the symptoms of mental illnesses. This chapter describes the different drugs used in various psychiatric disorders.

TYPES OF MENTAL ILLNESS

The treatment of psychiatric disorders can be considered in terms of three main types of disorders: psychosis, anxiety and depression (although there are other types of mental disorders discussed later).

Psychosis is a term used to describe disorders when the patient loses contact with reality. Features of psychosis may include hallucinations (perceptual disturbance), delusions (false fixed beliefs), altered behaviour, speech and thought disturbance.

Anxiety is a term often used to describe a condition of excessive worry or fear. It is featured by an emotionally inappropriate response to the patient's environment and to circumstances. Traditionally, patients were termed 'neurotic' but this term is no longer favoured. Commonly used professional terms to describe the symptoms of anxiety include social phobia, agoraphobia, panic disorder, generalized anxiety disorder, etc. Anxiety and depression can often coexist.

Depression is a term used for several disorders that are characterized by changes in mood, thoughts and behaviour. Professionals describe depression as an affective disorder. Symptoms can range from extreme sadness to suicidal intent. It can sometimes occur with manic disorder and then the condition is termed 'bipolar disorder'.

BRAIN NEUROTRANSMITTERS AND PSYCHIATRIC DISORDERS

Many of the drugs that have been introduced for the treatment of psychiatric disorders are known to interfere with the normal action of several of the brain neurotransmitters and their receptors. The major brain neurotransmitters that have been implicated in psychiatric disorders are:

- acetylcholine (ACh)
- adrenaline
- noradrenaline
- dopamine
- 5-hydroxytryptamine (5-HT; serotonin)
- GABA (gamma-aminobutyric acid)
- neuropeptides.

The amounts of adrenaline and noradrenaline are increased in the brain by giving drugs such as monoamine oxidase inhibitors (MAOIs), which are drugs that retard their breakdown. Tricyclic antidepressants (TCAs) inhibit the reuptake of catecholamines into the nerve terminals. Thus, an awakening and stimulating effect is produced, and these drugs are used as antidepressants. If the amounts of catecholamines in the brain are reduced, a tranquillizing or depressing effect is produced. 5-HT is also concerned with mood, whereas GABA exerts a sedating inhibiting effect. Dopamine stimulates more than one class of receptors: it causes nausea and vomiting, but also appears to be concerned with the psychotic state. In fact, the evidence suggests that the efficacy of many antipsychotic drugs can be correlated, approximately, with their ability to block dopamine D_2 receptors (see later).

ADMINISTRATION OF DRUGS TO PSYCHIATRIC PATIENTS

General Points

- In psychiatric units, many people with mental health problems are not confined to bed and drugs may be administered at a central point on the ward rather than having a 'drug round' around the ward.
- Two nurses should always be involved with drug administration.
- In psychiatric units, patient compliance may be a problem and it is necessary to ensure that medication is actually taken. For example, patients may put the tablets in their mouths, but spit them out when no longer observed by the nurse.
- In some patients, especially people suffering from schizophrenias, drugs may be given by injection as depot preparations to get round the problem of non-compliance.
- Occasionally, a patient's paranoia may extend to drugs they are given and they may think the staff are trying to poison them.
- Drug education for when the patient returns home is very important and relatives may have to be involved. Non-compliance is an important hazard as the patient's illness may relapse if treatment is stopped. It should also be possible for patients or relatives to have contact numbers to call for information if problems arise.
- The nurse should observe the effects and side-effects of drug treatment.
- On discharge, care should be taken not to prescribe excessive quantities of drugs, particularly if there is a suicide risk.

ANTIPSYCHOTIC DRUGS

Classification of Antipsychotic Drugs

Traditionally, antipsychotic drugs such as chlorpromazine (see later) have been referred to as *major tranquillizers*, while anxiety-suppressing drugs such as the benzodiazepines have been called *minor tranquillizers*. Antipsychotic drugs have also been called *neuroleptics*. These terminologies are generally no longer in favour and will not be used here. Antipsychotic drugs, because of their diverse chemical nature and wide range of pharmacological actions, are notoriously difficult to classify but the following classification may be helpful:

- **First generation antipsychotic (FGA) drugs**, which are generally those that have been in use for many years (often referred to as typical antipsychotics).
- **Second generation** antipsychotic (SGA) drugs, which are more recent additions to the repertoire of drugs available (often referred to as atypical antipsychotics).

Examples of first generation (typical) antipsychotic drugs:

- benperidol
- chlorpromazine
- flupentixol
- fluphenazine
- haloperidol
- levomepromazine
- pericyazine
- perphenazine
- pimozide
- pipotiazine
- prochlorperazine
- promazine hydrochloride
- sulpiride
- trifluoperazine
- zuclopenthixol acetate
- zuclopenthixol dihydrochloride.

Examples of second generation (atypical) antipsychotic drugs:

- amisulpride
- aripiprazole
- clozapine
- iloperidone
- lurasidone
- olanzapine
- paliperidone
- quetiapine
- risperidone
- sertindole.

This list is not exhaustive and other antipsychotic drugs are also licensed in some countries.

Mechanism of Action of Antipsychotic Drugs

Virtually all antipsychotic drugs have so many different pharmacological actions that it is very difficult to relate any one action to a therapeutic effect. The only statement that can be made with reasonable confidence is that most, if not all, effective antipsychotic drugs share the ability to block dopamine D_2 receptors in the brain.

These drugs are particularly useful in controlling the psychotic symptoms in disorders such as schizophrenia, schizoaffective disorder, mania and depression. Their exact mode of action in these conditions is not known but most of them block the action of dopamine on D_2 receptors in the mesolimbic system of the brain, which seems important in antipsychotic action and can cause sedation (Fig. 22.1). Therefore, some of these can be used for tranquillization and sedation. They also block the action of dopamine on the brain chemoreceptor trigger zone and can have antiemetic action. Some, such as haloperidol (see later), block the action of the dopaminergic nerves that run from the substantia nigra to the corpus striatum. Interruption of this system causes parkinsonism and such drugs may cause various disorders of movement and posture. There are new hypotheses emerging with ongoing research.

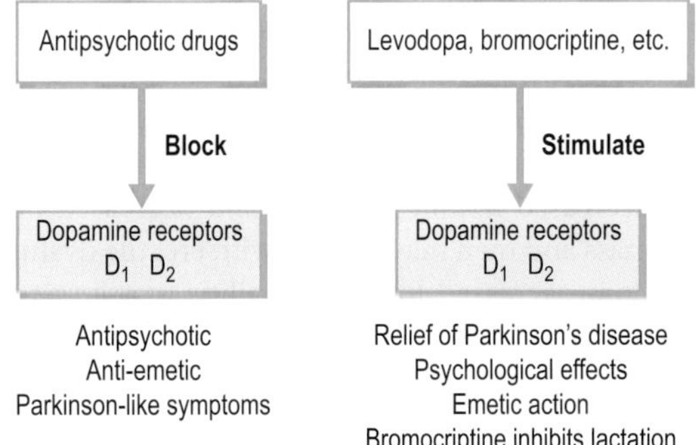

Fig. 22.1 ■ Effect of drugs on dopamine receptors in the brain. The exact part played by D_1 and D_2 receptors and other subgroups is not known.

FIRST GENERATION ANTIPSYCHOTIC DRUGS

The first generation antipsychotic drugs (FGA) are:

- phenothiazines
- thioxanthenes
- butyrophenones
- other antipsychotics.

Phenothiazines

Therapeutic Uses and Effects

Phenothiazines have an antipsychotic effect. Restlessness, agitation and hallucinations are reduced, and this has made this class of drug especially useful for treating schizophrenia. They can produce sedation with a feeling of detachment from external worries. Chlorpromazine is sometimes used to control persistent hiccup. Most of the phenothiazines are well absorbed after oral dosage. They are largely metabolized in the liver to numerous breakdown substances.

Like other antipsychotics, they can sometimes be used for tranquillization. They are, in addition, used as antiemetics, in severe pruritus and may be used in association with anaesthetic agents. A number of phenothiazines are now in use; some are preferred for one type of disorder and some for another. They have been classified according to their sedative, antimuscarinic and extrapyramidal symptoms (Box 22.1).

The doses of these drugs are very variable and depend on the disorder being treated, and on the response and age of the patient. In long-term administration, it is not worth altering the dose more than once a week, because of their variable and prolonged actions.

BOX 22.1
CLASSIFICATION OF PHENOTHIAZINES

GROUP 1

- Chlorpromazine
- Levomepromazine (methotrimeprazine)
- Promazine
  - Sedation ++++, antimuscarinic ++, extrapyramidal ++

GROUP 2

- Pericyazine
- Pipotiazine
- Thioridazine
  - Sedation ++, antimuscarinic ++++, extrapyramidal ++

GROUP 3

- Fluphenazine
- Perphenazine
- Prochlorperazine
- Trifluoperazine
  - Sedation ++, antimuscarinic ++, extrapyramidal ++++

Key: ++, few to moderate effects, ++++, marked effects.

In treating psychotic patients, large doses of phenothiazines are often used and if it helps in symptom control, then these drugs should be continued long term. This means that a careful watch must be kept for adverse effects, especially those involving the nervous system.

Adverse Effects

Adverse effects with phenothiazines are not uncommon and the incidence varies from drug to drug. Various phenothiazine derivatives may exhibit antihistaminic, adrenergic blocking, anticholinergic or metabolic-endocrine actions (Hollister, 1964). Some of the side-effects include:

- **Various disorders of movement**, commonly known as **extrapyramidal symptoms (EPS)**, due directly or indirectly to a dopamine-blocking action in the brain, are noted here:
  - Drug-induced **parkinsonism**, can present with symptoms like slow initiation of movement, tremor at rest, rigidness of muscles, shuffling gait and reduced facial expressions
  - **Akathisia**, which is a feeling of restlessness with an inability to stay still
  - Acute **dystonia**, which is uncontrolled abnormal body movements (sporadic and sustained muscle spasm) and often develops very soon after commencing the antipsychotic
  - **Tardive dyskinesia (TD)**, commonly consists of uncontrolled abnormal movements of facial parts but it can involve any other part of the body. It develops in some patients, usually after long-term antipsychotic use. Control is difficult and it may not stop even if the drug is withdrawn.

These extrapyramidal symptoms require a reduction of antipsychotic dose and/or change to an alternative antipsychotic with low propensity to cause EPS, if possible. Antimuscarinic drugs (i.e. procyclidine hydrochloride, trihexyphenidyl hydrochloride) can help with acute dystonia and parkinsonism.

- Rarely, **neuroleptic malignant syndrome (NMS)** may occur, which can be life-threatening and requires urgent treatment (often the general medical hospital setting). The research NMS diagnostic criteria in the *Diagnostic and Statistical Manual of Mental Disorders* (4th edition) are noted as follows: development of severe muscle rigidity and elevated temperature associated with the use of neuroleptic medication and two (or more) of the following: changes in level of consciousness ranging from confusion to coma, tachycardia, elevated or labile blood pressure, diaphoresis, dysphagia, tremor, incontinence, mutism, leucocytosis and laboratory evidence of muscle injury (e.g. elevated CPK).
- **Hyperprolactinaemia** (raised serum prolactin level). Women can present with symptoms of oligomenorrhoea, amenorrhoea, galactorrhoea, decreased libido, infertility and decreased bone mass and men may present with erectile dysfunction, decreased libido, infertility, gynecomastia, decreased bone mass but rarely galactorrhoea (Majumdar and Mangal, 2013).
- **Antiadrenergic and anticholinergic effects:** see Tricyclic antidepressants section, later.
- **Cardiac abnormalities.** Phenothiazines therapy has been attributed to surface electrocardiogram

(ECG) changes (lengthening of the QTc interval, ST-T wave changes, increased size of U waves and prolongation of the PR interval) and various arrhythmias, where numerous cases of sudden death as a result of fatal arrhythmia have been described (Elkayam and Frishman, 1980).
- **Antihistaminergic effects** such as body temperature dysregulation, sedation (greatest with chlorpromazine), increased appetite (causing weight gain), etc.
- Depressed leucocyte count.
- Skin rashes, including light sensitivity and contact dermatitis when the drug is handled. A sunscreen is advised with chlorpromazine.
- Jaundice, which occurs with chlorpromazine and is due to blocking of the bile canaliculi in the liver. It is presumed to be an allergic effect, and recovery occurs when the drug is stopped.

Antipsychotics may lower seizure threshold, may be linked to venous thromboembolism (including deep vein thrombosis, pulmonary embolism) and can cause NMS. Data from 10 meta-analyses indicate that the use of antipsychotics among individuals with dementia results in a greater number of adverse effects when compared with placebo-treated individuals, including cerebrovascular adverse events and deaths (Tampi et al., 2016).

CLINICAL NOTE

Staff should avoid contact with chlorpromazine (tablets should not be crushed) because of the risk of contact sensitization.

Thioxanthenes

These are somewhat similar to the phenothiazines. They are antipsychotic and antiemetic, and are mainly used in the treatment of schizophrenia. They are less sedative than the phenothiazines, but akathisia and some side-effects, noted earlier, are common. An example is **flupentixol**, which is used as an injected depot preparation every 2 weeks, or daily as tablets.

Butyrophenones

This group of drugs has actions similar to those of the phenothiazines. They are less sedative, but are liable to produce EPS and some of the side-effects noted under phenothiazines. **Haloperidol** is particularly useful in the management of psychotic, manic or delirious patients (see later). Before commencing haloperidol, baseline ECG should be obtained and regular ECG monitoring is required during treatment (for QTc interval and rhythm abnormalities).

Other Antipsychotics

Pimozide is an antipsychotic drug used in the treatment of schizophrenia and manic states. It is longer-acting and less sedative than chlorpromazine. Pimozide can cause dangerous cardiac side-effects and should not be given to those with cardiac abnormalities. An ECG should be taken before starting treatment and repeated periodically during treatment as required.

Sulpiride causes less EPS compared with other first generation antipsychotics, although some of the other side-effects noted earlier are common including hyperprolactinemia, weight gain, sedation and liver enzyme abnormality.

SECOND GENERATION ANTIPSYCHOTIC DRUGS

Second generation antipsychotic (SGA) drugs differ from first generation antipsychotic (FGA) drugs in a few ways. In some of these drugs, D_2-blocking action may be confined to those areas of the brain believed to be concerned with schizophrenia (the mesolimbic system), which results in a lower incidence of prolactin secretion from the pituitary gland. In addition, they may also block serotonin (5-HT) and adrenoreceptors. EPS are more common in FGA drugs compared with SGA drugs, although may occur with almost all antipsychotics at different doses. Many SGA drugs (and some FGA) are likely to cause metabolic syndrome (e.g. weight gain, diabetes, dyslipidaemia and hypertension) leading to higher risk of cardiovascular diseases. As noted in the NICE guidance on schizophrenia (see later), regular monitoring of all these parameters is required with antipsychotic treatment. FGA and SGA drugs have many other common side-effects (as noted in the phenothiazine section, previously). A brief description of some SGA drugs is given here.

Clozapine is used for patients who have not benefitted from other antipsychotic drugs and is very effective in the treatment of schizophrenia. Due to its significant side-effects, its use should be under the supervision of an appropriate specialist and reserved for specific patients where alternate treatment strategies are not available (and where there are no contraindications for its use). Prior to its initiation, comprehensive assessment and relevant investigations need to be undertaken, including a range of blood tests (especially leucocytes and absolute neutrophil count). Leucocyte and absolute neutrophil count should continue to be mandatorily monitored regularly during treatment.

It is essential to be mindful of concomitant use of other drugs, products (i.e. smoking, caffeine) or medical conditions, which can interact with clozapine or exacerbate its side-effects. Clozapine should be started with cautious titration and a divided dosage schedule to minimize the risk of side-effects. Measurement of clozapine blood levels should be considered as required (i.e. suspected potential interactions, symptoms of toxicity, inefficacy).

Constipation, hypersalivation, sedation, tachycardia and dizziness are very common adverse effects. Agranulocytosis, cardiovascular effects, seizure and fever are its most serious side-effects. A lot of the information and advice given here on clozapine has been noted from 'Clozaril 100 mg tablets – Summary of Product Characteristics (SPC) - (eMC)'; Medicines.org.uk, 2020. Please refer to this SPC to understand the suitable context of this information and advice and for further details.

Risperidone blocks several receptors in the brain, including dopamine receptors. It is useful in the treatment of schizophrenia, mania and short-term management of aggression in certain conditions. Some side-effects often witnessed include increased weight, hyperprolactinaemia, tachycardia and hypertension. EPS are dose-dependent and more likely at higher doses.

Olanzapine is an effective drug commonly used for treating schizophrenia and mania. Some of the frequent side-effects include drowsiness, weight gain, postural hypotension, dyslipidaemia and diabetes.

Aripiprazole has a different mode of action – it is a partial agonist of D_2 receptors. It is also helpful in treating schizophrenia and mania and has a better side-effect profile compared with the previously mentioned drugs. It is less likely to cause symptoms like sedation (can cause akathisia at start of treatment, as well as insomnia and anxiety), weight gain and hyperprolactinemia but quite a few of the antipsychotic side-effects noted earlier can occur.

Quetiapine and asenapine are also used in treatment of schizophrenia and mania. Iloperidone is related in structure to risperidone.

DEPOT INJECTIONS

Several antipsychotic drugs are given as depot injections (including fluphenazine, flupentixol, zuclopenthixol, haloperidol, aripiprazole, risperidone, paliperidone and olanzapine), because patients with severe mental disease often fail to take their pills regularly. It also gives the option of not taking oral drugs daily. Patients should be involved in the choice of taking depot medication as far as possible. The depot dosage scheme is inflexible and there is difficulty if a patient develops some adverse effect. Depot preparations are usually given by deep muscular injection in the gluteal muscle, lateral thigh or deltoid muscle, depending on the depot licence indication. The injection sites must be regularly changed, e.g. alternating between right and left side of the body and a Z-tracking technique should be used (see Chapter 2). A test dose should be given when advised in the drug SPC. These injections may be very painful, and seepage of fluid can result in inaccurate dosage unless the injection technique is well executed.

CLINICAL NOTE

Do not forget the adverse effects of this group of drugs, particularly those affecting the nervous system and the metabolic syndrome. With long-term use, careful surveillance is also required on withdrawal of treatment, as the re-emergence of psychiatric symptoms may be delayed for several weeks.

CLINICAL NOTE

Special care is needed if antipsychotics are given to:

- patients with Parkinson's disease, as symptoms may be increased

- patients with epilepsy or patients with alcohol withdrawal symptoms, as fits may be precipitated
- elderly patients, who may get postural hypotension and are more prone to other side- effects
- pregnant and lactating mothers.

TREATMENT OF SCHIZOPHRENIA

Introduction

The ICD-10 Classification of Mental and Behavioural Disorders identifies different schizophrenic disorders, e.g. paranoid schizophrenia, hebephrenic schizophrenia, catatonic schizophrenia, undifferentiated schizophrenia, etc. Paranoid schizophrenia is the most common type in most parts of the world. Its features (as noted in ICD-10) usually include paranoid delusions, auditory hallucinations and other perceptual disturbances. 'Negative' symptoms such as blunting of affect, reduced speech, apathy and impaired volition are often present but do not dominate the clinical picture.

Theories about Schizophrenia

There are several theories as to the cause of schizophrenia. It seems most likely that it is a complex biochemical disorder in the brain. The fact that symptoms can be relieved in many patients by dopamine-blocking drugs supports the view that it is due to overactivity of the dopaminergic system, probably involving D_2 receptors in the mesolimbic system of the brain. However, not all patients respond to D_2-receptor antagonists and other receptors are probably involved. The idea that it is a disorder of personality development due to faulty interaction with the family in early life is not valid, although it is probably made worse, or even precipitated, in susceptible individuals by periods of stress and difficulty, and possibly after using drugs of abuse such as ecstasy and cannabis.

Management of Patients with Schizophrenia

The comprehensive management of patients with schizophrenia has many facets, but the introduction of antipsychotic drugs has greatly improved treatment, enabling many patients to take their place in the community and lead a reasonable life. However, drugs alone are not enough, and very efficient psychosocial measures are required to ensure that patients are properly supported in the community. Psychological interventions that can be offered include cognitive behavioural therapy (CBT) and family therapy.

CLINICAL NOTE

- Psychiatric multidisciplinary team members play a very important role supporting patients with schizophrenia and their families.
- A patient with schizophrenia receiving appropriate drugs may well behave normally but there may be a catastrophic relapse if treatment is stopped suddenly.
- Diagnosis of a psychotic disorder is a specialized task and the dangers of misdiagnosis are highlighted in Case History 22.1.

NICE Recommendations for Schizophrenia

Some of the recommendations made in the National Institute of Health and Care Excellence (NICE) guidelines for the prevention and management of psychosis and schizophrenia in adults (NICE, 2014) are noted here (please refer to this NICE guidance to understand the suitable context for following recommendations and for further details):

- The choice of antipsychotic medication should be made by the patient and healthcare professional together, after providing information and discussing the likely benefits and possible side-effects of each drug. Medication review should happen subsequent to a trial of the medication at optimum dosage for 4–6 weeks.
- Before starting antipsychotic medication and during treatment, the following investigations need to be made: weight, waist circumference, pulse, blood pressure, fasting blood glucose, glycosylated haemoglobin (HbA_{1c}), blood lipid profile and prolactin levels. Consideration should be given for doing an ECG if required.
- Clozapine should be offered to people with schizophrenia whose illness has not responded adequately to treatment, despite the sequential use of adequate doses of at least two different antipsychotic drugs. At least one of the drugs should be a non-clozapine second generation antipsychotic.

CASE HISTORY 22.1

Marina, a 15-year-old girl, who previously had been quiet, cheerful and studious, began to act irrationally at home. She developed a bad temper and started stealing from home and from shops. She became violent and terrorized her family. This alternated with periods of relative calm. Her parents sought medical advice and a psychiatrist diagnosed schizophrenia. She was placed on olanzapine, which sedated her and she had excessive weight gain. Her family continued to remain concerned about Marina several years on and followed up with her general practitioner about her episodes of psychosis and her inability to lead a normal life. In addition, she was complaining of headaches, dizziness and memory loss, for which she was subsequently referred to a neurologist. Following further investigations with blood tests and an MRI brain scan, she was diagnosed with cerebral lupus. The neurologist informed the family that the disease was causing occlusion of blood flow in the brain. She was prescribed high-dose steroids along with an anticoagulant. Her symptoms improved, which subsequently resulted in a significant improvement in her quality of life.

LESSONS:

- Psychotic behaviour may not necessarily be due to a disorder of CNS origin.
- Lupus can present as psychotic behaviour.
- Continuing professional development is an important modern feature of clinical practice.

ACUTE CONFUSIONAL STATE

Acute confusional state (ACS) is also called 'delirium' by some practitioners. It is a state of impaired cognition, self-awareness and attention that is often superimposed on an underlying disease and is more common in elderly people.

Aetiology

Acute confusional state has many causes. This may be part of a psychiatric illness, but may also develop as a result of a serious 'organic' illness or it may be due to drug dependence, e.g. alcohol withdrawal. The symptoms of ACS may be worsened during periods of intense stress, sleep disruption or as part of adverse reactions to antipsychotic drugs, especially in older patients. Examples of underlying conditions and drugs that cause ACS are summarized here.

Examples of underlying conditions:

- anoxia
- hyperkalaemia
- hyperparathyroidism
- hypoglycaemia
- hypokalaemia
- hypothyroidism
- metabolic acidosis
- post-concussion
- post-ictal state (an ictus is a stroke or sudden seizure)
- transient ischaemia.

Drugs:

- anticholinergic drugs; antiemetics; drugs for Parkinson's disease
- alcohol and other CNS depressants, e.g. digoxin; antihypertensive drugs; benzodiazepines.

This list is far from comprehensive, but alerts the reader to the fact that several different classes of drug are able to cause ACS. It is therefore important to identify and manage the possible underlying cause or combination of causes.

Diagnosis

It is extremely important to diagnose ACS quickly and treat the underlying illness, as a considerable number of hospitalized elderly people who develop ACS die and patients who develop ACS are likely to stay longer in hospital than those who do not develop it.

The American Psychiatric Association's 5th edition of the *Diagnostic and Statistical Manual of Mental Disorders* (DSM-5) considers disturbance in attention, awareness and cognition as essential diagnostic factors. It is noted in DSM-5 that the disturbance develops over a short period of time (usually hours to a few days), represents an acute change from baseline attention and awareness and tends to fluctuate in severity during the course of a day. It is mentioned that these disturbances are not better explained by a pre-existing, established or evolving neurocognitive disorder and do not occur in the context of a severely reduced level of arousal such as coma. Also, there should be evidence from the history, physical examination or laboratory findings that the disturbance is a direct physiological consequence of another medical condition, substance intoxication or withdrawal (i.e. due to a drug of abuse or to a medication), or exposure to a toxin, or multiple aetiologies.

Treatment

NICE guidance on delirium (NICE, 2010) suggests that if a person with delirium is distressed or considered a risk to themselves or others, first use verbal and non-verbal techniques to de-escalate the situation. If the de-escalation techniques are ineffective or inappropriate, consider giving short-term haloperidol (usually for 1 week or less, started at the lowest clinically appropriate dose and titrated cautiously according to symptoms). Use of antipsychotic drugs is advised with caution, and avoidance is recommended for people with conditions such as Parkinson's disease or dementia with Lewy bodies. (Please refer to this NICE guidance to understand the suitable context for these recommendations and for further details.)

It is important that such patients are nursed in quiet surroundings. The nurse's approach must be calm and as much explanation given as is feasible, and the nurse should try to ascertain the patient's degree of awareness of the situation (Andersson et al., 2002). Patients may be highly agitated, especially if this is a temporary and unusual experience (Fagerberg and Jonhagen, 2002).

If possible, drugs should be given orally. Chlorpromazine should not be given intramuscularly (IM) as it forms deposits in the muscle and may also cause hypotension.

ANXIETY

Anxiety is a universal phenomenon and a certain amount is useful to the individual, acting as a stimulant and increasing efficiency. However, when it becomes disproportionate to the stimulus, an anxiety state develops, and this degree of anxiety may interfere seriously with the patient's life.

Types of Anxiety Disorders

The ICD-10 Classification of Mental and Behavioural Disorders classifies several different types of anxiety disorders, including:

- **Phobic anxiety disorders** feature anxiety evoked, predominantly by certain well-defined situation or objects, which are not currently dangerous. Agoraphobia pertains to fear of not only open spaces but also of related aspects such as presence of crowds and the difficulty to immediately escape to a safe place. Social phobia incorporates fear of scrutiny by other people in comparatively small groups, usually leading to avoidance of social situations. Specific phobias are restricted to highly explicit situations such as proximity to animals, heights, flying, closed spaces, etc.
- **Generalized anxiety disorder (GAD)** incorporates generalized and persistent anxiety which is not restricted to any particular environmental circumstance (e.g. it is 'free floating').
- **Panic disorder** features recurrent panic attacks (attacks of anxiety), which are not restricted to any particular situation or set of circumstances, and which are therefore unpredictable.
- **Obsessive compulsive disorder** is characterized by compulsive behaviours (repetitive stereotyped actions) and/or obsessional thoughts (repetitive stereotyped ideas, images or impulses). These are unpleasant and unsuccessfully resisted by the person. For example, the feeling that one needs to check things more than once, such as whether the front door was locked on going out or the light or the gas hob was switched off.
- **Post-traumatic stress disorder** is the anxiety that follows traumatic experiences, e.g. rape or warfare.

Apart from anxiolytic medication, psychological interventions (e.g. self-help strategies, psychoeducation, cognitive behavioural therapy, applied relaxation, exposure and response prevention therapy, etc.) are well-known treatments for many anxiety disorders. Depending on the disorder and individual circumstances, these can be offered on their own or in conjunction with drug treatment.

NICE Guidance on Pharmacological Treatment of Anxiety Disorders

NICE guidelines on generalized anxiety disorder (GAD) and panic disorder in adults (NICE, 2011) recommends the use of a suitable selective serotonin reuptake inhibitor (SSRI) as first-line treatment. In GAD, if SSRIs are ineffective (or cannot be used) then a serotonin–noradrenaline reuptake inhibitor (SNRI) can be offered, if appropriate. Pregabalin can be considered as the next line of treatment. In panic disorder, imipramine or clomipramine may be considered if SSRI is not helpful. NICE guidance on social anxiety disorder (NICE, 2013) recommends that for adults with social anxiety disorder, SSRI (escitalopram or sertraline) should be initially considered. If this is not tolerated or is ineffective, then an alternative SSRI can be used considering licence indications (fluvoxamine or paroxetine) or an SNRI (venlafaxine). NICE guidance on obsessive-compulsive disorder (NICE, 2005) suggests that SSRI should be the initial choice and if this is not effective then a different SSRI or clomipramine should be offered. (Please refer to these NICE guidelines to understand the suitable context for these recommendations and for further details.)

ANXIOLYTIC DRUGS

Anxiolytic drugs comprise:

- antidepressants
- benzodiazepines
- buspirone
- β-blockers.

Antidepressants

Antidepressants are dealt with in more detail later in this chapter. As noted earlier, there is a good evidence base for effectiveness of SSRIs in treating anxiety disorders. In the tricyclic antidepressants, clomipramine has a strong effect on serotonin reuptake inhibition. Venlafaxine is an antidepressant with serotonin and noradrenaline reuptake inhibition.

Benzodiazepines (BZDs)

Examples include:

- alprazolam
- chlordiazepoxide
- clorazepate
- diazepam
- lorazepam
- oxazepam.

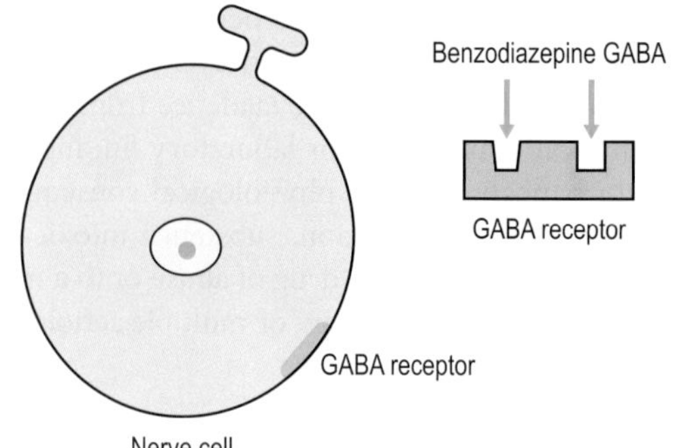

Fig. 22.2 ■ Gamma-aminobutyric acid (GABA) and benzodiazepine receptors are closely related. Benzodiazepines enhance the inhibitory action of GABA.

Mechanism of Action

It is believed that BZDs act on the reticular formation and limbic system in the brain. BZDs act at GABA receptors in the brain where they appear to enhance the action of this inhibitory neurotransmitter to depress brain function (Fig. 22.2).

Therapeutic Use of BZDs

In addition to their use as hypnotics (usually shorter-acting drugs), this group of drugs has been used for the treatment of anxiety (usually longer-acting drugs). Their use as hypnotics is described later. BZDs should only be used for acute agitation, panic attacks and for anxiety if it is severe and disabling, and the treatment should be at the lowest effective dose, preferably for no more than 2 weeks, and is often combined with other treatment. Previously, they have been used in the treatment of acute emotional crises, but, by preventing the patient from responding to the painful situation, they may delay psychological adjustment. Although the BZDs are effective in relieving anxiety, tolerance may develop with their use and they become less effective with prolonged use. They can lead to development of physical and psychological dependence. If the drug is stopped suddenly, even after a relatively short period of use (e.g. 2–3 weeks), about one-third of patients will develop some withdrawal symptoms. These can include anxiety and sleeplessness for a few days, but after prolonged and heavy dosage, may include symptoms like seizures, psychotic symptoms, muscle pains, twitching, etc.

They usually occur within a week of stopping the drug and earlier if it is short-acting. This suggests that dependence has developed and in severe cases, patients may take some months to recover. Patients, therefore, require slow and stepwise withdrawal of this drug class over several weeks.

Other Uses

BZDs have other uses:

- Diazepam and lorazepam can also be given intravenously (IV) for treating status epilepticus (see Chapter 21) and diazepam and midazolam have been used as sedatives before various invasive investigations, e.g. bronchoscopy.
- Diazepam has some muscle-relaxing properties and is used in combination with an analgesic to relieve pain and spasm in patients with lumbago and related disorders.
- Dentists sometimes use diazepam IV in patients when carrying out prolonged procedures.

The BZDs are metabolized in the liver and often produce further active compounds. For example, diazepam is partially converted to desmethyldiazepam, which also has a prolonged sedative action. Duration of action is also dependent on the dose and, to some degree, on the individual. Although the actions of many of these drugs are very similar, the price varies considerably.

Nitrazepam was the first BZD to be recommended as a hypnotic drug. Although it has been claimed that this drug is unlikely to confuse elderly patients, this is not necessarily true. In addition, some sedative effect may persist well into the following day.

Diazepam is more often used as an anxiolytic drug, but it is a fairly good hypnotic if there is some background anxiety and sedation lasting into the next day is needed.

Temazepam has a shorter half-life and length of action than most other BZDs and it does not produce metabolites that are also hypnotics. It is, therefore, less liable to cause drowsiness into the next day.

Flunitrazepam has a fairly prolonged action. Because it is tasteless, it can be added to drinks, etc. and sadly has gained a reputation for being used when rape is intended. It is not commonly prescribed in the UK.

Adverse Effects and Interactions

Common side-effects among all BZDs include drowsiness, lethargy and fatigue; at higher dosages – impaired motor coordination, dizziness, vertigo, slurred speech, blurry vision, mood swings and euphoria can occur, as well as hostile or erratic behaviour in some instances (Griffin et al., 2013). Controlled studies and systematic reviews have shown that BZD administration can result in dose-dependent effects such as sedation, drowsiness, anterograde amnesia (difficulty in forming new memories) and mental slowing (Baldwin et al., 2013). Elderly patients are more vulnerable to the cognitive and psychomotor effects of BZDs (they also eliminate long-acting drugs more slowly than younger patients), and an increased risk of falls should be considered when contemplating possible BZD prescription to such patients (Baldwin et al., 2013). Respiratory depression is more likely with IV administration and may also happen in an overdose of oral BZDs. Diazepam is an irritant when given IV and should be given as an emulsion (*Diazemuls*). Caution/contraindications should be considered when thinking of using BZDs with other CNS depressants (e.g. alcohol), in certain medical conditions (e.g. severe respiratory insufficiency, sleep apnoea syndrome) and other drugs that potentiate the action of BZDs as there may be worsening of BZD side-effects. They may cause fetal abnormalities when taken in pregnancy. Depending on the drug used, the patient should be given appropriate advice on driving.

Flumazenil is a BZD antagonist. It is given intravenously and reverses BZD-induced sedation in a few minutes. It has been used in the treatment of BZD overdose and to speed recovery in patients who have been anaesthetized with midazolam. However, its effect only lasts about 1 h, so repeated doses may be required with long-acting BZDs.

Buspirone

Buspirone is an anxiolytic belonging to the azapirone group of drugs, working at the 5 HT1A receptor. It has been used in GAD. Buspirone appears to have no sedative action or risk of dependence. Its adverse effects appear to include occasional nausea and headache. Its onset of action is delayed for about 2 weeks and it seems to be ineffective in treating the symptoms of BZD withdrawal.

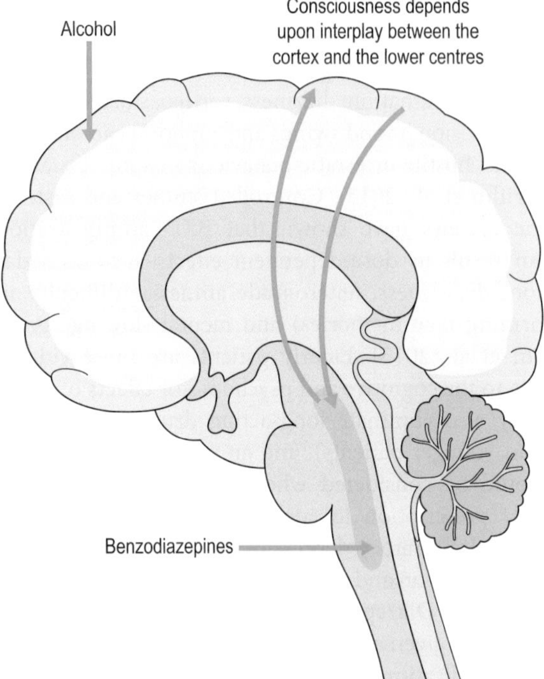

Fig. 22.3 ■ The mode of action of hypnotic drugs and tranquillizers.

β-Blockers

β-Blockers such as **propranolol** suppress some of the physical symptoms of anxiety (like tremor and palpitations) and have been used for this indication.

INSOMNIA

Anxiety and insomnia are, on the face of it, two different problems, and yet are treated in many cases by the same types of drugs. Insomnia can cause feelings of anxiety, inability to concentrate and general debility. Sleep requirements vary with age. Teenagers need about 10 h of sleep, adults about 8 h and the elderly about 6 h, but there is also considerable person variation.

Hypnotics are drugs that produce sleep comparable with normal sleep (Fig. 22.3). However, they do not relieve pain. Before prescribing hypnotics it is important to ascertain whether the patient is getting enough sleep and enquiring about the quality of sleep, since some people exaggerate their insomnia. The sleep disturbance should be occurring frequently and causing marked suffering or interference with day-to-day functioning. It is necessary to find out if there is some reason for failing to sleep. These reasons may include:

- anxiety and stress
- depression
- physical illness, e.g. heart failure, chronic lung disease and sleep disordered breathing
- pain
- use of caffeine, alcohol, nicotine or illegal drugs
- use of medications that may interfere with sleep (i.e. steroids).

If these problems are remedied, sleep should occur naturally. Various simple measures can be tried: e.g. a walk, a bath, a rather unexciting book before retiring or a glass of milk at bedtime may be sufficient. More comprehensive programmes to encourage sleep are detailed by Espie (1993).

Although hypnotic medicines may be required in some circumstances, e.g. during periods of stress or for certain chronic insomniacs, their use should be discouraged. Tolerance to their action often develops in 2–3 weeks with some degree of dependence. Withdrawal at this stage can lead to increasing wakefulness at night for a few days or longer. This is particularly important in hospitals, where they are sometimes too freely prescribed and where a lifetime of habituation to these medicines may start. Patients should not, as a general rule, be sent home from hospital with hypnotic medicines.

The Nature of Sleep

Sleep is not just a state into which one lapses on going to bed and from which one emerges on waking. It is a series of cycles, each lasting about 90 min. In a normal sleeping pattern, after falling asleep, a person becomes progressively more relaxed with slow pulse and respiration rate; this phase lasts about 80 min and ultimately the state of 'deep sleep' is reached. Then follows a phase lasting about 10 min, with dreaming, atonic skeletal muscles, rapid eye movements and increased heart rate, known as rapid eye movement (REM) sleep. The whole cycle is then repeated about six times per night. It has been shown that if a subject is deprived of REM sleep, he or she will show psychological changes during waking hours. Many centrally acting drugs and alcohol do in fact suppress REM sleep and thus do not really produce a completely natural sleep.

Treatment Guidelines for Insomnia

Some of the recommendations made in the European guideline for the diagnosis and treatment of insomnia (Riemann et al., 2017) are as follows (please refer to this guidance to understand the suitable context of following recommendations and for further details):

- Cognitive behavioural therapy for insomnia (CBT-I) is recommended as first-line treatment for chronic insomnia in adults of any age. Benzodiazepines and benzodiazepine receptor agonists are effective in the short-term treatment of insomnia (≤4 weeks) if CBT-I is ineffective or unavailable.
- Sedating antidepressants are effective in the short-term treatment of insomnia.

Hypnotic Drugs

Hypnotic drugs fall into the following categories:

- zaleplon, zopiclone and zolpidem
- benzodiazepines (BZDs)
- melatonin receptor agonists
- sedating antidepressants
- promethazine
- other hypnotics.

Zaleplon, Zopiclone and Zolpidem

These short-acting 'Z-drugs' are BZD receptor agonists. Although differing in structure from the BZDs, they also bind to the BZD receptors and increase the sedating activity of GABA in the brain. These drugs are equally effective as BZDs (see European insomnia guidelines in the previous section) and some of their side-effects are similar to BZD adverse effects. As mentioned earlier, they are recommended only for short-term insomnia treatment. The lowest effective dose should be utilized. These drugs are quite similar to each other. They may produce tolerance and dependence, and the risk of these (and withdrawal symptoms, rebound insomnia) is likely to increase with higher dose and treatment duration. They are not recommended for pregnant/breastfeeding women or children under 18. Increased drowsiness is experienced if used with other central depressants such as alcohol or BZDs. Depending on the drug used, the patient should be given appropriate advice on driving. The following is a brief description of these drugs:

Zopiclone has an elimination half-life of around 3.5–6.5 h and produces sleep lasting 6–8 h. Some common side-effects include somnolence the next day, bitter metallic taste and dry mouth.

Zolpidem has an elimination half-life of around 2.5 h. In a randomized placebo-controlled trial, the side-effects from zolpidem noted were excessive day-time drowsiness, tiredness, headache, body aches, nausea/vomiting, diarrhoea, constipation and dry mouth (Sharma et al., 2019).

Zaleplon has an elimination half-life of 1 h and is useful in insomnia where there is a problem falling asleep. Some of the side-effects are similar to those of the afore-mentioned drugs.

BZDs

Several members of this group of drugs can be used as a hypnotic. There is very little to choose between them in terms of efficacy, the main difference being in their duration of action. BZDs with a prolonged action may produce a hangover effect the next day if given in a dose sufficient to produce sleep. (See other details about BZDs in the Anxiety section.)

Melatonin Receptor Agonists

Melatonin is a hormone produced in the body, assisting in the body's sleep cycle. A synthetic version of melatonin is available in immediate release and sustained release form. In the UK, the sustained release form is licensed only for primary insomnia in people aged 55 years or over. Side-effects are not often encountered but some uncommon ones may include headache, drowsiness, dizziness, etc.

Sedating Antidepressants

Some examples include: trazodone, doxepin, mirtazapine, amitriptyline and trimipramine. (See further details about these later in this chapter.)

Promethazine

Promethazine is an H1 receptor antagonist and by blocking the action of histamine in the brain, it produces sleep. It is sometimes used as a hypnotic drug and is available without prescription in the UK. It is not a particularly good hypnotic, having rather a long action, with sedation the next morning. It also has some antimuscarinic side-effects. The evidence for its effectiveness is poor.

Other Hypnotics

The popularity of other hypnotics such as chloral hydrate and clomethiazole has declined over time and there appears to be poor evidence supporting their use.

CLINICAL NOTE

Dependence can occur with long-term use of some hypnotics. Use the minimum dose for the minimum time. Depression can cause insomnia.

SEDATIVES PRIOR TO MINOR PROCEDURES

Patients often require some sedation before invasive procedures, e.g. gastroscopy, bronchoscopy, etc. BZDs are useful because they are both sedative and also produce amnesia for the event. Diazepam is used intravenously, e.g. in dentistry. It is, however, irritant to the vein. A specially prepared non-irritant emulsion of diazepam (*Diazemuls*; see also earlier) is preferable.

Alternatively, **midazolam**, which has an action lasting about 2 h, can be given. Following injections of this type, the patient should be warned not to drive until the next day and to avoid alcohol and other CNS depressants. With regard to adverse effects and interactions, there have been a number of reports of respiratory depression and cardiac arrest after midazolam, especially in elderly patients, who do not eliminate the drug as rapidly as younger subjects. This is usually due to excessive dosage and care should be taken. The action of midazolam is increased when used with erythromycin.

DEPRESSION

Occasional sadness is a common and normal emotion and people naturally become sad as a result of unfortunate domestic and social conditions. Sometimes, however, the low mood and negative associated features are disproportionate to the precipitating factors (or there may be no obvious cause at all) and lead to depression. The ICD-10 Classification of Mental and Behavioural Disorders notes that depressed mood, loss of interest and enjoyment, and increased fatigability are usually regarded as the most typical symptoms of depression. Other common symptoms of depression identified in the ICD-10 are disturbed sleep, reduced appetite, ideas of guilt and self-harm, hopelessness, diminished concentration and reduced self-esteem. These symptoms can have characteristic features such as early morning awakening, weight loss, worsening of depression in the mornings, loss of libido and psychomotor agitation or retardation. Psychotic symptoms may be present in severe depression and suicide is a special risk in all depressed patients.

Psychosocial Causes of Clinical Depression

Clinical depression may possibly be an eventual result in some individuals who experience the following stressors:

- social, economic or relationship difficulties (i.e. family problems, bereavement, isolation, financial, accommodation or employment issues)
- substance misuse (i.e. alcohol, recreational drugs)
- chronic or severe physical health problems
- other triggers that adversely impact the individual and they find it hard to adapt to these difficulties.

Brain Neurotransmitters and Depression

The aetiology of depression is not known, but there is evidence that a major factor is a reduction in the amount of neurotransmitter amines such as 5-HT

(5-hydroxytryptamine; serotonin) or noradrenaline at the junctions between neurones in the brain. Many of the drugs used to treat depression increase the amount of these substances in the brain, thus providing some evidence that amines are connected with changes of mood. With research, there are other hypotheses emerging.

Management of Depression

A variety of psychological and behavioural treatments have been used in depression (including cognitive behaviour therapy, behavioural activation, interpersonal psychotherapy, problem-solving therapy and guided self-help). It is worth considering these in combination with pharmacological treatment or on their own, taking into account the patient's presentation and preference. Patients need to be reviewed regularly at the start of antidepressant treatment to assess effectiveness and side-effects of the drug. Mania/hypomania (see later) symptoms may be triggered by antidepressant treatment.

The following groups of drugs are used to relieve depression:

- selective serotonin reuptake inhibitors (SSRIs)
- tricyclic antidepressants (TCAs)
- tricyclic anxiolytics
- monoamine oxidase inhibitors (MAOIs)
- other antidepressants.

British Association for Psychopharmacology Guidelines for Depression Management

There follows some of the recommendations made in the revised version of the 2008 British Association for Psychopharmacology (BAP) evidence-based guidelines, specifically for treating depressive disorders with antidepressants. (Please refer to this BAP guidance to understand the suitable context of these recommendations and for further details; Cleare et al. 2015):

- There is most evidence for SSRIs which, together with other newer antidepressants, are first-line choices.
- In more severely ill patients, and in other situations where maximizing efficacy is of overriding importance, consider clomipramine, venlafaxine (≥150 mg), escitalopram (20 mg), sertraline, amitriptyline or mirtazapine, in preference to other antidepressants.

Selective Serotonin Reuptake Inhibitors

Serotonin (5-HT) is a neurotransmitter concerned with mood and behaviour, and a deficiency of serotonin in the brain is believed to be a factor in depression. Several SSRI drugs have been introduced, which specifically inhibit serotonin reuptake at nerve junctions and thus raise its concentration in the brain. They are recommended as first-line treatment in depression and many anxiety disorders. Their examples include:

- citalopram
- escitalopram
- fluoxetine
- fluvoxamine
- paroxetine
- sertraline.

Adverse Effects. Advantage of SSRIs lies in the lack of many of the adverse effects of the older tricyclics as they generally do not cause cardiotoxicity (therefore are less dangerous in overdose), hypotension, anticholinergic effects and weight gain.

In most studies, the commonest side-effects from SSRIs compared to placebo have been nausea, diarrhoea, tremor, sexual dysfunction, sweating and reduced appetite (Cookson, 1993). Some of the most frequently reported gastrointestinal side-effects associated with the use of SSRIs (and SNRIs) include nausea, diarrhoea, dyspepsia, gastrointestinal bleeding and abdominal pain (Carvalho et al., 2016). SSRIs can prolong QT interval, which can be a concern (Funk and Bostwick, 2013). Some other side-effects can be troublesome such as abnormal bleeding (including gastrointestinal bleeding), hyponatremia, headaches and insomnia. SSRIs can cause serotonin syndrome (see later), which may have varying presentation and severity, with clinical findings such as high blood pressure, tachycardia, akathisia, tremor, altered mental state, clonus, muscular hypertonicity, hyperthermia, etc. (Boyer and Shannon, 2005). Paroxetine can have prominent withdrawal symptoms

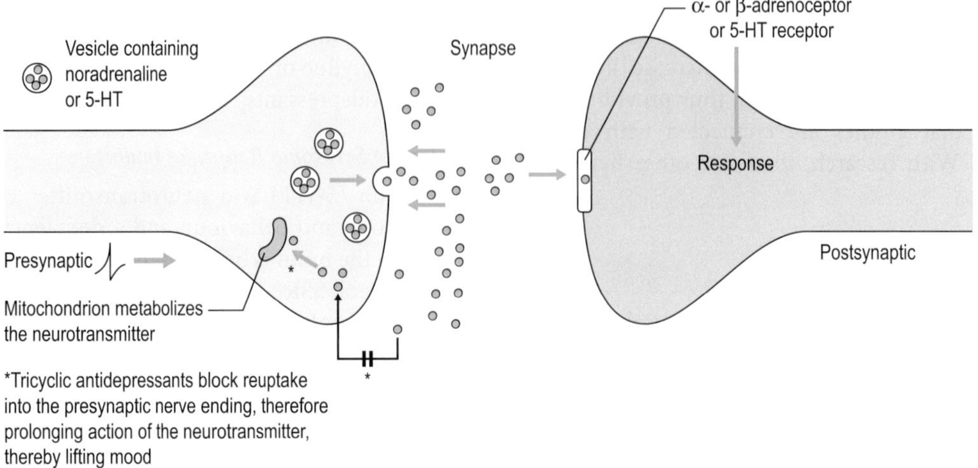

Fig. 22.4 Mechanism of action of the tricyclic antidepressants.

so has to be gradually discontinued. Various hypersensitivity reactions can occur with fluoxetine and may herald a serious vasculitis.

Contraindications, Interactions and Precautions. SSRIs should not be used if a depressed patient becomes manic. They should be used with caution in epileptic patients, since they can precipitate seizures, which may be prolonged with fluoxetine, particularly if the patient is receiving ECT. They may precipitate adverse reactions in diabetic patients and patients with cardiac disease or angle-closure glaucoma. They should be used with caution in patients with a history of gastrointestinal/other bleeding problems or who have renal or hepatic disease. SSRIs should not be prescribed with irreversible MAOIs and caution is advised in concomitant prescription (and switching prescriptions) with other serotonergic drugs, as that could cause serotonin syndrome.

Caution in SSRI prescription is required when there are other factors that can exacerbate these side-effects and risks.

Tricyclic Antidepressants

TCAs comprise:

- amitriptyline
- clomipramine
- desipramine
- imipramine
- lofepramine
- nortriptyline
- protriptyline.

There are several TCAs in use and there is not a great deal of difference between them. Therefore, a few representative drugs will be considered here. They are well absorbed after oral administration and undergo considerable breakdown in the liver; some of these metabolic products are therapeutically active. It is believed that they produce their therapeutic effect by preventing the reuptake of amines at nerve endings in the brain, which thus increases the concentration of these substances available for receptor uptake (Fig. 22.4).

Some members of the group (i.e. nortriptyline and desipramine) have a greater effect on noradrenaline concentration, and others (i.e. imipramine and amitriptyline) on 5-HT concentration. Clomipramine is closer in its action to SSRIs (predominant effect on 5-HT and much less on noradrenaline).

Imipramine and Amitriptyline

Imipramine was the first of these drugs to be used. Amitriptyline is very similar to imipramine, but is rather more sedating. If amitriptyline is given in the evening, its sedative action will help sleep, which is often disturbed in depression. Both these drugs have a long action (need only be given once a day) and have prominent anticholinergic effects. Imipramine is actually a prodrug and is metabolized to the active drug, namely, **desipramine** (see earlier).

Therapeutic Use. After starting treatment, the sleep disorders associated with depression usually respond fairly quickly, but it is important to remember that it may take several weeks before depression is relieved. Treatment should therefore be continued for around 6 weeks before deciding that treatment has failed, as about 80% of depressed patients will ultimately respond. TCAs are also used in the treatment of pain of obscure origin, such as atypical facial pain.

Bedwetting. Imipramine is used for nocturnal enuresis (bedwetting) in children. It is important to explain to the child's parents that:

- the effect may be delayed for 2–3 weeks
- the tablets must be stored in a childproof place
- treatment should not usually be given for more than 3 months.

Adverse Effects of TCAs

Some of the side-effects of TCAs are noted here:

- **Heart:** TCAs depress conduction in the heart, and a number of sudden deaths have been reported in patients with heart disease taking these medicines. It can have other cardiovascular side-effects and are therefore best avoided in this group of patients.
- **Antiadrenergic effects:** postural hypotension is a fall in blood pressure with occasional faintness, especially observed in elderly patients. Other problems can present like dizziness, tachycardia, etc.
- **Increased appetite**, **sedation** and **weight gain.**
- **Anticholinergic effects:** dry mouth can be troublesome and may be mitigated by lemon juice. Difficulty with micturition (especially in elderly), and constipation can be a problem, particularly in depressed patients already preoccupied with their bowels. Owing to a dilating effect on the pupil of the eye, TCAs should not be given to patients with glaucoma. There can be other symptoms, e.g. blurred vision, tachycardia, skin reactions.
- **Overdose:** TCAs are dangerous in overdose, producing a variety of symptoms including cardiovascular disturbance, seizures and coma.
- **Withdrawal symptoms** may develop if these drugs are stopped suddenly.
- As with some other antidepressants, it can precipitate hypomania/mania (especially when there is history of mania or bipolar disorder).

CLINICAL NOTE

Drug interactions. TCAs have interactions with other drugs, including antiepileptics, sympathomimetic drugs (but not local anaesthetics) and with other antidepressants and MAOIs. They may reverse the effect of some hypotensive agents and their action is enhanced by alcohol, so care should be taken when combining tricyclics with these drugs.

Tricyclic Anxiolytics

Doxepin and **dosulepin** are similar to the TCAs, but have a weaker antidepressant action and are particularly useful when anxiety complicates mild depression. They are also more rapidly effective than the standard tricyclics. Doxepin has been used for sleep problems (see earlier). Adverse effects are similar to those of the tricyclics, but generally can be less marked. They are still dangerous in overdose.

Maprotiline is not a tricyclic drug, but is an amine reuptake inhibitor. Its action and adverse effects profile is very similar to that of the tricyclics. It is also cardiotoxic.

SPECIAL POINTS FOR PATIENT EDUCATION

- Patients must understand that the response to treatment may be delayed by up to 6 weeks with tricyclics.
- They should be told of the possible adverse effects and how to make the best of them.
- They must be informed of the important interactions and how to avoid them.
- They must realize that most of these drugs are dangerous in overdose.

CLINICAL NOTE

Non-adherence is an important cause of treatment failure in the treatment of patients with depression. If accidental or deliberate overdose occurs, among other measures, a patient should be monitored using a cardiac monitor and regular full nursing observations.

Monoamine Oxidase Inhibitors

These drugs inhibit the enzyme monoamine oxidase (MAO) and lead to accumulation of noradrenaline and 5-HT in the brain.

Phenelzine and **isocarboxazid** are *irreversible inhibitors*, which means that they bind to MAO and do not detach themselves from the enzyme so the new MAO enzyme has to be biosynthesized to replace it.

Moclobemide, on the other hand, is a *reversible inhibitor*, as it binds to MAO and inhibits the action of this enzyme but detaches itself so that the enzyme can resume its normal function of metabolizing amines. This renders it somewhat safer than the irreversible inhibitors, since there is less chance of potentiating other drugs that are amines, or interfering with the normal metabolism of amines in the diet. Nevertheless, moclobemide is associated with many and potentially dangerous adverse effects.

Therapeutic Use. They can be used in the treatment of typical and atypical depression and some anxiety disorders. They are not the first-line treatment for depression. The long list of possible adverse effects limits their usefulness and they should only be prescribed by those who are familiar with the problems that may arise. All three drugs are taken orally in tablet form. They are initially usually given twice or three times daily and the dose reduced if possible, depending on the patient's response.

Adverse Effects. MAOIs can cause, among other problems, postural hypotension, insomnia, jaundice and sedation. Orthostatic hypotension can be managed with slow titration of the drug, divided dosing, or increased fluid intake; insomnia with adjustments in time of dosing and sedation (more likely with phenelzine) with dosing schedule alteration (Fiedorowicz and Swartz, 2004). Phenelzine can cause agitation and psychotic episodes with hypomania. All MAOIs can cause weight gain but phenelzine may have more of this adverse effect (Rabkin et al., 1984) and dietary advice may help. Sexual dysfunction, cardiovascular and hepatic complications may occur. There can be several side-effects observed with MAOIs but only some of these are mentioned here and this is not a comprehensive list.

Interactions. Interactions are important and can be dangerous. Some of these include:

- MAOIs may exaggerate the effects of centrally acting drugs such as the barbiturates, alcohol, cocaine, morphine and particularly pethidine (meperidine). If a surgical operation is to be undertaken, when it may be necessary to give such drugs as morphine or pethidine (meperidine), the MAOIs should be stopped 2 weeks previously.
- They lead to over action by vasopressors such as adrenaline (epinephrine) and amphetamine and a number of vasoconstrictor drugs, some of which are included in widely used 'cold-remedies', e.g. ephedrine and phenylephrine. The results may include symptoms such as headaches, hypertension, restlessness and even coma and death. Consequential hypertensive crisis (severe increase in blood pressure, which can cause damage to different organs in the body) is a dangerous possibility with such indirect sympathomimetic agents.
- Similar effects may also occur if these MAOIs are taken with various items of food, including cheese, meat, yeast extracts, some wines and beers, game, broad bean pods and pickled herrings. This is because these foods contain naturally occurring vasopressor substances that are normally broken down by MAO. If this breakdown is inhibited, the vasopressors accumulate and produce toxic effects such as a hypertensive crisis, as described previously.
- Their administration with serotonergic drugs such as SSRIs, TCAs and SNRIs can cause complications such as serotonin syndrome (see earlier).

There should be an adequate gap between these drugs and prescription of MAOIs (i.e. 5 weeks between treatment with fluoxetine and MAOIs).

- Similar to some other antidepressants, they may reduce seizure threshold.

Therefore, MAOIs should not be administered together with drugs/substances that increase the aforementioned risks. The utmost care must be taken in prescribing and administering MAOIs. Patients (and their carers) should be informed of the potential dangers associated with these drugs and their interactions with other substances (all relevant information in this regard is not provided here). Hospitals often have their own policies listing restrictions and cautions when administering MAOIs.

Other Antidepressants

There are several other antidepressants which act by modifying the amount of amines in the brain, but do not fit the previous pharmacological categories. These antidepressants are briefly described here.

Trazodone has a mixed action on 5-HT receptors. It is an antidepressant and also an anxiolytic. Among other things, postural hypotension and sedation can be problematic (although it is sometimes used as a hypnotic). It does not have significant cardiovascular side-effects but can increase QT interval.

Venlafaxine is a combined 5-HT and noradrenaline reuptake inhibitor that is effective in depression and some anxiety disorders (see earlier). Its benefits and side-effects are dose-dependent. Many of its side-effects are similar to SSRIs. Some of the most frequently reported gastrointestinal side-effects associated with the use of SNRIs include nausea, diarrhoea, dyspepsia, gastrointestinal bleeding and abdominal pain (Carvalho et al., 2016). Venlafaxine use has been associated with clinically significant increases in diastolic blood pressure of up to 15 mmHg from baseline (Carvalho et al., 2016); therefore regular blood pressure monitoring is required. It can have significant withdrawal symptoms (so gradual discontinuation required). It should not be prescribed with MAOIs due to risk of serotonin syndrome (see earlier).

Mirtazapine increases the concentration of noradrenaline and 5-HT in the brain and, by blocking some types of 5-HT receptors, has a more specific action on depression. It appears to be about as effective as the older antidepressants, but with a low incidence of side-effects. Among others, weight gain and sedation can be troublesome adverse effects.

CLINICAL NOTE

A persistent headache is often a warning of rising blood pressure in a patient taking MAOIs.

ELECTROCONVULSIVE THERAPY

ECT is the passing of electric current through the brain, which actually causes a convulsion or seizure. The modern method is to pre-treat the patient with a muscle relaxant and apply general anaesthesia so that the patient is not conscious during the procedure and the violence of the spasm is avoided. Electrodes are placed on the brain and the current is applied. The patient may experience side-effects, which include headache, confusion and loss of memory afterwards, but these effects usually soon wear off. Applying the electrodes unilaterally to the non-dominant hemisphere of the brain can reduce these after-effects. ECT is used for clinical depression and occasionally for mania or catatonia.

The combined use of drugs and ECT is illustrated in Case History 22.2.

MANIA/BIPOLAR DISORDER

The ICD-10 Classification of Mental and Behavioural Disorders notes the following major categories in this section. The hypomanic or manic episode involves symptoms including elevation of mood, increased energy and activity, disinhibition and disturbance of work and social activity. Details of depression symptoms have been mentioned in the depression section earlier. Bipolar disorder may have episodes (more than one) of hypomania, mania, depression and/or mixed episodes. The manic and severe depressive episodes can be with or without psychotic symptoms.

CASE HISTORY 22.2

Mr. G, aged 55, was made redundant by his company. He had been a highly energetic and successful executive, but was the casualty of a takeover by another company. He tried to get another job but was consistently unsuccessful. He gradually sank into a depression with anxiety symptoms and the presentation worsened over time. His general practitioner prescribed an SSRI antidepressant, which helped with his depressive symptoms to a certain extent, but he developed troublesome side-effects of sexual dysfunction and gastrointestinal bleeding, making his anxiety worse. He was referred to a psychiatrist, who requested psychotherapist input and replaced the SSRI with a sedating tricyclic antidepressant. In the meantime, he developed psychotic symptoms, becoming convinced that his stomach and intestines were rotting and stopped food and fluid intake. The psychiatrist admitted him to the psychiatric unit, added an antipsychotic to treat the delusions and several sessions of ECT were administered. Nursing staff (initially on the ward and then in the community) closely supported him in his recovery. Thanks to the input of his family and the coordinated efforts of the multidisciplinary team treating him, Mr. G gradually came through this trying period. After about a year since the onset of first psychiatric symptoms, with help from an occupational therapist, he became well enough to set up his own consultancy business. There was no reoccurrence of psychiatric symptoms and the psychotherapist and psychiatric team also discharged him after a year of community input.

LESSONS:

- Family and multidisciplinary professional support are possibly more important than drugs in helping people recover successfully from psychiatric disorders.
- Psychoactive drugs may cause further problems, exacerbate existing ones and cannot be expected to solve problems, such as those of Mr. G, without non-pharmacological measures and holistic care planning (such as psychotherapy, occupational therapy, family and nursing support).

Drugs such as antipsychotics, anticonvulsants (i.e. sodium valproate, lamotrigine and carbamazepine) and lithium have been used for treatment and relapse prevention of these disorders. Antidepressant drugs may pose a risk of triggering a hypomanic/manic episode in these disorders, so have to be used with great caution and in specific situations, under specialist supervision.

Antipsychotic drugs are mentioned earlier in this chapter and the anticonvulsant drugs mentioned here are described in Chapter 21.

Lithium

The body treats lithium in a similar way to sodium. It is believed to modify neurotransmission in the brain and increase levels of serotonin and choline, among other changes.

Therapeutic Use

Lithium salts are used prophylactically, i.e. as a preventative measure, for unipolar and bipolar depression and for prophylaxis or treatment of mania. Lithium will control acute mania, but is slow to produce a therapeutic effect and haloperidol (or some other antipsychotics) may be preferred in this situation. The decision to prescribe lithium is not taken lightly in view of its potential risks (see later) and specialist advice must be sought.

Preparations

The following preparations are used:

- lithium carbonate tablets
- lithium citrate liquid
- slow-release lithium carbonate tablets (i.e. *Priadel*).

Before starting lithium, and regularly during its use, it is important to carry out tests such as renal function and thyroid function (see later). Also monitoring of electrolytes, weight and cardiac function (i.e. ECG if required) is beneficial. If renal function is impaired, then lithium excretion is reduced, which may lead to toxicity symptoms (see later).

Whatever the preparation prescribed, the dose must be adjusted to achieve a safe yet effective lithium blood serum concentration. If the slow-release preparation is used, the tablet must be swallowed whole. Because lithium is excreted slowly, it takes some days of treatment before a steady plasma level is reached and it is usual to start measuring plasma levels 1 week after starting treatment. In clinical practice guidelines, there is consensus that the ideal lithium plasma concentration for maintenance and monitoring of lithium is 0.6–0.8 mmol/L (however, this consensus varies in atypical presentations and special populations), along with the need for regular monitoring of renal and endocrine function (Malhi et al., 2017). A blood sample is taken 12 h after the last dose (trough level) but the sample should not be collected in tubes that use lithium heparin as the anticoagulant. Lithium blood levels have to be monitored regularly during treatment, especially around initiation of the drug, dose changes or concerns about its effectiveness or side-effects. Lithium has a low therapeutic index, i.e. blood levels not much above therapeutic levels are dangerous. For example, plasma concentrations above 1.5 mmol/L are often linked to toxicity symptoms, which can include serious complications.

Abrupt lithium withdrawal may increase risk of relapse.

Adverse Effects. Table 22.1 shows some of the overdose and non-dose related side-effects of lithium. Few other possible adverse effects of lithium are noted here but this is not a complete list. Long-term lithium treatment is associated with gradual decline of renal functioning (eGFR) by about 30% more than that associated with ageing alone (Tondo et al., 2017). Goitre occurs in up to 40% and hypothyroidism in about 20% of the patients treated with lithium (Lazarus, 2009). Tremor, nausea, diarrhoea, thirst and excessive urination are common side-effects, that can be easier to manager, but weight gain and cognitive impairment tend to be more distressing to patients and more difficult to manage (Gitlin, 2016). In mild lithium toxicity, symptoms include diarrhoea, poor concentration, worsening tremor, mild ataxia and weakness (Gitlin, 2016). As Table 22.1 suggests, more severe symptoms can include drowsiness, confusion, etc. and even cause death. It can have teratogenic effects causing cardiac and other abnormalities, therefore women of child-bearing age should be advised of this and about effective contraception when taking lithium.

TABLE 22.1

Some Adverse Effects of Lithium

Overdose	Not Dose-related
Weakness	Thyroid deficiency
Drowsiness	Increased urine secretion
Confusion	Weight gain
Coma	

Drug Interactions

Only some of the drug interactions with lithium are described here. If a thiazide or loop diuretic is combined with lithium, the excretion of lithium by the kidney is reduced and toxicity may develop. Under these circumstances, the dose of lithium must be reduced and the plasma level carefully monitored. Interaction can occur with non-steroidal antiinflammatory drugs and angiotensin-converting enzyme inhibitors (causing increased lithium levels), and also with some other antidepressants (causing serotonin syndrome). Patients must be counselled and advised on how to avoid dietary regimens that unduly change sodium input or excretion, the importance of adequate fluid intake and other measures to reduce risk of lithium toxicity. Also, they should be informed about toxicity symptoms and how to get urgent help. Anything that depletes the body of sodium increases the chances of toxicity. This includes not only diuretics but also prolonged vomiting or diarrhoea.

SPECIAL POINTS FOR PATIENT EDUCATION

- Different preparations of lithium vary in their bioavailability and patients should receive only one preparation. They should also maintain a reasonable fluid intake.
- Record cards are available for patients taking lithium.

DEMENTIA

Dementia is the progressive loss of cognition and normal brain function. The most common cause of dementia is Alzheimer's disease. Some other forms of dementia are alcohol-related dementia, Lewy body dementia, Pick's disease and vascular dementias (including multi-infarct dementia, which is the most common vascular dementia). All these diseases damage and kill neurons and other cell types in the CNS.

In **Alzheimer's disease**, a protein called 'amyloid' forms plaques and Tau protein forms neurofibrillary tangles in the brain. The cause of Alzheimer's disease is unknown. Some forms of Alzheimer's disease that affect people under 65, and build-up of amyloid protein in the brain, may be inherited. The clue that led to a treatment with some modest alleviation of symptoms was the discovery that Alzheimer's disease is associated with the loss of neurons containing acetylcholine (the cholinergic system) in parts of the brain associated with memory. Glutamatergic neurotransmission is also affected in this disease.

Non-pharmacological treatment should be tried in dementia, including environmental interventions, psychosocial adjustments, staff/carer education and training in dementia. Data from 10 meta-analyses indicate that the use of antipsychotics among individuals with dementia results in a greater number of adverse effects when compared with placebo-treated individuals, including cerebrovascular adverse events and deaths (Tampi et al., 2016). Therefore, cautious prescription of antipsychotics is required in dementia, weighing risks and benefits. Due to their mode of actions, the majority of antipsychotics can lead to severe adverse reactions in people with Lewy body dementia and Parkinson's disease dementia.

Symptoms of Dementia

The symptoms of dementia reflect the area of the brain that is damaged.

In Alzheimer's disease, for example, the degenerative changes seem to target brain areas responsible for short-term memory, while initially sparing long-stored memories. Thus, patients may not remember something that has just happened, but will be able to retrace their steps to an address they had lived in 30 years ago. Often, Alzheimer's disease develops gradually over a long time. As the disease progresses, the memories fade progressively. Patients lose track of time and date and become confused and frightened. Slowly, they lose the ability to reason and to function at home and outside of it. This presentation may be accompanied with behavioural, affective and/or psychotic symptoms. Personality changes occur and these can be devastating for those nearest to the patient, who becomes more and more difficult to manage, and the primary carer is very often an elderly, and perhaps frail, partner. As time goes by, the patient will gradually lose the ability to perform simple everyday functions such as dressing, eating, washing and attending to their personal toilet. The disease can place unbearable strains on the home for perhaps 10 years or more. Eventually the patient has to be hospitalized or put into care.

There seems little doubt with the increased lifespan in most western countries that dementia is going to become a much more prevalent problem. Alzheimer's disease, for example, affects about one-quarter of those over 85 years of age. The healthcare system faces a large incipient demand on resources to treat the growing population of dementia sufferers, to assist those who have to care for patients at home, and to provide inpatient care when these patients reach the point when they need permanent hospitalization (Cummings et al., 2002; Hake, 2002). This makes the development of treatments and research into dementias a very high priority.

Medication Treatments in Alzheimer's Disease

There are no effective drugs for prevention or cure of this disease. The drugs that may have some palliative effect (i.e. slow the disease progression) are the acetyl cholinesterase inhibitors (which inhibit the breakdown of the neurotransmitter acetylcholine, e.g. donepezil, galantamine and rivastigmine) and NMDA receptor antagonist (memantine).

The NICE guidelines on dementia (NICE, 2018b) recommends that the three acetylcholinesterase (AChE) inhibitors (donepezil, galantamine and rivastigmine) are first-line options for managing mild to moderate Alzheimer's disease. Memantine is second-line choice in moderate Alzheimer's disease or first-line in severe Alzheimer's disease. For people with an established diagnosis of Alzheimer's disease, who are already taking an AChE inhibitor, memantine can be prescribed in addition to an AChE inhibitor if they have moderate or severe disease. (Please refer to this NICE guideline to understand the suitable context of these recommendations and for further details.)

Acetylcholinesterase Inhibitors

Donepezil seems to help some patients but it is unlikely to help significantly once the cholinergic nerves have been destroyed. It has a half-life of around 70 h. The most common side-effects of donepezil in Chinese Alzheimer's disease patients included dizziness, gastrointestinal symptoms (nausea, loss of appetite, vomiting, diarrhoea and constipation), insomnia, fatigue, sinus bradycardia, Q-T interval prolongation, abnormal liver function tests and agitation (Zhang and Gordon, 2018). Among other things, bradycardia needs to be closely monitored, as it can have dangerous consequences. Also weight loss and gastrointestinal bleeding may be of concern. Other drugs, which have cholinomimetic action, can augment cumulative adverse effects if prescribed with AChE inhibitors. This is not a comprehensive list.

Galantamine is quite similar to donepezil and **rivastigmine** is also in this category.

NMDA Receptor Antagonist

Memantine has a half-life of 60–100 h. The most common adverse events of memantine include dizziness, headaches, fatigue, diarrhoea and gastric pain, and in clinical experience the side-effects that are most likely to lead to discontinuation are restlessness and hyperexcitation (Overshott and Burns, 2005).

CLINICAL NOTE

There is continuous research into dementia and Alzheimer's disease and patients are attending memory clinics, as more information becomes available. Many patients take dietary supplements to aid memory function and nursing staff should be aware of this if a patient is admitted to hospital and has a diagnosis of dementia or Alzheimer's disease.

ATTENTION DEFICIT HYPERACTIVITY DISORDER

The main symptoms of ADHD in this category of hyperkinetic disorders, include hyperactivity, impulsive behaviour and/or inattention present in more than one setting, where other causes do not explain this. These symptoms can hinder a child's development and cause problems in different domains of life. It is important to carry out a comprehensive assessment and identify all bio-psycho-social needs of the patient. Non-pharmacological strategies are an important part of the holistic treatment (e.g. parent/carer training, CBT, etc.).

NICE Guidelines for ADHD

Some of the recommendations made in the NICE guidelines on ADHD (NICE, 2018a) are as follows (please refer to this NICE guidance to understand the suitable context of these recommendations and for further details):

- Prior to commencing treatment, there should be assessment of cardiovascular history/symptoms, height, weight, BP, pulse and ECG (if required), and these should continue during treatment. A close eye needs to be kept on emergence/worsening of sleep problems, deteriorating behaviour and tics.
- For children aged 5 years and over and young people with ADHD, methylphenidate is the first-line pharmacological treatment and dexamfetamine or lisdexamfetamine can be tried thereafter. Atomoxetine or guanfacine treatment is the next step.
- For adults, lisdexamfetamine or methylphenidate is the first-line pharmacological treatment and atomoxetine is the second-line drug (licence indications of these drugs vary compared with those for children).

ADHD Drugs

- methylphenidate
- dexamfetamine
- lisdexamfetamine
- atomoxetine
- guanfacine
- other drugs.

Although **methylphenidate and dexamfetamine** are CNS stimulants and increase dopamine levels in the brain, they are effective for treating ADHD symptoms (see also Chapter 4). Lisdexamfetamine converts to dexamfetamine in the body. Neither of these drugs are licensed in the UK for children under 6 years of age. These drugs have a risk of being misused and diverted, so need to be closely monitored. They also need to be monitored after prolonged use in case of increased heart rate, BP and reduced appetite (which can cause decreased height and weight). There can be numerous other side-effects. These drugs should be used cautiously in patients with epilepsy, as they may lower the seizure threshold. Methylphenidate comes in immediate release and extended release formulations and either can be used to have best treatment effect.

Atomoxetine is an inhibitor of the pre-synaptic noradrenaline transporter. It has low potential of abuse. It may cause side-effects including increased pulse and BP, decreased appetite, etc. Increase in suicidal thoughts is uncommon.

Guanfacine is a selective agonist of alpha2A adrenergic receptor. Among other side-effects, decreased BP and heart rate, sedation and weight gain can be problematic, so these need to be monitored.

Other Drugs

Clonidine is a drug quite similar to guanfacine. **Modafinil** is more often prescribed for narcolepsy and obstructive sleep apnoea syndrome, although it is also used to treat ADHD in some countries. It is associated with several adverse effects, including that on the cardiovascular system and the CNS and should be used with caution, if at all, in patients with cardiovascular disorders.

JET LAG

Long flights, crossing several time zones, give rise to fatigue and loss of concentration and appetite on arrival. Flights to the West lead to early wakening, and to the East, difficulty getting to sleep. This is due to the body clock becoming out of phase with its local time and it may take 2 or 3 days to adjust. Simple measures (e.g. having adequate rest and gradually changing sleep routine before travelling and trying not to sleep during the day on arrival by exposure to sunlight/bright light) to get back to a normal routine should help. It is best to avoid medication for this if possible. Short-term hypnotics can be prescribed if insomnia is a problem (see earlier). **Melatonin** (see hypnotics section) helps with this adjustment and there is some evidence that, if given orally in the evening, it helps sleep and reduces jet lag.

SUMMARY

- Two nurses should always be involved when a drug is administered. Nurses should be familiar with local policy and guidelines for administration of medication.
- Patient compliance can be a problem (e.g. patients may secretly spit out drugs), so they need explanation and reassurance when they are given drugs. Documentation of all drug non-compliance and its reasons should be precise.
- Drugs can be given by depot injection to overcome problems of compliance, e.g. when treating patients with schizophrenia.
- Antipsychotic drugs may have several adverse effects, since they affect CNS neurotransmitter activity, and these should be watched for, as confused and fearful patients may not be able to report them.
- Acute confusional state may be brought on by drugs.
- Apart from medication, psychological interventions are a well-known treatment for many anxiety and depressive disorders.
- Hypnotics should not be prescribed until diagnosis of insomnia is ascertained (including presence of marked distress or interference with ordinary activities of daily living).
- BZDs and Z-drugs may be associated with dependence and withdrawal symptoms, so short-term use is advised, and treatment discontinuation should involve a stepwise reduction.
- Suicide is a special risk in depressed patients.
- It may take time before depression is relieved by antidepressant drugs and treatment should therefore be continued for several weeks before deciding that it has failed.
- Compared with the older TCAs, SSRIs generally have less adverse effects and are less dangerous in overdose. Nevertheless, they can have prominent side-effects.
- SSRIs must be used with caution in patients with a history/risk of bleeding disorders, hyponatremia and cardiac conduction problems, to avoid these complications or with other serotonergic drugs (as risk of serotonin syndrome).
- TCAs, MAOIs and lithium have several adverse effects and interactions with other drugs, so should be used with caution.
- Cheese and other foods that contain tyramine are absolutely contraindicated with monoamine

oxidase inhibitors (MAOIs), as the combination can cause a fatal hypertensive crisis. This can also happen when indirect sympathomimetic agents are prescribed with MAOIs.

- The plasma levels of lithium must be monitored regularly.
- Antidepressant drugs have to be used with caution in bipolar disorder (may trigger a hypomanic/manic episode) or in epilepsy (can precipitate seizures).
- The family of a patient with dementia needs a great deal of practical and emotional support and the multidisciplinary team plays an invaluable role in this.
- People with ADHD should have a comprehensive and holistic shared treatment plan that addresses their bio-psycho-social needs.

Note: Please refer to the Summary of Product Characteristics of the drugs mentioned in this chapter for further description, as the information given may not summarize all essential details.

REFERENCES AND FURTHER READING

American Psychiatric Association, 1994. Neuroleptic Malignant Syndrome. Diagnostic and Statistical Manual of Mental Disorders, fourth ed. APA Press, Washington DC, pp. 739–742.

American Psychiatric Association, 2013. Diagnostic and Statistical Manual of Mental Disorders, fifth ed. APA Press, Washington, DC.

Andersson, E.M., Hallberg, I.R., Norberg, A., et al., 2002. The meaning of acute confusional state from the perspective of elderly patients. Int. J. Geriatr. Psychiatry 17, 652–663.

Antai-Otong, D., 2007. The art of prescribing. Monotherapy antidepressant: a thing of the past? Implications for the treatment of major depressive disorder. Perspect. Psychiatr. Care 43, 142–145.

Baldwin, D.S., Aitchison, K., Bateson, A., et al., 2013. Benzodiazepines: risks and benefits: a reconsideration. J. Psychopharmacol. 27 (11), 967–971.

Ballinger, B.R., 1990. Hypnotics and anxiolytics. BMJ 300, 456–458.

Beach, S.R., Celano, C.M., Noseworthy, P.A., et al., 2013. QTc prolongation, torsades de pointes, and psychotropic medications. Psychosomatics 54 (1), 1–13.

Boyer, E.W., Shannon, M., 2005. The serotonin syndrome. N. Engl. J. Med. 352 (11), 1112–1120.

Buckley, N.A., Dawson, A.H., Whyte, I.M., et al., 1995. Relative toxicity of benzodiazepines in overdose. BMJ 310, 219–221.

Camps, P., Munoz-Torrero, D., 2002. Cholinergic drugs in pharmacotherapy of Alzheimer's disease. Mini. Rev. Med. Chem. 2, 11–25.

Carvalho, A.F., Sharma, M.S., Brunoni, A.R., et al., 2016. The safety, tolerability and risks associated with the use of newer generation antidepressant drugs: a critical review of the literature. Psychother. Psychosom. 85, 270–288.

Cleare, A., Pariante, C.M., Young, A.H., et al., 2015. Evidence-based guidelines for treating depressive disorders with antidepressants: a revision of the 2008 British Association for Psychopharmacology guidelines. J. Psychopharmacol. 29 (5), 459–525.

Cookson, J., 1993. Side-effects of antidepressants. Br. J. Psychiatry 163 (S20), 20–24.

Culpepper, L., 2002. The active management of depression. J. Fam. Pract. 51, 769–776.

Cummings, J.L., Frank, J.C., Cherry, D., et al., 2002. Guidelines for managing Alzheimer's disease: Part II. Treatment. Am. Fam. Physician 65, 2525–2534.

Editorial, 1988. Benzodiazepines and dependence: a college statement. Bull. RCP 12 (03), 107–109.

Editorial, 1988. Tardive dyskinesia. BMJ 296, 150.

Editorial, 1994. Risperidone for schizophrenia. BMJ 308, 1311–1312.

Editorial, 1995. The drug treatment of patients with schizophrenia. Drug Ther. Bull. 33, 81–86.

Editorial, 1997. Donepezil for Alzheimer's disease. Drug Ther. Bull. 35, 75–76.

Editorial, 1999. Acetylcholinesterase inhibitors for Alzheimer's disease. BMJ 318, 615–616.

Edwards, J.G., 1994. Selective serotonin re-uptake inhibitors in the treatment of depression. Prescribers' J. 34, 197.

Elkayam, U., Frishman, W., 1980. Cardiovascular effects of phenothiazines. Am. Heart J. 100 (3), 397–401.

Espie, C.A., 1993. Practical management of insomnia. BMJ 306, 509–511.

Fagerberg, I., Jonhagen, M.E., 2002. Temporary confusion: a fearful experience. J. Psychiatr. Ment. Health Nurs. 9, 339–346.

Fiedorowicz, J.G., Swartz, K.L., 2004. The role of monoamine oxidase inhibitors in current psychiatric practice. J. Psychiatr. Pract. 10 (4), 239–248.

Funk, K.A., Bostwick, J.R., 2013. A comparison of the risk of QT prolongation among SSRIs. Ann. Pharmacother. 47 (10), 1330–1341.

Gitlin, M., 2016. Lithium side effects and toxicity: prevalence and management strategies. Int. J. Bipolar Disord. 4 (1), 27.

Gram, L., 1994. Fluoxetine. N. Engl. J. Med. 331 (20), 1354–1361.

Gray, R., Robson, D., Bressington, D., 2002. Medication management for people with a diagnosis of schizophrenia. Nurs. Times 98 (47), 38–40.

Griffin 3rd, C.E., Kaye, A.M., Bueno, F.R., et al., 2013. Benzodiazepine pharmacology and central nervous system-mediated effects. Ochsner. J. 13 (2), 214–223.

Hake, A.M., 2002. The treatment of Alzheimer's disease: the approach from a clinical specialist in the trenches. Semin. Neurol. 22, 71–74.

Henry, J.A., Alexander, C.A., Sener, E.K., 1995. Relative mortality from overdose of antidepressants. BMJ 310, 221–224.

Hollister, L.E., 1964. Adverse reactions to phenothiazines. J. Am. Med. Assoc. 189 (4), 311–313.

Hoskins, B., 2011. Safe prescribing for the elderly. Nurse Pract. 36 (12), 47–52.

Jefferson, J.W., 1998. Lithium. BMJ 316, 1330–1331.

Jordan, S., Gabe-Walters, M.E., Watkins, A., et al., 2015. Nurse-led medicines' monitoring for patients with dementia in care homes: a pragmatic cohort stepped wedge cluster randomized trial. PloS One 10 (10), e0140203.

Lader, M., 1994. Treatment of anxiety. BMJ 309, 321–3224.

Lazarus, J.H., 2009. Lithium and thyroid. Best Pract. Res. Clin. Endocrinol. Metab. 23 (6), 723–733.

Majumdar, A., Mangal, N.S., 2013. Hyperprolactinemia. J. Hum. Reprod. Sci. 6 (3), 168–175.

Malhi, G.S., Gessler, D., Outhred, T., 2017. The use of lithium for the treatment of bipolar disorder: recommendations from clinical practice guidelines. J. Affect. Disord. 217, 266–280.

Medicines.org.uk, 2020. Clozaril 100 Mg Tablets – Summary of Product Characteristics (SPC) - (EMC). https://www.medicines.org.uk/emc/product/10290/smpc.

NICE, 2005. Obsessive-compulsive Disorder and Body Dysmorphic Disorder: Treatment [CG31]. https://www.nice.org.uk/guidance/cg31.

NICE, 2010. Delirium: Prevention, Diagnosis and Management [CG103] (Updated 2019). https://www.nice.org.uk/guidance/cg103.

NICE, 2011. Generalized Anxiety Disorder and Panic Disorder in Adults: Management [CG113] (Updated 2019). https://www.nice.org.uk/guidance/cg113.

NICE, 2013. Social Anxiety Disorder: Recognition, Assessment and Treatment [CG159]. https://www.nice.org.uk/guidance/cg159.

NICE, 2014. Psychosis and Schizophrenia in Adults: Prevention and Management [CG178] (Updated 2014). https://www.nice.org.uk/guidance/cg178.

NICE, 2018a. Attention Deficit Hyperactivity Disorder: Diagnosis and Management [NG87]. https://www.nice.org.uk/guidance/ng87.

NICE, 2018b. Dementia: Assessment, Management and Support for People Living with Dementia and Their Carers [NG97]. https://www.nice.org.uk/guidance/ng97.

Nursing Times, 2014. Medicines Management: Reducing Antipsychotic Drugs in Care Homes. https://www.nursingtimes.net/clinical-archive/medicine-management/reducing-antipsychotic-drugs-in-care-homes-30-05-2014.

Overshott, R., Burns, A., 2005. Treatment of dementia. J. Neurol. Neurosurg. Psychiatry 76 (Suppl. 5), v53–v59.

Pathare, S.R., Paton, C., 1997. Psychotropic drug treatment. BMJ 315, 661–664.

Rabkin, J., Quitkin, F., Harrison, W., et al., 1984. Adverse reactions to monoamine oxidase inhibitors. Part IA comparative study. J. Clin. Psychopharmacol. 4, 270–278.

Relkin, N.R., 2007. Beyond symptomatic therapy: a re-examination of acetylcholinesterase inhibitors in Alzheimer's disease. Expert Rev. Neurother. 7, 735–748.

Riemann, D., Baglioni, C., Bassetti, C., et al., 2017. European guideline for the diagnosis and treatment of insomnia. J. Sleep Res. 26 (6), 675–700.

Robson, D., Gray, R., 2007. Prescribing psychotropic medication: what nurses need to know. NursePrescribing 5 (4), 148–152.

Sabella, D., 2017. Antipsychotic medications. Am. J. Nurs. 17 (6), 36–43.

Sage, J., 2006. Depression: a treatable condition that affects the whole person. NursePrescribing 4 (2), 65–68.

Sharma, M.K., Kainth, S., Kumar, S., et al., 2019. Effects of zolpidem on sleep parameters in patients with cirrhosis and sleep disturbances: a randomized, placebo-controlled trial. Clin. Mol. Hepatol. 25 (2), 199–209.

Swanberg, M.M., Cummings, J.L., 2002. Benefit–risk considerations in the treatment of dementia with Lewy bodies. Drug Saf. 25, 511–523.

Tampi, R.R., Tampi, D.J., Balachandran, S., et al., 2016. Antipsychotic use in dementia: a systematic review of benefits and risks from meta-analyses. Ther. Adv. Chronic Dis. 7 (5), 229–245.

Tondo, L., Abramowicz, M., Alda, M., et al., 2017. Long-term lithium treatment in bipolar disorder: effects on glomerular filtration rate and other metabolic parameters. Int. J. Bipolar Disord. 5 (1), 27.

WHO, 1992. The ICD-10 Classification of Mental and Behavioural Disorders: Clinical Description and Diagnostic Guidelines. World Health Organization. https://www.who.int/classifications/icd/en/bluebook.pdf.

Zhang, N., Gordon, M.L., 2018. Clinical efficacy and safety of donepezil in the treatment of Alzheimer's disease in Chinese patients. Clin. Interv. Aging 13, 1963–1970.

USEFUL WEBSITES

Alzheimer's Society. https://www.alzheimers.org.uk.

Attention Deficit Disorder Information and Support Service (ADDISS). http://addiss.co.uk.

British Association for Psychopharmacology. https://www.bap.org.uk/guidelines.

Depression Alliance. https://www.depressionalliance.org.

Electronic Medicines Compendium. https://www.medicines.org.uk/emc/product/10290/smpc#gref.

National Institute for Health and Care Excellence (NICE). https://www.nice.org.uk/guidance.

NICE. Medicines optimisation: the safe and effective use of medicines to enable the best possible outcomes [NG5]. https://www.nice.org.uk/guidance/ng5/resources/shared-learning.

Nurses Labs. https://nurseslabs.com/anxiolytic-hypnotic-drugs.

Nursing Times. https://www.nursingtimes.net/clinical-archive/dementia/a-guide-to-prescribing-anti-dementia-medication-30-05-2014.

Nursing Times. https://www.nursingtimes.net/clinical-archive/medicine-management.

Nursing Times. https://www.nursingtimes.net/news/research-and-innovation/new-drug-may-provide-relief-from-psychosis-in-dementia-14-02-2018.

Seasonal Affective Disorder Association (SADA). http://sada.org.uk.

World Health Organization (WHO). https://www.who.int/classifications/icd/en/bluebook.pdf.

23 DRUG DEPENDENCE AND DRUG ABUSE

CHAPTER OUTLINE

LEARNING OBJECTIVES

At the end of this chapter, the reader should be able to:

- explain the meanings of the terms psychological and physical dependence on medicine or recreational drugs
- give theories to explain why some people become dependent on medicine or recreational drugs
- describe the short- and long-term effects of alcohol, recommended level of alcohol intake and the dangers of alcohol and driving
- talk about alcohol withdrawal and its treatment
- list the risks associated with heroin dependence and describe the medicines used to treat opioid dependence
- give an account of the effects of cocaine, amphetamines and ecstasy and the dangers associated with their use
- discuss the use of cannabis, hallucinogens, solvent sniffing and new psychoactive substances
- describe the association between cigarette smoking and disease and mention what treatments are used to aid people to give up smoking
- list commonly used foods that contain caffeine

INTRODUCTION

Drug *dependence* may be defined as a state resulting from the interaction of a person and a drug in which the person has a compulsion to continue taking the drug to experience pleasurable psychological effects and sometimes avoid discomfort due to its withdrawal.

Drug *abuse* is the use of a drug for recreational rather than medical reasons, often in excessive quantities, although dependence on certain types of prescription medicines can also occur.

There are several groups of drugs of dependence:

- alcohol
- opioids
- cocaine
- amphetamines and ecstasy
- barbiturates
- cannabis
- volatile solvents (glue sniffing)
- hallucinogens
- new psychoactive substances
- nicotine
- caffeine.

Types of Drug Dependence

Dependence is usually divided into **psychological** and **physical** dependence.

In **psychological** dependence, the person exhibits compulsive drug-seeking behaviour. The drug often produces a pleasant feeling, usually relaxation, freedom from worry or heightened awareness and increased energy and sexual drive. The patient suffers mental anguish when it is withdrawn.

In **physical** dependence, repeated administration produces biochemical changes in the subject taking the drug. If the drug is withdrawn, very unpleasant symptoms and signs of a physical nature develop, which may last for a varying period but will finally disappear. During this period there is an intense craving for the drug, which if given, will temporarily relieve the unpleasant symptoms. Thus, after the establishment of physical dependence, the patient's drug-seeking behaviour is motivated chiefly by fear of the withdrawal symptoms.

Tolerance to Drugs

Tolerance is a phenomenon whereby more of a drug is needed to produce the same response. This often develops with drugs causing dependence, especially morphine and heroin. Tolerance usually (but not always) develops to the central, but not peripheral, effects of a drug (Adewumi et al., 2018). Morphine and heroin cause euphoria (central) and constipation (peripheral). Thus, with heroin or morphine, tolerance to the central effects develops invariably and the user will have to keep increasing the dose to get the euphoria, but will not develop tolerance to the drug's effect in causing constipation. As a consequence of taking ever increasing doses to achieve CNS effects, the person will become severely and chronically constipated.

Reasons for Drug Abuse and Drug Dependence

Drugs may be used intermittently for social or emotional reasons, e.g. to relieve a stressful situation. Those who are truly dependent take drugs continually and may reach a state in which their whole life centres around obtaining and using drugs. Dependence may not be confined to one drug or group of drugs. It is common to find dependent subjects who have escalated from 'minor' drugs (e.g. cannabis) to 'hard' drugs (e.g. heroin) and some subjects may alternate or combine drugs (e.g. cocaine and morphine would produce alternating stimulation and relaxation).

Why Do People Become Dependent?

This is a very difficult question and the answer is still incomplete. It appears that there is no single cause for drug dependence and no single set of circumstances. There is some evidence to support the theory that there are some special types of personality, which render the person more susceptible to becoming dependent. There follows here a list of possible motives.

Curiosity and the Need to Belong. Many young people start taking drugs because they want to know what it feels like. Pressure from peer groups may also play a part, particularly with drugs such as alcohol and cannabis, which are to some degree socially acceptable. This in turn may be tied up with the wish to belong to a group who have a common interest in drug-taking and there may be an element of rebellion against accepted values. This need to achieve social acceptance may well be symptomatic of an underlying personality disorder, so there are both social and psychological factors at work.

Chemical Props and Escapism. Some people take drugs to relieve mental tension and worries or to give themselves more energy and confidence. Most people have to face difficulties from time to time and some look for a prop to help them. This may include advice from a friend, religion, a holiday or the development of a psychiatric illness. The dependent person has taken what may be termed the 'chemical way out' and by altering his or her psychological state with drugs has partially escaped from reality. Unfortunately, this method brings only temporary relief as it does not solve anything and brings in its train a set of further problems, which are both physical and psychological.

Biological Make-up. It has long been suggested that people who become drug-dependent differ in their genetic or biochemical make-up from those who show no interest in drugs. This has been particularly suggested in alcoholism, which might be regarded as a disease of metabolism, one facet of which is craving for alcohol. This is an attractive hypothesis because it takes the 'sin' out of dependence and puts it in a medical setting, but so far there is little evidence to support it.

Availability. There is little doubt that the availability and price of drugs of dependence influence both the amount and pattern of dependence. For example, countries where alcohol is cheap, such as France and South Africa, have a high incidence of alcoholism and cirrhosis of the liver.

Pressure of Work. It has long been known that those who have to work long hours and do arduous jobs may turn to certain drugs to give them energy. In South America, for example, the natives who were pressed into service in the silver mines by the Spanish chewed coca leaves to give themselves energy. The use of cocaine among workers in high-pressure financial institutions and in the modern entertainment industry is well known. Doctors and nurses, through the stresses and pressures of their vocation have a long history of being particularly susceptible to the temptations offered by the use of stimulant drugs, especially given the long hours they have to work and the accessibility of drugs. The emotional involvement that comes with working with the very ill has driven many a health worker to the use of opioids at one time or another. Nowadays, access to these drugs is very strictly controlled and their use is (or should be) documented meticulously. The records are inspected regularly and those who seek to remove these drugs from stock risk heavy penalties, not least de-registration and loss of their career.

ALCOHOL

Alcohol presents a special problem, as moderate amounts are taken for social reasons by many people. However, dependence on alcohol is very common and its management is a difficult medical and social problem. It occurs most often in those countries where alcoholic drinks are cheap, for instance the USA and France. Not only does it frequently lead to moral and financial breakdown for the patient, but it is also a tragedy for the wider family.

Effects of Alcohol

Alcohol causes both acute and chronic disorders. Acute consumption of excessive amounts of alcohol produces a deterioration of brain function, with changes in behaviour progressing through slurred speech and unsteady gait to unconsciousness.

The relationship between plasma concentration and effect is given in Table 23.1, although there is considerable interpersonal variation.

One unit of alcohol raises the plasma alcohol level to about 10–20 mg/100 mL. Normally, alcohol is rapidly absorbed from the gastrointestinal tract, though food may slow absorption. Peak blood levels are reached in about 1 h. It is largely metabolized in the liver, though small amounts are excreted in the urine and breath.

Given the same dose of alcohol, women have a higher blood level and appear more prone to develop alcohol-related diseases. This is partly because they are generally smaller than men, so the volume of distribution is less, but also because, in women, less alcohol is

TABLE 23.1

Plasma Concentration and Effect of Alcohol

Plasma Level (mg/100 mL)	Effect
20	Relaxed
30	Talkative
50	A little uncoordinated (e.g. knocks over glass)
100	Fall about, vomiting
300	Stupor

broken down as it passes from the gastrointestinal tract via the liver to the circulation (greater bioavailability).

Hangovers

Hangovers follow excessive intake of alcohol, although there is considerable interpersonal variation in their severity. The symptoms of headache, thirst, anxiety and nausea are familiar. To some degree they depend on the type of alcoholic beverage consumed. Brandy is the worst culprit and vodka is the least likely to provoke symptoms. This is because brandy contains substances, other than alcohol, which are toxic. Other factors resulting from excessive alcohol intake include dehydration, hypoglycaemia, tachycardia, gastric irritability, excessive smoking and lack of sleep.

Chronic Alcoholism

Chronic alcoholism can damage several organs and cause numerous adverse effects. Examples of some adverse effects follow.

In the central nervous system (**CNS**), it can lead to dementia and other complications. **Wernicke's encephalopathy** (WE) is caused due to thiamine (vitamin B_1) deficiency, especially in conjunction with poor nutrition, and can present with a variety of symptoms. The clinical diagnosis of WE in alcoholics requires two of the following four signs: (1) dietary deficiencies; (2) eye signs (oculomotor abnormalities); (3) cerebellar dysfunction; and (4) either an altered mental state or mild memory impairment (Galvin et al., 2010). If this is not treated promptly then, due to brain damage, it can progress to **Korsakoff syndrome** (involving memory loss, confabulation, impaired concentration, difficulty attaining new memories/information, etc.).

The **liver** may be damaged, leading to multiple problems and ultimately to cirrhosis. It can cause pancreatitis and several types of cancer. The **stomach** may develop gastritis and alcohol can affect the **heart muscle**, resulting in atrial fibrillation and cardiomyopathy. In addition, high alcohol consumption raises **blood pressure** and may be a factor in precipitating strokes. Chronic alcoholics are especially prone to infection and have a high incidence of **tuberculosis**. Depression and alcoholic hallucinosis may occur. It is now recognized that excessive consumption of alcohol during pregnancy causes the fetal alcohol syndrome, with mild mental retardation, small head, turned-up nose and other facial abnormalities.

Alcohol Intake

The intake of alcohol is usually measured in terms of units per day or per week:

One unit = Half a pint of beer
One glass of wine
One glass of sherry or port
One measure of spirits.

Each of these contains about 8 g (10 mL) of alcohol.

The UK Chief Medical Officers' guideline advises that, for both men and women, it is safest not to drink more than 14 units a week on a regular basis to keep health risks from alcohol at a low level (DH, 2016). Even if the average intake of alcohol is within the safe range, a bout of high intake is associated with an increased risk of accident and injury.

There has been considerable evidence that moderate consumption of alcohol protects against coronary artery disease. The cardioprotective effect of moderate alcohol consumption is negated when light to moderate drinking is mixed with irregular heavy-drinking occasions (Rehm, 2011). Also, other cardiovascular adverse effects of alcohol intake have been noted earlier.

Alcohol Withdrawal

Alcohol withdrawal can present with various signs (elevated blood pressure, pulse and temperature, hyperarousal, agitation, restlessness, cutaneous flushing, tremors, diaphoresis, dilated pupils, ataxia, clouding of consciousness, disorientation) and symptoms (anxiety, panic, paranoid delusions, illusions, visual and auditory hallucinations) (Miller et al., 1998). Delirium tremens is a more serious withdrawal disorder where many of these signs and symptoms are witnessed with severe intensity. It is a medical emergency and best treated in a specialist general hospital setting. The mortality is around 5%.

Treatment Guidelines

Some of the recommendations made in the British Association of Psychopharmacology updated guidelines on pharmacological management of substance abuse (Lingford-Hughes et al., 2012) for management of alcohol withdrawal and detoxification are as follows (please refer to this BAP guidance to understand the suitable context for these recommendations and for further details):

- Benzodiazepines are efficacious in reducing signs and symptoms of alcohol withdrawal and carbamazepine has also been shown to be equally efficacious.
- During detoxification oral or parenteral (depending on risk/suspicion of WE) thiamine should be given.
- Acamprosate can be used to improve abstinence rates.

Benzodiazepines have been described in detail in Chapter 22 and **carbamazepine** in Chapter 19. Disulfiram inhibits the breakdown of alcohol, producing toxic substances, which cause flushing, nausea and headaches, and thus the patient is discouraged from further drinking. **Acamprosate** is a centrally acting drug that modifies the GABA system.

Alcohol and Driving

Increasing doses of alcohol produce a progressive deterioration in physical and mental performance. This is particularly important as it may cause road traffic accidents. Drunk in charge of a car is a serious offence, but the definition of drunkenness is difficult. In the UK, it is an offence to have 80 mg or more of alcohol per 100 mL of blood while in charge of a vehicle (the limit is 50 mg or more in Scotland). There are currently several techniques available for monitoring the levels of alcohol in the blood, although sometimes urinary levels are used to confirm whether a person has imbibed excessive amounts of alcohol.

OPIOIDS

- **Heroin (diamorphine)**
- **Morphine**

There are many people dependent on opioids in the UK at present, and the number is increasing. Most members of the opioid group of drugs are to a greater or lesser extent drugs of dependence. The most frequently used is heroin, which is extremely potent. Heroin passes through the blood–brain barrier much more readily than morphine, and in the brain it is converted into morphine. The user thus gets a larger dose than if the equivalent doses of morphine were used, and the duration of the effect is shorter than with morphine.

Withdrawal and Other Risks of Dependence

Heroin may be injected intravenously, taken orally or smoked, and produces a feeling of euphoria and relaxation. Dependence is both psychological and physical, and a few hours after withdrawal of the drug the person develops a craving for a further dose, combined with increasing restlessness, anxiety and distress. After 48 h, physical withdrawal symptoms such as nausea, vomiting and muscle/stomach cramps become prominent. Some of the other symptoms that may occur include cold skin, gooseflesh ('cold turkey'), raised pulse rate and blood pressure. The withdrawal symptoms last for about a week.

In addition to the hazards of withdrawal the patient runs further risks:

The Possibility of Overdosage. The drug is often adulterated with other powders and preparations may vary considerably in potency. In addition, the development of tolerance will increase the dose required for the desired effect and can lead to respiratory depression.

Sepsis and Blood-borne Viruses. There is a frequent occurrence of sepsis due to injection under non-sterile conditions. This may take the form of septicaemia or endocarditis. In addition, the sharing of injection needles greatly increases the risk of being infected with hepatitis B or C, or the HIV causing AIDS. A high proportion of intravenous drug users are carrying HIV and will eventually develop AIDS.

Effects on Baby. Babies born to an addict may have a low birth weight and, among other complications, can suffer acute withdrawal symptoms after birth with a mortality rate of 50%.

Crime. An addict may go to any length, even serious crime, to obtain further supplies of the drug.

NICE Guidance on Opioid Detoxification

Some of the recommendations made in the NICE (2007) guidance on opioid detoxification are noted below (please refer to this NICE guidance to understand the suitable context for these recommendations and for further details):

- Pharmacological approaches are the primary treatment option for opioid detoxification, with psychosocial interventions providing an important adjunct, including involvement of families and carers.
- Methadone or buprenorphine should be offered as the first-line treatment in opioid detoxification.
- Lofexidine may be considered for people with mild or uncertain dependence. It may be offered when a person has made a clinically appropriate informed decision to not use methadone or buprenorphine and/or to detoxify within a short time period.

Treatment of Opioid Dependence with Drugs

The basic aims of treatment are to keep the craving for drugs and the unpleasant withdrawal symptoms at bay so that the patient does not seek to obtain heroin or morphine illegally.

The drugs used to treat opioid dependence are:

- methadone
- buprenorphine
- naltrexone
- clonidine
- lofexidine.

Methadone

Methadone is a full μ-receptor agonist and used orally as a substitute for morphine or diamorphine in the treatment of drug dependence (see also Chapter 20). As noted earlier, it is one of the first-line treatments and is commonly used. When taken orally, the drug prevents the severe symptoms of withdrawal from heroin, while not producing the euphoria. It is usually given once daily. Methadone is potentially a drug of abuse and should be prescribed only to patients who are dependent on opioids.

Buprenorphine

Buprenorphine is a partial μ-receptor agonist that is also frequently used. Due to its partial agonist action, it can precipitate withdrawal symptoms (but has lesser side-effects than a full agonist), so caution is required in its choice and administration timing. It is usually given as a sublingual tablet.

Naltrexone

Naltrexone is an orally active opioid antagonist. It is inadvisable to give antagonists to very dependent patients, as this will precipitate withdrawal symptoms. However, it is more important to supply patients who have been withdrawn from heroin for at least 7–10 days with naltrexone, as this helps to prevent relapse into heroin use. Naltrexone is supplied as oral tablets.

Clonidine

Clonidine blocks presynaptic α_2 adrenoceptors on adrenergic nerve terminals, thus reducing the release of the neurotransmitter noradrenaline, and thereby reducing blood pressure. Clonidine prevents the rise of noradrenaline in the brain, which occurs when opioids are withdrawn and which is responsible for many of the unpleasant withdrawal symptoms. Its use in these circumstances requires careful monitoring, combined with full support. It is important to tell the patient that the relief of symptoms may be delayed for 12–24 h.

Lofexidine

Lofexidine is similar to clonidine, but does not lower blood pressure.

Whichever method of opioid withdrawal is used, the main aim is to prevent relapse and a great deal of support is needed. The aforementioned drugs can have side-effects, interactions and contraindications, so have to be used with caution and only when appropriate to do so.

Case History 23.1 gives a representative example of the presentation of opioid overdose and both emergency and longer-term treatment.

COCAINE

Cocaine dependence is still on the increase. The drug produces a strong feeling of elation, increased self-confidence and appears to temporarily increase physical capacity. In South America, the leaves of the coca tree, which contain cocaine, are chewed for this purpose. Cocaine can be given orally; also it is

CASE HISTORY 23.1

Her boyfriend brought Miss L, a 21-year-old woman with a known dependence on heroin, into A&E. She was comatose, pale, had pinpoint pupils and shallow breathing. Her fingers and fingernails were blue and she had abscesses on both arms. She was immediately intubated to assist her breathing and given an injection of an opioid antagonist to block the action of any heroin still in her body. After she regained consciousness, she was admitted to an inpatient ward and prescribed methadone liquid to prevent the occurrence of withdrawal symptoms. Fortunately, she tested negative for blood-borne viruses, despite her confession that she had shared needles with other addicts. After discharge, she was referred to the local addiction service, where she commenced pharmacological opioid detoxification and participated in psychosocial interventions offered at the service. The nursing and occupational therapy team (with input from her family) supported her rehabilitation in the community and she enrolled on to a hair dressing course at the college. Her comprehensive treatment plan was continued for a year and she remained abstinent and was discharged without any detoxification medication.

absorbed through mucous membranes and may be sniffed, which can produce ulceration of the nasal septum. More rapid effects are obtained by giving cocaine intravenously, when it may be mixed with heroin. 'Crack' is the free 'base' of cocaine. If this is vaporized and the fumes inhaled, the drug is absorbed through the lungs, producing a rapid and intense effect. Because the action of cocaine is short-lived, it often is taken in repeated doses every 30 min or so and there is risk of dangerous overdose. It constricts the blood vessels, which can lead to some of its adverse effects. It can cause numerous short-term side-effects including increased temperature, hypertension, tachycardia, confusion, paranoia, perceptual disturbance and disturbed sleep. Cocaine use may be associated with adverse effects linked to cardiac, cerebrovascular, neurological, psychiatric, obstetric, pulmonary, dermatological and gastrointestinal systems (Cregler, 1989). Dependence is largely psychological and withdrawal symptoms include depression, sleepiness, reduced energy levels, increased appetite, etc.

AMPHETAMINES AND ECSTASY

Effects and side-effects of these drugs are somewhat similar to cocaine. For many years, amphetamines were used as appetite suppressors and for increasing wakefulness (widely used by soldiers in World War II). In large doses, amphetamines are powerful stimulants, producing increased energy levels, feelings of confidence and elation, but also, numerous adverse effects. There is considerable psychological dependence, but the withdrawal symptoms are usually not severe. Except for special circumstances (see Chapter 22, ADHD treatment), amphetamines are now rarely used in medical practice.

Ecstasy (MDMA) is an amphetamine derivative that produces feelings similar to those produced by amphetamines and feelings of 'togetherness'. In the UK, it is used largely as a dance drug at 'rave' parties. It is manufactured illegally and the strength of tablets is variable. The lethal dose also varies considerably, depending on the individual. The danger is that with vigorous dancing, hyperpyrexia, dehydration and electrolyte disturbances can develop rapidly, and a person who has taken ecstasy runs the risk of seizures, collapse, renal failure and death. Many side-effects are as noted in the cocaine section earlier and other symptoms may occur. Ecstasy appears to have a low addictive potential, but long-term use may cause problems, e.g. psychosis, depression and sleep problems. It is a far-from-safe drug.

BARBITURATES

Until sometime after World War II, barbiturates were the most commonly used hypnotic and sedative drugs. It is now realized that prolonged use, particularly in large doses, can lead to dependence. The drug abuser on barbiturates experiences symptoms including drowsiness, ataxia and nystagmus (on examination). Sudden withdrawal produces well-marked symptoms such as anxiety, vomiting and epileptic seizures (that can be fatal in the elderly).

CANNABIS (MARIJUANA)

Cannabis is a resin obtained from a plant that is widely grown in America, Africa and Asia. It is usually smoked. It produces mild excitement combined with a feeling of relaxation and peace. Perception of time is distorted, the passage of time is slowed ('spaced-out') and the subjects may be hungry ('the munchies'). The conjunctivae appear red due to vasodilatation.

Cannabis-based products and cannabinoids have medicinal use for indications including chronic pain, some treatment-resistant epilepsies and nausea and vomiting caused by chemotherapy (Freeman et al., 2019). Cannabis is illegal in the UK, but whether it is more addictive and socially more undesirable than alcohol is a matter of debate. Some main arguments against its legalization are:

- Repeated use, particularly in high doses, can reduce motivation and interfere with the person's life.
- Rarely, it can cause a psychotic state with hallucinations and disorientation.
- The use of cannabis may lead a person on to take more seriously addictive drugs such as heroin. Although this happens infrequently, most heroin addicts have passed through a phase of using cannabis.
- Cannabis is a drug of dependence in that there are withdrawal symptoms (anxiety and sleeplessness) and tolerance develops.

The argument has also been put forward that cannabis destroys personal motivation in society and the user 'opts out'.

Unfortunately, many so-called recreational drugs are resorted to as remedies for symptoms produced by other drugs, and Case History 23.2 illustrates the plight of an otherwise healthy individual who experimented with these drugs.

VOLATILE SOLVENTS

Various substances contain organic solvents, which are volatile and highly fat-soluble and therefore easily penetrate the brain, causing depression of cerebral function with euphoria. There are numerous kinds of volatile solvents and they can produce a variety of effects depending on the product used and its dose, but often produce effects similar to alcohol consumption. They can cause multiple organ damage and serious complications and sudden death has been reported even after first use because of cardiac arrhythmia. It can cause dependence and withdrawal symptoms. The problem of 'glue sniffing' has become serious among teenagers and is difficult to control, as the use of these solvents has become more widespread and these preparations are widely available.

HALLUCINOGENS

Lysergic Acid Diethylamide

LSD is a synthetic derivative of lysergic acid, which occurs naturally in ergot (see Chapter 21, migraine section). It produces vivid hallucinations that disorientate the taker, causes heightened appreciation of colours and sounds, and the taker may experience a feeling of complete detachment from the body. It can produce so-called 'bad trips' that consist of highly terrifying images and experiences and can lead to suicide attempts, although successful suicides from LSD are rare. It can produce autonomic effects such as sweating and digestive upsets. The drug is believed to exert its effects mainly as an agonist at central 5-HT_2 receptors. It is illegal to possess, use or distribute the drug, except under a Home Office licence.

Psilocybin ('Magic Mushrooms')

These are mushrooms that produce hallucinations and unusual sensations rather like those produced by LSD, although not as powerfully, nor for as long. The chief danger with harvesting mushrooms from the wild is the very real possibility of picking the wrong species and poisoning oneself. The UK Drugs Act 2005 made all magic mushrooms illegal (fresh, dried or prepared).

Mescaline

Mescaline is a chemical found in the dried tops of certain Mexican cacti, including one called *Lophophora williamsii*. It produces vivid hallucinations and a condition that resembles inebriation (drunkenness). It has no therapeutic value.

NEW PSYCHOACTIVE SUBSTANCES

In recent years, a new class of synthetic psychoactive substances has been widely available in the market, as they have effects similar to many of the previously mentioned illicit drugs. A wide variety of such substances

CASE HISTORY 23.2

Miss C, a 26-year-old receptionist, complained to her general practitioner about palpitations, anxiety, insomnia, low mood and loss of appetite. The doctor questioned her about her lifestyle and it became apparent that she was using an array of illicit drugs.

Apparently, Miss C had been out clubbing with friends regularly on Friday nights. In order to be able to enjoy the music and dancing and to forget about stress and problems at work, she took a couple of amphetamine capsules. Later the same evening, when the effect of the drug eased off, she took more amphetamines and ecstasy pills to restore her energy and make her feel good. When she got hot and thirsty, she drank beer. At the end of the night, in order to calm down and relax, she shared a joint (cannabis cigarette) with a friend. Afterwards at home, when she could not sleep, she smoked another joint to fight against an upcoming low mood.

The doctor explained that the cocktail of drugs had affected her and caused insomnia and anxiety. The amphetamine and ecstasy tablets had the short-term effect of her feeling more energetic and confident. Ecstasy caused sweating and a dry mouth and throat, and it also encouraged her to drink; in her case, alcohol. Alcohol intensified the effects of the substances taken. Once the body's energy supplies were exhausted, the predominant feelings in her case were anxiety, confusion, low mood and restlessness. To combat these unpleasant feelings, she self-medicated with alcohol and cannabis in order to be able to relax and cheer herself up.

The doctor gave her leaflets to explain the dangers of drug and alcohol misuse and referred her to local services to support her in stopping recreational drug use and moderating her intake of alcohol.

LESSONS:

- The substance-use behaviour of Miss C is very similar to other young people on a night out.
- Substances used as mood enhancers can increase existing feelings of depression and anxiety.
- When substances are taken as a cocktail of drugs, particularly when coupled with alcohol, the effect of the individual drug may be stronger. Substance use therefore is likely to get out of control.
- Energy retrieved through the use of amphetamines or ecstasy is only borrowed energy. The body usually needs days to recover and restore its energy levels.
- Insomnia and loss of appetite over several days debilitates the body and makes the user vulnerable to diseases and infections.
- Substance use can lead to panic attacks, anxiety, confusion and drug-induced psychosis. Mostly, these symptoms cease when substance use is stopped.
- The nurse can give information on the effects of substance use and/or refer to specialist drug treatment services.

have been manufactured to be sold in high street shops and over the internet across countries. They have caused serious adverse effects including many deaths. It has been difficult for law enforcement agencies to keep a check on this and although the legislation is catching up, it is still tricky to control as new types of substances are constantly being synthesized. They were misleadingly called 'legal highs' as they were initially legal in the UK. The Psychoactive Substances Act 2016 in the UK made these so-called 'legal highs' illegal.

NICOTINE

Incidence of Diseases, Mortality and Withdrawal

Nicotine is a constituent of tobacco smoke. It stimulates the autonomic nervous system (raised blood pressure and pulse rate) and has a mild cocaine-like stimulant action on the brain. It causes both psychological and physical dependence. Unfortunately, its use is associated with an increased incidence of several diseases, most notably:

- **cancer of the lung, lip and tongue**
- **chronic bronchitis and emphysema**
- **coronary artery disease**
- **peripheral vascular disease.**

The death rate among smokers is about twice that of non-smokers and the figure is higher for heavy smokers, whose life expectancy is reduced by about 5 years. There is a progressive improvement in prognosis after giving up smoking.

Withdrawal symptoms include craving for nicotine, constipation and increased appetite.

NURSING NOTE

All patients should be given quit smoking advice when being assessed. Healthy choices around nicotine and smoking are encouraged and prescriptions for quit smoking aids is encouraged.

Treatment Guidelines

Some of the recommendations made in the British Association of Psychopharmacology updated guidelines on pharmacological management of substance abuse (Lingford-Hughes et al., 2012) for management of nicotine addiction are as follows (please refer to this BAP guidance to understand the suitable context for these recommendations and for further details):

- Nicotine replacement therapy (NRT), varenicline, bupropion, nortriptyline and cytisine are all effective in aiding smoking cessation. Prescriptions for one of these should be offered to all smokers.
- All smokers should also be encouraged to use behavioural support where this is available (e.g. in the UK NHS, all smokers should have access to a trained stop-smoking practitioner), but unwillingness to use behavioural support should not preclude prescribing pharmacotherapy.

Nicotine replacement therapy:

- includes substances that are used to provide a nicotine dose in a safer way, to help people quit smoking
- there are several formulations available, e.g. chewing gum, lozenges, inhalers, spray, skin patches, electronic cigarettes (e-cigarettes).

E-cigarettes belong to a family of products that have been widely available in recent years as alternatives to cigarettes. E-cigarettes are an example of an electronic nicotine delivery system, whereby the user inhales an aerosol (vapours) containing pure nicotine. This is sometimes referred to as 'vaping' and there are now different types of vaping devices that can be obtained without prescription, sometimes containing nicotine solutions that are flavoured, to make them more palatable. While these products are often considered as part of aiding people to quit smoking, and certainly do not contain the thousands of chemicals generated on burning tobacco in conventional cigarettes, there is increasing concern about the free availability of these products and the health hazards of having unrestricted regular access to nicotine. A number of Regulatory Agencies have now taken an interest in these products and the claims that are made about them by the manufacturers.

Bupropion

Bupropion is a drug that was originally introduced as an antidepressant. It has been found useful as an aid to help smokers give up the habit. It is taken orally in tablet form. Its mechanism of action, both as an antidepressant and for giving up smoking, is unknown. Its use is associated with some dangers and contraindications.

Adverse Effects of Bupropion. The drug has several adverse effects, some of the most common being insomnia, rashes, urticaria and depression.

Contraindications. Bupropion lowers the threshold for seizures. This makes it dangerous for epileptics or anyone who has ever had a seizure for any reason. It has several other contraindications.

Varenicline is a partial agonist of nicotine receptors. Clinical trials have consistently demonstrated that varenicline is a safe and effective agent for smoking cessation (Burke et al., 2016). **Cytisine** action is similar to varenicline and has a low cost. **Nortriptyline** is a tricyclic antidepressant (see Chapter 22).

CAFFEINE

Although caffeine is not a serious drug of addiction, transient symptoms of headaches, sleepiness and general depression occur when it is withdrawn from the diet. It is perhaps not generally realized that most people are taking caffeine regularly, because it is found not only in coffee, but also in other dietary components such as tea, chocolate, cocoa and some proprietary colas. Occasionally, exclusion of caffeine from the diet will cure sleeplessness, anxiety and palpitations.

SUMMARY

- Peer group pressure, tension, work pressure, chronic illness and domestic upheaval are important factors in drug misuse.
- Overdose is a continual danger with street buying of drugs, which have unknown potency and purity.
- Injection under non-sterile conditions is an important source of sepsis among drug misusers. Shared needles is a significant cause of the rise in blood-borne virus infections like HIV and hepatitis.
- Alcohol causes both acute and chronic disorders. Taking large amounts of alcohol during pregnancy may result in the birth of a mentally retarded baby with a small head and facial deformities.
- Alcohol withdrawal can present with various signs and symptoms and, in severe cases, can be lethal.
- Opioid users become tolerant to the central, but not to the peripheral actions of the drugs, and the continual increases in dose means they will suffer from chronic constipation.
- It is not unusual for opioid dependence to develop if the user has escalated to opioids from more minor drugs such as cannabis.
- Babies born of opioid addicts can suffer acute withdrawal symptoms after birth.
- Ecstasy can and has proved fatal due to variable tablet quality of manufacture (consequent unpredictability of dose) and the circumstances under which it is usually taken (rave parties).
- From the UK NHS, all smokers should have access to a trained stop-smoking practitioner.
- There are several drugs that can be offered to aid smoking cessation.

Note: Please refer to the Summary of Product Characteristics of the drugs mentioned in this chapter for further description, as the information given may not summarize all essential details.

REFERENCES AND FURTHER READING

Adewumi, A.D., Staatz, C.E., Hollingworth, S.A., et al., 2018. Prescription opioid fatalities: examining why the healer could be the culprit. Drug Saf. 41 (11), 1023–1033.

Burke, M.V., Hays, J.T., Ebbert, J.O., 2016. Varenicline for smoking cessation: a narrative review of efficacy, adverse effects, use in at-risk populations, and adherence. Patient Prefer. Adherence 10, 435–441.

Cregler, L.L., 1989. Adverse health consequences of cocaine abuse. J. Natl. Med. Assoc. 81 (1), 27–38.

DH, 2016. UK Chief Medical Officers' Low Risk Drinking Guidelines. Department of Health, UK. https://assets.publishing.service.gov.uk/government/uploads/system/uploads/attachment_data/file/545937/UK_CMOs__report.pdf.

Dixon, P., 2007. Managing acute heroin overdose. Emerg. Nurse 15 (2), 30–35.

Freeman, T.P., Hindocha, C., Green, S.F., et al., 2019. Medicinal use of cannabis based products and cannabinoids. BMJ 365, l1141.

Galvin, R., Bråthen, G., Ivashynka, A., et al., 2010. EFNS guidelines for diagnosis, therapy and prevention of Wernicke encephalopathy. Eur. J. Neurol. 17 (12), 1408–1418.

Häuser, W., Finn, D.P., Kalso, E., et al., 2018. European Pain Federation (EFIC) position paper on appropriate use of cannabis-based medicines and medical cannabis for chronic pain management. Eur. J. Pain 22 (9), 1547–1564.

Lingford-Hughes, A.R., Welch, S., Peters, L., Nutt, D.J., 2012. BAP updated guidelines: evidence-based guidelines for the pharmacological management of substance abuse, harmful use, addiction and comorbidity: recommendations from BAP. J. Psychopharmacol. 26 (7), 899–952.

Miller, N.S., Gold, M.S., 1998. Management of withdrawal syndromes and relapse prevention in drug and alcohol dependence. American Family Physician. 58 (1), 139–46.

NICE, 2007. Drug Misuse in over 16s: Opioid Detoxification [CG52]. https://www.nice.org.uk/guidance/cg52.

Pilling, S., Strang, J., Gerada, C., NICE, 2007. Psychosocial interventions and opioid detoxification for drug misuse: summary of NICE guidance. BMJ 335 (7612), 203–205.

Rehm, J., 2011. The risks associated with alcohol use and alcoholism. Alcohol Res. Health 34 (2), 135–143.

Vadivelu, N., Singh-Gill, H., Kodumudi, G., et al., 2014. Practical guide to the management of acute and chronic pain in the presence of drug tolerance for the healthcare practitioner. Ochsner J. 14 (3), 426–433.

USEFUL WEBSITES

British Association for Psychopharmacology. https://www.bap.org.uk/docdetails.php?docID=7.

Electronic Medicines Compendium (EMC). https://medicines.org.uk/emc.

National Institute for Health and Care Excellence (NICE). https://nice.org.uk.

NHS. https://www.nhs.uk/live-well/healthy-body/drug-addiction-getting-help.

Nursing Times. https://www.nursingtimes.net/clinical-archive/substance-misuse/caring-for-problem-drug-users-16-05-2006.

World Health Organization (WHO). https://who.int/classifications/icd/en/bluebook.pdf.

24 DRUGS USED FOR DERMATOLOGICAL CONDITIONS

CHAPTER OUTLINE

LEARNING OBJECTIVES

At the end of this chapter, the reader should be able to:

- describe the basic principles of dermatological treatment
- understand the importance of emollients
- list the different bases used for topical preparations
- identify the relevant base to use for a medication, depending on the acuteness of the skin condition
- identify the main treatments for common skin diseases
- list the potential sensitizers used in topical preparations
- describe different potencies of topical corticosteroids
- demonstrate the correct way to apply the different forms of topical medications
- describe the recognized methods for applying the prescribed amounts of corticosteroids
- identify the drugs that may cause a reaction on the skin

DERMATOLOGICAL DIAGNOSIS AND TREATMENT

In primary care settings, nurses and allied professionals are increasingly the first practitioners to see patients with common dermatological conditions. The expectation is that they will be able to diagnose and treat these conditions. Most undergraduate courses teach very little dermatology and so the subject can seem mysterious and difficult. It is not the place of a text such as this to teach the details of diagnosing and managing skin conditions, but there are important principles that can go some way to helping practitioners understand the essentials of diagnosis and management. A primary care practitioner can then build their knowledge through seeing patients and how they respond to the treatments prescribed, and through contextualized learning. Colour atlases in book form are popular, but on-line resources are more convenient. *DermNet NZ* and the *Primary Care Dermatology Society (PCDS)* are excellent resources for both diagnosis and treatment of skin conditions. Dermatological diagnosis is often provisional and is refined through (intelligent) trials of treatment, with regular review.

It has been said, not entirely in jest, that the principles of dermatological management are:

> *If it's wet, then dry it; if it's dry, then moisturize it and if you don't know what it is, put steroids on it!*

If this is modified to 'if it's inflamed, consider topical steroids', then this is not a bad initial approach, as it emphasizes the importance of emollients.

EMOLLIENTS

Emollients are essential to the management of most dry and inflamed skin conditions and warrant a section although they contain no pharmacologically active ingredients. Almost the only dry and inflamed skin condition that is not helped – but rather worsened – by emollients is the condition *perioral dermatitis.* **Practitioners should learn to recognize this condition, which is also worsened by the application of topical steroid preparations.**

Emollients can be ointments, creams or lotions, as discussed later, and can have a liquid paraffin base or a base of plant fats such as cocoa butter, or be based on colloidal oatmeal. Some products contain hydrous wool fat (lanolin), which is an excellent emollient ingredient, but can occasionally lead to allergy. The base of the emollient is very much a matter of personal preference, and it is important to realize that different products will suit people differently, and if they are to apply them regularly, then it needs to be a product that they like. Having said this, for many people, a liquid paraffin-based cream is a good starting point.

Greasier emollients (ointments) tend to be more effective than creams, which are themselves more effective than lotions. However, there is a trade-off between effectiveness and acceptability, as greasy products are more difficult to apply and make the skin shiny and slippery. Again, a cream is often the best choice, but for very dry, cracked skin, a greasy ointment may be the only product that works. Sometimes it may be possible to apply the greasy product at night and use a lighter product during the day.

Although patients will often feel that a particular emollient is not working for them, and a change of product may be helpful, the most common reason for treatment failure is to not use enough of the emollient, and to not use it frequently enough. Regular emollient use is time consuming and it is not surprising that patients rebel against the routine. Concordance will be helped by explaining the rationale for use, showing empathy for the tedium of the routine of skin maintenance, and by trying to find a product that is acceptable.

Emollients should be used at least twice a day and often need to be used much more frequently. Use after bathing helps trap moisture in the skin. They should be used liberally and smoothed into the skin in the direction of hair growth. They should be used even after the initial condition has settled, although the frequency of use may be reduced.

Emollients may be all that is required to settle mild to moderate eczema, particularly in children, and are of vital importance in the initial management of severe psoriasis, where potent steroids may actually destabilize the condition.

Preparations such as **aqueous cream** and **emulsifying ointment** can be used as soap substitutes for handwashing. They are rubbed into the skin and then rinsed off.

Urea in proportions of around 10% may be added to emollients for an additional water trapping (humectant) effect. It may also enhance the penetration of other active ingredients. In concentrations of 20% or more, it has a *keratolytic* action, breaking down the hard outer layer of the epidermis. This can be useful, when there is overgrowth of this layer, particularly on the feet.

Nicotinamide may be added to emollients and has an antiinflammatory effect that may be useful in mild eczema and other inflammatory conditions.

SAFETY POINT

All emollients, but particularly paraffin containing ones, can build up on clothing, dressings and bedding and present a real fire risk. Serious injury has occurred. All patients should be warned of this risk and should avoid any sources of ignition, such as cigarettes. A hot wash of clothing and bedding will reduce the risk, but not completely remove it.

TYPES OF SKIN APPLICATIONS

When drugs are applied to the skin, the term *topical treatment* is often used. A topical application generally consists of an active application, the drug, in a base or vehicle. The type of topical application that is used depends on the type and stage of the skin disease, and it is just as important to use the correct base as it is to use the correct active agent. The base consists of one or more of the following: powder, water and grease. The most commonly used bases or vehicles are as described in the following sections.

Ointments

The distinction between modern ointments and creams is no longer so obvious because of the wide range of bases that are used. Ointments are generally greasier and creams are thinner. The main classes of base are:

- **Water-soluble bases:** these bases have the advantage that they do not stain.
- **Emulsifying bases:** these emulsify with water. An example of these is lanolin. These bases are useful for retaining active agents in contact with the skin for as long as possible.
- **Non-emulsifying ointments:** these do not mix with water. The paraffins form the basis of most of the very greasy ointments. With the addition of a suitable active agent they are a good treatment for chronic, dry skin disorders such as chronic atopic eczema, psoriasis, ichthyosis (dry skin with fish-like scales) and for common disorders such as chapped hands.

Greasier ointment bases for corticosteroids and other drugs are generally more effective than creams, particularly for dry skin conditions like eczema and psoriasis. However, the greasiness makes them more difficult to apply and less cosmetically acceptable. This may limit concordance with treatment. If a treatment is not used, then it will not work, and so it may be more appropriate to prescribe a cream in some cases.

Creams

Creams are emulsions which are either water dispersed in oil (i.e. oily cream) or oil dispersed in water (i.e. aqueous cream). The latter are generally very acceptable to patients cosmetically and are used to moisten and soften the skin surface. Appropriate active agents can be added. Barrier creams protect the skin against physical agents such as water or sunlight.

Pastes

Pastes can be greasy or drying and they contain a large amount of powder. They are particularly useful for localized lesions, e.g. in psoriasis. Pastes can also be used to protect inflamed or excoriated skin and can be applied very freely.

Lotions

Water lotions are used to cool acutely inflamed skin and may have to be frequently reapplied. Potassium permanganate lotion can be helpful for acute exuding lesions of the hands and feet. Lotions should generally not be used when the acute phase has subsided.

Lotions such as **calamine lotion** cool by evaporation and leave an inert powder on the skin surface. They are a traditional symptomatic treatment for sunburn and the lesions of chickenpox (varicella). It is not clear whether they are particularly effective for either of these conditions.

Dusting Powders

These are drying agents and increase the effective evaporating surface. They are particularly useful in the folds of the skin. Talc, starch and zinc oxide are commonly used powders. Active agents can be added as needed, e.g. antiseptics for bacterial infections and antifungal agents for athlete's foot (tinea pedis).

INGREDIENTS IN PREPARATIONS

The Base

When formulating a skin preparation, the first decision to make is the type of base that will be used. This will depend on the type and severity of the skin disease. Many conditions often derive more benefit from the base than from the active agent. A decision on the active ingredient to be added generally implies at least a provisional diagnosis of the skin disorder. Ointments prepared by pharmaceutical companies have complicated formulae, but it is very important to know the active ingredients and their strength in these preparations.

TABLE 24.1

Examples of Potential Skin Sensitizers in Topical Preparations

Beeswax	Isopropyl palmitate
Benzyl alcohol	Polysorbates
Butylated hydroxyanisole	Propylene glycol
Chlorocresol	Sorbic acid

It is also important to check for additives in topical preparations, which may be associated with sensitization (Table 24.1).

Active Ingredients for Topical Treatment

Some of the most commonly used or otherwise important active ingredients are described here. Others are described in the section on specific skin disorders.

Corticosteroids

These are probably the most widely prescribed and useful ingredients to be added to the various bases as treatments for various inflammatory dermatoses. They are often overprescribed and in particular *they should not be used alone where the cause of the skin disease is a bacterial, fungal or viral infection as they may cause spread of the infection by lowering host defence mechanisms.* They are very useful for acute and subacute disorders such as the eczemas and they are excellent for reducing itching (pruritus).

Topical corticosteroids are classified according to their potency (Table 24.2). In the UK and Australia there are four categories, in the USA there are seven. Table 24.2 also includes common UK brand names for these drugs, as they are very often referred to by these.

The choice of a topical corticosteroid should be the least potent preparation for the shortest treatment duration *which is effective.* There is, however, no benefit in prescribing a preparation that is too weak to be effective or prescribing it for too short a period.

Hydrocortisone cream or ointment (0.5%–1%) is a useful, standard preparation. Nothing stronger than this should routinely be used in infants or on the face. These preparations can be applied up to twice a day. In certain cases, a short course of a more potent corticosteroid preparation may be prescribed for use on infants or on the face by practitioners with dermatological experience, but such courses need regular clinical review.

TABLE 24.2

Topical Corticosteroid Potencies

Potency	Examples	Common UK Brand Name
Mild	Hydrocortisone 1%	–
Moderately potent	Clobetasone butyrate 0.05%	Eumovate
Potent	Betamethasone valerate 0.1%	Betnovate
	Mometasone furoate 0.1%	Elocon
Very potent	Clobetasol propionate 0.05%	Dermovate

More potent corticosteroids such as **betamethasone valerate** can achieve a much more intense effect than hydrocortisone, but can lead to atrophy of the skin, telangiectasia, striae and steroid rosacea following prolonged use. They are, however, valuable for thick, dry skin disorders, such as the chronic eczemas and psoriasis, or with some special disorders such as lupus erythematosus. The absorption of these preparations is enhanced by occlusive dressings, but the unwanted effects are also increased, and the systemic absorption may even be sufficient to cause pituitary suppression if treatment is prolonged. As patients become familiar with their skin condition, they may find that short courses of moderately potent topical steroids used for a few days at a time, followed by a week or two of maintenance with just emollients is sufficient to control their condition.

Mometasone furoate in cream or ointment form is a useful potent corticosteroid, with very low systemic absorption and a low risk of local adverse reactions. It may be the preferred choice if a potent corticosteroid needs to be used for longer periods. It also has the benefit of only requiring once daily use.

Clobetasol propionate is the most potent topical steroid commonly available. It should normally only be used by specialist dermatologists, except in the treatment of plantar and palmar dermatoses such as pompholyx eczema, which are common conditions, distinctive in appearance and which require short courses of very potent agents to settle them.

CLINICAL NOTE

Clobetasol propionate (*Dermovate* in the UK) and clobetasone butyrate (*Eumovate* in the UK) have very similar generic names and very different potencies. It is important not to confuse them when prescribing.

Sometimes corticosteroids are combined with an antibacterial or antifungal agent and used to treat dermatoses with superimposed bacterial or fungal infections. A popular preparation is a combination of hydrocortisone and miconazole in a cream base. It is often used when the practitioner is not quite sure if a rash is eczematous or has a fungal component. Sometimes it can be difficult to decide, and a short course of such a preparation may be justified. However, a definite diagnosis should always be the aim.

Some preparations are available containing a corticosteroid *and* an antifungal *and* an antibacterial agent. To prescribe one of these preparations is an admission of diagnostic defeat, and it is far better to seek the opinion of a colleague than to do so.

Calcineurin Inhibitors

Tacrolimus and **pimecrolimus** are powerful anti-inflammatory drugs in a class known as 'calcineurin inhibitors'. They were initially developed as immunosuppressant drugs for transplant surgery, but in topical form are useful treatments for inflammatory skin conditions where maximal topical corticosteroid therapy is ineffective, or not possible – such as on the face. They should only be initiated by experienced practitioners and should be used sparingly, for the shortest period of time that is effective. They may be irritant when first started and the quantity and frequency of use may be increased over a few days to minimize this. They should not be applied to malignant or possibly malignant or infected lesions. Local infection is the most common adverse effect.

Calcitriol and Vitamin D Analogues

Topical applications of vitamin D in the form of **calcitriol** or the vitamin D analogues **calcipotriol** and **tacalcitol** are used for long-term treatment of psoriasis. They work through an effect on skin-cell division and differentiation. Calcitriol and tacalcitol are less irritant than calcipotriol and more suitable for sensitive areas. They are absorbed systemically and affect calcium metabolism in the same way as oral vitamin D. Total weekly use needs to be controlled to prevent hypercalcaemia. For instance, no more than 60 g of calcipotriol ointment should be used in any week.

Retinoids

The retinoids are chemically related to vitamin A. They are used in oral form to treat severe acne and psoriasis and topically to treat mild to moderate acne. They are all teratogenic, and pregnancy must be avoided even with topical use. Skin irritation and dryness is their major unwanted effect. They may take several months to achieve maximal effect. Topical **tretinoin** and **isotretinoin** were the first drugs in this class. The retinoid-like drug **adapalene** is less irritant.

Keratolytics and Anti-comedonal Agents

Keratolytics break down the hard keratin material of the epidermis and are useful treatments for hard skin, callus and warts. As previously noted, urea is a useful keratolytic in higher concentrations and is helpful for hard skin on the feet. Salicylic acid, lactic acid, allantoin, glycolic acid, and trichloroacetic acid are all keratolytic agents, used for various indications in various bases. **Salicylic acid** is probably the most commonly used agent, on its own and in combination with other ingredients in various bases. For the treatment of warts, it is commonly used as a paint or in a base of collodion, which dries to form a transparent water-resistant film. At the end of the day, the film is removed, and the softened keratin may be rubbed or pared away before more of the treatment is applied. Wart treatment generally takes weeks of patient (in both senses!) treatment.

Anti-comedonal agents have the effect of unblocking pores and thus reducing comedones (blackheads and whiteheads). These agents are important acne treatments. Several drugs have anti-comedonal properties, often combined with other antiinflammatory properties. **Benzoyl peroxide** is a widely available topical anti-comedonal agent, available in various strengths, as skin dryness and irritation may be a problem in use, in which case lower strengths can be used. It is also a bleaching agent that can take the colour out of pillowcases if the patient rests their face on them after applying the drug. **Azelaic acid** has marked antiinflammatory activity but is also useful as an anti-comedonal agent. Compounded preparations of salicylic acid are also anti-comedonal.

Coal Tar

Coal tar is less used than in previous times, but when applied to the skin is an antiinflammatory agent and is also effective in reducing thick scale. Crude coal tar is most effective in concentrations up to 10%. It is smelly and staining. The more refined preparations smell and stain less than the crude tars but are also less effective. Shampoos and liquids containing refined tars are useful for the treatment of mild flaky and itchy scalp conditions. Tar containing creams may be helpful for mild psoriasis. Tar containing bath additives are also available. The use of more potent tars is now generally restricted to severe hyperkeratotic and scaly scalp conditions (such as severe scalp psoriasis). Here compound preparations of coal tar, salicylic acid, precipitated sulfur and coconut oil (*Cocois; Sebco* in the UK) can be very effective. They are applied to the scalp and shampooed off after an hour. They are, however, greasy, smelly and staining.

Dithranol

Dithranol was widely used to treat chronic plaques of psoriasis on extensor surfaces only. It is relatively rarely used now. It is an irritant and application must be limited to the psoriatic areas as it burns normal skin, particularly if the skin is fair or has previously been treated with corticosteroids. It should not be used if there is evidence of infection. If used, then treatment should begin with the weakest strength available and gradually increased in strength as required: 0.1%–0.5% can be applied and left overnight before washing off; 1%–3% cream should be left for short contact periods of between 5 and 60 min. Gloves must be worn when applying it and it must not be used on acute or pustular psoriasis.

Antibacterial Agents

Many infections of the skin are best treated with systemic rather than topical antibacterial agents. This is particularly true for cellulitis and erysipelas. Minor skin infections may respond to topical antibiotics, but the prolonged use of drugs such as neomycin on the skin carries a high risk of sensitization to the drug, so that a bacterial infection may be replaced by a contact dermatitis. If topical antibacterial agents are used, the treatment should be determined by the known (or likely) sensitivity of the organism. Swabs can therefore be very helpful in determining sensitivity. Minor staphylococcal infections including mild cases of impetigo can be treated with topical **fusidic acid** cream. Sulphonamides and penicillin should never be used on the skin owing to the high risk of sensitization.

Topical antibiotics have a particular role in the treatment of acne, where it seems likely that an anti-inflammatory activity not directly related to their antibacterial action is important. **Clindamycin** or **erythromycin complexed with zinc acetate** (*Zineryt* in the UK) are the most commonly used drugs.

Antifungal Agents

Fungal skin infections are hugely over-diagnosed. Most suspected fungal skin infections are actually eczema or psoriasis. A UV (Wood's) light can help in diagnosis as some fungal infections fluoresce brightly in UV light. Similarly, skin scrapings to identify the fungus can be helpful and should always be taken before considering systemic treatment. Systemic treatment is used for widespread infections and for nail (tinea unguium) and scalp ringworm. Treatment may need to be for several months in the case of nail and scalp infections. In adults, **itraconazole**, **fluconazole** and other triazole antifungals are the drugs of choice for systemic use. **Griseofulvin** remains the preferred choice in children.

Itraconazole may precipitate heart failure in patients at high risk of this condition. It may also, very rarely, lead to reversable liver dysfunction. It is not known if this is also a problem with the other triazole antifungals.

CLINICAL NOTE

Patients prescribed oral itraconazole (and possibly other triazoles) should be warned how to recognize signs of liver disorder and to seek prompt medical attention if symptoms such as nausea, vomiting, abdominal pain, jaundice or dark urine develop.

Topical treatments are usually adequate for most localized infections. Effective preparations commonly used are the imidazoles **clotrimazole**, **econazole** and **miconazole**. These are widely available without prescription and are also useful for candidal infections, such as vaginal thrush. Their disadvantage for use elsewhere is that they need to be used for several weeks to be effective. Newer, more active agents are now available, which need only be used for a week for conditions such as athlete's foot (tinea pedis). These include **terbinafine** and **amorolfine** creams. Amorolfine is also available as a lacquer for fungal nail infections.

Antiviral Agents

Aciclovir cream is the treatment of choice for herpes simplex of the skin. It is important that the cream should be applied as early as possible, 5 times a day, for 5 days.

Cytotoxic Agents

Topical cytotoxins are sometimes used in the treatment of malignant and pre-malignant skin conditions. They require extra care in their application as they are very irritant and damage normal skin. Written information on their use should always be provided with clear instructions on application and duration of use. **5-Fluorouracil cream** (or a cutaneous solution combined with salicylic acid) is the most commonly prescribed preparation, mainly used to treat actinic (solar) keratoses. It was originally developed as a systemic cancer chemotherapy drug of the antimetabolite class. Gloves must be worn while using it. It is applied once or twice a day for 3–4 weeks for actinic keratoses and longer for some skin malignancies.

Podophyllotoxin is used in cream or paint form to treat soft (non-keratinized) anogenital warts. It is used in short, repeated courses, the durations of which depend on the preparation used. Large warts should be treated under medical supervision.

Imiquimod cream is not a cytotoxic, but an immune modifier, and may also be used to treat anogenital warts and also some cancerous and pre-cancerous skin lesions. An extract of green tea (*Camellia sinensis*) is also available in cream form for the treatment of anogenital warts. Its mechanism of action is unknown.

Systemic Treatment of Skin Conditions

Although most dermatological conditions require topical treatment, some require systemic treatment either as an adjunct to, or instead of, topical therapy. Skin infections may require oral antibiotics or antifungals, but the most common oral treatments are specific antibiotics used by dermatologists in long (months) periods of treatment to manage acne, rosacea, peri-oral dermatitis and a number of other conditions. These are not principally treating infections but have antiinflammatory and immune-modulating activity. The tetracyclines are most commonly used. Of these, **lymecycline** is the most satisfactory, as it has a once daily dose regimen. **Minocycline** was very widely used and effective, but its use is not recommended as it can lead to irreversible slate grey discolouration of skin, eyes and nails, and a reversable lupus-like syndrome. Low-dose **erythromycin** is sometimes used when tetracyclines are not tolerated or are ineffective.

Oral **isotretinoin** is used by specialists only, to treat severe acne and other severe inflammatory conditions. It is a toxic and highly teratogenic drug and women must use effective contraception while using it. It causes severe skin and mucosal dryness and nose-bleeds are relatively common. There is concern that its use may be associated with the development of or worsening of depression, sometimes with suicidal thoughts. Careful monitoring for this is required. The related oral retinoid **acitretin** is used by specialists to treat very severe psoriasis. It is extremely teratogenic, and women are advised to avoid pregnancy for up to 3 years after treatment ends, and men and women should avoid donating blood for 3 years after treatment finishes.

Immunosuppressant drugs, such as ciclosporin and methotrexate are sometimes used in severe skin conditions, and disease-modifying antirheumatic drugs (DMARDs) and biologics are used to treat psoriasis with associated arthropathy.

A fixed-dose combination of ethinylestradiol and the anti-androgen cyproterone acetate is known as **co-cyprindiol** (*Dianette, Diane*) and is widely used to treat acne in women. It is used as a contraceptive, and the anti-androgen effect reduces sebum production. It is very effective in many cases, but the oestrogen dose is higher than most modern contraceptives and the risk of serious adverse events – particularly venous thrombosis and pulmonary embolism – may be raised. It has been withdrawn from some markets as a consequence. It should not continue to be used after the worst of the acne has resolved.

TREATMENT OF SOME COMMON SKIN CONDITIONS

The conditions now discussed are commonly seen in primary care clinics around the world.

Eczema

The mainstay of eczema treatment is the use of emollients. This cannot be overemphasized. Topical corticosteroids in appropriate strengths and suitable treatment course lengths are the next step up in treatment. Patients may be able develop a regimen of brief courses of topical corticosteroids repeated as required. Topical calcineurin inhibitors may help if steroids are ineffective or contraindicated. Occasionally, oral steroids are required for severe flares. Oral or topical antibiotics should be used to treat local infection. Antihistamines may be needed to relieve itch. Oral immunosuppressants such as azathioprine or ciclosporin are occasionally prescribed by specialists to treat very severe eczema.

Food (and other) allergies are a relatively rare cause of eczema, but cow's milk protein allergy in infants can lead to difficult to manage, widespread eczema, that improves when cow's milk is temporarily excluded.

Psoriasis

Emollients are also the mainstay of psoriasis treatment but are often neglected. Mild flares of psoriasis can be treated with a moderately potent corticosteroid cream or scalp application. For longer-term treatment, vitamin D analogues are more appropriate in cream or scalp application form. These can be combined with corticosteroids as a single preparation, if required. A cutaneous foam presentation of betamethasone and calcipotriol has proved useful in patients with widespread and resistant psoriasis. Coal tar preparations have a role, particularly for the scalp, and can be very helpful when thick scale is present. Dithranol is little used now but has a role in the treatment of resistant extensor psoriasis. Systemic treatments are used by specialists to treat severe disease and psoriatic arthropathy.

Acne

Acne is common and can be very distressing. It requires a stepwise approach, depending on the severity of the condition. Patients should be advised that treatments are prolonged – at least 6 months and often longer – and take time to work, and a treatment needs to be used for at least a month to judge its effectiveness. Very mild acne may only require gentle skin washes, perhaps containing an antiseptic such as resorcinol. Benzoyl peroxide is often effective for slightly more severe acne and may be combined with a topical antibiotic appropriate for acne treatment. If acne is widespread or more severe, oral antibiotics should be used, perhaps combined with a topical retinoid. In women, co-cyprindiol is often effective as an adjunct to other treatments, but carries some risks, that should be discussed with the patient. Regular review is important, and it should be established that the patient has actually been using the treatment prescribed. Oral isotretinoin, prescribed by a specialist, will often work when other treatments have failed, but relapse is quite common, and further courses are then needed. Fortunately, most patients grow out of their acne.

Rosacea

Although sometimes called 'acne rosacea', this is not acne. It has two main manifestations: inflammatory papules with occasional pustules, and erythema and telangiectasia. The papules respond to topical **azelaic acid** or to **ivermectin cream** (ivermectin may exert its effect through reducing the population of a particular skin mite). **Metronidazole gel** is less effective than these preparations. Oral tetracyclines are effective for more widespread or resistant disease. Recurrence is common. The erythema and telangiectasia do not respond very well to these treatments. A topical application of the vasoconstrictor **brimonidine tartrate** will reduce the redness, but the effect is temporary. Camouflagers may help hide the condition. Pulsed dye laser treatment is effective for telangiectasias. Severe rosacea is sometimes treated with oral isotretinoin.

Scabies

The itch caused by the mite infestation underlying scabies can be intolerable. Unfortunately, it persists for some weeks after treatment, and antipruritics such as **crotamiton cream** and antihistamines may be needed.

The infestation is best treated with **permethrin dermal cream** applied carefully to every nook and cranny of the body below the ears. One careful application is sufficient. No new burrows should appear after successful treatment.

Pityriasis Versicolor

This is a common condition causing discoloured or depigmented, mildly inflamed 'geographic' patches, often on the back. It is caused by a yeast infection and responds to some antifungals. While topical application of ketoconazole shampoo can be effective, the rash is often difficult to get at, and a 1-week course of oral itraconazole is generally effective and safe. Selenium sulphide shampoo is still sometimes advocated but is less effective than the other treatments. Patients should be advised that the altered pigmentation may take some months to resolve, but no new patches should appear after successful treatment.

Seborrhoeic Dermatitis

Seborrhoeic dermatitis is a common inflammatory skin condition affecting the scalp, nasolabial folds, eyebrows and chest. In infants, the scalp is most commonly affected ('cradle cap'). Yeast overgrowth in the skin is thought to be part of the cause. Infantile seborrhoeic dermatitis usually resolves by 4 months of age.

Management of seborrhoeic dermatitis in infants involves advice on simple measures such as softening of scales with almond oil and washing of the scalp with baby shampoo. An imidazole cream can be used if also needed.

In adults, ketoconazole 2% shampoo or an anti-dandruff shampoo (containing coal tar or salicylic acid) is often effective. Ketoconazole shampoo can be used on the face, beard and chest. The shampoo should be left on for 5 min before rinsing off. If the body is mainly affected, then ketoconazole cream or an imidazole cream can also be used. A mild corticosteroid cream can be used for itchy and inflamed lesions, and a more potent application can be used for short period on very itchy scalps.

CLINICAL NOTE

Skin conditions can have marked psychological effects and clinicians should be aware that quality of life can be severely affected by conditions such as acne, eczema and psoriasis (Cengiz and Gürel, 2020). Teenagers and young adults are most affected and specialist psychological support in addition to pharmacological treatment have shown to have a positive effect on people with dermatological conditions (De Vere Hunt et al., 2019).

APPLICATION OF SKIN PREPARATIONS

Use of Gloves by Nurses. Drugs can be absorbed through the intact skin. It is therefore very important that the person applying cream wears gloves when applying any preparation to the skin, particularly one containing active ingredients.

Patient Education. Many patients will be required to apply their skin preparations over long periods, so they must be taught the correct technique. Adverse effects, such as redness and soreness, and relapse may require a change of treatment. They need to know how many times a day to apply the preparation, how much to apply and if more than one topical preparation is necessary, how to use them in conjunction with one another. Many skin conditions fluctuate in severity and it is useful if patients can be taught to identify trigger factors so they can be avoided.

Skin conditions are easily observable to other people and can be very distressing. Patients may need considerable psychological support if symptoms persist long term.

Wet Wraps. Wet wraps are warm, wet occlusive dressings made up from elasticated viscose stockinette. They are used for children in the treatment of atopic eczema to rehydrate the skin using emollients, treat inflammation with appropriate corticosteroids, cool the skin and promote skin healing. The dressings are usually applied daily for about a week. The procedure for use is as follows:

1. Lengths of the tubular bandage are used to make two body suits. They are measured and cut to fit the patient.
2. The prescribed medication is applied to the skin.
3. The first layer is soaked in warm water, squeezed out and applied to the body while still warm and wet.
4. The second dry layer is applied over the wet layer.
5. The child then can put on normal clothing.
6. The process is repeated after 24 hours.

CLINICAL NOTE

Wet wraps should not be used on infants under 6 months of age because of the risk of hypothermia. Children and parents need support and education from specially-trained nurses when wet wraps are used on children.

Medicated Baths.

- The bath water should be approximately 36°C.
- Stir in the medication and mix well to ensure an even concentration.
- The patient should soak for about 10 min.

Creams and Ointments.

- Most active agents should be applied sparingly.
- Do not rub unless specifically directed.
- Smooth the preparation on gently in the direction of the hair fall (Fig. 24.1).

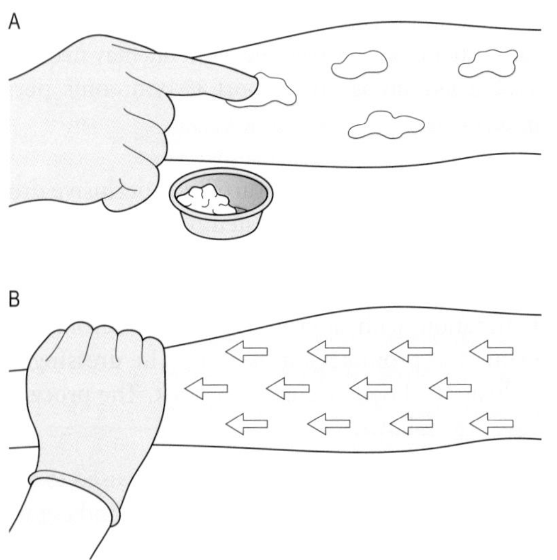

Fig. 24.1 Application of creams and ointments: smooth on in the direction of the hair fall.

- A 10 cm strip of cream or ointment from a standard nozzle of a tube of medication is the equivalent of 2 g (Fig. 24.2).

Application of Corticosteroids.

- Corticosteroids are best applied to hydrated skin.
- Apply an emollient 20 min before the steroid to increase its effectiveness.
- Care should be taken to apply only the prescribed amount of corticosteroid to avoid potential side-effects. The **Rule of Nines** is a recognized method for assessing the quantity of the preparation to be applied (Fig. 24.3).
- Patients may also be advised on how to use the '**fingertip method**' to apply their topical preparations in safe quantities (Fig. 24.4).

DRUG ERUPTIONS

A skin eruption following a drug treatment is quite common and therefore this cause must always be considered whenever a patient is seen with an unusual rash. However, patients are often receiving more than one drug, and it may be difficult or impossible to determine which one is responsible.

The skin can only react in a certain number of ways, which are known as reaction patterns. A good example is *urticaria*, which can be provoked by a number of different drugs and is the most likely reaction pattern following ingestion of aspirin or related drugs. The angiotensin-converting enzyme (ACE) inhibitors

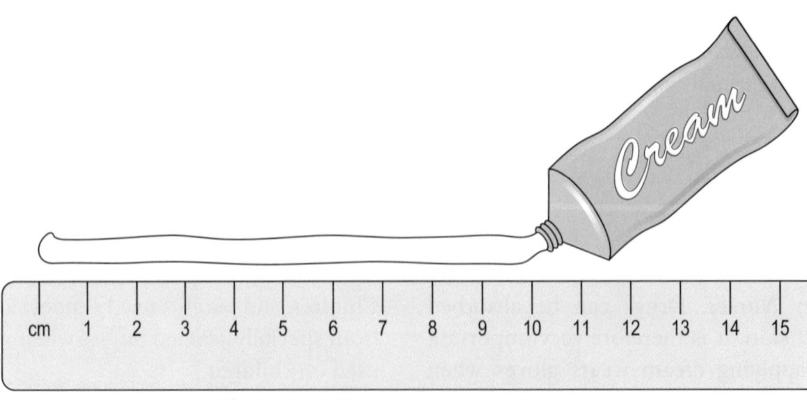

Fig. 24.2 Measuring ointment/cream.

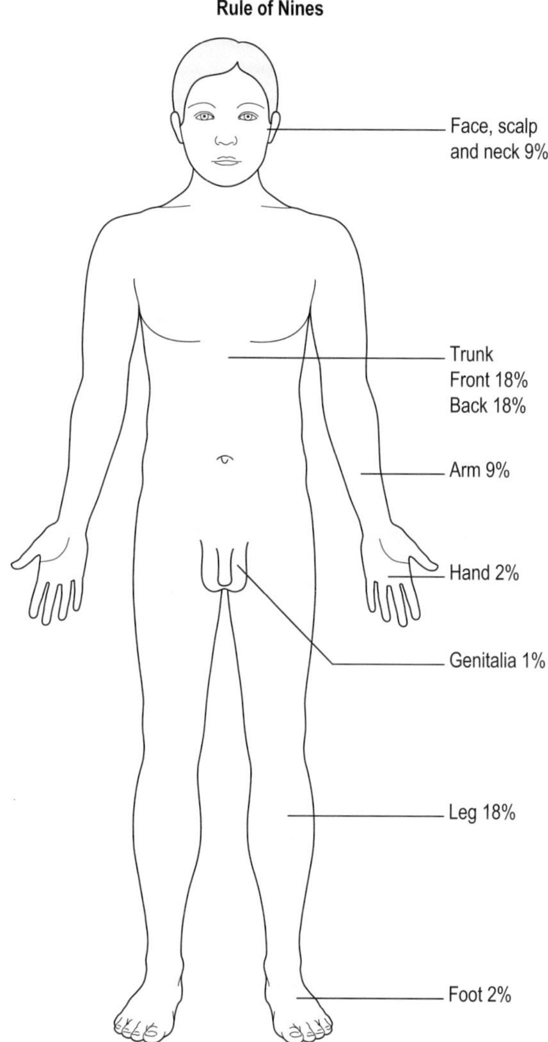

Fig. 24.3 ■ Rule of Nines. This shows the percentage of the total body surface area made up of the various parts of the body. It can be seen that the percentages are usually 9% or a multiple of 9%. In general, no more than 2 g of steroid ointment per 9% of body surface should be applied at any one time, i.e. 4 fingertip units per 9% of body surface (measured by the male finger) or 5 fingertip units per 9% of body surface (measured by the female finger).

are an important cause of urticarial rashes. Other drug classes can produce different types of reaction: furosemide can cause a purpuric rash, glutethimide can induce a generalized erythema and sulphonamides can elicit a measles-like rash.

Some drugs can cause many different types of skin eruption. Gold can provoke a generalized exfoliative erythroderma, which may be fatal, or a rash resembling pityriasis rosea, or just a nondescript erythema associated with a stomatitis. Penicillin can cause a severe erythema in some patients, and this may be so marked that a diagnosis of erythema multiforme may be considered.

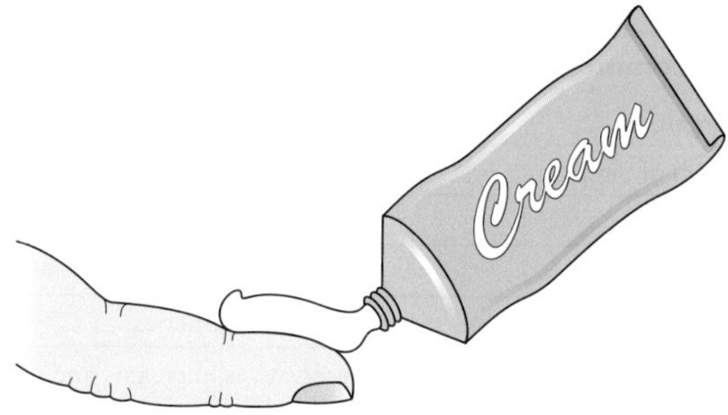
Cream
1 g ointment/cream = 2 fingertip units (males)
2.5 fingertip units (females)

Fig. 24.4 ■ Fingertip units (males and females for 1 g of cream).

In a few cases, adverse drug reactions including Stevens–Johnson syndrome and toxic epidermal necrosis (TEN) may be so severe that they become life-threatening. The following is a list of drugs most frequently associated with Stevens–Johnson syndrome and TEN:

- Sulfadoxine
- Sulfadiazine
- Sulfasalazine
- Co-trimoxazole
- Phenytoin
- Carbamazepine
- Barbiturates
- Phenylbutazone
- Piroxicam
- Allopurinol
- Aminopenicillins.

CLINICAL NOTE

Patients should be asked about allergies and sensitivities when topical preparations are recommended or prescribed. These allergies should be documented clearly on the medication chart and or in the patient's clinical notes. It is all healthcare workers' responsibility to document an allergy, including the updating of allergy cards.

TABLE 24.3

Common Allergens in Contact Dermatitis

Allergen	Sources
Balsam of Peru	Perfumes, citrus fruit
Colophony	Sticking plaster, collodion
Neomycin	Topical medicaments
Benzocaine	Topical anaesthetics
Parabens	Preservatives in creams and cosmetics
Wool alcohols	Lanolin, creams and cosmetics
Imidazolidinyl urea	Preservative in creams and cosmetics
Formaldehyde (aqueous)	Cosmetics, clothing, glues, paper

Contact Dermatitis

Contact dermatitis is an eczematous eruption produced by external agents, including some medicines (Table 24.3). Some emollients and paste bandages contain preservatives and many preparations have fragrance additives, both of which are known sensitizers. The BNF and pharmaceutical company data sheets list any additives that may be present in topical preparations.

CLINICAL NOTE

Medicated agents such as antiseptics can cause contact dermatitis. This is an occupational health hazard in nursing and may increase the risk of contracting parenteral viral infections such as HIV due to the production on the skin of micro-abrasions.

Light Sensitization

Some drugs sensitize the skin to ultraviolet light. A skin eruption occurs when the photosensitive person has taken or applied the medication and then been exposed to sunlight. Two subtypes of reactions occur, phototoxic and photoallergic (Table 24.4).

Phototoxic reactions develop a few hours after exposure to sunlight and often resemble severe sunburn. In photoallergic reactions the onset is delayed, and the rash is eczematous in nature. Table 24.5 lists some more agents causing photosensitivity.

TABLE 24.4

Drugs Causing Phototoxic and Photoallergic Reactions

Phototoxic	Photoallergic
Topical	
Coal tar	Halogenated salicylamides
Psoralens	
Furocoumarins, e.g. bergamot oil	
Systemic	
Demeclocycline	Sulphonamides
Doxycycline	Phenothiazines
Chlorpromazine	Griseofulvin

TABLE 24.5

Agents Causing Photosensitivity

Agent Type	Examples
Drug reactions	
Antibiotics	Sulphonamides, tetracycline
NSAIDs	Azapropazone
Hypoglycaemics	Chlorpropamide, glibenclamide
Sedatives	Chlorpromazine
Diuretics	Amiloride, thiazides
Contact sensitivity	
Drugs	Chlorpromazine
Sunscreens	Para-aminobenzoic acid (PABA)
Cosmetics	Perfumes, especially musk ambrette
Plants	Chrysanthemums, St. John's Wort

Treatment of Adverse Skin Reactions

Treatment is generally simple in that all medicines which are the likely cause photosensitivity should be withdrawn. However, sometimes symptomatic treatment may be required, with calamine cream for pruritus or oral H_1 receptor antagonists (antihistamines) to make the patient more comfortable. It should be noted that the topical application of antibiotics, H_1 receptor antagonists (antihistamines) and local anaesthetics should be avoided, as they often cause sensitization rashes themselves.

CLINICAL NOTE

Photosensitive patients, including those with disorders such as systemic lupus erythematosus, porphyria and chronic actinic dermatitis, must be advised to wear sunscreens and protective clothing when outdoors.

SUMMARY

- Emollients are the mainstay of management for both eczema and psoriasis.
- Prolonged use of lanolin can lead to skin sensitization.
- Pastes are particularly useful for localized lesions, e.g. psoriasis.
- Dusting powders are particularly useful in the folds of the skin.
- The choice of a topical corticosteroid should be the least potent preparation at the lowest strength that is effective.
- No corticosteroid stronger than hydrocortisone ointment (0.5%–1%) should routinely be used in infants or on the face.
- Aciclovir cream is the treatment of choice for herpes simplex of the skin and should be applied as early as possible.
- With hyperkeratotic conditions the skin should be hydrated before applying emollients.
- Nurses should wear gloves when applying any preparation to the patient's skin.
- Patients should be taught the correct technique for applying skin preparations.
- Steroids are best applied to hydrated skin.
- The Rule of Nines is a recognized method for assessing the quantity of the steroid preparation to be applied.
- Topical application of antibiotics, antihistamines and local anaesthetics should be avoided, as they often cause sensitization rashes.
- Make-up should always be removed at night.

REFERENCES AND FURTHER READING

Aldredge, L.M., Higham, R.C., 2018. Manifestations and management of difficult-to-treat psoriasis. J. Dermatol. Nurs. 10 (4), 189–197.

Bahrani, E., Nunneley, C.E., Hsu, S., Kass, J.S., 2016. Cutaneous adverse effects of neurologic medications. CNS Drugs 30 (3), 245–267.

Brandon, A., Mufti, A., Gary Sibbald, R., 2019. Diagnosis and management of cutaneous psoriasis: a review. Adv. Skin Wound Care 32 (2), 58–69.

Cengiz, G.F., Gürel, G., 2020. Difficulties in emotion regulation and quality of life in patients with acne. Qual. Life Res. 29 (2), 431–438.

De Vere Hunt, I., Chapman, K., Wali, G., et al., 2019. Establishing and developing a teenage and young adult dermatology clinic with embedded specialist psychological support. Clin. Exp. Dermatol. 44 (8), 893–896.

Erdil, D., Koku Aksu, A.E., Falay Gür, T., Gürel, M.S., 2020. Hand eczema treatment: change behaviour with text messaging, a randomized trial. Contact Dermatitis 82 (3), 153–160.

Jheeta, A., Fawcett, J.M., de Berke, D., 2016. Topical treatments for scalp psoriasis. Prescriber 27, 38–41.

Lavers, I., 2014. Diagnosis and management of acne vulgaris in aesthetic practice. J. Aesthet. Nurs. 3 (10), 482–489.

Lawton, S., 2013. Safe and effective application of topical treatments to the skin. Nurs. Stand. 27, 42–56.

Lawton, S., 2014. Childhood atopic eczema: adherence to treatment. Nurse Prescribing 12, 226–231.

Lawton, S., 2014. Managing difficult and severe eczema in children. Nurse Prescribing 12, 26–31.

Mochizuki, H., Lavery, M.J., Nattkemper, L.A., et al., 2019. Impact of acute stress on itch sensation and scratching behaviour in patients with atopic dermatitis and healthy controls. Br. J. Dermatol. 180 (4), 821–827.

Penzer, R., 2013. Prescribing for dry skin conditions. Nurse Prescribing 11, 276–283.

Peters, J., 2006. Exploring the use of emollient therapy in dermatology nursing. Br. J. Community Nurs. 11, 194–201.

Roujeau, J.C., Stern, R.S., 1994. Severe adverse cutaneous reactions to drugs. N. Engl. J. Med. 331, 1272–1285.

Stone, L.A., Lindfield, E.M., Robertson, S., 1989. A Colour Atlas of Nursing Procedures in Skin Disorders. Wolfe Medical, London.

Stone, L.A., 2000. Medilan: a hypoallergenic lanolin for emollient therapy. Br. J. Nurs. 9, 54.

Watkins, J., 2014. Effective management of atopic eczema in adults. Nurse Prescribing 12, 430–435.

Watkins, J., 2014. Overview of the treatment of psoriasis in adults. Nurse Prescribing 12, 174–179.

Woo, T.E., Somayaji, R., Haber, R.M., Parsons, L., 2019. Scratching the surface: a review of dermatitis. Adv. Skin Wound Care 32 (12), 542–549.

Woolever, D.R., 2020. Skin infections and outpatient burn management: fungal and viral skin infections. FP Essent. 489, 16–20.

25 DRUGS USED FOR EAR, NOSE AND THROAT DISORDERS

CHAPTER OUTLINE

LEARNING OBJECTIVES

At the end of the chapter, the reader should be able to:

- Describe the drug and non-drug treatment of otitis externa
- Describe the drug and non-drug treatment of otitis media
- Describe how to apply nose drops
- Explain the uses of steroid drops and sprays
- Describe the treatment of sore throats

THE EAR

The use of ear drops will be considered under individual disorders of the ear.

Instillation of Drops

1. The head is turned so that the affected ear is uppermost.
2. Discharge is gently mopped away.
3. Two or three drops are instilled, and the head is held in position for 1–2 min.

Wax in the Ear

Wax may become hard and impacted in the ear. It only need be removed if it is affecting hearing. This only occurs if the whole ear canal is obstructed. Otherwise, wax is a normal, physiological substance and should be left alone. If removal is needed, then before syringing (irrigation), and ideally before microsuction, wax should be softened. Over-the-counter wax softening agents often seem to irritate the ear canal. A 5.0% solution of sodium bicarbonate or warm almond or olive oil instilled for a few days will usually soften wax without causing irritation.

Ear wax 'candles' are sometimes promoted as a means of removing wax. A type of long tubular wick is inserted into the ear and is lit and allowed to smoulder. A wax-like substance appears at the end of the wick, which is taken as 'proof' that ear wax has been removed. Unfortunately, it is easy to prove that these devices are completely useless (and sometimes dangerous), which still does not stop some people from buying them and some 'therapists' from offering them.

Otitis Externa

Severe infection is best managed with expert guidance, as regular aural cleansing and medication are required. An absorbent wick may be inserted into the ear canal to promote drainage of debris and allow medication access.

Ear drops will only be effective if the canal is cleared of debris. Most commonly, drops containing a combination of antibacterial and antiinflammatory substances are used. The following preparations are often used to treat mild to moderate infective otitis externa:

- **Clioquinol 1% with flumetasone 0.02%** has a mild antibacterial and antifungal action but stains the skin and clothes.
- **Gentamicin 0.3% with hydrocortisone 1%** is antibacterial and antiinflammatory.
- **Dexamethasone with glacial acetic acid and neomycin sulfate** is available as a spray, which may simplify application. Glacial acetic acid is antibacterial (particularly against *pseudomonas* species) and antifungal. It is also available as a spray without steroids or antimicrobials.
- **Aluminium acetate** drops are often effective for mild infections and inflammation of the ear canal.

Other combinations of antibacterial drugs with corticosteroids are available.

However, the following precautions should be observed when using such medicines:

- Treatment with antibiotic ear drops should not be continued for longer than 1 week owing to the risks of drug sensitization and the development of fungal infection.
- Gentamicin or neomycin ear drops should not be used if the eardrum is perforated, as these drugs are ototoxic and may affect hearing. Some specialists do use these drugs in the presence of a grommet or perforation, to treat chronic infection. In this case, patients must be counselled about the risks and benefits of treatment.

CLINICAL NOTE

A rare, but serious, complication of otitis external is necrotizing otitis externa, which, if left untreated, may result in permanent cranial nerve palsy or death. People with poorly-controlled diabetes may be at particular risk and a recently published clinical guideline recommends that people who present with this condition and with poor diabetic control should be referred to diabetes specialists to optimize glycaemic control (Hopkins et al., 2020).

Eczema of the ear canal is a common problem, even in patients with no eczema elsewhere. The itch provokes most people to poke at the ear, often with all manner of unsuitable instruments, risking ear drum damage and wax impaction. Cotton buds are often used, but are little better, and their use should be discouraged. Local corticosteroid drops can be used to reduce irritation and inflammation. Prednisolone 0.5% and betamethasone 0.1% work well and can be used intermittently.

Otitis Media

If the eardrum is not perforated, the instillation of antibiotics into the external ear is useless, as it will not reach the site of infection. Most infections are viral and require only an analgesic to reduce symptoms. There is good research evidence to show that even with proven bacterial otitis media in children, the use of antibiotics has a minimal effect on the duration of symptoms and does not reduce the risk of glue ear, ear drum perforation or mastoiditis (a rare infection of the mastoid bone of the skull). In trials, 60% of children with otitis media recovered within 24 h, whether they were given an antibiotic or a placebo. Given the need to reduce antibiotic prescribing in order to slow the progress of antibiotic resistance, most children with otitis media should not be prescribed an antibiotic. Among parents, there remains a high level of expectation for an antibiotic prescription. Careful explanation accompanied by printed information can reduce this expectation.

Antibiotics should be prescribed for otitis media in people of any age who are significantly unwell. Current UK guidance suggests that antibiotics should be considered in children under the age of 2 years who have bilateral otitis media, and people of any age with otitis media with discharge. Clinical judgement should be exercised in these cases. For instance, there is some evidence that antibiotics reduce the duration and severity of pain very slightly. In most cases, this is of minimal benefit but may be of great value in a child who is screaming with pain and has a bright red, bulging eardrum. If a decision is made to treat, then oral antibiotics should be used. Infections are usually due to *Streptococcus pneumoniae* or *Haemophilus influenzae*. Amoxicillin is usually effective, and erythromycin can be used for those who are sensitive to penicillin. A delayed prescription may be considered in some cases, i.e. a prescription is given, but the patient is asked not to have it dispensed unless the condition does not resolve within 3 days or seems to worsen.

Glue Ear

Chronic secretory otitis media, often referred to as 'glue ear', is a common sequel of acute otitis media in children and in adults. Following an infection, an effusion of fluid forms in the middle ear and interferes with the normal function of the tiny bones associated with hearing. A degree of loss of hearing is a consequence. In most cases, it is mild and resolves over 6–12 weeks. In some cases, hearing loss is more severe, and the effusion takes longer to resolve. If this occurs in early childhood, language development may be affected. Until quite recently, many children with glue ear were treated by surgical insertion of grommets to ventilate the middle ear. It is now recognized that most of these treatments were unnecessary, as the condition was not causing problems with speech or school progress and is self-limiting. Grommets are now used far more sparingly in situations where there are language or school problems and the condition is not resolving or keeps recurring.

Most children with glue ear can be manged expectantly. There is evidence that the use of devices that allow children to perform the Valsalva manoeuvre (expiration against a closed airway) can help resolution, by encouraging the eustachian tubes to open and ventilate the middle ear. Such devices include one which enables children to blow up balloons, using their noses (*Otovent* in the UK). In adults, chewing gum and performing the Valsalva manoeuvre can help resolution. While congestion of the eustachian tubes seems to be part of the cause of glue ear, there is no good evidence to support the use of topical or systemic decongestants, antihistamines, mucolytics, corticosteroids or antibiotics to help relieve this congestion. Despite this, their use remains popular in some countries.

Vertigo

Vertigo is a sensation of spinning movement and unsteadiness, often associated with nausea. It is caused by an upset to the sense of balance, either due to viral infection or age-related processes. It is a common condition in primary care situations and relatively rarely seen in hospital clinics. It can be very distressing, but most episodes are benign and self-limiting, although they can take some weeks to resolve completely.

Drugs have very little role in the management of vertigo, although they are often prescribed despite this.

Antiemetic drugs such as **prochlorperazine** may help if nausea is severe. They also have a sedative effect on the balance mechanism and can relieve the symptoms of vertigo. However, there is evidence that using these drugs may prolong the resolution of the attack. They also can cause sedation in the elderly. They are better avoided unless the symptoms are very severe.

Ménière's disease is a condition characterized by episodes of vertigo, with tinnitus and progressive hearing loss. **Betahistine** is a tablet licensed for treatment of this condition yet there is limited evidence on its efficacy (Devantier et al., 2020). It appears to lower pressure in the inner ear which may be helpful. There is little evidence of benefit in using this drug for other types of vertigo.

CLINICAL NOTE

People living with Ménière's disease report a profound effect on quality of life, with vertigo being the most problematic symptom. Clinicians supporting people with the condition should consider the psychosocial as well as the physical effects of the conditions. Recent in-depth qualitative research reports loss of control and having to make adjustments to lifestyle to live with the condition (Bell et al., 2017; Talewar et al., 2020).

THE NOSE

Drugs may be instilled into the nose. However, medication with strong solutions of antibiotics or vasoconstrictors can stop the nasal mucous membranes' cilia beating and thus impede rather than help the clearance of infected material from the nasal cavities. The use of topical nasal decongestants for more than a short period runs the risk of rebound congestion (see later). In general, the only agents that should be applied topically to the nose for extended periods, if needed, are the corticosteroid sprays.

Applying Nose Drops

Nose drops should always be given in a way that enables the apex of the nasal cavity to be reached and to bathe the openings of the sinuses. A fairly easy way of doing this is the 'head down position': the patient lies back on a couch or bed with the head extended over the end and the opening of the nostrils pointing towards the ceiling. The appropriate drops are instilled into each nostril, the patient being instructed to breathe through the mouth, thus holding the nose drops in the nasal cavities. This position should be maintained for at least 1 min. If the neck cannot be extended fully or the position is too uncomfortable, then other positions may be tried (Fig. 25.1).

While nasal drops are needed to treat severe congestion, polyps and sinusitis, nasal sprays are far more convenient for milder cases of allergic rhinitis.

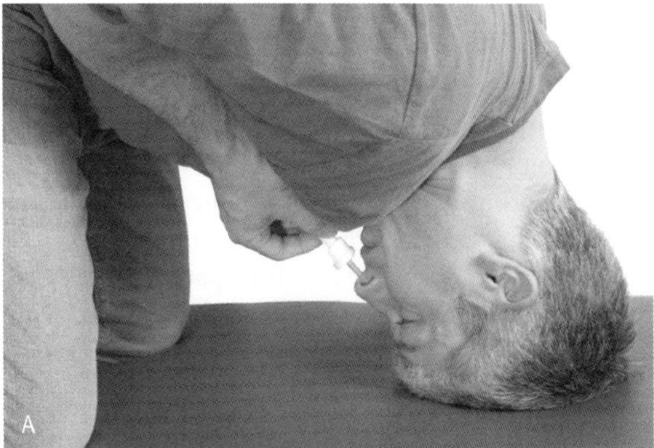

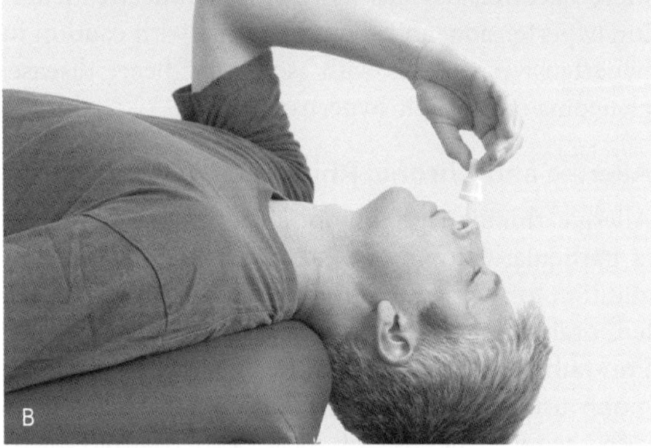

Fig. 25.1 ■ Correct positions for delivery of nasal drops in the 'head down' position. (A, B) Either of these positions ensure that drops find their way to the openings of the facial sinus spaces.

Nasal Congestion

Nasal congestion is a common experience. It is often acute, as a consequence of an upper respiratory tract infection (URTI), or a seasonal allergy (allergic rhinitis; 'hay fever'). It may be chronic, either as a result of chronic allergy, often to house-dust mites, or constitutional (vasomotor rhinitis). Long-term allergy may result in the formation of nasal mucosal polyps, which further obstruct the nasal passages. The symptoms of nasal congestion include both difficulty in breathing through one or both nostrils and rhinitis (a 'runny nose'). Acute or chronic nasal congestion may interfere with the normal drainage of the sinuses, resulting in discomfort and pain in the face. Sometimes the sinuses fill with secretions that may become secondarily infected, causing severe pain and constitutional upset.

Decongestant Nose Drops, Sprays and Tablets

Sympathomimetic drops and sprays work by constricting blood vessels in the nasal mucosa, causing them to shrink, reducing congestion and rhinitis. They are useful for temporary relief of symptoms in URTI and may help relieve the symptoms of acute sinusitis. **Ephedrine** drops are sometimes used, while **oxymetazoline** and similar agents are available without prescription, in spray form. These products should never be used regularly for more than a few days, as they run the risk of rebound congestion with continued use. Here the mucous membranes become more swollen and the congestion worsens as the medication wears off. If use is then continued, chronic severe congestion develops – a condition known as *rhinitis medicamentosa*.

Systemic decongestants such as **pseudoephedrine hydrochloride** and **phenylephrine hydrochloride** are available in tablet form and have limited role in short-term treatment of severe congestion. Rebound congestion is less likely to occur. Pseudoephedrine is more effective, but has more adverse effects, including hypertension, and should be used with caution in hypertensives, people with ischaemic heart disease, glaucoma or prostatic hypertrophy.

Allergic and Chronic Rhinitis

Allergic rhinitis is common, and seasonal hay fever is particularly common and can be debilitating. In addition to advice about minimizing exposure to pollen, oral antihistamines are effective in milder cases. **Loratadine, cetirizine** and **fexofenadine** are commonly used non-sedating antihistamines. More severe cases require the use of local corticosteroid nasal sprays. **Beclomethasone**, **fluticasone**, **budesonide** and **mometasone** sprays are all commonly used. They are of similar efficacy in clinical use, but differ in frequency of application, delivery system and cost. Patients should be advised that they take a few days to take effect and they should be used continuously throughout the season. Antihistamine sprays, such as **azelastine** may be helpful in addition or instead of corticosteroids and are rapid acting. A nasal spray preparation of the mast cell stabilizer **sodium cromoglycate** is also available for the prophylaxis of allergic rhinitis. Cromoglycate is more commonly used as an eye drop to relieve the itchy eyes associated with hay fever.

Chronic allergic rhinitis can be managed by allergen reduction, if possible, and by a combination of any of the above treatments, although nasal corticosteroids are generally most effective. In addition, **ipratropium bromide**, more commonly used in the treatment of chronic obstructive pulmonary disease, can be used as a nasal spray, to relieve chronic rhinitis. It should be used with caution in patients with glaucoma. The oral asthma drug **montelukast** (see Chapter 9) can also help relieve the symptoms of acute and chronic allergic rhinitis.

Non-allergic chronic rhinitis (vasomotor rhinitis) can be difficult to treat. Any of the previously mentioned treatments may be tried alone or in combination, and corticosteroids and ipratropium bromide seem to be the most effective choices.

Chronic rhinitis is often accompanied by nasal polyps. Bilateral nasal polyps may be greatly reduced by the use of corticosteroid nose drops for several weeks. The improvement can then be maintained using corticosteroid sprays. Recalcitrant polyps need surgical removal, and a lone polyp should always be biopsied, in case of malignancy.

Sinusitis

Sinus pain and discomfort is unpleasant but does not usually imply significant infection. Most cases should be managed with analgesia, decongestants, steam inhalations and nasal douches with saline solution. More prolonged cases benefit from the use of nasal steroids in drop or spray form. If there is evidence of infection, such as fever, systemic upset and purulent nasal discharge, then antibiotics should be used. A 5-day course of phenoxymethyl penicillin, doxycycline or clarithromycin may be used.

Chronic sinusitis or frequently recurrent acute attacks may be helped by long-term use of corticosteroid sprays. If not, then functional endoscopic sinus surgery may be effective. There is no role for the old practice of sinus washouts.

CLINICAL NOTE

Patients with sinusitis may request antibiotics; however, a recent systematic review reported marginal efficacy when they were prescribed (Lemiengre et al., 2018). This review states there is no indication for prescribing antibiotics in this condition in the adult population and, if prescribed, may increase the risk of antimicrobial resistance.

Local Antibiotics

Local antibiotics have little place in the treatment of nasal infections, but a cream containing **chlorhexidine and neomycin** (*Naseptin*) can be applied locally to Little's area in the nasal vestibule in patients whose recurrent nosebleeds are caused by chronic low-grade infection in this area. Naseptin is also useful in patients who are carriers of staphylococci, especially MRSA. It may be used as part of a decontamination procedure in these patients before they undergo surgery, since it may reduce the risk of cross-infection to other patients and the transfer of the bacteria from the nose to the wound. **Mupirocin** ointments are also used for the eradication of MRSA prior to surgery.

THE THROAT

Treatment of Sore Throats

Most sore throats are caused by viral illnesses and get better on their own over a few days. The common bacterial causes are *group A streptococci*. Most of these infections are also mild and self-limiting and probably do not require antibiotics. There is no substantial evidence to suggest that the widespread use of antibiotics to date is the reason for the decline in the incidence of feared complications of streptococcal infection, such as rheumatic fever or kidney damage. In general, adults and children who are not significantly unwell, with a sore throat of less than 3 days duration, particularly if it is in the context of an URTI, can be managed with analgesia. If the sore throat is severe and persistent, or if it is accompanied by systemic upset, then antibiotics should be considered. Various clinical scoring systems such as the modified CENTOR criteria or FeverPAIN score can be used to guide the decision about antibiotic use. These use clinical signs, symptoms and the patient's age to produce a score that can be helpful but should not be a substitute for clinical judgement. If antibiotics are given (and once again, a delayed prescription can be considered), phenoxymethyl penicillin is the antibiotic of choice, given for 10 days, as recurrence is common with shorter courses. Clarithromycin is an alternative if there is penicillin allergy.

CLINICAL NOTE

A sore throat may be a pointer to a blood dyscrasia such as neutropenia (low white cell count). This is a rare but serious condition and is most commonly associated with treatment with certain drugs. Chemotherapy drugs for cancer, DMARDs in rheumatoid disease and immunosuppressive drugs for transplants are the most common causes, but other drugs can also cause neutropenia, including carbimazole and the selective serotonin reuptake inhibitor antidepressants. If there is any suspicion of this, a full blood count (FBC) must be urgently arranged.

THE MOUTH

Dry Mouth

Dry mouth (xerostomia) is a feature of some rheumatic disorders, such as Sjogren's disease and may also be a consequence of radiation therapy in the head and neck area. Any drug with an anticholinergic (antimuscarinic) effect can cause some degree of dry mouth. Such drugs include tricyclic antidepressants and gut and bladder antispasmodics. Xerostomia can be very unpleasant, and the absence of normal saliva also increases the risk of dental decay. Patients can be advised to sip iced water or suck ice-cubes, and sucking sugar free sweets or chewing sugar free gum can stimulate residual salivary function. The drug **pilocarpine** can also help if there is some residual salivary function. If these measures are insufficient, then various thickened liquids in mouthwash and spray form can act as artificial saliva. Fluoridated mouthwashes and toothpastes are also important to try to preserve the teeth.

Mouth Ulcers

Many mouth ulcers are caused by minor trauma and resolve in a few days. Many mildly analgesic, antiinflammatory products are available without prescription and may aid healing. Some of these products also coat the exposed ulcer bases and thus relieve pain.

Some people get recurrent painful mouth ulcers without trauma. These can be very debilitating. Some may be a consequence of rheumatic disorders such as Behçet's disease, but many appear to have an autoimmune cause and are known as *aphthous ulcers*. These may respond to improved oral hygiene measures and antiseptic mouthwashes. Some may be improved by the use of a topical corticosteroid. A preparation of hydrocortisone in a tablet form that sticks to mucous membranes is available (hydrocortisone 2.5 mg mucoadhesive buccal tablets). These may be applied on or near to the ulcer 4 times a day.

Halitosis

Halitosis (bad breath) is a common complaint. It rarely indicates any kind of serious illness, but it may be distressing. Obsessional complaints of bad breath in the absence of any evidence to support it may indicate psychiatric illness, sometimes serious. Most halitosis is the result of poor dental hygiene or smoking and food habits. Appropriate advice, dental treatment and regular dental hygiene is most helpful. Mild antiseptic mouthwashes can help.

SUMMARY

- Strong solutions of antibiotics or vasoconstrictors will cause cilia to stop beating in the nose and will therefore impede the clearance of infected material from the nasal cavities.
- Decongestant nasal drops or sprays should not be used for more than 1 week.
- Nasal drops should always be administered in the 'head down' or similar positions.
- Nasal steroids have a major role in many conditions.
- Antibiotics should not routinely be used to treat acute sinusitis.
- Treatment with antibiotic ear drops should not be continued for longer than 1 week owing to the risks of drug sensitization and the development of fungal infection.
- Gentamicin or neomycin ear drops should not be used if the eardrum is perforated, as deafness may result.
- In otitis media, instillation of ear drops is useless if the eardrum is not perforated.
- Antibiotics have a very limited role in the management of otitis media. Analgesia is usually sufficient.
- Glue ear does not normally require drug or surgical treatment.
- Vertigo should not normally be treated with drugs, but prochlorperazine can sometimes be useful to relieve severe symptoms.
- Most sore throats do not require antibiotics.
- A sore throat can be a sign of a drug-related blood dyscrasia.
- Hydrocortisone pellets can help aphthous mouth ulcers.

REFERENCES AND FURTHER READING

Bell, S.L., Tyrrell, J., Phoenix, C., 2017. A day in the life of a Ménière's patient: understanding the lived experiences and mental health impacts of Ménière's disease. Sociol Health Illn. 39 (5), 680–695.

Devantier, L., Hougaard, D., Händel, M.N., et al., 2020. Using betahistine in the treatment of patients with Ménière's disease: a meta-analysis with the current randomized-controlled evidence. Acta. Otolaryngol. 140 (10), 845–853.

Granath, A., 2017. Recurrent acute otitis media: what are the options for treatment and prevention? Curr. Otorhinolaryngol. Rep. 5 (2), 93–100.

Hopkins, M.E., Bennett, A., Henderson, N., et al., 2020. A retrospective review and multi-specialty, evidence-based guideline for the management of necrotizing otitis externa. J. Laryngol. Otol. 134 (6), 487–492.

Hossenbaccus, L., Linton, S., Garvey, S., Ellis, A.K., 2020. Towards definitive management of allergic rhinitis: best use of new and established therapies. Allergy Asthma Clin. Immunol. 16, 39.

Lemiengre, M.B., van Driel, M.L., Merenstein, D., et al., 2018. Antibiotics for acute rhinosinusitis in adults. Cochrane Database Syst. Rev. 9 (9), CD006089.

Mildenhall, N., Honeybrook, A., Risoli Jr., T., et al., 2020. Clinician adherence to the clinical practice guideline: acute otitis externa. Laryngoscope 130 (6), 1565–1571.

Schwartz, S.R., Magit, A.E., Rosenfeld, R.M., et al., 2017. Clinical practice guideline (update): earwax (cerumen impaction). Otolaryngol. Head Neck Surg. 156, S1–S29.

Talewar, K.K., Cassidy, E., McIntyre, A., 2020. Living with Ménière's disease: an interpretative phenomenological analysis. Disabil. Rehabil. 42 (12), 1714–1726.

26 ANTIBACTERIALS

CHAPTER OUTLINE

LEARNING OBJECTIVES

At the end of this chapter, the reader should be able to:

- explain how the bacterial cell wall is a target for antibiotics
- define the terms Gram-positive and Gram-negative bacteria
- discuss how an antibiotic is chosen
- distinguish between the different classes of antibiotics and give important examples of each
- give an account of what TB is, how it is diagnosed and treated with drugs, and about immunization
- describe resistance to antibiotics, and how it happens with penicillins as an exemplar
- explain how antibiotics are used to treat common infections
- state the practicalities and precautions of antibiotic handling and administration

INTRODUCTION

The term 'antimicrobial' includes all agents that act against all types of microorganisms: **bacteria** (antibacterial), **viruses** (antiviral), **fungi** (antifungal) and **parasites** such as **protozoa** (antiparasitics). Many microorganisms live in or on our bodies and are normally harmless and can be beneficial. However, they can cause infectious disease under certain conditions, which is not completely understood. This is important to acknowledge because in clinical practice, it helps to appropriately act on investigation results, which requires knowledge and understanding of, e.g. commensal organisms that would not normally cause harm but normally do inhabit us. 'Antibacterials' and 'antibiotics' are commonly used terms that can sometimes be used interchangeably. 'Antibiotic' is a term used to describe any substance produced by or derived from an organism which inhibits the growth of or destroys another organism, usually a bacteria.

Antibacterial drugs have revolutionized the treatment of infection, and many diseases such as bacterial meningitis, which previously were often fatal, are now usually curable, but it must be realized that the battle against pathogenic bacteria is by no means over. Many organisms have become resistant to antibacterial drugs and this requires a continuing search for new drugs and modification of those already in use. It also means that they should never be used unnecessarily.

CLINICAL NOTE

According to the World Health Organization, the global burden of antimicrobial resistance costs 700,000 deaths annually (WHO, 2016). It is the health professionals' responsibility to be vigilant about appropriate antibiotic use. Advise patients about completing a full course of prescribed antibiotics, and challenge overuse or long-term use of antibiotics.

HOW ANTIBACTERIAL SUBSTANCES WORK

Antibiotics exert their effects in two main ways:

- Bactericidal agents kill bacteria rapidly (e.g. aminoglycosides, polymyxin).
- Bacteriostatic agents prevent bacteria from replicating, but do not kill them (e.g. sulphonamides, tetracyclines, chloramphenicol).

The distinction between these two categories is not clear. Many antibiotics that operate principally as bacteriostatic agents can become bactericidal under favourable circumstances. Factors affecting the mode of action include the concentration of the drug and the number and type of organisms. When relatively modest numbers of bacteria are present and the drug is given in high doses to highly sensitive organisms, a normally bacteriostatic agent such as penicillin may become bactericidal.

Antibiotics and the Bacterial Cell Wall

Each of the main groups of antibiotics has a different molecular structure and this is the factor that determines its mode of action. Many antibiotics exert their effects directly on the bacterial cell wall or must pass through it before disrupting bacterial metabolism at the intracellular level. The cell walls of all bacteria are composed of layers of protein molecules bound together by cross-linkages, resulting in large, complex chemical aggregates, but their fine structure depends on whether they are **Gram-positive** or

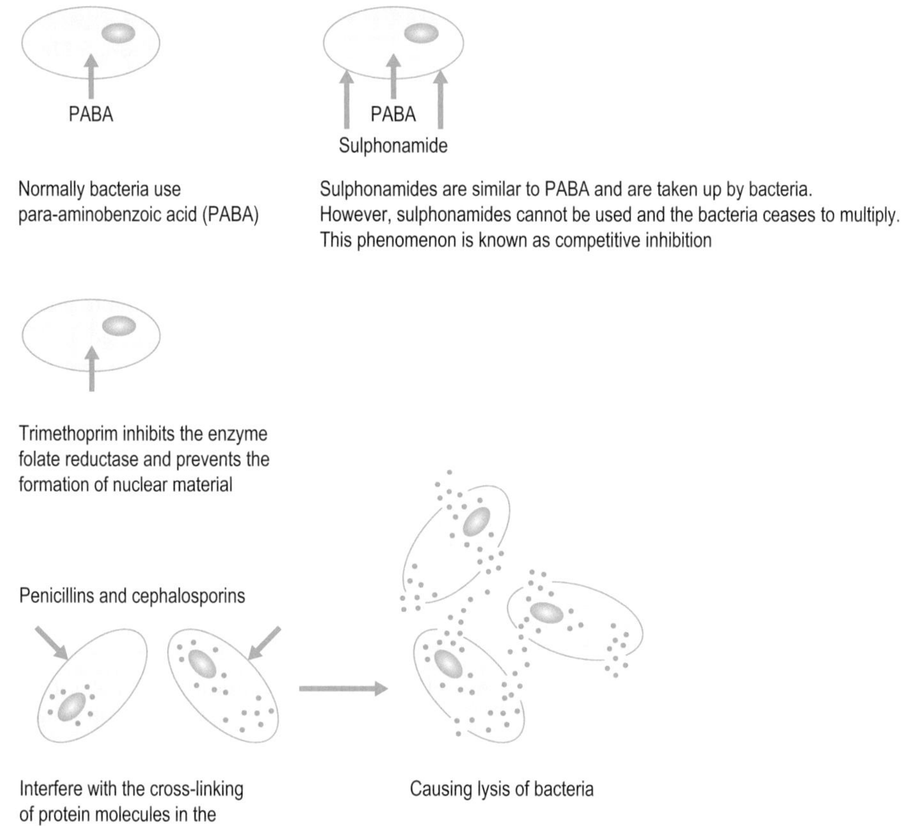
PABA
PABA
Sulphonamide
Normally bacteria use para-aminobenzoic acid (PABA)
Sulphonamides are similar to PABA and are taken up by bacteria. However, sulphonamides cannot be used and the bacteria ceases to multiply. This phenomenon is known as competitive inhibition
Trimethoprim inhibits the enzyme folate reductase and prevents the formation of nuclear material
Penicillins and cephalosporins
Interfere with the cross-linking of protein molecules in the cell walls of dividing bacteria
Causing lysis of bacteria

Fig. 26.1 ■ Some of the modes of action of antibacterial drugs.

Gram-negative. The fine structure of the cell wall influences susceptibility to the different groups of antibiotics. Some of the diverse ways in which the different groups of antibiotics exert their effects are illustrated in Fig. 26.1.

GRAM-POSITIVE AND GRAM-NEGATIVE BACTERIA

With few exceptions, bacteria may be classified as Gram-positive or Gram-negative, according to a staining technique used in laboratory identification that distinguishes different features of the cell wall. Generally, Gram-positive bacteria are able to withstand desiccation better than Gram-negative bacteria, and many form spores that resist drying. Gram-negative species multiply rapidly in the presence of moisture even when provided with minimal nourishment. Several Gram-positive and Gram-negative bacteria have had a long association with hospital infection and, because they can be carried on the hands, may be spread by cross-infection in any healthcare setting (Table 26.1). Prevention of spread of bacteria is strongly reinforced in healthcare settings using simple measure of handwashing.

Anaerobes

This term refers to bacteria that can live and multiply in the absence of free oxygen. In the laboratory, they require special conditions before they will grow in culture, but they are able to cause severe infections given the correct circumstances. Anaerobic bacteria naturally inhabiting the gut may cause severe sepsis following abdominal surgery.

TABLE 26.1

Gram-positive and Gram-negative Organisms in Hospitals

Gram-positive	Gram-negative
Staphylococcus aureus *Streptococcus pyogenes* *Streptococcus viridans* *Streptococcus pneumoniae* (*Pneumococcus*)	*Haemophilus influenzae* *Neisseria gonorrhoeae* (*Gonococcus*) *Neisseria meningitides* (*Meningococcus*) *E. coli* *Proteus* *Pseudomonas* *Klebsiella*

CLINICAL NOTE

If *Clostridium tetani* gains access to a penetrating wound that is free of oxygen, the organism multiplies and produces a toxin that causes tetanus. Tetanus vaccinations are effective and the WHO report an 88% reduction in the incidence of tetany since 1990, with 38,000 deaths in 2017. The widespread vaccination programme in Europe resulted in no deaths.

CHOOSING AN ANTIBIOTIC

When faced with a patient with an infectious disease, the first consideration is whether an antibiotic is required. Many infections (e.g. a mild sore throat) get better quickly without specific treatment. If antibiotic treatment is needed, the following points should be considered:

- The infecting organism: this is often suspected from the nature of the disease, and initial treatment is usually based on this suspicion. The nature of the organism should ideally be confirmed by culture of blood, sputum, urine, etc., although in practice this is not always possible or economically viable.
- The correct antibiotic to be used to eradicate the infection.
- The ability of the antibiotic to penetrate the site of infection (e.g. in meningitis not all drugs enter the cerebrospinal fluid, CSF).
- The route of administration: some antibiotics are ineffective orally and injection may be required for rapid action.

TABLE 26.2

Available Sulphonamides

Drug	Important features
Sulfasalazine	Used in ulcerative colitis. It is particularly useful for long-term maintenance treatment
Silver sulfadiazine	Applied locally as a cream to prevent infection in severe burns

- A drug history is essential to ensure that the patient has not previously had an adverse reaction to the chosen antibiotic, or that the antibiotic will not compromise any other drug being used, e.g. rifampicin and the contraceptive pill (see later).
- Possible complicating factors such as pregnancy, renal or hepatic failure.
- Cost implications of the drug balanced against its clinical effectiveness.

SULPHONAMIDES

This is one of the oldest groups of antibacterial agents. They differ to some extent in the range of organisms they attack, but most of their pharmacological properties are similar. They have been largely replaced because of the development of bacterial resistance and adverse side-effects, and most have disappeared from use. They are, with few exceptions, well and rapidly absorbed from the intestinal tract. They circulate widely in the body fluids and cross the meningeal barrier to enter the CSF.

After absorption, the liver begins to acetylate the sulphonamides. The acetylated drugs together with unaltered sulphonamide are excreted in the urine. The acetylated sulphonamides are very poorly soluble and therefore there is a danger that they will precipitate in the urine unless an adequate flow is maintained. Most of the sulphonamides are effective against a fairly wide range of bacteria, although unfortunately, certain of these bacteria have become resistant to treatment with these drugs. Table 26.2 gives a number of available sulphonamides.

Co-trimoxazole (Trimethoprim and Sulfamethoxazole)

Mechanism of Action. Sulphonamides affect bacteria by interfering with their use of para-aminobenzoic acid (PABA), a precursor of folic acid, which is ultimately essential in cell division (see Fig. 26.1). Trimethoprim interferes with folic acid metabolism at the phase when folic acid is changed to folinic acid to build up the cell nucleus. This requires the action of an enzyme, and, by combining with that enzyme, trimethoprim stops the reaction and the cell dies. The combination of a sulphonamide with trimethoprim is used because of their synergistic activity and is particularly effective in preventing bacterial cell division and is also bactericidal.

Therapeutic Use. The combined tablet of trimethoprim plus sulfamethoxazole, co-trimoxazole, is used for the treatment of urinary tract infection and exacerbation of chronic bronchitis if there is bacteriological evidence of sensitivity to this agent. Because of increased bacterial resistance and its adverse-effect profile, it is largely used in the treatment and prophylaxis of pneumocystis pneumonia. It is also used for nocardiasis (infections primarily in the lungs from bacteria found in soil and water) and toxoplasmosis (infection due to a parasite which can be found in cat faeces or undercooked meat). It has unlicensed indication for the use of *Burkholderia cepacia* (e.g. found in patients suffering with cystic fibrosis).

Adverse Effects. These can be nausea and vomiting, and occasionally blood disorders. More serious is the occasional development of Stevens–Johnson syndrome, with a bullous rash, mouth ulceration and fever, which can be fatal.

Trimethoprim

Trimethoprim can also be used alone. At present, it is largely used to treat urinary tract infections, but it can also be used to treat respiratory tract infection as well as acne.

Adverse effects. These include nausea, rashes and, rarely, depression of the blood count.

Contraindication. It should not be used in the first 3 months of pregnancy as it is as a folate antagonist so can predispose to increased risk of neural tube defects.

NITROFURANS

This group of drugs has been investigated sporadically for over 30 years. However, the only one currently used is **nitrofurantoin**.

Nitrofurantoin has a fairly wide antibacterial spectrum and is considerably concentrated in the urine. It is therefore particularly useful in the treatment or prophylaxis of urinary tract infection. Nitrofurantoin is often the first-line treatment for urinary tract infections, rather than trimethoprim, due to increased incidence of bacterial resistance against trimethoprim. Nausea sometimes occurs, but this can be minimized by giving the drug after food. Other adverse effects include rashes and fever. It should not be used in patients with renal failure, as accumulation will occur with the potential for toxicity.

CLINICAL NOTE

Drug counselling: nitrofurantoin may colour urine yellow/brown. This is harmless.

QUINOLONES

The Medicines and Healthcare products Regulatory Agency (MHRA) has issued a warning against quinolones that they can cause long-lasting or potentially irreversible adverse reactions affecting musculoskeletal (tendinitis or tendon rupture) and nervous system (e.g. peripheral neuropathy). The quinolones comprise:

- Ciprofloxacin
- Levofloxacin
- Moxifloxacin
- Nalidixic acid
- Norfloxacin
- Ofloxacin.

Ciprofloxacin

Therapeutic Use. Ciprofloxacin acts against a wide range of organisms, but is not very effective against some Gram-positive organisms, particularly pneumococci. It is given orally twice daily or by infusion. At present, its use should be confined to patients for whom older antibacterial drugs are unsatisfactory, particularly for the treatment of urinary tract infections and gonorrhoea. It is the preferred drug in adults as a prophylactic in patients having close contact with patients having meningococcal meningitis. However, there has been a large increase in resistance to ciprofloxacin in recent years.

Adverse Effects. These include gastrointestinal upsets and rashes. Ciprofloxacin should be avoided, if possible, in patients with epilepsy, as it has a potential to cause seizures, and in children it may cause damage to developing weight-bearing joints. It can also cause pain and inflammation of tendons, especially in older people.

Drug Interactions. Ciprofloxacin raises the blood levels of theophylline, while the action of warfarin is increased.

Other Quinolones

Ofloxacin is similar to ciprofloxacin. **Levofloxacin** is more active against *Streptococcus pneumoniae* and can be used in community-acquired pneumonia, but offers no real advantage over the usual antibiotics.

Norfloxacin and **nalidixic acid** are effective in the treatment of uncomplicated urinary tract infections and are used when the infecting organism is resistant to the older antibacterial drugs. For an uncomplicated infection, a 3-day course is adequate, but prolonged treatment is required for severe or recurrent infections. They should be avoided in children and pregnancy, in cases of porphyria and renal impairment. Moxifloxacin is a more recently introduced orally active broad-spectrum fluoroquinolone. It has greater activity against Gram-positive organisms compared with ciprofloxacin.

CLINICAL NOTE

Absorption of quinolones (excluding nalidixic acid) is reduced by concurrent administration of indigestion remedies, or medicines containing iron or zinc. This can result in sub-therapeutic drug concentrations and prolonged infection. They should therefore be taken 2 h before or after any of the agents mentioned. In addition, ciprofloxacin and norfloxacin should not be taken at the same time as milk or milk-containing products.

β-LACTAM ANTIBIOTICS

The β-lactam antibiotics can be divided into:

- The penicillins
- The cephalosporins
- Others.

The β-lactam antibiotics all contain the β-lactam ring, which is a chemical structure essential for their antibacterial activity. The family of β-lactams is summarized in Fig. 26.2.

Penicillins

The penicillins comprise:

- Amoxicillin
- Ampicillin
- Azlocillin
- Benzylpenicillin
- Co-amoxiclav
- Flucloxacillin
- Phenoxymethylpenicillin
- Piperacillin
- Pivampicillin.

The penicillins were the first antibiotics to be isolated. Over the years, their structure has been repeatedly chemically modified to deal with the problem of

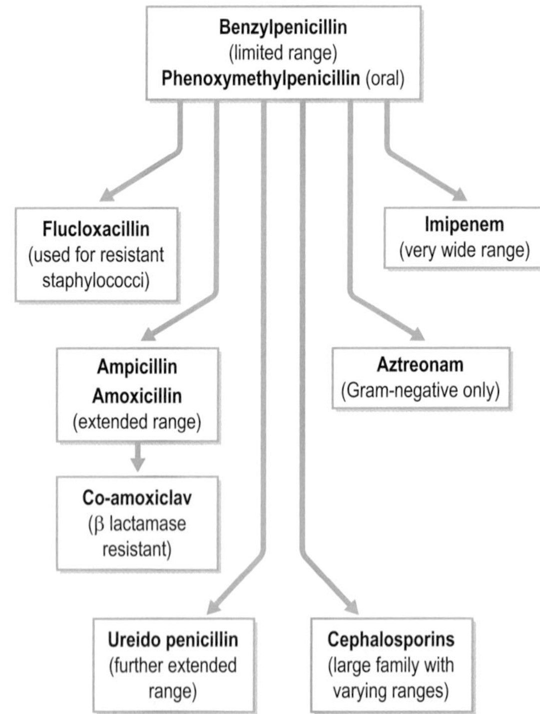

Fig. 26.2 ■ The β-lactam family of antibiotics.

resistance and to extend the range of organisms that they can inhibit. This class of drugs are still probably the most widely used family of antibiotics.

Benzylpenicillin

Benzylpenicillin was the first penicillin to be used clinically. It is usually given by deep intramuscular injection, which is painful. If a large single dose is needed, it should be given intravenously. It enters the circulation rapidly and spreads through the body. It does not, however, cross into the CSF in any great quantity, although this may be increased if the meninges are inflamed.

Elimination of Penicillins. All penicillins are excreted by the kidneys, partially through the glomeruli, but the major part via the renal tubules. The excretion is rapid and blood levels fall nearly to zero 4 h after injection. If benzylpenicillin is given orally, it is partially broken down by the gastric acid, and is not now given by this route.

Range of Benzylpenicillin. Benzylpenicillin is effective against a fairly wide range of organisms. Table 26.3 lists the most common.

Penicillins are bacteriostatic and in higher doses are bactericidal. When treating an infection, it is ideal to maintain the blood level of penicillin continually at bactericidal levels, and this requires injections every 4 h. In milder infections, however, it is often adequate to give less frequent injections. Even after the blood levels of penicillin have dropped below bactericidal or bacteriostatic levels, the organism may take some time to recover and by that time the blood level of penicillin has risen again following a further injection.

TABLE 26.3

Main Uses of Benzylpenicillin

Organisms	Disease
Streptococcus pyogenes	Tonsillitis, scarlet fever, septicaemia
Streptococcus viridans	Subacute bacterial endocarditis
Staphylococcus aureus[a]	Carbuncles, osteomyelitis, septicaemia, boils
Streptococcus pneumoniae	Pneumonia
Neisseria gonorrhoeae	Gonorrhoea
Neisseria meningitidis	Meningococcal meningitis
Treponema pallidum	Syphilis
Clostridium perfringens	Gangrene
Clostridium tetani	Tetanus
Actinomyces	Actinomycosis

[a]Note that a high proportion of staphylococci found in hospital are now resistant to benzylpenicillin.

Procaine Benzylpenicillin

Numerous attempts have been made to prolong the action of benzylpenicillin after injection by slowing down its release from the injection site. A successful method is to combine benzylpenicillin with procaine. The combination is called 'procaine benzylpenicillin' and will maintain a satisfactory blood level for at least 12 h. This preparation is, however, rather slow to produce a satisfactory blood level, so that if a rapid effect is required, benzylpenicillin should be given as well.

The action of penicillin can be augmented and prolonged by slowing down its excretion. This can be done by giving **probenecid**, a drug that blocks the tubular secretion of penicillin, thus allowing penicillin to accumulate in the body.

Penicillin Resistance: Penicillinase and the β-Lactam Ring

Certain organisms develop resistance to the action of penicillin. Organisms which were originally sensitive appear to adapt themselves to the penicillin by producing an enzyme called **penicillinase**, which inactivates penicillin by attacking part of the penicillin molecule known as the **β-lactam ring**. This structure is an essential part of penicillins and cephalosporins, and the family of enzymes involved is sometimes known as the **β-lactamases**. This is particularly so in the case of staphylococci, and strains of this organism, which are resistant to penicillin and other antibiotics, are now a serious clinical problem. There is at present a considerable degree of alarm because of the rapidly reducing number of effective antibiotics, and there is growing realization that we may be in danger of entering a period analogous to that before antibiotics were originally introduced.

Other Penicillins

These include:

- Phenoxymethylpenicillin
- Flucloxacillin

- Broad-spectrum penicillins
- Extended-spectrum penicillins (ureido penicillins).

CLINICAL NOTE

Antibiotics can be time-sensitive; ensure drugs are given appropriately either before, after or with a meal.

There are a number of penicillins that are similar to benzylpenicillin, but these drugs are effective by mouth. Some of the examples given here are not destroyed by the acid in the stomach and are fairly well absorbed from the intestinal tract.

Phenoxymethylpenicillin. Adequate absorption with a satisfactory therapeutic response usually occurs with oral penicillin. This is a time-sensitive medication and should be prescribed and administered appropriately. The patient must be carefully observed in case the drug is ineffective due to vomiting or inadequate absorption. Penicillin must then be given by injection.

Flucloxacillin. The elucidation of the structure of the penicillin pharmacophore has made it possible to produce penicillins that are not broken down by penicillinase and are therefore effective against organisms, particularly staphylococci, which have become resistant to benzylpenicillin. Flucloxacillin is a commonly used example. It is used almost exclusively for treating staphylococcal infections.

CLINICAL NOTE

A specific strain of staphylococcal species has emerged and become resistant to penicillin. It is called 'methicillin-resistant *Staphylococcus aureus*' (MRSA) and responds to alternative treatment using vancomycin or teicoplanin, linezolid and doxycyline.

Broad-spectrum Penicillins. These include ampicillin, amoxicillin and pivampicillin.

Ampicillin is effective against a number of bacteria, including salmonellae, *E. coli*, *Shigella* and *H. influenzae*, which are little affected by benzylpenicillin. Ampicillin has proved particularly useful in the treatment of chronic bronchitis and urinary tract infections. It can be given orally or by injection.

Amoxicillin is very similar to ampicillin but is better absorbed, so a smaller dose is required. For this reason it is perhaps to be preferred to ampicillin.

Pivampicillin consists of ampicillin linked to another molecule that facilitates absorption. As it passes through the gut wall, pivampicillin is split and ampicillin is released. It therefore has no advantage over ampicillin except that it is better absorbed.

Co-amoxiclav. Some bacteria produce β-lactamases capable of breaking down both ampicillin and amoxicillin together with other antibiotics. Antibiotics can be combined with a substance called clavulanate, which prevents this breakdown and thus enables it to destroy β-lactamase-producing bacteria. The combined preparation of amoxicillin and clavulanate is called 'co-amoxiclav'.

Extended-spectrum Penicillins (Ureido Penicillins). These include azlocillin and piperacillin. This group of extended-spectrum penicillins (ureido penicillins) have much the same antibacterial spectrum as ampicillin but are also effective against *Pseudomonas aeruginosa* and *Proteus morganii*. They are, however, inactivated by some β-lactamases and are therefore not active against penicillin-resistant staphylococci and, in addition, are not very effective against other Gram-positive organisms (e.g. *Streptococcus pneumoniae*). They are not absorbed from the gut and must be given by injection. They are reserved for serious infections with pseudomonas or when the causative organism is not known. In this case, due to deficiencies in their antibacterial spectrum, they are usually combined with an aminoglycoside, *but must not be mixed in the same infusion or syringe.* They are very expensive.

Azlocillin is the most effective of the three against *Pseudomonas*, but is not so effective against other microorganisms. **Piperacillin** has good broad-spectrum activity and is available combined with tazobactam, a β-lactamase inhibitor.

As these drugs are excreted via the kidney, the dose should be reduced in patients with renal failure.

Adverse Effects of Penicillins

Considering the wide use of penicillin, it is remarkably free from toxic effects. Pain and, rarely, abscess formation may be seen at the site of injection. More commonly, sensitization rashes occur as a result of contact with the drug either during or after systemic administration. The rash is often urticarial and is sometimes resistant to treatment. With ampicillin or amoxicillin the rash is sometimes erythematous and is particularly liable to occur if they are given to a patient with glandular fever or lymphoma. It may also appear after the drugs have been stopped. Rarely, penicillin causes an acute anaphylactic reaction with collapse, which can be fatal.

NURSING NOTE

Always ask about previous medicine reactions before giving a patient a penicillin, cephalosporin or any drug. Record all episodes of allergy with a medicine on the medicine prescription and in the medical records. Use local allergy notifications immediately for all medicine-related allergies reported by the patient, other healthcare worker or patient's relative or carer. This may be an allergy band, allergy sticker, allergy card or electronic alert on the prescription chart.

Drug allergy recording is the healthcare professional's responsibility.

Other adverse effects include diarrhoea. Penicillins may reduce the efficacy of the contraceptive pill. Co-amoxiclav can cause jaundice.

Patients should be monitored closely after the first administration of an antibiotic, particularly an injection of penicillin. Monitor for signs of allergy, especially if there is a history from the patient suggesting food allergy (e.g. eggs) or drug allergy.

Cephalosporins

This is a large group of antibiotics that structurally bear some relationship to the penicillins in that they both contain a β-lactam ring. They have a broad spectrum of antibacterial activity, although there are differences in this respect between the older cephalosporins and the newer drugs. Most of the cephalosporins can be given only by injection. Although they are efficient antibiotics, they are rarely the drugs of first choice, as for many infections there are cheaper, effective substitutes.

Cephalosporins can be divided into three groups:

- The older cephalosporins
- The newer, recently introduced cephalosporins
- Oral cephalosporins.

The Older Cephalosporins

The older cephalosporins (Table 26.4) are active against:

- *Staphylococcus aureus* (including some strains resistant to penicillin)
- *Streptococcus pyogenes*
- *Streptococcus pneumoniae*
- *E. coli* (most strains)
- *Klebsiella* (most strains)
- *Proteus* (most strains)
- *H. influenzae* (variable).

They may be inactivated by β-lactamases and are excreted by the kidneys.

The Newer Cephalosporins

These are an improvement on the older members of the group. They are more β-lactamase-resistant and are therefore effective against some resistant strains.

In general, they act against:

- *Streptococcus pyogenes*
- *Staphylococcus aureus*
- *H. influenzae*
- *Neisseria (N.) meningitidis*
- *E. coli*
- *Proteus*

Some of them also have activity against *Pseudomonas* and *Bacillus fragilis*, which are important organisms in many abdominal infections. The latest drugs do, however, show some falling off in their activity

TABLE 26.4
The Older Cephalosporins[a]

Drug	Important Features
Cefazolin	Some biliary excretion, so used before surgery on the bile duct
Cefradine	Fairly β-lactamase-stable

[a]This group is being superseded.

against certain Gram-positive organisms. There are now so many of this group available that only a selection is shown in Table 26.5.

The main uses for these new cephalosporins are:

- to treat severe infection (septicaemias, etc.) when the causative organism is not known or other antibiotics are contraindicated
- cefotaxime and ceftriaxone penetrate well into the CSF and are effective in meningococcal meningitis
- possibly in hepatobiliary or abdominal sepsis
- rarely in resistant urinary tract infections
- cefuroxime is effective in most chest infections, including those caused by Gram-positive organisms, i.e. *Streptococcus pneumoniae.*

Some of the newer drugs in this group are expensive.

Oral Cephalosporins

Cefadroxil is given every 12 h and has a similar antibacterial range to the older cephalosporins. It can be used in the treatment of urinary and respiratory tract infections. **Cefixime** is similar, but rather long-acting, and more effective against *H. influenzae.* Although **cefuroxime** is ineffective if given orally, a derivative of it, **cefuroxime axetil**, is absorbed from the gastrointestinal tract and is now available.

CLINICAL NOTE

Cross-sensitivity with penicillin: Approximately 10% of patients who are allergic to penicillin will also be allergic to a cephalosporin. In general, this excludes the use of cephalosporins in penicillin-sensitive patients, although exceptions may be made in special circumstances. Refer to local allergy policies.

TABLE 26.5

The Newer Cephalosporins

Drug	Important Features
Cefuroxime	Good all-round activity
Cefoxitin	Active against *Bacteroides fragilis*
Cefotaxime	Good all-round activity against Gram-negative organisms
Ceftazidime	Useful in pseudomonal infection
Ceftriaxone	Long-acting

Carbapenems

Carbapenems are β-lactam antibacterials, and generally have a broad-spectrum of activity.

Imipenem with cilastatin has the widest antibacterial range of any antibiotic, including not only the usual Gram-positive and Gram-negative bacteria, but also pseudomonads and anaerobes. It is administered via an intravenous infusion. It is excreted via the kidney and is inactivated in the renal tubule by an enzyme; the urinary concentration is therefore very low. Combining imipenem with cilastatin, which inhibits the enzyme, prevents this. At present, the use of this combination is confined to patients in whom older antibiotics are contraindicated or ineffective.

Meropenem is similar to the other two drugs, but is not broken down in the kidneys and therefore does not need to be combined with cilastatin. It is given by intravenous injection or infusion.

Ertapenem is similar in activity to other carbapenems; however, it is ineffective against *Pseudomonas.* An advantage of ertapenem is that it has a long duration of action and can be given once a day.

CLINICAL NOTE

Cross-sensitivity with penicillin: Carbapenems can show cross-sensitivity with penicillin; caution with use in patients with penicillin allergy.

Other β-Lactams

Aztreonam has a relatively narrow spectrum of antibacterial action. It can be used against infections caused by *N. gonorrhoeae* and *H. influenzae,* but is ineffective against the common Gram-positive organisms. It is given by injection.

CLINICAL NOTE

Cross-sensitivity with penicillin: Aztreonam can show cross-sensitivity with penicillin; caution with use in patients with penicillin allergy.

AMINOGLYCOSIDES

Aminoglycosides include:

- Amikacin
- Gentamicin
- Neomycin
- Netilmicin
- Spectinomycin
- Streptomycin
- Tobramycin.

This group of antibiotics interferes with protein synthesis in the bacteria and they are bactericidal, i.e. they kill the bacteria rather than preventing them from multiplying. They have a fairly broad antibacterial range and one of them (streptomycin) is also effective against *Mycobacterium tuberculosis* (Table 26.6).

Effectiveness of Aminoglycosides

This drug class has a number of common properties:

- They are all given by injection if a systemic effect is required.
- They are all primarily excreted via the kidneys and accumulation occurs with impaired renal function.
- They are all, to a greater or lesser degree, ototoxic (they impair hearing and/or balance) and nephrotoxic.
- Their antibacterial spectrum differs a little, but they are generally active against a range of organisms.

TABLE 26.6
Main Uses of Aminoglycosides

Organism	Disease
Staphylococcus aureus	Septicaemia, abscesses, endocarditis
Streptococcus viridans	Endocarditis
Haemophilus influenzae	Pneumonia, meningitis
Brucella abortus	Brucellosis
E. coli	Renal and other infections
Proteus	Various infections, largely abdominal
Pseudomonas	Pneumonia
Klebsiella	Pneumonia, urinary tract infections
Mycobacterium tuberculosis[a]	All forms of tuberculosis; they are not particularly effective against *Streptococcus pneumoniae* or *Streptococcus pyogenes*

[a]Streptomycin only.

Gentamicin

Therapeutic Use. This antibiotic is widely used, especially in treating severe infection caused by staphylococci and by various Gram-negative organisms. It is given intravenously or intramuscularly. Once-daily administration is convenient, and provides adequate serum concentrations, and has largely superseded multiple daily dosing regimens (with the exception of the treatment for endocarditis).

NURSING NOTE

1. It is essential to monitor the blood levels of gentamicin as accumulation of the drug can cause ototoxicity and nephrotoxicity when levels are above the therapeutic range. Refer to local guidelines for monitoring of gentamicin levels. The dose is adjusted to produce these levels. If the blood level is too low, the antibiotic may not be effective, but if it is above 10 mg/L for long, ototoxicity will result. It should be remembered that toxicity depends not only on the blood level, but also upon the length of treatment.
2. Ensuring appropriate monitoring of gentamicin levels will guide safe and effective dosing.
3. Renal function may deteriorate in the course of a serious illness and, if impaired, accumulation and toxicity will occur.
4. Gentamicin is incompatible with a number of drugs and care should be taken to ensure the line is appropriately flushed before and after administration of gentamicin.

Excretion. Gentamicin is excreted via the kidneys, and accumulation and toxicity will occur if the drug is given to patients with impaired renal function. In these circumstances, a lower dosage will be required, and information is available which relates the dose necessary to the degree of impairment of renal function. Reduced dosages are also usually given to elderly patients.

Drug Interactions and Adverse Effects. Renal damage may occur if gentamicin is combined with furosemide. Gentamicin is ototoxic, causing disorders of balance and hearing, which are dose related. Gentamicin also augments the action of curare-like neuromuscular blocking agents. It should be avoided in patients with myasthenia gravis as it may exacerbate symptoms. Gentamicin should be avoided during pregnancy, as it is ototoxic to the fetus.

Tobramycin, **amikacin** and **netilmicin** are very similar to gentamicin; however, they are sometimes effective against Gram-negative organisms that are resistant to gentamicin. They should only be used in this situation, as they offer no other advantage. Side-effects are similar, except that netilmicin is perhaps a little less toxic.

Spectinomycin has only one use, namely the treatment of gonorrhoeal infection due to organisms that have become resistant to penicillin. Adverse effects include rashes and vomiting.

Neomycin

Neomycin is an antibiotic that is bactericidal against a wide range of Gram-positive and Gram-negative organisms, and against *Mycobacterium tuberculosis*. It is very poorly absorbed from the intestinal tract and because of toxicity is not given systemically. It is chiefly used to sterilize the gut before surgery. It can also be applied locally as ear or eye drops.

Extensive local application to areas such as burns should be avoided, as enough absorption can occur to cause ototoxicity.

Streptomycin

Streptomycin is derived from one of the *Actinomyces* group of fungi.

Therapeutic Use. Streptomycin is usually given by intramuscular injection. The maximum concentration in the blood is reached after about 1–2 h and excretion is not completed for 24 h or more. Streptomycin is excreted in the urine. It is not absorbed after oral administration, so this route is not used except for treating gut infections. Streptomycin is now rarely used for infections other than drug-resistant tuberculosis. It may be combined with doxycycline in the treatment of brucellosis.

Resistance. The development of resistance to streptomycin is relatively common. Combining streptomycin with some other drug class to which the organism is sensitive may largely prevent this. With such treatment, the development of resistance is delayed or even prevented altogether.

TETRACYCLINES

Following the discovery of penicillin and streptomycin, a large-scale investigation was carried out into substances that were produced by various fungi. Two important antibiotics, namely the tetracyclines, were discovered. They are very similar in chemical structure, have similar toxic effects, and are effective against the same wide range of organisms. They are:

- Oxytetracycline
- Tetracycline.

The properties of these drugs are so similar that they may be considered together.

Properties of the Main Tetracyclines

Administration. They are usually given orally, are quite well absorbed from the intestinal tract, and 6-hourly dosage is satisfactory.

Distribution and Excretion. After absorption, the tetracyclines spread widely through the body. The penetration across the meningeal barrier into the CSF is variable, being greatest in the case of tetracycline itself. The greater part of these drugs is excreted in the urine; the fate of the remainder is unknown.

Therapeutic Use. The tetracyclines are very broad spectrum across a very wide range of bacteria, which includes not only true bacteria, but also some of the larger viruses and some other groups of organisms. However, with some bacteria, resistant strains have emerged, which limit their use. The main uses for the tetracyclines at present are shown in Table 26.7.

TABLE 26.7
Main Uses of Tetracyclines

Organism	Disease
Haemophilus influenzae	Bronchitis
Streptococcus pneumoniae	Bronchitis
Mycoplasma	Pneumonia
Chlamydia	Non-specific urethritis
Rickettsia	Typhus Q. fever, etc.
Brucella abortus	Brucellosis

They are also used over long periods in the treatment of acne. Whether their efficacy in this disorder is due to their antibacterial action or is due to some other factor is not known.

Other Tetracyclines

These comprise:

- Demeclocycline
- Doxycycline
- Lymecycline
- Minocycline.

Demeclocycline is similar to the others in the group, but rather smaller doses are required and its action is more prolonged. Doxycycline is similar to the older tetracyclines, but is excreted slowly, so only one dose is required daily. Doxycycline is used in the treatment of *Chlamydia*, respiratory infections and genital infections. The other important difference is that, unlike tetracycline, it can be used when renal function is impaired (see later). It is also used in Lyme disease and the prevention of malaria. Minocycline has a broader spectrum than the other tetracyclines, and is active against *Neisseria meningitidis*. It is less commonly used for treatment of acne now, due to causing potentially irreversible slate-grey hyperpigmentation.

Adverse Effects of the Tetracyclines.

- A certain amount of nausea, vomiting and epigastric disturbance due to a direct irritant effect often follows administration of the tetracyclines.
- Because of their broad antibacterial spectrum the tetracyclines cause considerable changes in the bacterial flora both in the intestine and elsewhere. This often results in diarrhoea, which usually recovers quickly when the drug is stopped. Occasionally, they may cause serious enteritis due to the multiplication of a resistant organism, usually a staphylococcus. *Candida* is the other troublesome organism that may emerge in those receiving tetracyclines, causing 'thrush' in the mouth or vaginal candidiasis.
- Tetracyclines damage and discolour developing teeth and should be avoided, if possible, from the fourth month of pregnancy until the child is 12 years old.
- Other toxic effects are rare, but include skin rashes and other sensitization phenomena.

Contraindications. Tetracyclines (except doxycycline) should not be given when renal function is impaired, as they cause increased tissue breakdown with a subsequent rise of breakdown products in the blood, and exacerbation of the renal failure.

NURSING NOTE

Tetracycline tablets should be swallowed whole with the patient sitting or standing and washed down with plenty of water. Absorption is reduced by concurrent administration of iron, calcium or magnesium compounds (including milk).

CHLORAMPHENICOL

Chloramphenicol is a broad-spectrum antibiotic closely related in its action to the tetracyclines. It has, however, serious, but rare, toxic effects on the bone marrow; this limits its use to those patients who cannot obtain benefit from any other form of treatment.

Therapeutic Use. Chloramphenicol is given by mouth and is rapidly absorbed from the intestine. It diffuses widely and crosses the meningeal barrier into the CSF. It is excreted via the kidneys. Like the tetracyclines, it is effective against a wide range of organisms with the important addition of *Salmonella typhi* and the paratyphoid group.

Bone marrow toxicity limits its use, but it can be used for the treatment of meningitis and acute epiglottitis due to *Haemophilus influenzae*. It is also very effective in the treatment of typhoid and paratyphoid fevers, although resistant strains are emerging and ciprofloxacin may be preferred. It is also commonly used topically as eye and ear drops.

Adverse Effects. The most serious toxic effects of chloramphenicol are on the bone marrow. Although they are rare, they are nearly always fatal when they occur. The most common effect is aplastic anaemia; the other reported change is depression of the numbers of leucocytes and platelets in circulating blood.

Toxic effects are more common after prolonged or repeated courses of chloramphenicol and their appearance may be delayed for up to 2 months after receiving the drug.

In newborn infants, chloramphenicol is less rapidly broken down, so accumulation may occur, producing the so-called 'grey syndrome', with circulatory collapse and shock.

MACROLIDES

These comprise:

- Erythromycin
- Clarithromycin
- Azithromycin.

Erythromycin

Erythromycin was first introduced in 1952. It is absorbed rather erratically after oral administration and diffuses widely, but does not enter into the CSF very well. It is bacteriostatic and acts against a wide range of organisms, including:

- *Streptococcus pyogenes*
- *Staphylococcus aureus*
- *Mycoplasma pneumoniae*
- *Legionella pneumophila*, which causes Legionnaires' disease.

It is not, however, always effective against *Haemophilus influenzae*, a common cause of respiratory infection.

Resistance. Bacteria readily become resistant to erythromycin, but do not show cross-resistance to other antibiotics.

Therapeutic Use. Erythromycin has a similar range of activity to penicillin and can be used instead of that drug in those who are allergic to penicillin. It is used for the treatment of various respiratory diseases, including those caused by *Mycoplasma pneumoniae* and Legionnaires' disease. To reduce nausea, it is best taken with food. Erythromycin can be given by infusion as the preparation **erythromycin lactobionate**.

Adverse Effects. These are rare and include diarrhoea and vomiting, and rarely jaundice, if injected. Intravenous administration rarely, is liable to cause thrombophlebitis.

Clarithromycin

Clarithromycin has a similar antibacterial spectrum to erythromycin, but higher concentrations are found in the tissues and it has a greater effect than erythromycin against *H. influenzae*. It is also used for the eradication of *Helicobacter pylori* (see Chapter 10). Gastrointestinal upsets are less frequent but can commonly cause taste disturbance.

CLINICAL NOTE

Erythromycin and clarithromycin interfere with the breakdown of certain drugs, drug interactions should be assessed prior to administration. Statins can commonly interact with them resulting in myopathy or rhabdomyolysis (Hougaard Christensen et al., 2020). As a result it is advised that are withheld while a course of the antibiotics are completed, and can be re-initiated following completion.

Azithromycin

Azithromycin appears to be similar, but with a long half-life; one daily dose is adequate.

GLYCOPEPTIDES

These comprise of:

- Vancomycin
- Teicoplanin.

Vancomycin

Vancomycin has bactericidal activity against Gram-positive bacteria and is particularly useful for treating severe staphylococcal infections resistant to other antibiotics. It is also given orally in the treatment of pseudomembranous colitis, which occasionally follows the use of some antibiotics and is due to infection of the colon with *Clostridium difficile*. It is given by slow intravenous infusion and blood levels are measured to control the dose.

Adverse Effects. It is ototoxic and nephrotoxic and is often given into a central vein as it can cause venous thrombosis.

CLINICAL NOTE

Vancomycin should be used with caution with anyone with renal impairment and drug levels should be carefully monitored if prescribed in this group (Filippone et al., 2017). Due to poor absorption if given enterally, it is prescribed intravenously.

Teicoplanin

Teicoplanin is similar to vancomycin, but with considerably fewer adverse effects and a longer duration of action. It is indicated for potentially serious infections such as *Staphylococcus aureus*, and for dialysis-associated peritonitis and endocarditis. It is also useful in orthopaedic surgery where there is a risk of infection with Gram-positive organisms.

Adverse Effects. Several adverse effects have been reported, including angio-oedema, anaphylaxis, various blood disorders, mild hearing loss and injection-site abscesses. Both liver and kidney function should be assessed during treatment. Contraindications include pregnancy, breastfeeding and renal impairment. If a patient has adverse effects with vancomycin, then teicoplanin should be used.

MISCELLANEOUS ANTIBIOTICS

Clindamycin

Clindamycin is effective against many Gram-positive organisms and can be used to treat infections caused by anaerobic organisms, particularly those that complicate bowel surgery. It is well absorbed when taken orally and appears to penetrate into bone and thus can be used successfully to treat osteomyelitis and diabetic foot infections.

Adverse Effects. These are not common; diarrhoea may be a problem and rarely takes the form of a serious colitis (pseudomembranous colitis).

Polymyxin

Polymyxin is effective against a wide range of Gram-negative organisms. It is particularly useful when applied topically for resistant infections caused by such organisms as *Pseudomonas*, e.g. otitis externa.

Sodium Fusidate

Sodium fusidate is effective against resistant staphylococci. When used, it is usually combined with other antibiotics in the treatment of severe staphylococcal infections. It is relatively free of side-effects, although high doses may cause jaundice, which recovers when the drug is stopped.

Linezolid

Linezolid is a newer type of antibiotic that interferes with protein synthesis in the bacteria. It is effective against *Staphylococcus aureus* and *Streptococcus pneumoniae*, and in the treatment of pneumonia and soft-tissue infections caused by Gram-positive bacteria. It is given orally or intravenously and has a relatively short half-life. It is also a monoamine oxidase inhibitor (MAOI).

Adverse Effects. These include disturbances of taste, tongue discoloration, hypertension, tinnitus and various blood dyscrasias. Prolonged use has been noted to have a rare issue with severe optic neuropathy resulting in visual symptoms which patients should be warned about.

Contraindications. These include breastfeeding and, as mentioned earlier, other MAOIs. The MHRA has published guidelines for the use of linezolid, particularly with respect to its effects on the blood (see the *British National Formulary*, BNF).

Colistin and Polymyxin B

Colistin is an example of a polymyxin antibiotic active against Gram-negative bacteria such as *Pseudomonas aeruginosa*. It is a toxic substance that is not absorbed when taken orally, and is usually administered together with the antifungal nystatin (see Chapter

27), for bowel sterilization in neutropenic patients. It should not be used to treat gut infections. Polymyxin B is another antibiotic potent against Gram-negative bacteria; it is used in topical applications for the eye and ear infections.

Dalfopristin with Quinupristin

This is a mixture of two so-called streptogramin antibiotics to treat Gram-positive infections. The preparation is recommended only for patients who have failed to respond to any other antibiotics or who cannot take any others. It is indicated for serious infections such as soft-tissue and skin infections, infections caused by vancomycin-resistant *Enterococcus faecium* and some forms of hospital-acquired pneumonia. It is ineffective against *Enterococcus faecalis*.

The preparation consists of a powder for reconstitution to give a mixture of quinupristin/dalfopristin and is administered via an intravenous infusion into a central vein.

Adverse Effects. These include myalgia, rashes, pruritus, nausea and vomiting, blood dyscrasias and electrolyte disturbances.

Contraindications. It is contraindicated in severe liver disease and should be used with caution in patients with renal or heart disease, and during pregnancy and breastfeeding.

The antibacterial activity of some of the major antibiotics is summarized in Table 26.8.

TUBERCULOSIS

In the past, tuberculosis (TB) was a common and frequently fatal disease. In the UK in the first half of the last century, its incidence declined rapidly due to improved living conditions and effective drug treatment. However, where the resistance of the population is lowered by poverty, malnutrition and, more recently, by HIV, TB is becoming a major health problem again.

TB is an infectious bacterial disease caused by *Mycobacterium tuberculosis*. A person can become infected by inhaling the aerosol from an infected person's sneezing or coughing, but it is caught usually only after prolonged close proximity to an infected person. It is more often spread by contaminated hands. According to World Health Organization (WHO) estimates, about a third of the world's population is infected with TB, mainly in Africa and Asia, where incomes and standards of living are poor, coupled with genetic susceptibility. The most at risk are:

- alcoholics and drug misusers
- immunocompromised patients, especially those with HIV disease
- doctors, nurses and other health workers in continual contact with patients who have pulmonary TB, unless protected by immunization (see later)
- patients on immunosuppressive chemotherapy
- populations living or working in overcrowded conditions
- patients suffering from concomitant debilitating diseases such as diabetes, or those recovering from serious surgery, e.g. operations on the gastrointestinal tract.

Common Symptoms of Tuberculosis

TB can cause pulmonary disease if it infects the lungs or it can also spread to other parts of the body to cause extrapulmonary disease. Common presenting TB symptoms can include swollen lymph glands, especially in the neck, loss of weight and appetite, tiredness, chronic non-productive cough, pleurisy, sweating at night and, in advanced TB, haemoptysis (coughing up blood).

Testing for Tuberculosis

The tuberculin test consists of the injection into the skin of very small amounts of the tuberculin protein, which is extracted from cultures of *M. tuberculosis*. A strong patch of inflammation on the skin about 48–72 h later indicates a positive reaction. There may be a mild reaction, which is not unusual, but does not necessarily signify TB. The test is called the 'Mantoux test', and a positive skin reaction is confirmed by testing a sample of sputum.

An alternative newer test is called the 'QuantiFERON-TB Gold test', which is a blood test to detect *M.*

TABLE 26.8

The Antibacterial Activity of Antibiotics and Chemotherapeutic Agents

Organism	Diseases	Macrolides	Benzylpenicillin	Gentamicin	Ampicillin, Amoxicillin	Others
Staphylococcus aureus	Purulent infection	++	++[a]	++	++[a]	Vancomycin ++ Erythromycin ++ Flucloxacillin ++ Sodium fusidate ++
Streptococcus pyogenes	Tonsillitis, scarlet fever	++	++	0	++	
Streptococcus viridans	Infective endocarditis	++	++	+	++	
Streptococcus pneumoniae	Pneumonia	++	++	0	++	
Neisseria meningitidis	Meningitis	0	++	0	++	Newer cephalosporins ++
Neisseria gonorrhoeae	Gonorrhoea	0	++	++	++	Spectinomycin ++ 4-Quinolones ++
E. coli	Urinary tract infection	0	0	++	++	Trimethoprim Nitrofurantoin ++
Shigella	Dysentery	0	0	+	++	Ciprofloxacin ++
Salmonella typhi	Typhoid	0	0	+	++	Chloramphenicol ++ Trimethoprim ++
Haemophilus influenzae	Meningitis and pneumonia	+	0	+	++	Chloramphenicol ++
Treponema pallidum	Syphilis	++	++	0	0	
Pseudomonas aeruginosa	Various infections, septicaemia	0	0	++	0	Ureido penicillins ++ Some new cephalosporins +
Chlamydia	Nonspecific urethritis	++	0	0	++	Doxycycline ++

Very effective, ++; sometimes effective, +; little or no action, 0.
[a]Owing to resistance – flucloxacillin, ++

tuberculosis. However, like the Mantoux test it cannot detect between active or latent TB infection.

Immunization

Large-scale immunization of a population can control the spread of TB. In the UK, the BCG (bacille Calmette–Guérin) vaccine is used. It is administered at birth in high-risk situations, which includes living in areas with high rates of prevalence or if they have a parent or grandparent who was born in a country where there is a high rate of TB. The vaccine is not recommended for those over the age of 45 unless there is a high risk of infection. Immunization usually lasts for at least 15 years.

Main Drugs Used in Tuberculosis

Anti-tuberculous drugs include:

- Isoniazid
- Rifampicin

- Ethambutol
- Pyrazinamide
- Rifabutin
- Capreomycin
- Cycloserine
- Streptomycin.

Isoniazid

Therapeutic Use. Isoniazid is bacteriostatic and possibly bactericidal to *M. tuberculosis*. It is rapidly absorbed from the intestine and largely excreted by the kidneys. It diffuses widely through the body and it crosses the meningeal barrier to the CSF in amounts adequate to inhibit the growth of *M. tuberculosis*.

Isoniazid is metabolized in the liver. It is possible to divide people into two groups: those who break isoniazid down rapidly and those who break it down slowly. As a result of this, the rapidly inactivating group will have lower concentrations of the drug in their blood than the slow inactivators. In the dosage schemes used in the UK, this is of no importance, but in less developed countries where the drug may be given less frequently to save cost, rapid inactivators are in danger of getting less than a full therapeutic effect from the drug.

Adverse Effects. Neuropathy can develop in slow inactivators who are given large doses and in those at special risk of nerve damage (patients with diabetes, alcoholics). Giving pyridoxine can prevent this. Another serious adverse effect can be hepatotoxicity; a small percentage of patients can subsequently develop severe liver injury as a result.

Rifampicin

Rifampicin is effective against several Gram-positive and Gram-negative organisms and in particular against *M. tuberculosis*. Its use is largely confined to TB, but it can also be used in the treatment of Legionnaires' disease and to prevent infection in subjects who have had close contact with meningococcal meningitis. It is well absorbed orally and is taken once daily before breakfast in standard treatment regimen for TB. It is mainly excreted in the bile. It is useful in the treatment of TB, but must be combined with other antituberculous drugs to prevent resistance developing.

Rifampicin is a potent enzyme inducer of the cytochrome P450 system. Care should be taken when coadministering other drugs that are metabolized by this system, as rifampicin may increase their metabolism and reduce their activity.

Adverse Effects. These are uncommon, but it should not be used in patients with liver disease, as it can cause changes in liver function tests and, rarely, severe liver damage. It may cause red discoloration of the urine and sputum. By increasing the rate of breakdown of oestrogen, rifampicin may reduce the effectiveness of oral contraceptives.

Rifabutin

Rifabutin is similar to rifampicin. However, it is a less potent enzyme inducer. Rifabutin may be considered as an alternative option if rifampicin is contraindicated due to potential drug interactions.

CLINICAL NOTE

Medication counselling: may colour urine or sputum orange/red. This is harmless.

Rifampicin is a powerful enzyme inducer and reduces the effect of many drugs, e.g. benzodiazepines and antidiabetic drugs (Niemi et al., 2003). Hence, it is important to check for potential drug interactions if rifampicin or rifabutin are prescribed.

Ethambutol

Ethambutol is usually satisfactory, but is now rarely used unless there is a possibility of resistance to other antituberculous drugs. The most important side-effect is damage to the optic nerve, leading to deterioration of visual acuity and colour vision. Correct dosage reduces this risk, but vision should be tested before starting treatment and at 6-monthly intervals.

Pyrazinamide

Pyrazinamide is powerful and effective, with good penetration into tuberculous lesions and the CSF. Its use is limited by adverse effects, but is justified, particularly in the treatment of tuberculous meningitis, provided that the correct dose is given and the course lasts no longer than 2 months. During treatment, liver function tests should be performed and alcohol avoided.

Adverse Effects. These include liver damage with jaundice, light sensitization (use a barrier cream) and attacks of gout.

Streptomycin

Streptomycin is less commonly used in the UK and is an unlicensed indication for TB. However, it can be considered in TB treatment where there is resistance to the commonly prescribed combination. It is very effective against *M. tuberculosis*, but resistant strains develop in about 6 weeks if it is used alone. This is prevented if it is combined with other antituberculous drugs. It is given by injection once daily. Because it has to be injected and adverse effects can be troublesome, it has now been largely replaced by other drugs.

Adverse Effects. These are not uncommon with streptomycin. The most important are those affecting the eighth cranial nerve. The symptoms include high-pitched tinnitus and vertigo. This may be followed by varying degrees of deafness. Sensitization phenomena also occur with streptomycin. These may affect not only the patient, but also the person injecting the drug. Swelling of the eyelids is an early sign. Care should be taken when giving the drug to avoid contamination of the hands and face, which may occur when the syringe is held at eye level to measure the exact dose. The wearing of plastic gloves and a mask is advisable for those who handle large quantities of streptomycin.

Combined Preparations

Preparations that combine isoniazid, rifampicin and pyrazinamide are available and they improve compliance. Examples include Rifater and Rifinah; however, these fixed dose combination preparations are unlicensed in children.

Drug Regimens for the Treatment of Tuberculosis

There are now a number of drugs that are effective against *M. tuberculosis*. It is important, however, that:

- at least two drugs are used at the same time to prevent the emergence of resistant organisms
- treatment is continued for a long time (months) to eradicate the infection completely.

The choice of drugs is determined by the sensitivity of the infective *M. tuberculosis* bacillus. Ethambutol is only used if resistance is a possibility.

Variation in the drugs used is due to their differing penetration of tissue, their effectiveness against dividing organisms and their ability to sterilize a lesion. The excellent penetration of isoniazid and pyrazinamide into the CSF makes them particularly useful in the treatment of meningeal tuberculosis. Resistance by *M. tuberculosis* to one or other drug may require a change of regimen.

CLINICAL NOTE

Although the discovery of these drugs has revolutionized the treatment of TB, it must be realized that they form only part of the treatment. A major barrier to treatment is poor adherence and a key factor associated with non-adherence is people living with TB may stop treatment once they start to feel better (Gebreweld et al., 2018). Optimal adherence can be achieved using outreach teams to observe treatment, particularly in people with active, rather than latent disease (Pradipta et al., 2020).

BACTERIAL RESISTANCE TO ANTIBIOTICS

Antimicrobial Resistance

Resistance may be produced in several ways. In any population of bacteria there are usually a few organisms that are resistant to an antibiotic, and when all the sensitive organisms have been destroyed, the resistant ones are left to flourish and multiply. These resistant organisms have often been produced by mutations (changes in their genetic make-up). It has also been shown that certain bacteria can transmit resistance to each other and even to different types of bacteria by incorporating foreign DNA, which induces resistance. For example, genes carrying resistance can be spread from staphylococci to different species of bacteria. It follows therefore that wherever antibiotics are widely used, resistant strains will appear. Antibiotic resistance has been declared a global problem by the WHO and many countries have drawn up national guidelines in an attempt to reduce it. These are based on the following principles:

- Antibiotics should only be used when really necessary to treat a specific infection or provide prophylaxis against a known risk of infection (e.g. after some types of surgical procedure).
- Antibiotics should be given in adequate doses and patients must be warned to finish the course and not to give or take antibiotics (or any other prescribed medication) from other people.
- The use of antibiotics prophylactically should be carefully selected and at appropriate time intervals reassessed for their continued use to help limit resistance developing. For example 3–6 months' use of prophylactic antibiotics for recurrent UTI, following which a review should be considered for continued use, which not only helps to reduce potential harm caused by unnecessary use but will also help combat antibiotic resistance.
- In certain circumstances, e.g. the treatment of tuberculosis, the use of several antibiotics together may prevent resistant strains developing.
- The use of antibiotics by farmers to promote animal growth should be strictly controlled, as it has promoted the emergence of resistant strains of bacteria.

Research is now being undertaken to reduce risks of antibiotic resistance in primary care settings by educating prescribers and patients about the risks associated with the unnecessary, inappropriate and excessive use of antibiotics. Improving standards of hygiene and making sure that infection control precautions are implemented in all care settings is also receiving renewed attention as part of the drive to reduce the risks of antibiotic resistance.

Multidrug Resistance

In recent years, the problem of patients infected with *M. tuberculosis* resistant to one or more antibiotics has emerged. This happens most often in patients who have relapsed, as they may have received inadequate treatment. Patients infected with HIV disease have poor resistance to infection (see Chapter 27); this makes treatment difficult and may add to the number of resistant organisms. Such patients require individually designed combinations of drugs and the treatment is prolonged. Among the drugs used are: streptomycin, capreomycin, cycloserine and clarithromycin.

The aminoglycosides, e.g. capreomycin, kanamycin and amikacin, and the newer quinolones, e.g. ciprofloxacin and ofloxacin, are used only in patients who are resistant to other drugs. Combinations of a β-lactam antibiotic with a β-lactamase inhibitor appear to improve the effectiveness of treatment.

SPECIAL POINTS FOR PATIENT EDUCATION

It is imperative that patients realize the importance of taking their medication regularly as directed. Poor adherence or failure to finish the course of treatment is common in tuberculosis and is a major factor in the emergence of resistant strains.

CLINICAL NOTE

Patients with tuberculosis should cease to be infectious after 1 week of treatment provided that the organism is sensitive. When nursing patients with open tuberculosis, nurses must be careful to avoid open infection. This is particularly important if the patient has a multidrug-resistant infection, when the infectious period may be prolonged.

ANTIMICROBIAL STEWARDSHIP

Policies have been developed to encourage the efficient, safe and economical use of antimicrobials (antimicrobial stewardship). The aims of stewardship are to improve the safety and quality of patient care and to reduce the emergence of antimicrobial resistance and healthcare-associated infections. These can be achieved by improving antimicrobial prescribing through implementation of an organized antimicrobial stewardship programme. Many hospitals include the following in their stewardship programme:

- an antimicrobial stewardship team/committee which is multidisciplinary
- antimicrobial guidelines based on evidence and local microbiology sensitivity patterns
- ward-based antimicrobial team
- audits and feedback of antimicrobial prescribing practice
- education and training.

Additionally, most hospitals have a local formulary drawn up to reserve the use of particular antibiotics. Most local policies adopt the following general format:

- A section that includes a single member of each of the main groups of antibiotics. Each of these can be prescribed without formality. These drugs may be held as ward stock.
- A restricted section containing alternatives, including the most newly developed antibiotics. These are not usually prescribed without liaison with the microbiology team and need to be prescribed and ordered for single patient administration.

Policies need regular updating. In many countries, this important work is undertaken by Pharmacists who specialize in antimicrobial drugs, but who work closely with medical and nursing staff.

NURSING NOTE

Role of the nursing team in antimicrobial stewardship

- Support the multidisciplinary team to ensure that antimicrobial use is appropriate and follows local guidelines/policies.
- Understand and support appropriate taking of microbiological samples for patients with infection.
- Ensure timely administration of antimicrobials.
- Monitor duration and route of antimicrobial therapy and prompt review of course length and switching from intravenous to oral therapy.
- Monitor patients for adverse reactions to treatment (allergies or side-effects).
- Support appropriate therapeutic drug monitoring.
- Engage in education and training on antimicrobials.
- Support patients understanding of appropriate antibiotic use.

ANTIBIOTIC DRUGS IN THE TREATMENT OF COMMON INFECTIONS

The Common Cold

The treatment of the common cold is the relief of symptoms with non-steroidal antiinflammatory drugs (NSAIDs), paracetamol (to reduce fever), decongestants and steam inhalation. Although antibiotics are often prescribed, they are usually of *NO* value in healthy adults or children, as the common cold is usually caused by viral, rather than bacterial infections. **It is important to note that antibiotics are ineffective against viruses**; thus the inappropriate use of antibiotics in this circumstance increases the risk of resistant organisms emerging. Furthermore, they are expensive. Various antiviral agents have been tried against the common cold, including interferons, but so far there is no evidence that they are of any clinically significant benefit, although new antiviral approaches are under development.

Sore Throat

Minor sore throats are self-limiting and usually caused by viral infections; therefore antibiotic treatment is not appropriate. Symptoms can last for approximately a week, but generally, most people will get better within this time without antibiotics. In some circumstances a sore throat may be caused by streptococcal infection. It is recommended that a **FeverPain** or **Centor Score** is used to identify those who are more likely to benefit from an antibiotic and managed with phenoxymethylpenicillin. If vomiting is a problem, benzylpenicillin should be given by injection. This drug is also used in smaller doses over long periods to prevent throat infection in those who have had rheumatic fever and thus decrease the chance of recurrence.

Bronchitis

A mild attack of acute bronchitis in an otherwise healthy adult does not usually require antibiotic treatment and is frequently due to a viral infection. It can take 3 weeks for symptoms to resolve. Antibiotic therapy should be considered for a severe attack or an acute exacerbation of chronic bronchitis in patients who meet certain criteria, and is best treated with amoxicillin or doxycycline, as the infection in these circumstances may be due to *H. influenzae*, *Streptococcus pneumoniae* or *Moraxella catarrhalis*.

Pneumonia

Pneumonia is common and has a high mortality rate. Patients who present with lower respiratory tract symptoms are risk assessed for mortality using the

CURB-65 Severity Score in conjunction with clinical judgement. Patients are then stratified into either low-, moderate- or high-severity disease. The grade of severity will usually correspond to the risk of death. The difficulty with pneumonia is that various bacteria with different antibiotic sensitivities may be the cause. Choice of antibiotic therapy will be based on the severity score. Sputum and blood cultures may be considered for moderate- or high-severity pneumonia to determine appropriate choice of antibiotic when results are available. Penicillin-resistant *Streptococcus pneumoniae* has appeared and in the future, this may alter the choice of antibacterial treatment.

Urinary Tract Infections

Urinary tract infections (UTIs) are usually due to *E. coli* and respond satisfactorily to nitrofurantoin. It should, however, be avoided at term of pregnancy. Trimethoprim and cefalexin can also be considered; however, in some areas, the organism has become resistant to these antibacterial drugs and pivmecillinam, a type of penicillin, can be used as an alternative. It is sometimes necessary to use antibacterial drugs prophylactically, particularly in children. Trimethoprim or nitrofurantoin at night is usually adequate. Patients with indwelling urethral catheters are not usually treated with antibiotics unless they develop symptoms. If the catheter is removed, bacteria disappear from the urine.

NURSING NOTE

Where appropriate, take a urine sample prior to commencing antibacterial therapy. Remember to check urine culture and susceptibility results (including previous results) to ensure choice of antibacterial therapy is still appropriate.

Meningitis

Meningitis may be caused by a variety of organisms and its treatment is complicated because certain antibiotics penetrate poorly into the CSF. Drugs that penetrate poorly have to be given intrathecally (Table 26.9).

TABLE 26.9

Drug Penetration

Good Penetration	Poor Penetration
Sulphonamides (particularly sulfadiazine)	Penicillin
Chloramphenicol	Streptomycin
Tetracycline	
The newer cephalosporins	

Meningococcal Meningitis

This should be treated with a dose of benzylpenicillin intravenously. Enough penicillin will diffuse through the inflamed meninges to eradicate the infection. If the bacterial diagnosis is in doubt, ceftriaxone should be used, as it has a broader antibacterial spectrum. Immediate treatment is important, as sometimes a very dangerous state of shock develops.

Prevention. Those in close contact with patients with meningococcal meningitis should be given rifampicin twice daily for 2 days for children, or ciprofloxacin as a single dose for adults.

NURSING NOTE

If meningococcal disease is suspected, then antibiotic therapy should be administered as soon as possible. Sepsis bundles and sepsis treatment should never be delayed. Ensure you are familiar with local sepsis policies and guidelines and act quickly with medication administration.

Meningitis in Neonates

This is usually due to Gram-negative organisms. The most common cause in neonates in the UK is *Group B streptococcus*. Other causes in neonates for meningococcal disease include *E. coli* and *Listeria monocytogenes*. The initial empirical therapy in neonates (aged under 3 months) is intravenous cefotaxime and amoxicillin.

Streptococcus Pneumoniae *Meningitis*

This does not usually respond so well as meningococcal infection. The usual treatment is with cefotaxime, as some strains of *Streptococcus pneumoniae* are penicillin-resistant.

Haemophilus Influenzae *Meningitis*

This is treated with cefotaxime or ceftriaxone, administered intravenously. The condition is now uncommon in countries where vaccination has been introduced.

Infective Endocarditis

This is an infection of damaged heart valves, and used to be commonly due to *Streptococcus viridans*, which can still account for about 20% of the cases; however, *Staphylococcus aureus* is now the most common cause of the disease. At-risk patients include those who abuse intravenous drugs. Because the organisms are buried in the thick microbiome and biofilms on the valves, they are difficult to reach and kill with antibiotics, so that prolonged treatment with high doses is needed. Usually initial 'blind' therapy is with amoxicillin and low dose gentamicin, which are given together for 2 weeks and penicillin continued for another 2 weeks. If the organism is less sensitive, then a prolonged period of treatment may be recommended. Other organisms may require other regimens and the management should be worked out with the microbiology team.

Antibiotic prophylaxis is not routinely recommended for the prevention of infective endocarditis in patients undergoing procedures involving dental, upper and lower respiratory tract, genitourinary tract and upper and lower gastrointestinal tract. While these procedures can cause bacteria to enter the blood, there is no clear association with developing infective endocarditis.

Staphylococcal Infections

These cover a wide range, including boils and carbuncles, and extending to severe and sometimes fatal septicaemias, pneumonias and osteomyelitis. Mild infections that once responded to phenoxymethylpenicillin, are often now resistant; in addition, the severe infections are often due to organisms that have also become resistant to penicillin. In these circumstances, flucloxacillin by mouth or by injection is given. Other useful antibiotics in staphylococcal infections are gentamicin, erythromycin, clindamycin, sodium fusidate and vancomycin or teicoplanin. One or other of these is often combined with flucloxacillin.

Infection due to MRSA will require special infection control precautions in line with local policy. A high degree of hygiene practice should be maintained. Wounds will require cleaning and the local application of antibacterial agents such as *Iodosorb*. In addition, an appropriate antibiotic (usually vancomycin) should be employed.

Chlamydial Infection

Organisms of the *Chlamydia* group can cause various infections. *Chlamydia trachomatis* is responsible for most cases of nonspecific urethritis and cervicitis, which are the most common sexually transmitted diseases in the Western world. Acute infections may lead to chronic pelvic pain in women and epididymo-orchitis in men. Treatment is with doxycycline or azithromycin and both sexual partners must be treated.

Intestinal Infections

Intestinal infections can be caused by various organisms, the most common in the UK being Salmonellae and Shigellae. Although these organisms are sensitive to a number of antibiotics, it has been found that their use does not hasten recovery and may lead to an increased number of chronic carriers of these infections. Antibiotic treatment is usually not indicated, except in the dangerous systemic infection induced by *Salmonella typhi* (typhoid or paratyphoid fever) or severe gut infection, which is treated with ciprofloxacin.

Septicaemias

The UK has more than 250,000 episodes of sepsis annually, with at least 44,000 deaths, 14,000 of which could be prevented. Sepsis claims more lives than breast, bowel and prostate cancer together and costs the NHS £2 billion per year. Many lives and £160 million could be saved every year through better diagnosis and treatment of sepsis.

Sepsis is a life-threatening condition that arises when the body's response to an infection injures its own tissues and organs. It is caused by an abnormal or dysregulated host response to an infection that causes organ failure. Sepsis can be triggered by any infection, but most commonly, it occurs in response to bacterial infections of the lungs, urinary tract, abdominal organs, skin and soft tissues or from infections acquired in healthcare settings. Anyone who develops an infection can develop sepsis.

Sepsis is a medical emergency and is frequently underdiagnosed at an early stage when it is still potentially reversible. It often presents as the clinical deterioration of common and preventable infections. If not recognized early and managed promptly, it can lead to septic shock, multiple organ failure and death. The key to reducing deaths from sepsis is early detection and initiation of treatment. The **Sepsis 6**, as recommended by the UK Sepsis Trust, is a set of interventions that may reduce mortality by 50% if they are implemented within 60 min of diagnosis of sepsis. Refer to local sepsis guidelines and policies.

PREVENTION OF SURGICAL SITE INFECTION

Antibiotic prophylaxis is often given prior to certain surgical procedures. The goals of surgical antibiotic prophylaxis are to reduce the incidence of surgical site infection, use antibiotics in a manner supported by evidence of effectiveness and minimize adverse effects (e.g. *C. difficile*-associated infection, antibiotic resistance or allergy reaction). Antibiotic prophylaxis administered too early or too late increases the risk of surgical site infection. Intravenous antibiotics must be fully administered within 60 min prior to skin incision in the anaesthetic room.

Choice of surgical antibiotic prophylaxis should be directed against specific organisms relevant to the type of surgery with predictable sensitivities. Refer to local guidelines.

Practical Points in the Administration of Antibiotics

- Oral flucloxacillin and tetracyclines are time-sensitive and should be taken on an empty stomach to facilitate absorption. This means 1 h before food or 2 h after food.
- Erythromycin, sodium fusidate and metronidazole should be given with or just after food, to minimize nausea.
- In general, intravenous antibiotics should be given as a bolus. A few, e.g. piperacillin, are given as short-term infusions. If long-term infusions are used, remember that some antibiotics are unstable in certain solutions and rapidly lose their potency. Among the most important are:
  - ampicillin – loses activity in dextrose solutions
  - gentamicin – unstable in solution and inactivated if combined with penicillins.
- Do not, as a rule, mix drugs in an infusion bottle; if this is necessary, first check their compatibilities with the pharmacist.
- Do not mix **ureido penicillins** with **aminoglycosides** in the same infusion or syringe.
- When making up solutions for injection, avoid contamination of hands, etc., due to the risk of contact dermatitis. Hands should be washed after as well as before giving injections, and gloves should be worn for intravenous injections due to risks of contaminated blood. When patients are taking antibiotics at home, compliance must be assured by full explanation of its importance, particularly with reference to taking the full course prescribed.

ROUTINE SURVEILLANE OF HEALTHCARE-ASSOCIATED INFECTIONS

In the UK and many other countries, healthcare providers are required to report the number of infections caused by key organisms responsible for healthcare-associated infection to the public health bodies (e.g. Public Health England) as part of a major surveillance programme intended to reduce risks of infection. These figures are available to the public and to health professionals to enable them to compare local infection rates with national ones. Mandatory reporting of infection caused by MRSA and *Clostridium difficile* in the UK has demonstrated that since 2000, when stringent infection prevention policies were implemented, rates of infections caused by these bacteria have declined. Similar initiatives have been effective in many other countries. Healthcare-associated infection remains an important challenge to the quality of patient care however, and there is evidence in many countries including the UK, that the number of infections caused by Gram-negative bacteria resistant to antibiotics is increasing.

CLINICAL NOTE

Ensure you are aware of all local policies relating to antimicrobial stewardship, MRSA including patient identification and screening and *Clostridium difficile* including isolation for infected patients and infection control precautions.

REFERENCES AND FURTHER READING

Aziz, M., 2013. Nursing management of *Clostridium difficile* infection. Nurse Prescribing 11, 21–27.

Daum, R.S., 2007. Clinical practice. Skin and soft-tissue infections caused by methicillin-resistant *Staphylococcus aureus*. N. Engl. J. Med. 357 (4), 380–390.

Department of Health and the Health Protection Agency, 2008. *Clostridium difficile* Infection: How to deal with the Problem. Department of Health, London.

Dye, C., Watt, C.J., Bleed, D.M., et al., 2005. Evolution of tuberculosis control and prospects for reducing tuberculosis incidence, prevalence and deaths globally. J. Am. Med. Assoc. 293, 2767–2775.

Filippone, E.J., Kraft, W.K., Farber, J.L., 2017. The nephrotoxicity of vancomycin. Clin. Pharmacol. Ther. 102 (3), 459–469.

Gebreweld, F.H., Kifle, M.M., Gebremicheal, F.E., et al., 2018. Factors influencing adherence to tuberculosis treatment in Asmara, Eritrea: a qualitative study. J. Health Popul. Nutr. 37 (1), 1.

Giuliano, C., Haase, K.K., Hall, R., 2010. Use of vancomycin pharmacokinetic-pharmacodynamic properties in the treatment of MRSA infections. Expert Rev. Anti. Infect. Ther. 8 (1), 95–106.

Greener, M., 2012. Antiviral drugs: an important part of the defence against flu. Nurse Prescribing 10, 446–450.

Hawking, M., Ashira-Oredope, D., Northeast, S., McNulty, C., 2014. Antimicrobial stewardship: how can nurses contribute? Nurse Prescribing 12, 536–537.

Health Foundation. 2015. Infection prevention and control: lessons from acute care in England. Towards a whole health economy approach. Health Foundation Learning Report, Health Foundation. https://www.health.org.uk/about-the-health-foundation.

Hougaard Christensen, M.M., Bruun Haastrup, M., Øhlenschlaeger, T., et al., 2020. Interaction potential between clarithromycin and individual statins – a systematic review. Basic Clin. Pharmacol. Toxicol. 126 (4), 307–317.

Maartens, G., Wilkinson, R.J., 2007. Tuberculosis. Lancet 370 (9604), 2030–2043.

Ness, V., Price, L., Carrie, K., Reilly, J., 2014. Antimicrobial resistance and prescribing behaviour. Nurse Prescribing 12, 248–235.

NICE. 2006. Tuberculosis. Clinical diagnosis and management of tuberculosis, and measures for its prevention and control [CG33]. https://www.nice.org.uk/guidance/cg33.

Niemi, M., Backman, J.T., Fromm, M.F., et al., 2003. Pharmacokinetic interactions with rifampicin: clinical relevance. Clin. Pharmacokinet. 42 (9), 819–850.

Picard, M., Robitaille, G., Karam, F., et al., 2019. Cross-reactivity to cephalosporins and carbapenems in penicillin-allergic patients: two systematic reviews and meta-analyses. J. Allergy Clin. Immunol. Pract. 7 (8), 2722–2738.e5.

Pradipta, I.S., Houtsma, D., van Boven, J.F.M., et al., 2020. Interventions to improve medication adherence in tuberculosis patients: a systematic review of randomized controlled studies. NPJ Prim. Care Respir. Med. 30 (1), 21.

Stewart, K., 2016. New guidance on the prevention and management of tuberculosis. Prescriber 27, 16–22.

WHO. 2016. The evolving threat of antimicrobial resistance. Options for action. http://apps.who.int/iris/bitstream/10665/44812/1/9789241503181_eng.pdf.

USEFUL WEBSITES

Health and Social Care Act 2008. Code of practice for the NHS on the prevention and control of health care associated infections and related guidance. https://www.legislation.gov.uk/ukpga/2008/14/contents.

HM Government 2014. UK 5 Year Antimicrobial Resistance (AMR) strategy 2013–2018. Annual Progress Report and Implementation Plan, 2014. https://www.gov.uk/government/uploads/system/uploads/attachment_data/file/385733/UK_AMR_annual_report.pdf.

NICE Guideline [NG109]. Urinary tract infection (lower): antimicrobial prescribing. https://www.nice.org.uk/guidance/ng109.

NICE Guideline [NG15]. Antimicrobial stewardship: systems and processes for effective antimicrobial medicine use. https://www.nice.org.uk/guidance/ng15.

NICE Guideline [NG24]. Sore throat (acute): antimicrobial prescribing. https://www.nice.org.uk/guidance/ng84.

NICE Guideline [NG51]. Sepsis: recognition, diagnosis and early management. https://www.nice.org.uk/guidance/ng51.

NICE Quality Standard [49]. Surgical site infection. https://www.nice.org.uk/guidance/qs49/resources/surgical-site-infection-2098675107781.

O'Neill Report, March 2016. Review on antimicrobial resistance: tackling drug-resistant infections globally. Infection prevention, control and surveillance: limiting the spread and development of drug resistance. http://amr-review.org/sites/default/files/Health%20infrastructure%20and%20surveillance%20final%20version_LR_NO%20CROPS.pdf.

Public Health England. Antimicrobial stewardship: Start smart, then focus. https://www.gov.uk/government/publications/antimicrobial-stewardship-start-smart-then-focus.

SIGN. National Clinical Guideline 104. Antibiotic prophylaxis in surgery. https://www.just.edu.jo/DIC/ClinicGuidlines/Antibiotic%20prophylaxis%20in%20surgery.pdf.

The UK Sepsis Trust. https://sepsistrust.org.

27 ANTIVIRALS
Treatments for HIV, Hepatitis and Influenza

CHAPTER OUTLINE

LEARNING OBJECTIVES

At the end of this chapter, the reader should be able to:

- explain how cytomegalovirus is treated and list the names of important drugs used to treat HIV disease and explain how they work
- describe what is meant by reverse transcriptase inhibitors and give examples
- discuss the importance of combined therapy for HIV disease
- state the danger of needle-stick injuries and provide examples of drugs that are used to try to prevent infection with HIV after a needle-stick injury
- give an account of fungal infections and explain that they may be superficial or systemic
- list the main antifungal drugs and their uses
- give an account of the treatment of candidiasis
- discuss the growth in incidence of systemic fungal infections due to AIDS and organ and tissue transplantation

THE VIRUS

Viruses cause a number of diseases, some of which are serious and potentially fatal, although most are of minor importance (e.g. the common cold). In subjects who are immunosuppressed – e.g. by the human immunodeficiency virus (HIV) or treatment with cytotoxic drugs – a relatively benign viral infection may become virulent.

It is difficult to produce effective antiviral agents for several reasons:

- Viruses live within human cells and they use processes in those cells to multiply. They are not therefore readily accessible.
- They are very sophisticated structures and are not easy to destroy.
- A great deal of virus replication occurs before the patient develops symptoms.
- Viruses mutate rapidly and this can render vaccines and many drugs useless. Many viruses, e.g. influenza virus, are subject to antigenic drift.

ANTIVIRAL AGENTS

Antiviral agents include:

- Aciclovir
- Famciclovir
- Valaciclovir
- Amantadine
- Ribavirin
- Foscarnet.

Aciclovir

This agent is effective against the herpesviruses. It enters the infected cells, where it is changed into a powerful antiviral agent.

Therapeutic Use.

- Aciclovir is prescribed for herpes zoster (shingles). If the ophthalmic branch of the trigeminal nerve is affected, review by an ophthalmologist is pertinent as it can affect the eyes in several ways such as corneal ulcers and serious inflammation. This can result in reduction of vision. As shingles can result in prolonged neuralgia and damage to the eye, antivirals should be started within 48 h of the symptom onset to help reduce complications. Oral aciclovir is usually given for 7 days in uncomplicated cases of shingles in adults.
- In generalized herpes simplex infection in immunosuppressed patients or in herpes meningoencephalitis, it is given by intravenous infusion. This may cause a deterioration of renal function, which should be monitored. Patients with impaired renal function will require smaller doses.
- It can be applied as a 3% ointment 5 times daily to treat ulceration of the cornea due to the herpes simplex virus and should be continued for 3 days after healing.
- Given orally 5 times daily for 5 days, it accelerates the healing of genital herpes. Very severe attacks may require parenteral treatment.
- A 5% cream of aciclovir is only effective in labial herpes if used in the prodromal period when there is only a local burning sensation.
- It also shortens the course of varicella (chickenpox), but its use in this disorder should be confined to those at special risk (i.e. immunosuppressed patients).

Adverse Effects. These include rashes, nausea and vomiting.

Contraindication. Pregnancy.

Famciclovir and **valaciclovir** are similar and are given orally to treat herpes simplex and herpes zoster (shingles). They have the advantage of only needing to be administered 2 or 3 times daily.

Amantadine (see later) has some action against the influenza virus but is not recommended for treatment of influenza due to antiviral resistance. **Ribavirin** is used in the treatment of respiratory tract viruses, particularly respiratory syncytial virus, which causes bronchiolitis in infants. It is given by nebuliser or aerosol inhalation.

CYTOMEGALOVIRUS

Cidofovir, **foscarnet**, **ganciclovir** and **valganciclovir** are used for the treatment of serious infections by the cytomegalovirus. The disease is usually mild, except in immunosuppressed patients (e.g. those with AIDS) and as a risk to the fetus in pregnancy. All except valganciclovir, which is administered in oral tablet form, are given by intravenous infusion.

The most serious adverse effect is suppression of the leucocyte count and of the platelets, which usually recover when the drugs are stopped. They are contraindicated during pregnancy, and patients should be warned to take effective contraceptive measures during treatment. Men should take contraceptive measures during treatment and for at least 90 days afterwards.

Valganciclovir is a prodrug of ganciclovir. It is used for the treatment of cytomegalovirus retinitis in people with AIDS. The precautions for use are as for ganciclovir.

Foscarnet is reserved for cytomegalovirus infection in immunocompromised patients. It is given by intravenous infusion and is highly nephrotoxic.

Cidofovir is prescribed for the treatment of cytomegalovirus retinitis in AIDS patients when the use of other antiviral agents is not appropriate. It should not be used in patients with impaired renal function. It is a nephrotoxic drug.

HUMAN IMMUNODEFICIENCY VIRUS (HIV) AND ACQUIRED IMMUNODEFICIENCY SYNDROME (AIDS)

In 2019, there were 38 million people worldwide living with HIV (WHO, 2020), and this number is likely to rise. So far, no cure is available but treatment is becoming more successful and the progression of the disease can be successfully halted.

There are two main variants of HIV virus: HIV-1 and HIV-2. However, both of these major variants are subdivided further. HIV-1 is responsible for the majority of cases of AIDS worldwide and HIV-2 seems to be the more common variant in West Africa. HIV-2 is thought to have a lower transmission rate and is less pathogenic. It is felt this variant has a slower progression to AIDS.

After infection with HIV there is a latent period when the patient is symptom-free. During this time, the virus enters the cells of the immune system (CD4 T cells) and, using the host cells metabolic processes, multiplies and finally destroys the cells, releasing further virus. When the immune system has been sufficiently depleted of T cells, the patient becomes susceptible to a variety of opportunistic infections that ultimately prove fatal (Fig. 27.1). The latter stages when the patient is susceptible to these infections is referred to as AIDS, which is usually clinically characterized by a CD4 cell count of <200 cells/μL or presence of an AIDS-defining condition. AIDS-defining conditions are opportunistic infections, which present more frequently due to immunosuppression. Commonly occurring illness due to immunosuppression include *Pneumocystis jirovecii* pneumonia, oesophageal candidiasis, Kaposi sarcoma and tuberculosis. The median latency between infection with HIV and the onset of these opportunistic infections is about 10 years in the UK.

HIV Treatment

The aim of treatment is to reduce the numbers of virus particles as much as possible (reduce viral load) for as long as possible. This creates two problems: the patient will take toxic drugs for a long time and the virus develops resistance to the drugs. The use of single agents against HIV leads to the emergence of resistance and failure of treatment. It is now apparent that

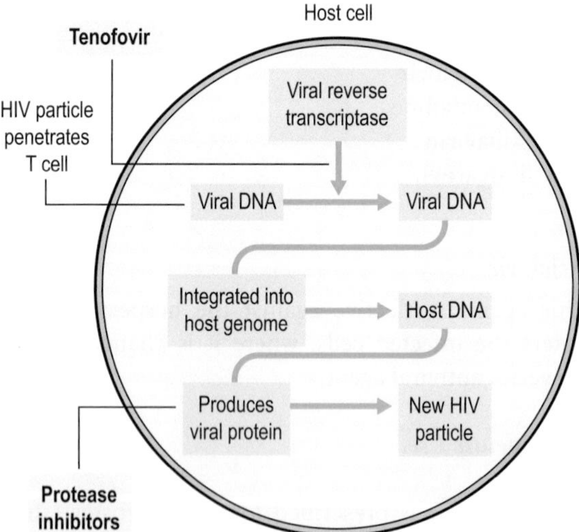

Fig. 27.1 Intracellular cycle of an HIV particle and site of action of tenofovir, which inhibits the enzyme reverse transcriptase, and protease inhibitors, which prevent the formation of new virus particles.

using antiretroviral therapy (ART) agents simultaneously, particularly if they affect different phases in the viral life cycle, is more effective.

Patients diagnosed with HIV should be reviewed and managed by an HIV specialist. It is now standard practice that patients diagnosed with HIV should be offered immediate treatment irrespective of their CD4 count. Previously, the treatment was initiated once the CD4 counts had dropped to 350; however, subsequent studies have found that, in doing this, there was a higher chance of patients developing AIDS-related illness.

There are six main classes of HIV drugs:

- Nucleoside reverse transcriptase inhibitors (NRTIs)
- Non-nucleoside reverse transcriptase inhibitors (NNRTIs)
- Protease inhibitors (PIs)
- CCR5 antagonists
- Integrase inhibitors (INIs)
- Fusion and entry inhibitors.

The British HIV Association (BHIVA) have developed guidelines on treatment for patients with HIV to suit the individual health needs of patients. Adherence to ART is crucial to help reduce viral load to undetectable levels (viral load below 20 copies/mL), which helps to reduce transmission of the virus as well as reducing the damage to the patient's immune system, hence reducing the progression of the disease. The preferred treatment initiation for HIV patients are a combination containing two NRTIs (e.g. emtricitabine and tenofovir disoproxil) and either a ritonavir-boosted protease inhibitor (e.g. atazanavir), an NNRTI (e.g. rilpivirine), or an integrase inhibitor (e.g. dolutegravir).

CLINICAL NOTE

Treatment optimization and adherence to HIV medication is vital. Studies suggest that 95% adherence achieves effective reductions in viral load. To achieve this, a shared understanding between the clinician and person with HIV of the disease, treatment and strategies to optimize adherence is important. A Cochrane review carried out in 2006 (Rueda et al., 2006) concluded that practical medicines management skills and interventions delivered over 12 weeks were most effective.

Nucleoside Reverse Transcriptase Inhibitors

NRTIs are similar in structure to the cellular chemicals used as building blocks by the viral enzyme reverse transcriptase when it makes viral DNA from its own viral RNA in the host cell. The enzyme is 'fooled' into trying to incorporate the drug into the strand of growing viral DNA. Once the drug is incorporated into the DNA, it stops the reaction from going any further, and the virus can no longer replicate itself in the host cell. Examples of licensed NRTIs in the UK are:

- Abacavir
- Tenofovir
- Emtricitabine
- Lamivudine
- Stavudine
- Zidovudine.

Zidovudine, an analogue of thymidine, was the most widely used drug of this group but now the most commonly used NRTIs are **tenofovir** and **abacavir.**

Tenofovir disoproxil can be given orally in combination with other ART. It inhibits the reverse transcriptase of both HIV and hepatitis B virus; therefore it is useful also for patients with co-infection with hepatitis B. Common **adverse effects of tenofovir disoproxil** include renal insufficiency and decrease in bone mineral density (thus increasing risk of fractures).

Abacavir is converted to its active metabolite carbovir triphosphate, which inhibits the effect of HIV reverse transcriptase. Abacavir is associated with immunologically mediated systemic hypersensitivity reaction. The symptoms of this includes fever, rash, flu-like syndrome, gastrointestinal disturbance and respiratory compromise. If this occurs, abacavir should be promptly discontinued and not re-challenged.

Non-nucleoside Reverse Transcriptase Inhibitors

Non-nucleoside reverse transcriptase inhibitors (NNRTIs) are non-competitive inhibitors of reverse transcriptase resulting in decreased action of this enzyme. NNRTIs are typically administered along with dual NRTI combination.

Licensed NNRTIs for HIV treatment in the UK include:

- Doravirine
- Etravirine

- Rilpivirine
- Nevirapine
- Efavirenz.

Doravirine, **etravirine** and **rilpivirine** are newer generation NNRTIs than the early NNRTIs efavirenz and nevirapine, which interfere with the action of viral reverse transcriptase. The newer generation of NNRTIs have longer half-lives, fewer side-effects and fewer drug interactions.

Rilpivirine has a once-daily dosing regimen. It is associated with Qt-prolongation and as it requires gastric acid to be effective, its use with proton pump inhibitors is contraindicated.

Efavirenz has significant side-effect profile, including neuropsychiatry toxicity, hyperlipidemia and abnormal liver function. Nevirapine is also not recommended for treatment-naive patients due to its significant side-effect profile, including liver toxicity and serious cutaneous reactions, e.g. Stevens–Johnson syndrome.

Protease Inhibitors

These drugs (PIs) act at a later stage in the formation of virus particles by inhibiting viral proteases, which are necessary for the formation of viral proteins. This class of ART generally requires multiple mutations to occur for resistance to develop.

Licensed PIs in the UK comprise of:

- Atazanavir
- Darunavir
- Fosamprenavir
- Lopinavir
- Ritonavir
- Saquinavir
- Tipranavir.

Therapeutic Use. **Atazanavir** and **darunavir** is usually prescribed together with **ritonavir**, which helps boost their levels in the body. All of these drugs are to be used in combination with other antiviral drugs. Ritonavir is prescribed specifically in advanced HIV infection together with NRTIs.

Adverse Effects. These include metabolic abnormalities including dyslipidemia (in particular hypertriglycerides), insulin resistance, hyperglycaemia and lipodystrophy. All of these protease inhibitors should be used with caution in patients with renal problems.

Contraindications. All protease inhibitors are contraindicated in patients who are breastfeeding, and ritonavir is contraindicated in patients with hepatic impairment.

CCR5 Antagonists

Maraviroc is the only CCR5 antagonist approved for use in HIV treatment. It binds to human CCR5 receptors on the cell membrane blocking the interaction of HIV gp120 (glycoprotein, which is essential as it helps facilitate HIV entry into the host cell) and CCR5 receptors.

Integrase Inhibitors

INIs block the integrase enzyme so that bonds between host and viral DNA do not form and thus preventing the incorporation of viral DNA into the host chromosome. There are three licensed INIs in the UK:

- Dolutegravir
- Elvitegravir
- Raltegravir.

INIs are generally well-tolerated but have the potential of interacting with products such as antacids. An ART regimen for naive patients can include two NRTIs and an INI. **Dolutegravir** is quite well-tolerated, with headache and insomnia being the most common adverse effects reported in less than 5% of patients in clinical trials.

Fusion Inhibitors

Enfuvirtide is an HIV fusion inhibitor. This means it blocks the initial fusion of the HIV virus with the target CD4-1 white blood cells of the patient. It is a newer approach to the treatment of HIV infection and AIDS. It is usually prescribed together with other antiviral agents for patients who have not responded to other treatment regimens, therefore it is generally reserved for patients with multiple drug class resistance. It is given by subcutaneous injection twice a day and, because it is a large molecule, may produce hypersensitivity reactions. It is best used under specialist supervision. Enfuvirtide seems to be most potent against HIV-1.

CLINICAL NOTE

Two or three drugs are given together (nucleoside analogue + protease inhibitor). Most experts believe that it is best to start treatment when the infection is first diagnosed rather than when symptoms develop. Although it is too early to talk of a cure, active life can be prolonged and complications minimized. Adherence to the prescribed regimen is vital for optimizing health and quality of life and studies have shown it to reduce mortality and morbidity (Paterson et al., 2000). Interventions to optimize adherence are varied and include reducing dose frequency, text message reminders and behavioural interventions such as motivational interviewing and cognitive behavioural therapy (Mbuagbaw et al., 2015).

Antiviral agents are expensive, and considering the widespread nature of HIV infection, much of it is in the Third World, the cost of treatment is enormous. In addition, when the disease is controlled, some maintenance treatment may be necessary to prevent relapse.

Monitoring Treatment

It is important to measure the extent of HIV infection in a patient in order to decide on optimal treatment and to assess progress. This can be achieved by:

- counting the number of CD4 T cells in the blood – the lower the count, the more advanced the disease
- measuring the concentration of RNA derived from the HIV in the plasma (viral load) – the higher the load (which is a measure of viral multiplication), the more active the disease.

CLINICAL NOTE

People living with HIV have a high prevalence of depressive symptoms and anxiety (Lowther et al., 2014); therefore, monitoring of viral load should also be combined with assessment of psychological symptoms and, where present, appropriate management. This will assist in optimizing adherence and reducing adverse events relating to the disease and prescribed medicines.

Mother-to-Infant Transmission of HIV

There is consensus that treating the pregnant mother with ARTs in pregnancy can considerably reduce mother-to-infant HIV transmission from an infected mother. Zidovudine is the only antiretroviral agent with a licence for use in pregnancy. However, non-pregnant adults are rarely now prescribed this due to its toxicity risks. The BHIVA recommends all pregnant women are started on ART by week 24 of pregnancy (first trimester is avoided due to the risk of congenital abnormality secondary to exposure from ART). BHIVA (2020) currently recommends that the best safety data in pregnancy are for efavirenz or atazanavir and thus these should be considered first-line in pregnancy.

The safest way for a mother with HIV to feed her baby is using a bottle using formula milk. However, according to the BHIVA, the mum may be supported with breastfeeding if her viral load is undetectable and using the 'safer triangle', which consists of 'no virus + happy tums + healthy breasts for mums' (see: www.bhiva.org). The mum should be informed that so far, our understanding is that breastfeeding is not as safe as using formula in women with HIV.

Needle-stick Injuries

Accidental infection of health professionals is very rare and the possibility of becoming HIV-positive after a needle-stick injury is about 1:400. Occupational exposure, e.g. via needle-stick injuries with a patient is a medical emergency and needs appropriate immediate referral for post-exposure prophylaxis (PEP) to greatly reduce the risk of infection. PEP must be taken within 72 h and ideally within 24 h. It is usually taken for 28 days and the medication commonly used for PEP is a combination of Truvada and raltegravir (Terrence Higgins Trust, 2020).

PEP is not recommended following a human bite, as the risk of transmission is extremely low – less than 1 in 10,000.

Pre-exposure Prophylaxis

Pre-exposure prophylaxis (PrEP) is a drug taken by people who are HIV-negative before sex, which reduces the risk of getting HIV. This is currently under trial in England. PrEP is made up of two drugs, namely **tenofovir** and **emtricitabine**. In the future, this may be more widely available if the trial results show success and can help reduce transmission and incidence of HIV in people who are considered to be at high risk of HIV.

Complications of HIV Infection

Pneumocystis carinii pneumonia is common and is treated by high-dose co-trimoxazole or by intravenous pentamidine in severe disease. Relapse can be prevented by long-term treatment with co-trimoxazole, inhaled pentamidine or dapsone. Patients with HIV disease are also susceptible to various fungal and viral infections and to tuberculosis.

The Search for Vaccines

At the time of writing, vaccines against HIV and cytomegalovirus have not been introduced, although a huge scientific effort is currently being made.

SUMMARY

- The aim of treatment of HIV disease is to reduce the numbers of virus particles as much as possible for as long as possible.
- It is generally considered better to start treatment as soon as HIV is diagnosed.
- The extent of HIV infection can be assessed by counting the numbers of CD4 T cells in the blood and by monitoring HIV RNA in the blood (the viral load).
- Mother-to-infant transmission of HIV can be considerably reduced during pregnancy by treating the infected mother with suitable ART and encouraging formula rather than breastfeeding.
- Occupational hazards associated with the HIV and hepatitis can be minimized by using scrupulous techniques when dealing with possible sources of infection.

HEPATITIS B AND HEPATITIS C VIRUS

Two other viral infections to which healthcare workers may be exposed in their occupation are of particular concern. These are:

- **Hepatitis B virus (HBV)**
- **Hepatitis C virus (HCV).**

Transmission is usually via contaminated blood or blood products. Other body fluids may be involved, because these are so often contaminated with blood. Infection occurs most commonly by needle-stick injury. Often it is through a break in the skin or via a mucous membrane. It does not occur through intact skin, but even a minute abrasion will let in the infection.

Prevention and Management

The most important preventative measure is avoidance of risk and scrupulous techniques when dealing with possible sources of infection.

Active immunization is available against HBV, but not against HCV. Immunization against HBV is given to children at 2, 3 and 4 months of age as part of the UK immunization schedule (see Chapter 28). At-risk groups should also be vaccinated, including healthcare workers, close family contacts of individuals with HBV, babies born to mothers infected with hepatitis B, sex workers and intravenous drug users. Approximately 10% of adults fail to respond to the three doses of the vaccine. Following primary immunization, healthcare workers should have an antibodies for hepatitis B check, which should be after 1–4 months following the vaccination.

If exposure to the virus has occurred, the following steps are advised, though it is possible that advances may alter these procedures:

- **Hepatitis B:** determine the immune status of the exposed person – if susceptible, give HBV immunoglobulin and immunize with vaccine. Hepatitis B immunoglobulin is given intramuscularly ideally within 48 h of exposure and at the same time as the first dose of the vaccine.
- **Hepatitis C:** there is no effective protection yet, but the subject must be followed up for evidence of infection, as there is a chance of developing chronic active hepatitis, as there is with HBV.

The Interferons

This is a family of protein-like substances produced by various cells in the body in response to viral infections. Interferons have the ability to act on cells and increase their resistance to viral infections and may also modify the immune response. In addition, they control the growth and differentiation of cells.

Interferons can now be produced synthetically and have been used in both neoplastic and infective disease in humans. Their main success has been in treating leukaemias, particularly the hairy-celled types, and to a lesser degree, in some other forms of cancer. In the control of viral infections their usefulness is limited, but they are used with some success in hepatitis B and C infections (see later).

Interferon beta is now being used in the relapsing/remitting form of multiple sclerosis, with some benefit. It is given by intramuscular injection. Adverse effects are fever and nausea.

A steroid that has been reported possibly to help sufferers with multiple sclerosis is oestriol, which is one of the oestrogens secreted in large amounts during pregnancy, and which is also used for hormone replacement therapy (HRT).

Readers will encounter reference to pegylated interferons. These are interferons to which are attached molecules of polyethylene glycol. This slows their rate of elimination from the body after administration.

Treatments for Viral Hepatitis

Hepatitis B is often eliminated by the patient's immune system without drugs, without the patient's awareness of its presence, and in any event, many cases are not diagnosed for the first few months after infection with the virus. Drugs are available to treat chronic hepatitis B; none will cure it, but they may block viral replication. **Pegylated interferon** **α-2A** (peginterferon-α) is the recommended first-line treatment of hepatitis B after diagnosis. The drug should be used with caution, if at all, in patients with decompensated liver disease. This is cirrhosis of the liver with a build-up of fluid in the abdomen (ascites). Other antivirals used in hepatitis B are **entecavir** or **tenofovir disoproxil** as initial treatments of chronic hepatitis B. **Lamivudine** and **adefovir** inhibit reverse transcriptase, the enzyme which can convert viral single-stranded RNA into single-stranded DNA, thus allowing the virus to incorporate its replicating code into the host cell. **Entecavir** is a drug which inhibits all the steps in viral replication.

Chronic hepatitis C is a more complicated problem and the genotype (genetic composition) of the infecting virus will determine the length of treatment. Hepatitis C may be caused by genotypes G_1, G_2, G_3, G_4, G_5 or G_6. Prior to treatment initiation, the genotype of the hepatitis C virus should be undertaken as well as measuring the viral load, to help plan the course of individualized treatment for the patient. Treatment will also depend on how well patients respond to it. Combinations of two drugs, e.g. **peginterferon**-α and **ribavirin**, which inhibits viral nucleic acid synthesis, may be used, or substituted for other options depending on the patient's response.

INFLUENZA

Treatment of Influenza

Apart from the more conventional drugs, such as ibuprofen and paracetamol, which reduce temperature and pain, there are antiviral drugs, which block the action of the virus, by blocking the action of the viral enzyme neuraminidase that normally makes possible the budding off of the virus from the host cell, e.g. **oseltamivir** and **zanamivir**, or which block viral ion channels, e.g. **amantadine**. Amantadine is also useful in the treatment of Parkinson's disease (see Chapter 21). These drugs may, under some circumstances, be used prophylactically to prevent influenza ('flu') taking hold, although, in the UK, National Institute for Health and Care Excellence (NICE) has recommended that these drugs are not a substitute for the annual vaccination against flu. The flu vaccination needs to be reviewed and updated each year to keep up with the evolving influenza viruses. **Antigenic drift**, which is a genetic variation in the virus caused by mutations, helps the virus evolve over time. It is also the reason why people can catch the flu more than once.

SUMMARY

- Healthcare workers should be immunized against HBV.
- If a worker is exposed to HBV, HBV immunoglobulin should be given and the worker vaccinated.

- Treatment with antivirals for flu is not recommended by NICE and instead vaccination against the flu in the at-risk group should be encouraged.
- The influenza virus undergoes antigenic drift.

ANTIFUNGAL AGENTS

Introduction

Fungi are simple organisms that lack chlorophyll; they were originally considered as plants. Fungi include mushrooms, moulds, yeasts and rusts. Some live commensally with a human, which means that neither organism harms the other. Some, however, cause disease when they infect. Fungal infections, at least in temperate countries, do not usually pose serious threats to health, and have largely been superficial in nature. The most common problems have been, e.g. athlete's foot and vaginal or oral thrush.

Systemic fungal infections in the UK were rare, but are now on the increase. This is due to the widespread use of broad-spectrum antibiotics, which destroy the non-pathogenic bacteria, especially in the gut, which compete with ingested fungi for food. Another exacerbating factor is the higher incidence of patients with reduced immune competence, due to diseases such as HIV disease and the use of immunosuppressive treatments such as irradiation and anticancer drugs.

Classification of Fungal Infections

Fungal infections are collectively called **mycoses**. They can be classified for convenience as superficial infections and systemic infections.

Superficial Infections

Superficial infections have not been traditionally serious in nature. They involve skin, mucous membranes, scalp and nails. They can be classified as candidiasis (thrush) and dermatomycoses.

Candidiasis infections are caused by a yeast-like fungus that infects mouth, skin and vagina.

Fungi called **dermatophytes** cause dermatomycoses infections. A dermatophyte feeds on keratin. The most common and therefore best known are the tinea fungi, which cause what is commonly called 'ringworm':

- tinea capitis is ringworm of the scalp
- tinea pedis is athlete's foot
- tinea cruris affects the thighs and groin
- tinea barbae affects the skin under a beard.

Systemic Infections

In the UK, systemic candidiasis is the most common fungal infection. Examples of others are:

- Cryptococcal meningitis: causes a serious infection of the brain and can occur in people with HIV. The fungus *Cryptococcus neoformans* is commonly found in pigeon droppings.
- Pulmonary aspergillosis is caused by aspergillus mould. This can be found in soil, damp buildings or air conditioning systems. Patients with respiratory conditions such as cystic fibrosis, asthma, chronic obstructive pulmonary disease, previous history of tuberculosis or those who are immunosuppressed, are more prone to the condition.
- Invasive pulmonary aspergillosis, which is an important cause of death in patients who have received bone marrow transplants (see explanation of aspergillosis later)
- Rhinocerebral mucormycosis (*Mucor* is a genus of fungus found on decaying organic matter) is a rare infection of the sinuses, oral cavity and the brain. It can affect individuals with diabetes or those who are immunosuppressed.

These conditions are still comparatively rare in the UK.

Aspergillosis refers to infection with the fungal genus *Aspergillus*, usually *A. fumigatus*. Infection occurs quite often in patients with pre-existing lung disease and three forms occur:

- an allergic reaction in asthma
- a colonizing form that forms a fungus ball in a lung cavity, e.g. a healed tuberculous cavity
- a form that may spread from the lungs to the rest of the body, usually in patients with compromised immune systems (e.g. in HIV patients or after bone marrow transplantation).

Drugs Used to Treat Fungal Infections

These include:

- Amphotericin
- Clotrimazole

- Fluconazole
- Flucytosine
- Griseofulvin
- Itraconazole
- Ketoconazole
- Miconazole
- Nystatin
- Terbinafine
- Voriconazole.

Many of these preparations can be sold without the need for a prescription and the pharmacist can advise.

Nystatin binds to the wall of the fungus, disrupting its integrity. It is very poorly absorbed after oral administration and is therefore used to treat infections of the intestinal tract or is applied locally. It is particularly used in *Candida* infections. Oral infections respond to nystatin drops placed inside the mouth four times daily.

Clotrimazole and **miconazole** are most effective if applied locally as pessaries in the treatment of vaginal candidiasis. Miconazole is available as a gel for treating oropharyngeal infection. Both can be applied to the skin as a 1% or 2% ointment for dermatophytoses.

Ketoconazole is now largely used in treatment of skin conditions such as seborrhoeic dermatitis in the form of a shampoo. Although oral forms of ketoconazole are available, the Committee for Medicinal Products for Human Use (CHMP) in 2013 concluded that the risks of hepatoxicity associated with it were greater than its benefit in treating fungal infections, therefore alternative treatment should be sought.

Fluconazole is effective in candidiasis and cryptococcal infection. Serious adverse effects, particularly liver damage, have been reported. For vaginal candidiasis and for oropharyngeal infections, a single oral dose is adequate.

Itraconazole is used in systemic candidiasis and dermatophyte infections, in particular if other antifungals have been ineffective. The dose is variable and the capsules should be taken immediately after food to ensure maximum absorption. It should not be used in patients with liver disease and there is risk of congestive heart failure.

Griseofulvin is administered orally in the treatment of various fungal infections. It is used in most types of fungal infection of the skin, particularly in ringworm of the scalp where local treatment is inadequate. It is slow-acting and may be continued for several weeks. As regards adverse effects, gastrointestinal upsets may occur when it is used, and griseofulvin may enhance the action of alcohol taken at the same time as the drug.

Terbinafine is applied locally for fungal infection of the skin and nails. It can also be given orally for dermatophyte infections of the toenails. Liver function tests should be closely monitored on provision of oral treatment for this, which may require 3 months or longer oral treatment, and the patient should be counselled about liver toxicity prior to prescribing.

Amphotericin is used in severe systemic infection with fungal organisms – namely, systemic candidiasis, cryptococcal meningitis and histoplasmosis. After an initial test dose, it is given by intravenous infusion, the dose being increased gradually. The MHRA (2020) reported serious harm and fatal overdoses following confusion between liposomal, pegylated-liposomal, lipid-complex and conventional formulations of the same drug. Although the various formulations may contain the same drug, these are **not** interchangeable.

Flucytosine is an antifungal agent effective against *Candida albicans* and cryptococcus and is usually an adjunct to amphotericin B. It is given intravenously, four times daily. The kidney excretes it and therefore reduced dosage may be required in patients with impaired renal function. Side-effects are rare, but depression of the blood count has been reported.

Voriconazole is an antifungal agent; the preferential treatment for aspergillosis. It can be given orally or via intravenous infusion. Close monitoring of renal function is required and if the eGFR is less than 50 mL/min per 1.73 m^2, the risk–benefit ratio needs to be reanalyzed if using intravenous infusion, and consideration given to switching it to an alternative or using the oral route considered.

CLINICAL NOTE

Clinicians may see a reduced effect of antifungals when prescribed with a proton-pump inhibitor drug, e.g. omeprazole. Antifungals require a high gastric Ph to promote absorption, which may be compromised if the two drugs are given concurrently (Dodds Ashley et al., 2006).

Candidiasis

Candidiasis is a common and troublesome problem. It can occur for no apparent reason but is particularly common in:

- Ill or immunocompromised patients, particularly those receiving broad-spectrum antibiotics
- Those receiving drugs which suppress immunity (i.e. cytotoxic drugs and steroids)
- Patients with HIV disease
- Patients with diabetes
- Infants
- Pregnancy
- Healthy women.

It may affect the mouth (thrush), the vagina or other mucous membranes. Rarely, it enters the bloodstream and becomes a systemic infection.

Treatment

Oral Candidiasis.

- Acute: nystatin drops or miconazole gel
- Oropharyngeal: fluconazole or itraconazole daily for up to 14 days
- Children: miconazole gel. The gel is not licensed for children under 4 months of age due to choking risk. It is commonly used and recommended by paediatricians in particular, as application is far easier than with the use of nystatin drops. However, due to its licensing, this should be discussed with the parents and documented in the clinical notes.

Oesophageal, Intestinal or Systemic Candidiasis.

- Fluconazole.

Vaginal Candidiasis.

- Fluconazole, a single oral dose, or itraconazole twice daily for 1 day
- Clotrimazole vaginal pessaries, one inserted at night as a single dose. For recurrent or persistent candidiasis immunosuppressive disorder/diabetes needs to be excluded and may require treatment with prolonged courses of antifungals.

CLINICAL NOTE

1. In oral candidiasis, remove dentures (if any) during treatment. They should be soaked in sodium hypochlorite overnight and rinsed thoroughly before being worn again.
2. People taking beclomethasone inhalers may be prone to oral candidiasis and they should be advised to brush their teeth or use an oral mouthwash after taking their inhaler. A spacer device may also reduce the incidence of thrush in this group.
3. In vaginal candidiasis, the partner (if any) must receive treatment.

Systemic Fungal Infections

These are increasing problems because of the large number of immunocompromised subjects due to HIV, cancer chemotherapy and other causes. In the past, amphotericin and flucytosine were the only drugs available, but now fluconazole and itraconazole are commonly used. The correct drug for a particular fungal infection is still being researched and the choice of treatment requires expert guidance.

SUMMARY

- Systemic fungal infections are on the increase because of widespread use of broad-spectrum antibiotics.
- Nystatin is particularly useful in *Candida* infections.
- Clotrimazole and miconazole are most effective if applied locally in the treatment of vaginal candidiasis.
- Ketoconazole is commonly used topically for treating fungal skin and scalp infections.
- Fluconazole can cause serious liver damage.
- Griseofulvin is administered orally for treating ringworm of the scalp.
- Terbinafine is useful by oral administration for treating tinea skin or nail infections and can be administered topically to the nails over long periods.
- Amphotericin B is used in severe systemic fungal infections.
- The dose of flucytosine should be reduced in patients with impaired kidney function.

REFERENCES AND FURTHER READING

Benitez, L.L., Carver, P.L., 2019. Adverse effects associated with long-term administration of azole antifungal agents. Drugs 79 (8), 833–853.

Dodds Ashley, E.S., Lewis, R., Lewis, J.S., et al., 2006. Pharmacology of systemic antifungal agents. Clin. Infect. Dis. 43 (Suppl. 1), S28–S39.

Esté, J.A., Telenti, A., 2007. HIV entry inhibitors. Lancet 370, 81–88.

Fukushima, C., Matsuse, H., Tomari, S., et al., 2003. Oral candidiasis associated with inhaled corticosteroid use: comparison of fluticasone and beclomethasone. Ann. Allergy Asthma Immunol. 90 (6), 646–651.

Lowther, K., Selman, L., Harding, R., Higginson, I.J., 2014. Experience of persistent psychological symptoms and perceived stigma among people with HIV on antiretroviral therapy (ART): a systematic review. Int. J. Nurs. Stud. 51 (8), 1171–1189.

Mbuagbaw, L., Sivaramalingam, B., Navarro, T., et al., 2015. Interventions for enhancing adherence to Antiretroviral Therapy (ART): a systematic review of high quality studies. AIDS patient care and STDs 29 (5), 248–266.

MHRA, 2020. Drug Safety Update. Volume 13 Issue 12. https://assets.publishing.service.gov.uk/government/uploads/system/uploads/attachment_data/file/905690/July-2020-DSU-PDF.pdf.

NICE. 2017. Candida – oral: Summary. https://cks.nice.org.uk/topics/candida-oral.

Paterson, D.L., Swindells, S., Mohr, J., et al., 2000. Adherence to protease inhibitor therapy and outcomes in patients with HIV infection. Ann. Intern. Med. 133 (1), 21–30. Erratum in: Ann. Intern. Med. 2002; 136(3):253.

Pau, A.K., George, J.M., 2014. Antiretroviral therapy: current drugs. Infect. Dis. Clin. North Am. 28 (3), 371–402.

Rai, M.A., Pannek, S., Fichtenbaum, C.J., 2018. Emerging reverse transcriptase inhibitors for HIV-1 infection. Expert Opin. Emerg. Drugs 23 (2), 149–157.

Rueda, S., Park-Wyllie, L.Y., Bayoumi, A., et al., 2006. Patient support and education for promoting adherence to highly active antiretroviral therapy for HIV/AIDS. Cochrane Database Syst. Rev. 3, CD001442.

Webster, D.P., Klenerman, P., Dusheiko, G.M., 2015. Hepatitis C. Lancet 385 (9973), 1124–1135.

WHO, 2020. HIV/AIDS. https://www.who.int/news-room/fact-sheets/detail/hiv-aids.

Zhong, J., Khanna, R., 2007. Vaccine strategies against human cytomegalovirus infection. Expert Rev. Anti Infect. Ther. 5, 449–459.

USEFUL WEBSITES

AVERT. Global information and education on HIV and AIDS. http://www.avert.org.

BHIVA. 2020. https://www.bhiva.org/pregnancy-guidelines.

NICE Oseltamivir, amantadine (review) and zanamivir for the prophylaxis of influenza [TA158] https://www.nice.org.uk/guidance/TA158.

NICE. Interferon alfa (pegylated and non-pegylated) and ribavirin for the treatment of chronic hepatitis C [TA75]. http://guidance.nice.org.uk/TA75.

Terrence Higgins Trust. 2020. https://www.tht.org.uk.

28 VACCINES

CHAPTER OUTLINE

LEARNING OBJECTIVES

At the end of this chapter, the reader should be able to:

- list the basic components of the immune system
- explain humoral and cell-mediated immunity
- explain active and passive immunization
- describe how these immunizations are achieved
- state the dangers and precautions associated with the administration of serum
- state what is meant by antiserum
- describe the immunization schedules used to protect against hepatitis A and B

THE IMMUNE REACTION

The human body is continually subjected to the risk of infection by microorganisms (bacteria, viruses, fungi) and to damage by toxins produced by these organisms. These organisms express proteins on their surface that are recognized by the immune system as 'foreign'; these are called **antigens**.

The cells that recognize and react to antigens are called **lymphocytes**. They are distributed throughout the body in blood, lymph and lymphoid tissues (spleen, lymph nodes, tonsils and adenoids). All lymphocytes originate in the bone marrow, but there are two main groups, the B and T cells, which mature differently and help to defend the body against foreign antigens in different ways (Fig. 28.1).

Humoral Immunity

B lymphocytes are a major component of humoral immunity as they are the only cell type in the body that can make antibodies. B lymphocytes, which mature in the spleen and lymph nodes after they leave the bone marrow, produce antibodies specific for particular antigens and the body can produce hundreds, possibly thousands, of types of B lymphocytes, each able to respond to a different specific antigen associated with a particular microorganism. When an antigen gains access to the tissues, the B lymphocytes become activated, dividing many times to form a clone of identical plasma cells. The plasma cells then make specific proteins that recognize specific antigens called **antibodies**; also known as 'immunoglobulins'. Antibodies circulate in the blood and react with antigens on microorganisms and this facilitates the destruction of the microorganism by other parts of our host defence system. Once the microorganisms have been removed, the antigen levels in the body drop and most of the plasma cells making antibodies specific for this antigen disappear, but a few persist as so-called 'memory cells'. If a second exposure occurs, the memory cells multiply rapidly and release antibodies even more swiftly than during the first exposure. This establishment of 'memory' by the B lymphocytes forms the basis of active immunization against infectious organisms and the harmful toxins they produce (see later).

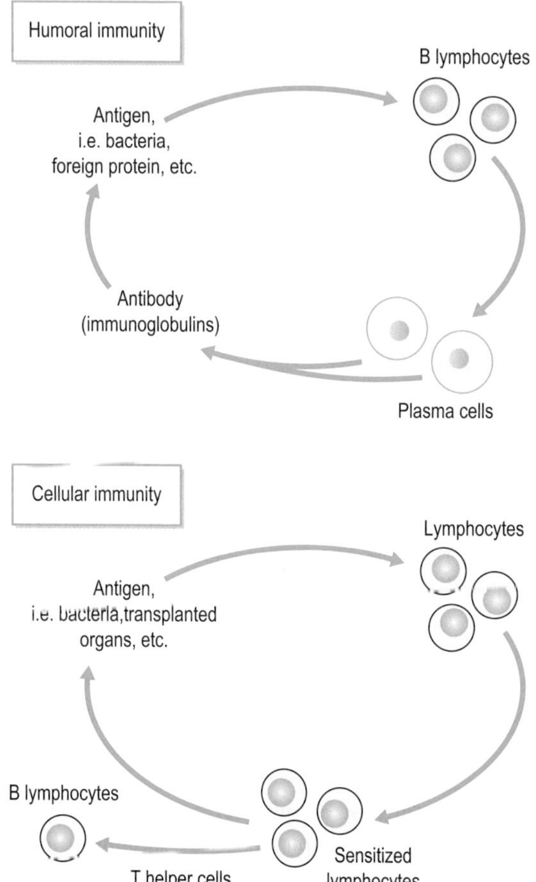

Fig. 28.1 ■ The sequence of events in the production of humoral and cellular immunity.

Cell-mediated Immunity

T lymphocytes play a major role in cell-mediated immunity and are sometimes referred to as being akin to 'Conductors of an orchestra' such is their importance to host defence. T lymphocytes mature in the thymus gland before they enter the circulation. They do not produce antibodies, but are an essential component of the immune response, as some T lymphocytes (T helper cells) appear to play an important part by 'switching on' the immune response when antigens invade, while others 'switch off' the immune response when the body no longer requires it. However, cell-mediated immunity is not just an important component of host defence against invading organisms, but can be inappropriately activated to contribute to pathological situations such as rejection of foreign materials, e.g. transplanted organs and medical devices, in autoimmune conditions such as myasthenia gravis, and in chronic infections such as tuberculosis. People whose cell mediated immunity is impaired by HIV infection, which destroys the T helper cells, become very prone to opportunistic bacterial, viral, fungal and protozoan infections that the T lymphocytes would normally keep in check (so-called 'acquired immunosuppression syndrome' or AIDS).

ACTIVE IMMUNIZATION

The principle of this method is to promote the immune system to produce specific antibodies towards antigens expressed on pathological organisms before a person has been infected. If the patient then becomes infected, the antibodies are quickly produced and are capable of rapidly dealing with the infecting organism or its toxin thus preventing or minimizing the disease.

Antibodies are usually produced by injecting the patient with killed or modified organisms, which, although harmless, still express certain antigens and are therefore still capable of eliciting antibodies. These preparations are known as a vaccine. A good example of this method is the widespread immunization against poliomyelitis by the oral polio vaccine, Sabin vaccine, which is a live virus that has been attenuated (rendered harmless).

Similarly, bacterial toxins may be modified to produce toxoids which are no longer harmful but which are capable of acting as antigens. They are then injected and protect against future damage from the particular toxin. Good examples of toxoids are the various diphtheria toxoids that produce immunity to the very dangerous toxin produced by the diphtheria organism (*Corynebacterium diphtheriae*).

Following injection of the antigen, whether vaccine or toxoid, there is usually an interval of a few days before antibodies appear. These antibodies may then persist for varying periods, from a few months up to many years. It is often the practice to give two or more booster injections of the antigen to produce a higher level of immunity.

Active immunization is used in the prevention of the following diseases:

measles	pertussis
rabies	polio
pneumococcal infections	rotavirus
anthrax	whooping cough
meningococcal disease	tetanus
influenza	typhoid (not often)
	typhus
mumps	tuberculosis
rubella	cholera
diphtheria	yellow fever
haemophilus influenza type b (Hib)	hepatitis A and B
human papillomavirus (certain serotypes)	varicella

Active immunization may take several weeks before enough antibodies are produced to be effective. This is satisfactory as a prophylactic measure, but this approach is not effective as a way to treat established disease. Under these conditions, passive immunization is used.

PASSIVE IMMUNIZATION

In this method of immunization, the appropriate antibody against the invading organism or toxin is injected. In the past, this antibody was produced on a large scale in animals, by injecting an antigen, either vaccine or toxoid, until a high blood level of antibody was obtained. Some of the blood was then removed and the antibody extracted and stored until required. Following the injection of antibody, immunity will last about 2 weeks. This method suffers from the disadvantage that it is not possible to purify the antibodies produced completely and there is therefore a risk of a hypersensitivity reaction to the injected antibody proteins by the body recognizing these foreign proteins and producing antibodies against the injected antibody. Nowadays, advances in genetic engineering and cloning procedures mean that antibodies can often be manufactured on a large scale industrially *in vitro*.

Certain types of antibody can be obtained from human blood, either after the subject has been actively immunized or has suffered a particular infection. These antibodies, usually called 'human immunoglobulins', are safer and rarely produce a serious reaction, although there may be discomfort at the injection site.

Common examples of animal- and human-derived antibodies are, respectively, diphtheria antitoxin, which was obtained from horse serum, and anti-tetanus immunoglobulin obtained from human blood.

ADMINISTRATION OF SERUM

Antitoxin raised in animals, often called 'antiserum', carries a real risk of a hypersensitivity reaction. This is particularly liable to occur in patients who have had previous serum injections or who suffer from allergic disorders (e.g. asthma). The reaction occurs because the antibody in the serum reacts with antigens already present in the patient, releasing histamine and other substances. Serum reactions take two forms:

- **Immediate or anaphylactic reaction:** within a few minutes of injection, the patient collapses with difficulty in breathing, low blood pressure and, sometimes, widespread urticaria. Rarely it can be fatal.

- **Serum sickness** occurs about a week after injection of serum. This is a delayed reaction. The patient is pyrexial with a rash and arthritis. It usually clears up in a few days.

CLINICAL NOTE

Sera and vaccines should be kept in a refrigerator at the correct temperature. Guidelines are given in *Immunisation against infectious disease* (DH, 2014). Temperature of these refrigerator's should be monitored daily and a temperature recorded so that the chain of cold storage is able to be assessed.

Precautions when Injecting Serum

Ask the patient:

- Have you had serum before?
- Have you had asthma or eczema?
- Do you suffer from allergies?

If all answers are negative, give a test dose of serum subcutaneously; if there is no reaction in 30 min, the rest may be given and the patient kept under observation for a further 1 h.

These precautions may well be unnecessary if human immunoglobin is used, but are mandatory for diphtheria antitoxin, which is raised in animals.

CLINICAL NOTE

Whenever serum is injected by any route, a syringe containing 1:1000 of adrenaline (epinephrine), an H1 receptor antagonist (antihistamine) and hydrocortisone should be ready at hand in case of immediate anaphylactic reaction.

ANTISERA

Diphtheria antitoxin is an antiserum raised in animals and there is a real risk of a hypersensitivity reaction. Due to this, diphtheria antitoxin is no longer used for prophylaxis.

- Therapeutic dose – not less than 10,000 units of antitoxin intramuscularly or intravenously.

Tetanus antitoxin is an immunoglobin prepared from human sources, with little or no risk of a hypersensitivity reaction. Following injury, immunized patients require a booster dose of vaccine to stimulate immunity. Penetrating and contaminated wounds may need, in addition, tetanus immunoglobin plus antibiotic cover. Non-immunized patients require 250 units of tetanus immunoglobin (post-exposure prophylaxis) and a course of tetanus vaccine should be started. These should not be given in the same syringe or into the same site. This should be combined with antibiotic cover.

VACCINES

Examples of vaccines:

- Adsorbed diphtheria vaccine
- Adsorbed tetanus vaccine
- Haemophilus influenzae type b (Hib)
- Diphtheria, tetanus and pertussis (DTP) vaccine
- Typhoid vaccine
- Bacille Calmette–Guérin (BCG) vaccine
- Poliomyelitis vaccine
- Rubella vaccine
- Measles, mumps and rubella (MMR) vaccine
- Meningococcal A and C vaccine
- Pneumococcal vaccine
- Influenza vaccine.

Adsorbed diphtheria vaccine for adults and adolescents is prepared by adsorbing toxoid onto aluminium phosphate. In addition to single vaccines, combined vaccines stimulating immunity to diphtheria, whooping cough and tetanus are available, and are routinely used for immunizing infants.

Hib is a vaccine against *H. influenzae* type b. Immunization is not required after the age of 4 years as infection is much less likely. Protocols for the immunization of children are shown in Table 28.1. *H. influenzae* was the most common cause of meningitis in the under 4s prior to the vaccination.

People at risk from **tetanus** should receive a booster dose of toxoid every 5 years. For **typhoid**, both oral and injected vaccines are available for those visiting a high-risk area. They are effective for about 3 years.

TABLE 28.1

Immunization of Children (UK Schedule 2020, Public Health England)

Age	Vaccine	Disease Protection
8 weeks old	DTaP/IPV/Hib/HepB	Diptheria, tetanus, pertussis, polio, *Haemophilus influenza* type b and hepatitis B
	MenB	Meningococcal group B
	Rotavirus	Rotavirus gastroenteritis
12 weeks old	DTaP/IPV/Hib/HepB	Diptheria, tetanus, pertussis, polio, *Haemophilus influenza* type b and hepatitis B
	PCV	Pneumococcal
	Rotavirus	Rotavirus gastroenteritis
16 weeks old	DTaP/IPV/Hib/HepB	Diptheria, tetanus, pertussis, polio, *Haemophilus influenza* type b and hepatitis B
	MenB	Meningococcal group B
1 year old	Hib and MenC	*Haemophilus influenza* type b and Meningococcal group C
	PCV booster	Pneumococcal
	MMR	Measles, mumps and rubella
	MenB	Meningococcal group B
3 years, 4 months	dTaP/IPV	Diptheria, tetanus, pertussis and polio
	MMR	Measles, mumps and rubella
12–13 years	HPV (2 doses 6–24 months apart)	Genital warts by types 6 and 11 and cancer caused by types 16 and 18
14 years old	Td/IPV	Tetanus, diptheria and polio
	MenACWY	Meningococcal groups A, C, W and Y
Eligible children	Live attenuated influenza	Influenza (annually from September)

At birth, the BCG vaccine should be administered if the baby is thought to be at increased risk of tuberculosis.

The controversy regarding the use of **pertussis (whooping cough) vaccine** has waxed and waned during the last 30 or so years over the issue that pertussis was suspected of causing brain damage. In the 1970s, many parents in the UK (over 50%) opted to omit the pertussis component of the diphtheria, tetanus and pertussis (DTP) vaccine and, consequently, several thousand children were admitted to hospital and over 100 died of whooping cough. In countries such as Sweden and Hungary, which actively adopted a strategy to drop the pertussis vaccine, childhood deaths from pertussis rose 10–100 fold. Most countries have now dropped anti-pertussis campaigns (Gangarosa et al., 1998).

Nevertheless, controversy continues and, unfortunately, children's issues are very emotive, and fears can be raised that may result in unwise measures. The fears over the MMR vaccine provide another example of the difficulty that is caused by extreme responses to sometimes ill-advised publication of emotive research reports, particularly those which do not have sufficient hard data to support their theses.

CLINICAL NOTE

- Children who develop a fever after receiving the MMR vaccine can be given paracetamol, which can be repeated once, if necessary, after 4–6 h.
- In the past, there have been fears that brain damage might, rarely, follow the use of pertussis vaccine and, although the frequency was difficult to assess, a figure of less than 1:80,000 was given. More recently, even this risk is considered unlikely. The dangers attached to having whooping cough, especially in infancy, are considerably greater.

BCG vaccine is a suspension of living bacilli that will produce tuberculosis antibodies.

Poliomyelitis vaccine may be either inactivated poliomyelitis viruses type 1, 2 and 3 (Salk vaccine) or attenuated live virus (Sabin vaccine); the latter is to be preferred as it avoids injections, provides a more prolonged immunity, and by producing antibodies in the intestine, it prevents the spread of infection.

Rubella vaccine should be offered to seronegative women of childbearing age. It is important to exclude pregnancy when giving the vaccine and to avoid it for 1 month thereafter.

CLINICAL NOTE

All nurses should be immunized to ensure that they are immune to rubella.

The combined **measles, mumps and rubella (MMR) vaccine** can be given as a single dose by intramuscular or deep subcutaneous injection to children aged 12–15 months, followed by a booster dose before starting school (i.e. age 3.5 years). This vaccine occasionally produces malaise, fever, a rash and parotid swelling about 1 week after injection. Meningitis due to the mumps component occurs in about 1 in 1,000,000 doses. There is no convincing evidence that MMR vaccine is a cause of autism or bowel disease (Editorial, 2002a).

Meningococcal vaccines (meningococcal group B; meningococcal group C and meningococcal conjugate MenACWY) can help prevent meningococcal disease. In the UK, *Neisseria meningitidis* serogroups B and C are the most common culprit causing meningococcal disease in childhood. See Table 28.1, which illustrates when these vaccines are provided in childhood. The risk of meningococcal disease declines with age and therefore are not usually given to people aged 25 years or older.

Pneumococcal vaccine is given to people who are at special risk from pneumococcal infection, including those with chronic lung and heart disease, diabetes, patients who have had a splenectomy, and those who are immunosuppressed or have sickle cell disease.

Influenza vaccine protects against the 'flu' viruses, although these are continually changing. The World Health Organization (WHO) recommends which strains of virus should be included in the vaccine for a particular year. The vaccine only protects about 70% of subjects for about 1 year and its use was confined to those at special risk, e.g. the elderly, those with heart, lung or renal disease and patients with diabetes. The NHS influenza vaccination programme for children was announced in 2013, whereby the vaccine can be administered intranasally to children. The first dose being given at age 2–3 years old. The intranasal route is thought to be more effective than the injected route but the latter may be used if the patient is immunosuppressed.

When families have immigrated, it is helpful to undertake an immunization history. Those travelled from areas of conflict or hard to reach population groups may not have been fully immunized. In such cases where the history of immunization is not reliable, it should be assumed that they are unimmunized and the full UK immunization schedule should be followed.

CLINICAL NOTE

Vaccination against infectious disease has made one of the most significant contributions to preventing disease globally. However, in industrial countries, parents and those who advise them no longer witness the debilitating and sometimes fatal infections that vaccines protect against. As a result, parents can develop concerns about vaccination that over-ride fears of infection or become apathetic about the risks posed by such infections. Providing information about the importance of vaccination is an important nursing responsibility.

CLINICAL NOTE

Oseltamivir (*Tamiflu*) medication has been found to reduce the incidence of flu significantly in some patients in nursing homes, and to reduce its duration, if the patient does get flu. However, it is not recommended as a replacement for vaccines (Editorial, 2002b), but has been used to protect contacts and for those affected during outbreak situations. A number of other drugs are under development for the prophylaxis of viral infections such as influenza.

CONTRAINDICATIONS TO IMMUNIZATION

1. Acute illness.
2. Live vaccines should not be given to those who have reduced immunity owing to:
   a. treatment with high doses of steroids or cytotoxic drugs
   b. the presence of active lymphomas, including Hodgkin's disease
   c. other causes of immunosuppression.
3. Pregnancy. Rarely, the risk of infection outweighs this precaution.
4. HIV-positive subjects should NOT receive oral typhoid vaccination, but may receive yellow fever vaccination and MAY in some cases be given BCG vaccination, but only after expert review; response to vaccination may be reduced.

Immunization programmes are constantly reviewed and altered from time to time. In case of doubt, nurses are referred to *Immunisation against infectious disease* (DH, 2014) or to the current edition of the *British National Formulary* (BNF).

Immunization Against Viral Hepatitis

Hepatitis A virus is spread by poor hygiene, and infection is usually due to contaminated food and water. A vaccine is now available and is given as a single injection with a booster dose after 6 months. It appears to be very effective in preventing hepatitis A, but the duration of protection is not yet known. There may be local soreness at the site of injection. Alternatively, normal human immunoglobulin, given by intramuscular injection, confers passive immunity for up to 2 months.

Hepatitis B viral infection is of particular importance to the health professional as it can be spread by infected body fluids (blood and saliva) and precautions should be enforced when nursing all patients, as it is impossible to predict who are carriers from the patient's history alone.

A vaccine prepared from the surface antigen of the virus is available (H-B-Vax). Three injections are given into the deltoid muscle; the first and second are given 1 month apart, and the third after 6 months. Immunity persists for at least 2 years. Passive immunization is also possible using a special serum containing large amounts of antibody against the hepatitis B virus.

CLINICAL NOTE

Nurses who work in primary care and private practice may be required to give advice regarding immunization to those travelling abroad, and must keep abreast of the latest information, which is available via the Public Health England website.

Anaphylaxis is very rare with active immunization, but treatment should be immediately available (see earlier).

COVID-19

Covid-19 first emerged as a severe respiratory infection in Wuhan, China in December 2019 (WHO 2020). Over time different variants of the virus have emerged. Covid-19 has high transmissibility and therefore strict measures to avoid spread included social distancing, mask wearing, handwashing, early quarantine and contact tracing.

Patients maybe asymptomatic or can report symptoms including cough, fever, loss of smell or altered taste. However, symptoms can also be more varied and non-specific such as myalgia, headache and runny nose. Children often exhibit mild disease and gastrointestinal symptoms are also common (Waterfield et al, 2020).

Vaccines for Covid-19 were developed with accelerated pace and trying to ensure maintenance of thorough testing and safety standards. In various countries mass vaccination campaigns to vaccinate the population are underway. Over 300 different Covid-19 vaccines are in various stages of development and in the UK at the time of writing there are three Covid-19 vaccines currently in use for the vaccination programme. These include Covid-19 mRNA vaccine BNT162b2 (manufactured by Pifzer); AstraZeneca and Moderna (Public Health England, 2021). Currently, each of these authorised vaccines require two doses for completion, current recommendations being with the same vaccine and can have efficacy as high as 95% following two doses. Currently there are plans on introducing the booster programme in the UK from September 2021.

Avian Flu

Avian flu is a viral disease that kills birds through a potent respiratory infection. There are several strains of the virus. One in particular, H5N1, a subtype of the influenza A virus, is passed from bird to bird (and presumably to humans) via the bird's faeces, saliva and nasal secretions, and has proved fatal in some human patients. In 2004, a pandemic was feared and strenuous efforts initiated to produce a vaccine. Fortunately, H5N1 is rarely, if ever, transmitted by air-borne infection, but through direct contact, e.g. eating infected birds. In 2006, the first human-to-human transmission was thought to have occurred when several members of a family in Sumatra became infected after contact with a family member who had worked with infected poultry.

A number of H5N1 vaccines have been approved, e.g., one produced by Sanofi Pasteur Inc. which has been approved by the National Institutes of Health (NIH) in the USA. In the UK, Glaxo-Smith-Kline has produced what appears to be a potent H5N1 vaccine, and the Chinese, in 2006, reported the development of a potent H5N1 vaccine.

Immunization Against the Human Papilloma Virus

The relationship between the human papilloma virus (HPV) and squamous cell carcinoma is well established. Cervical cancer is the fourth most common cause of cancer worldwide. Transmission is by direct contact and there is evidence that condoms do not offer complete protection. Vaccination is therefore an important public health measure. Two vaccines are licensed: Gardasil and Cervarix. Both are well tolerated. The only reported side-effects are mild local reactions at the injection site. Gardasil vaccine has been used since 2012 for the NHS immunization programme, as it protects against more types of HPV (6, 11, 16 and 18). HPV types 6 and 11 cause 90% of genital warts, thus the vaccine can help to reduce disease burden from this in addition to cancer risks. The target cohort were initially girls aged 12–13 years but since September 2019, both girls and boys are offered the HPV vaccine. Uptake of HPV vaccination is almost 90% in the UK (gov.uk).

Immunization Against Herpes Zoster (Shingles)

A live attenuated vaccine (Zostavax) has been offered to people aged 70–79 in the UK since 2013. A 'catch up' programme is also being offered. Individuals who are eligible can obtain the vaccine from their GP or pharmacist. There are similar arrangements in other countries. The vaccine does not eliminate the risks of developing herpes zoster completely but the pain associated with herpes zoster is reduced. Only a single dose is necessary: there is no need for boosters. Apart from minor discomfort at the injection site, no significant side-effects have been reported

DRUGS THAT BLOCK THE IMMUNE REACTION

The immune response can be blocked in two ways:

- **by interfering with the effects of immunity with drugs**
- **by suppressing cells involved in cellular or humoral immunity (immunosuppression).**

These effects, particularly suppression of the cells involved in cellular and humoral immunity, are extremely important when considering the treatment of autoimmune diseases, e.g. rheumatoid arthritis, which is covered in Chapter 13, and cancer, which is covered in Chapter 29.

SUMMARY

- Active immunization can protect the patient for years.
- Active immunization will not be used to treat an established disease, whereas passive immunization is sometimes used for this purpose.
- Passive immunization does not last long (usually, perhaps weeks or a few months at most).
- Antitoxins (antiserum) raised in animals carry the risk of a hypersensitivity reaction.
- Patients must be questioned about previous hypersensitivity reactions and about any allergies before administering them serum.

- Even if answers are negative, inject a small test dose first, and if there is no reaction by 30 min, the remainder may be given, and the patient should be kept under observation for another 1 h.
- When injecting serum into a patient by any route, always have ready a syringe with 1:1000 adrenaline (epinephrine), an H1 receptor antagonist (antihistamine) and hydrocortisone for emergency use.
- Keep antisera refrigerated at the correct temperature.
- Children may be given paracetamol if they develop fever after receiving the MMR vaccine.
- Although there has been controversy, there is no convincing evidence that the MMR vaccine causes autism in children (Editorial, 2002a).
- All nurses should ensure that they are immunized against rubella, especially if they are working in an obstetric role.
- Rubella vaccine should be offered to seronegative women of childbearing age, but to exclude pregnancy first, and to avoid pregnancy for at least 1 month after receiving the vaccine.
- Nurses should be familiar with the adverse effects of vaccines.
- For the nurse's own protection, precautions must be taken when nursing all patients since it is not possible to ascertain from the patient's history alone which patients may be carriers of hepatitis B.
- Adrenaline (epinephrine) is very effective in acute anaphylaxis.

REFERENCES AND FURTHER READING

Bedford, H., 2015. Updates to the UK adolescent vaccine schedule. NursePrescribing 13, 120–125.

Cadman, L., 2014. Human papilloma virus vaccine and public health. NursePrescribing 12, 180–183.

Chiodini, J., 2014. Safe storage and handling of vaccines. Nurs. Stand. 28, 45–52.

Clutterbuck, E., 2015. The biology of vaccine responses. NursePrescribing 13, 384–389.

DH, 2014. Immunisation against Infectious Disease. Department of Health, uk. https://www.gov.uk/government/collections/immunisation-against-infectious-disease-the-green-book.

Duncan, D., Boulton, J., 2012. Rabies: vaccination, symptoms and diagnosis. NursePrescribing 10, 179–183.

Duncan, D., 2015. Preventing and treating influenza in primary care. NursePrescribing 13, 556–561.

Editorial, 2002a. No correlation between MMR vaccination and autism. Pharmaceut. J. 266, 209.

Editorial, 2002b. Use Tamiflu for prevention not treatment of flu, says DTB. Pharmaceut. J. 270, 6.

Gambotto, A., Barratt-Boyes, S.M., de Jong, M.D., et al., 2008. Human infection with highly pathogenic H5N1 influenza virus. Lancet 371 (9622), 1464–1475.

Gangarosa, E.J., Galazka, A.M., Wolfe, C.R., et al., 1998. Impact of anti-vaccine movements on pertussis control: the untold story. Lancet 351 (9099), 356–361.

Gawthrop, M., 2014. Prescribing malaria chemoprophylaxis. NursePrescribing 12, 437–441.

Gould, D., 2014. Varicella zoster virus: chickenpox and shingles. Nurs. Stand. 28 (33), 52–58.

Heneghan, C.J., Onakpoya, I., Jones, M.A., et al., 2016. Neuraminidase inhibitors for influenza: a systematic review and meta-analysis of regulatory and mortality data. Health Technol. Assess. 20 (42), 1–242.

Ogden, J., 2016. Offering advice on immunization to UK patients traveling abroad. Prescriber 27, 16–22.

Peiris, J.S., de Jong, M.D., Guan, Y., 2007. Avian influenza virus (H5N1): a threat to human health. Clin. Microbiol. Rev. 20, 243–267.

Public Health England, 2021. COVID-19 Vaccination Programme Information for Healthcare Practitioners. Version 3.9 republished 6th July 2021. https://assets.publishing.service.gov.uk/government/uploads/system/uploads/attachment_data/file/999527/COVID-19_vaccination_programme_guidance_for_healthcare_workers_6July2021_v3.9.pdf.

Thakker, Y., Woods, S., 1992. Storage of vaccines in the community. BMJ 304, 756–758.

Umeed, M., 2016. Prescribing vaccines in travel health consultation. NursePrescribing 12, 484–491.

Waterfield, T., Watson, C., Moore, R., et al., 2021. Seroprevalence of SARS-CoV2 antibodies in children: a prospective multicentre cohort study. Arch Dis Child. 106 (7), 680–686.

WHO, 2020. Novel Coronavirus (2019-nCoV) Situation Report -1. https://www.who.int/docs/default-source/coronaviruse/situation-reports/20200121-sitrep-1-2019-ncov.pdf.

29 DRUGS USED IN THE TREATMENT OF MALIGNANT DISEASES

CHAPTER OUTLINE

LEARNING OBJECTIVES

At the end of this chapter, the reader should be able to:

- summarize the natural history of cancers and how drugs treatment may affect this
- describe the main stages of the cell cycle
- explain how the main types of drugs for cancer are classified
- give some examples of each class and which cancers they are used for
- give an account of the important adverse effects of anticancer drugs, e.g. myelosuppression
- describe the advantages of combination chemotherapy
- define the terms palliative and adjuvant therapy
- appreciate the problems of administering drugs, e.g. extravasation and dangers to staff
- give an account of the nurse's involvement in cancer chemotherapy, and patient counselling and care

INTRODUCTION

The Mechanisms and Natural History of Cancer

In most parts of the world, infectious diseases have been controlled and much cardiovascular disease prevented and treated. People are living longer, and cancers are very much diseases of older age (although not entirely restricted to older people). Cancers are an important cause of morbidity and mortality and finding treatments for them have become increasing priorities.

The development of more effective treatments for cancers has been facilitated by the tremendous growth in understanding of cellular function at the level of biochemical pathways, and a parallel growth in understanding the genetic basis of changes in cellular function that may lead to cancer. This knowledge has driven an explosion in new treatments, generally referred to as 'targeted', which aim to target abnormal biochemical pathways in specific types of cancers. The hope, which has been realized to some extent, is that these treatments may be both more effective and more tolerable than older treatments.

While '*a cure for cancer*' used to be hoped for, the reality is that cancers have a multitude of causes and require a multitude of treatments. In recent years, cancer survival rates have greatly increased in high-income countries, and it is reasonable to hope to cure many types of cancer. However, some cancers still remain difficult to treat and the search for better treatments continues.

Underlying all cancers are failures in the normal cellular machinery that controls the growth of cells, when and how often they divide, and how they then differentiate into different body tissues. These failures are nearly always due to an accumulation of mutations in the cells' DNA, which affect the function of particular proteins involved in this cellular machinery. The mutations occur for many reasons, including contact with *carcinogenic* substances and radiation. An accumulation of mutations is usually required for a cell to become cancerous, which is why cancers tend to occur in older people. Frequently dividing cells and metabolically active cells are also more prone to errors in transcription or replication of DNA that leads to mutations, which is why metabolically active tissues such as glands (breast, thyroid, prostate) have a higher risk of cancer than less active tissues such as fat. It has been recognized that some genes in the cells' DNA are particularly associated with cancer development if they sustain particular mutations that affect the protein for which they code. These are known as *oncogenes* and many have been identified. Identifying a particular oncogene mutation in a cancer may help guide treatment with a targeted therapy. An example of this is treatment with **trastuzumab**, which targets a protein called 'HER2', which is present in too high a quantity (*overexpressed*) in some types of breast cancer, due to a mutation in the gene that codes for HER2. Trastuzumab is effective in these cancers, but not in breast cancers where the mutation is not present. A biopsy of the cancer is needed to find out if it is HER2 positive.

When a cell becomes cancerous it is often referred to as *malignant*. Malignant cells do not differentiate in an orderly fashion and take their place in the formation of a tissue, but instead, multiply in a haphazard way leading to the formation of a tumour, which may then metastasize. Metastasis is when tumour cells leave the primary organ and invade distant structures in the body. Metastatic tumour cells can travel in the blood or lymphatic circulation to be carried to distant parts of the body, take root and set up further tumours, known as 'secondary deposits' or 'metastases'. Tumours kill by damaging normal body anatomy and so disrupting essential bodily functions. A tumour is sometimes referred to as a *neoplasm* and the cells that make it up are known as *neoplastic*, although strictly speaking, not all neoplasms are malignant.

The disordered cell division and altered function of cellular machinery in cancers offers the possibility of various approaches to their treatment with drugs. Before discussing treatment with cytotoxic drugs, it is important to understand the phases of the life cycle of cells.

The Cell Cycle

The cells of the body vary enormously in appearance and function, but all share some common characteristics. With very few exceptions (such as erythrocytes), cells consist of a nucleus surrounded by cytoplasm. The most vital component of the nucleus is DNA, which consists of two chains of molecules arranged into a double helix. DNA contains the code which,

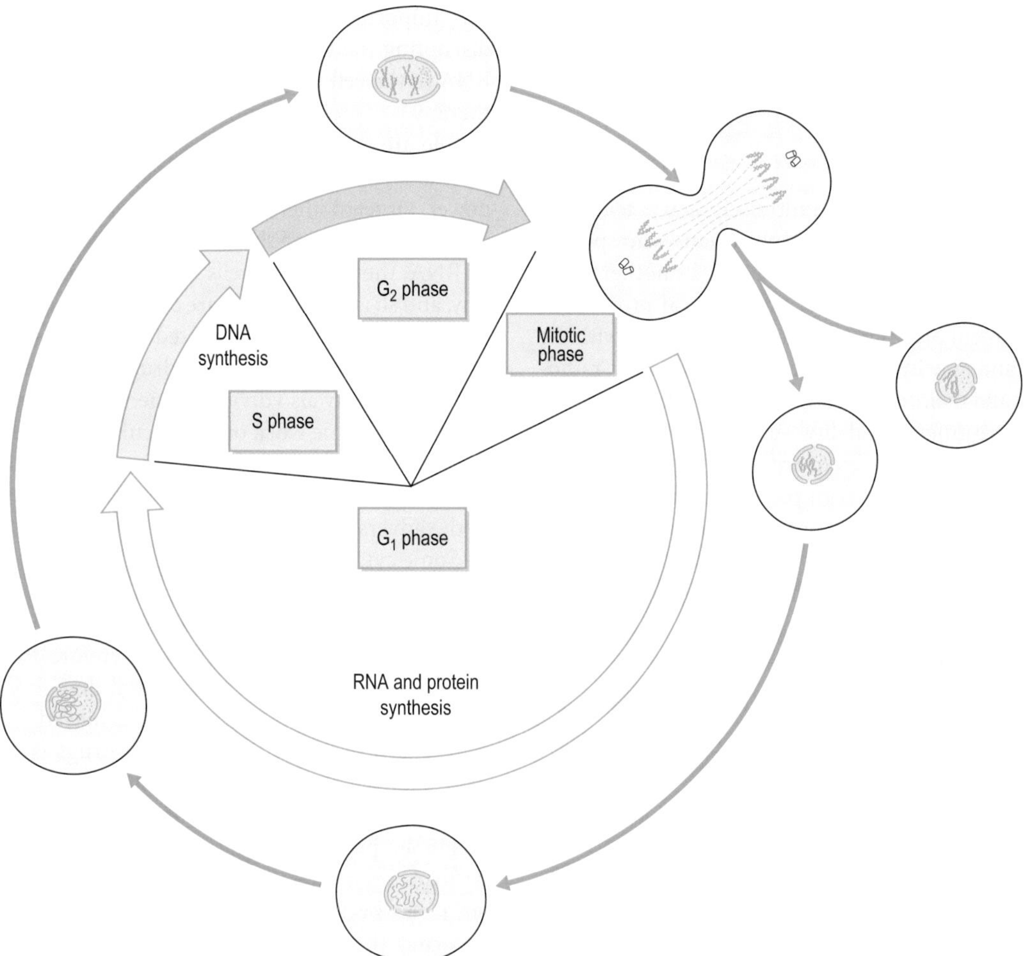

Fig. 29.1 ■ Phases of the cell cycle.

through production of messenger RNA, determines the types of proteins that are made by the cell and thus ultimately how the cell functions.

The cell goes through the following phases:

- **G_1 phase**
- **S phase**
- **G_2 phase**
- **mitotic phase.**

During its life, the cell passes through a series of changes. The newly formed cell enters the **G_1 phase**, which is a period of protein synthesis and intense metabolic activity. This may last for a variable time, from a few hours to many years. Many cells remain in this phase throughout the life of the organism, but some undergo division and enter the **S phase**. This phase is short and is concerned with DNA and RNA synthesis, so that the DNA strands may split when cell division occurs. It is also a period of great metabolic activity. The **G_2 phase** that follows is a short period of consolidation before cell division occurs. In the **mitotic phase**, the DNA spiral splits longitudinally so that each daughter cell has its full complement of DNA, which is exactly the same as that in the parent cell (Fig. 29.1). This splitting involves the production of particular cellular structures called 'microtubules', which are targeted by some cytotoxic drugs. A proportion of the cells in normal tissues and in cancers are in a resting phase, sometimes called the **G_0 phase**, when they are not dividing. This is important because at this stage, they are very resistant to chemotherapy with cytotoxic drugs.

APPROACHES TO CANCER TREATMENT

Cancers are treated by multidisciplinary teams of nurses, surgeons, oncologists (physicians who specialize in cancer treatment), pharmacists, radiotherapists, medical physicists and other paramedical professionals. Treatment plans are agreed in conjunction with the patient and may involve surgery, chemotherapy, radiotherapy and maintenance adjuvant therapy. Sometimes a single treatment modality, such as surgery, may be curative, but often different treatment modalities will be combined in a treatment package individualized to the patient. When cure cannot be achieved, then palliative treatments may involve any of the treatment modalities and may extend life or improve quality of life.

DRUG TREATMENTS FOR CANCER

The major classes of drugs used to treat cancers are:

- cytotoxic drugs
- targeted therapy
- immunotherapy
- hormone antagonists, sex hormones and corticosteroids.

Each of these classes has numerous subclasses, and there is some overlap between classes in this classification. It is nonetheless a useful way of thinking about cancer drugs. The major classes of drug are now discussed, with examples of some of the most important drugs in the class. There are so many drugs available now that it is impossible to describe all of them in this text and reference to more detailed material will be required if a practitioner is specializing in the field of oncology (cancer treatment).

Cytotoxic Drugs

While all treatment of cancers with drugs can strictly be referred to as *chemotherapy*, this word is most commonly reserved for drug treatment with cytotoxic drugs (*cyto = cell*; *toxic = poison*). These were the earliest types of drug treatment for cancer and remain very important. They all work by directly or indirectly disrupting the transcription or replication of DNA or RNA in the cell nucleus. In the popular mind, chemotherapy is associated with severe side-effects and many people are very afraid of treatment with these drugs. Not all cytotoxic drugs have severe side-effects (the newer targeted therapies can also have severe side-effects), but because they disrupt the copying of DNA or RNA, they affect all cells in the body in a profound way, and so adverse effects are common. Rapidly dividing cells are particularly affected, which is why cancer cells are very sensitive to these drugs, but some normal cells in the body also divide frequently to replace those that have become worn out, particularly the cells of the bone marrow, the lymphatic system and the lining of the intestinal tract, and these are particularly sensitive to the adverse effects of cytotoxic drugs.

Some cytotoxic drugs will affect cells at any phase in their life cycle; others will only act at a single phase of the cell cycle, usually when the cell is dividing, and are called **phase-specific**. It follows therefore that when using phase-specific drugs, repeated dosage is necessary if the maximum effect is to be achieved.

The aim of treating cancer with drugs is to find a drug that will kill the cancer cells while leaving the normal cells of the body unharmed. However, the metabolic processes of neoplastic cells are very similar to, or even the same as, that of normal cells and so far, it has been impossible to reach this ideal. Nearly all drugs that have so far been discovered, although having a marked toxic effect on neoplastic cells, have some adverse effect on the normal cells of the body, and this is particularly true of cytotoxic drugs. The best that can be done is to give the cytotoxic drug, or drugs, at repeated intervals so arranged that the recovery of normal cells can occur, but with as little recovery of cancer cells possible. It may then be possible progressively to reduce the number of malignant cells without unduly reducing the normal cells, until ultimately all the malignant cells are eradicated (Fig. 29.2). Recently, combination therapies of cytotoxic drugs and targeted drugs have been introduced, which may speed up this process and reduce adverse effects. However, it is also important to realize that the growth rate of cancers vary considerably, and the development of clinical symptoms and signs can occur at a late stage in the disease process (Fig. 29.3). Note particularly the long subclinical period and the fact that after chemotherapy, although the patient is apparently in full clinical remission, a small amount of tumour may remain.

As a result of these considerations, certain general principles and features of treatment have emerged:

- Cytotoxic drugs are usually given in intermittent high-dose treatments over long periods.
- The smaller the mass of tumour treated, the better the result, because small tumours have fewer resting cells that are insensitive to chemotherapy. Therefore, debulking the tumour by surgery or radiotherapy is often undertaken.
- Suppression of the bone marrow is very common, as cytotoxic drugs have to be given at the maximum tolerated dose.

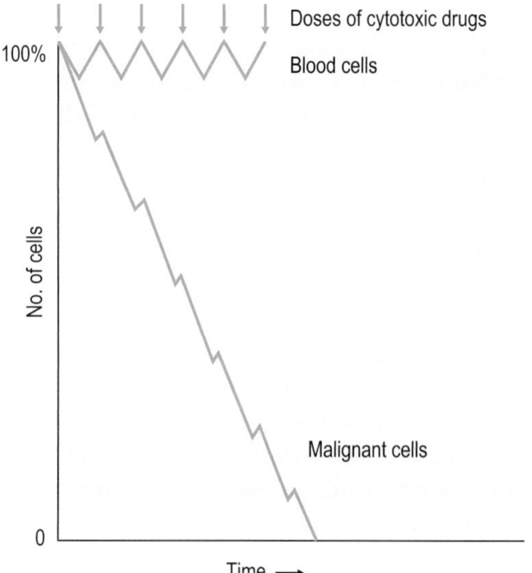

Fig. 29.2 ■ Progressive reduction in the number of malignant cells produced by repeated doses of a cytotoxic drug, with recovery of the normal blood cells. An ideal therapeutic response.

The cytotoxic drugs are divided into several important groups. There are too many individual drugs to discuss them all here, but key examples of each group are mentioned. The groups are:

- alkylating agents
- antimetabolites (antifolates and others)
- nucleoside analogues
- topoisomerase I inhibitors
- topoisomerase II inhibitors
- anthracyclines
- taxanes
- vinca alkaloids
- platinum compounds
- others.

Alkylating Agents

These are chemically very active substances that add alkyl groups to the DNA in the cell nucleus (*alkylate*), and thus damage or kill the cell. Unfortunately, although these substances have a marked effect on

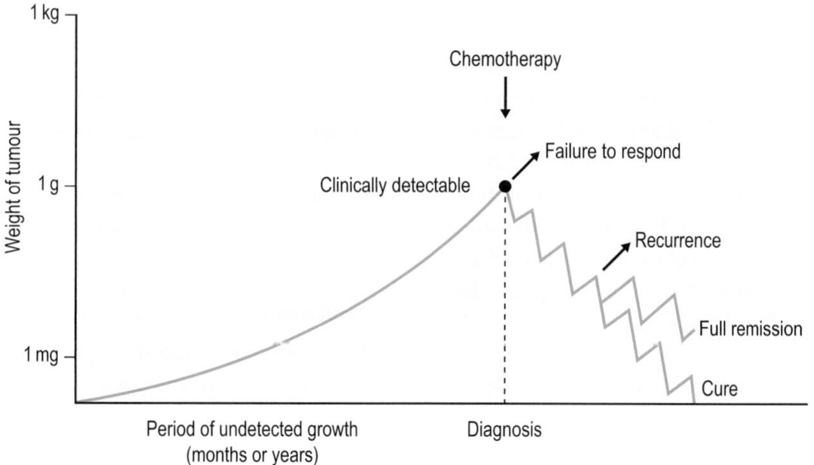

Fig. 29.3 ■ Tumour growth and possible responses to chemotherapy. (Modified from Ritter, J.M., et al., 2000. A Textbook of Clinical Pharmacology, third ed. Edward Arnold, London.)

certain types of malignant cells, they also damage normal cells, particularly those of the bone marrow (*myelosuppression*) and gastrointestinal tract. There are many alkylating agents and they are used to treat many different cancers, but particularly chronic leukaemias and some types of lymphoma and certain malignant brain tumours. They are not phase-specific. They have many adverse effects, of which myelosuppression is common, and pulmonary fibrosis is uncommon, but serious. There are some important sub-groups within the alkylating agents. Examples include:

- cyclophosphamide
- ifosfamide
- chlorambucil
- busulfan
- melphalan
- lomustine
- carmustine.

The mustines (nitrogen mustards) were derived from mustard gas. The original drug in the class, **mustine**, is also a Schedule 1 chemical weapon and is now rarely used therapeutically. Myelosuppression, hair loss and vomiting are common adverse effects of most of these drugs and monitoring of the blood count is essential. Pulmonary fibrosis can occur with many of these drugs. Important drugs in this group include:

Cyclophosphamide

Is itself non-toxic, but in the liver it is split by enzymes, which release cytotoxic metabolites. It can be given orally or intravenously, either daily or weekly, and is frequently combined with other cytotoxic agents. The therapeutic effect is usually delayed for a week or more. It is particularly used for blood and lymphatic cancers and also for serious autoimmune disorders. It is used in high doses to 'condition' the bone marrow before bone marrow transplantation. Here it destroys all the cancerous cells along with most of the normal cells and prepares the immune system for the transplant. **Ifosfamide** is a very similar drug.

Adverse Effects. A metabolite called 'acrolein' is excreted in the urine, which can cause severe cystitis. This may be avoided by giving a high fluid intake (4 L/day) or combining it with the drug **mesna**, which binds to acrolein and neutralizes it.

Chlorambucil

This is effective by mouth and although depression of the bone marrow can occur, vomiting is unusual.

Therapeutic Use. Chlorambucil is given orally over long periods. It is one of the few cytotoxic drugs that is used continuously rather than as high-dose intermittent treatment. It has been used on an outpatient basis, but community chemotherapy is now being introduced. Nevertheless, the patient should have regular blood counts; if severe bone marrow suppression occurs, recovery may be slow. It is effective against various forms of Hodgkin's disease and non-Hodgkin's lymphoma, and is probably the drug of choice in the treatment of chronic lymphatic leukaemia (often in combination with prednisolone).

Busulfan

This is an alkylating agent that is not a mustine. It is used particularly in chronic myeloid leukaemia, where it has a selective depressing action on the abnormal white cells. Excessive dosage will produce dangerous depression of normal white cells and platelets. It is used in high doses to condition the bone marrow before bone marrow transplants. It is given orally over weeks or months.

Adverse Effects. In addition to bone marrow depression, it can cause pigmentation and fibrosis of the lungs.

Melphalan

This is used particularly in the treatment of multiple myelomas. It is usually given daily for a week and may be repeated if the blood count is satisfactory. Melphalan is a powerful depressant of white cells and platelets and so is also used to condition the bone marrow prior to bone marrow transplant.

Lomustine

This is similar in many ways to the mustines but its lipid solubility means it crosses the blood–brain barrier. This makes it particularly useful for treating brain tumours. It is given orally as a single dose and this must not be repeated for 6–8 weeks, as depression of white cells and platelets may be long-lasting.

Adverse Effects. Nausea and sometimes vomiting is common for about 12 h after dosage.

Carmustine

This is similar to lomustine.

CLINICAL NOTE

When alkylating agents are prescribing, full blood count and renal function should be monitored. Fluid balance should be regularly monitored and a high fluid intake encouraged. This helps to minimize the risk of renal damage or, in the case of cyclophosphamide, cystitis. To optimize drug efficacy, Melphalan should be taken on an empty stomach 1–2 h before eating.

Antimetabolites

These agents resemble substances used by the cells for their metabolic processes. These drugs therefore become incorporated into the cells and because they cannot be metabolized, they normally cause the cell to die. Malignant cells often have a very rapid metabolic turnover and thus incorporate antimetabolites more rapidly than do normal cells. It is thus possible to kill the majority of malignant cells without interfering too drastically with normal cells. However, they will also inhibit normal cell division, particularly in the bone marrow. The main type of antimetabolites are those which interfere with the metabolism of folic acid (***antifolates***); however, some other types exist, and the nucleoside analogues (see later) are also sometimes classed as a type of antimetabolite. Examples of antimetabolite include:

- methotrexate (antifolate)
- raltitrexed (antifolate)
- pemetrexed (antifolate)
- hydroxycarbamide (DNA replication inhibitor).

Methotrexate

This is similar in structure to folic acid and it blocks one of the chemical processes necessary for the production of DNA from ***folate***.

Therapeutic Use. Methotrexate can be given orally, intravenously or by injection into the cerebrospinal fluid (intrathecally), but large doses are not well absorbed from the intestine and must be given by injection. Dosage schedules depend on the type of cancer being treated. It is excreted via the kidney and it is essential that renal function is measured before starting treatment. With impaired renal function, the dose needs to be reduced. Methotrexate is prescribed together with folic acid as a supplement.

In certain types of malignant disease, a large dose of methotrexate is given; then, after 24 h, giving folinic acid reverses the action of the drug. It is extremely important that this is carried out precisely. This method is known as folinic acid rescue.

Adverse Effects. In addition to bone marrow suppression, methotrexate can cause liver damage and mouth ulceration.

Methotrexate in low doses is also used as an immunosuppressant in rheumatoid arthritis and psoriasis. Regular blood monitoring is required.

Raltitrexed

This blocks several of the enzymes involved in ***folate*** metabolism and thus inhibiting DNA synthesis. It is administered intravenously to treat advanced colorectal cancer when drugs such as fluorouracil cannot be used. It is usually well tolerated by patients but can cause gastrointestinal upsets and myelosuppression (a reduction in blood cell production by the bone marrow).

Pemetrexed

This is similar to raltitrexed and is used to treat mesothelioma and some lung cancers.

Hydroxycarbamide

This is an antimetabolite with a different general mode of action to those previously described. It is orally active, and much used in haematological malignancies and other haematological disorders, including sickle cell anaemia. It holds cells in the G_1 phase, where they are sensitive to radiotherapy. It may therefore be used as an adjunct to improve the success of radiotherapy.

CLINICAL NOTE

Before commencing treatment full blood count, liver and renal function should be assessed and monitored frequently throughout treatment. If, at any point during treatment, leukopenia (low white cell count) or thrombocytopaenia (low platelets) should occur, treatment should be reduced or stopped altogether.

Nucleoside Analogues

These cytotoxics either resemble the *purines or pyrimidines*, which are the building blocks of DNA; or affect their synthesis in such a way as to unbalance their production. These are generally known as 'purine' or 'pyrimidine' analogues, and collectively as 'nucleoside analogues'. They affect the growing strand of DNA and stop the process of DNA synthesis. They are generally phase-specific cytotoxics. Examples include:

- fluorouracil (pyrimidine analogue)
- capecitabine (pyrimidine analogue)
- tegafur (pyrimidine analogue)
- cytarabine (pyrimidine analogue)
- gemcitabine (pyrimidine analogue)
- mercaptopurine (purine analogue)
- tioguanine (purine analogue)
- fludarabine (purine analogue).

Fluorouracil (5-fluorouracil; 5FU) blocks the synthesis of the ***pyrimidine*** molecule thymidine, and so prevents DNA formation. It is used in the treatment of a wide variety of tumours, including those of the gastrointestinal tract. It is given by intravenous infusion or as a bolus; the dose varies with circumstances. Fluorouracil can also be applied locally to certain skin cancers. Leukopenia and mouth ulceration are common with systemic use. **Capecitabine** is metabolized to fluorouracil and can be taken by mouth to treat breast, gastric and colorectal cancers. **Tegafur** is a similar oral prodrug of fluorouracil. All of these three drugs are metabolized by an enzyme known as DPD. Genetic variations in DPD activity exist, and people with complete or partial lack of DPD activity have an increased risk of severe adverse effects, particularly myelosuppression and neurotoxicity.

Cytarabine is a molecule that closely resembles the ***pyrimidine*** known as cytosine. It is incorporated into DNA and blocks further DNA synthesis. It is a key drug in the treatment of acute leukaemias and lymphomas. It is given intravenously or intrathecally. Bone marrow depression is a common adverse effect. In high doses it can cause damage to many organs, including the cerebellum, which may lead to ataxia.

Gemcitabine is an important prodrug that leads to production of a ***pyrimidine*** analogue. It is given intravenously and is particularly used to treat pancreatic cancers although it has many other uses. Its side effects are similar to other cytotoxics.

Mercaptopurine is closely related chemically to adenine and hypoxanthine, two substances used in the formation of DNA. It is a ***purine*** analogue cytotoxic. Mercaptopurine has several actions in biochemical pathways that lead to DNA synthesis; however, its precise mode of action is not known. Mercaptopurine is used in combination with other drugs in the treatment of acute and chronic leukaemias.

Therapeutic Use. Mercaptopurine is given daily by mouth, and the course of treatment is determined by the response of the patient. Excessive or prolonged treatment will produce depression of normal white cell counts.

Tioguanine (thioguanine; 6-TG) is a ***purine*** analogue, given orally to treat acute and chronic leukaemias, inflammatory bowel disease and severe psoriasis. As well as the side effects common to cytotoxics, serious liver toxicity is a dose-dependent problem. This has limited its use, despite its efficacy and rapid onset of action.

Fludarabine is a ***purine*** analogue, active orally and intravenously. It is very effective in treating chronic lymphocytic leukaemia (CLL) and is used in combination with other agents to treat some lymphomas and acute myeloid leukaemia. As it suppresses lymphocyte production so markedly, the risk of opportunistic infections is particularly high when it is used. The damage it causes to the lymphoid system is long lasting and can make any future blood transfusions dangerous. Any transfused blood must be irradiated to destroy any lymphocytes that it contains. Due to this serious disadvantage, it has been replaced by the targeted therapy drug **ibrutinib** for the treatment of CLL, if treatment is required (and if this very expensive drug is available).

Topoisomerase I Inhibitors (Camptothecins)

These include:

- irinotecan
- topotecan.

These inhibit the enzyme DNA topoisomerase I, which has a fundamental role in the transcription of DNA. By their action, they induce multiple breaks in DNA, which then triggers cell death (apoptosis). They are derived from a natural plant chemical called 'camptothecin'. They are effective drugs, given intravenously. Diarrhoea and myelosuppression are the most common side-effects.

- **Irinotecan** is used to treat colorectal cancer.
- **Topotecan** is used to treat ovarian, cervical and small cell lung cancers.

Topoisomerase II Inhibitors (Podophyllotoxins and Others)

Many important drugs inhibit this other topoisomerase enzyme, which controls the overall shape of DNA molecules. Inhibition of this enzyme again leads to an accumulation of DNA damage and triggers apoptosis. Some inhibitors of this enzyme have both cytotoxic anti-cancer activity and antibiotic activity.

There are some cytotoxic drugs that work only through inhibition of topoisomerase II. These are the podophyllotoxins:

- etoposide
- teniposide.

Etoposide is given orally or intravenously and is used to treat many cancers, including testicular and ovarian and sarcomas.

Teniposide is used to treat lymphomas, acute lymphoblastic leukaemia and neuroblastoma.

Myelosuppression and hypersensitivity reactions are the most common early adverse effects, but secondary cancers, particularly acute myeloid leukaemia, are late adverse effects that occur more often with these drugs than with some other cytotoxics. They are important drugs, but this adverse effect does seem particularly cruel.

Another major group of long established and important cytotoxics inhibit topoisomerase II, but also have other cytotoxic actions. These are the anthracyclines.

Anthracyclines (Cytotoxic Antibiotics)

These drugs also have antibiotic activity, although they are too toxic to use for this purpose. They are sometimes referred to as *cytotoxic antibiotics*. Examples include:

- daunorubicin
- doxorubicin
- idarubicin
- mitoxantrone
- pixantrone.

There are several other drugs in this important group. They all work by binding to DNA and interfering with its replication, in part by interfering with the function of the topoisomerase II enzyme, and by other means as well. **Idarubicin** is the only drug in the group that can be given orally. All these drugs are irritant to tissues, some extremely so, and generally are given via an implanted central venous line. As well as myelosuppression, all can cause serious cardiotoxicity, including late onset cardiomyopathies. As with the other drugs that interfere with topoisomerase II, secondary malignancies can occur. They may also cause a condition called *radiation recall*, which is a severe skin rash in the area where radiotherapy has previously been administered. These drugs are generally used in combination with other anti-cancer drugs.

Daunorubicin was the first of these drugs and is used to treat acute leukaemias. It may be less cardiotoxic than doxorubicin. **Doxorubicin** is closely related and is used to treat many cancers, including breast cancer and lymphomas, but also difficult to treat tumours such as sarcomas and neuroblastomas. It can be directly instilled into the bladder to treat bladder cancers. It has been reformulated into a *liposomal* form in which it is encapsulated in a lipid globule, which prolongs its time in the bloodstream. In this form it is particularly useful in the treatment of AIDS-associated Kaposi's sarcoma. Daunorubicin and doxorubicin are bright red liquids that colour urine red and may cause discolouration of other tissues. They are very irritant (although the liposomal formulation is less so), and when given intravenously need to be given with care to avoid extravasation into the tissues, where they can cause severe necrosis.

SAFETY POINT

Inadvertent intrathecal injection of these drugs is likely to be fatal.

Idarubicin is used to treat acute leukaemias. Although it is orally active, gastrointestinal side effects are common.

Mitoxantrone is used to treat acute leukaemias, especially acute myeloid leukaemia. It is given by intermittent infusion. It is also used to slow the progression of secondary progressive multiple sclerosis, although its cardiotoxicity limits the total lifetime dose that can be given. Apart from this it is reasonably well tolerated. It may colour urine blue-green for a few days.

Pixantrone is a new mitoxantrone analogue that was developed with the intention of reducing the cardiotoxicity. Initial experience suggests it is effective for the treatment of non-Hodgkin's lymphoma and does seem to be less cardiotoxic and less irritant than other drugs in this class.

CLINICAL NOTE

- Cytotoxic drugs, especially the anthracyclines, can cause tissue necrosis if they leak into extravascular compartments. Therefore, when given intravenously, only specially trained staff should administer them.
- Intravenous cannulas should be checked frequently (as per local policies) to ensure the cannula is patent and with no redness, swelling or pain. A cannula should be re-sited immediately if it causes pain, or there is redness or swelling. It may be that patients require a more permanent vascular access device to receive chemotherapy and this will reduce discomfort and the trauma of repeated intravenous cannulation (Farrell et al., 2017).

Taxanes

These diterpene agents were originally identified from the yew (*Taxus*) family. They inhibit cell division in the G_2 and M phase and are given intravenously. The most widely used examples are:

- paclitaxel
- docetaxel.

Taxanes prevent cell division by acting as mitotic inhibitors. They do this by interfering with the function of the intracellular microtubules that are essential for mitosis. They also appear to increase sensitivity to radiotherapy.

Paclitaxel was the first of this class and is extracted from the bark of the Pacific Yew. It is used to treat a variety of solid tumours and is first-line treatment for ovarian carcinomas. It tends to be used for recurrent and metastatic disease, particularly in the breast, and may be used in conjunction with other agents. It is also used in the treatment of Kaposi's sarcoma. Side-effects are common, and as well as nausea and vomiting and myelosuppression, there is a risk of severe hypersensitivity reactions with flushing, rashes, dyspnoea and collapse. An antihistamine and glucocorticoid are often administered to prevent this. Much of the hypersensitivity seems to come from the solvent in which the drug is dissolved before administration. This substance is known as *Kolliphor EL* (previously known as *Cremophor EL*). An albumin bound version of paclitaxel (*Abraxane*) has been developed and has greater tolerability.

Docetaxel is a semi-synthetic extract of the leaves of the European Yew and is slightly better tolerated than paclitaxel, but significant bone marrow suppression is very common, and serious side effects seem more common in people with disordered liver function. Its solvent is less allergenic than that of paclitaxel, but hypersensitivity can occur. It is also used to treat a wide variety of tumours, most commonly metastatic or locally recurrent and is often used as palliative chemotherapy, where it can lead to a meaningful increase in quantity and quality of life in some patients.

Vinca Alkaloids

The vinca alkaloids are an important group of drugs originally derived from the Madagascan Periwinkle. Examples include:

- vincristine
- vinblastine
- vindesine
- vinorelbine.

Apart from **vinorelbine**, which is a semi-synthetic vinca alkaloid that can be given orally, all the vinca alkaloids may only be given intravenously. **Vincristine** and **vinblastine** were the first to be used clinically and several others have now been developed.

SAFETY POINT

Vinca alkaloids must **never** be given intrathecally. Severe neurotoxicity will result and is almost always fatal.

These drugs are used in the treatment of leukaemias and lymphomas, generally in combination with other drugs. They are also used to treat solid tumours, particularly breast and lung cancer. Like the taxanes they are cell cycle-specific mitotic inhibitors that work by inhibiting microtubule function, although by a different mechanism. As well as the side-effects common to most cytotoxics, neurotoxicity is very common and may be severe and permanent. Peripheral neuropathy with pain, numbness, tingling and foot drop is the most common manifestation and may limit the use of the drugs. This occurs because long, thin nerve cells rely on microtubules for their integrity. The neuropathy is dose-dependent and generally more severe with vincristine than vinorelbine. Other nerve dysfunction can occur, including blindness, with vincristine treatment. Hyponatraemia, constipation and hair loss are also particularly common. Once again, the potential for severe adverse effects needs to be balanced against the severity of the diseases that they are used to treat.

Platinum Compounds (Organoplatinum Compounds; 'Platins')

The platinum-based anti-cancer drugs are very widely used, with around half of all people on chemotherapy receiving one of them, often in combination with other drugs. They are effective, relatively inexpensive, but have common adverse effects that can be severe. They are given by intravenous injection. Examples include:

- cisplatin
- carboplatin
- oxaliplatin
- nedaplatin.

They cross-link DNA strands together, preventing them from separating in mitosis. The damaged DNA cannot be repaired by normal cellular mechanisms and apoptosis is therefore triggered.

Cisplatin and **carboplatin** are particularly useful in the treatment of testicular cancers, where they have had a dramatic effect in reducing mortality from this disease. They are also used in the treatment of ovarian cancers, lung cancers (including small cell carcinomas) and head and neck tumours. **Oxaliplatin** is used, in combination with other drugs, to treat metastatic colon cancer, and on its own as an adjuvant therapy for colon cancer after surgery. These are powerful drugs, used to treat difficult to treat cancers, but they have many adverse effects:

- Vomiting is the most severe initial adverse effect, and the platins are worse than any other chemotherapy drugs for this. Carboplatin is better tolerated than cisplatin. The introduction of the 5-HT$_3$ antagonist antiemetic drugs such as **ondansetron** made a major difference to the tolerability of treatment with platins. Ondansetron is usually combined with dexamethasone for this purpose, and ideally also with the NK1 (tachykinin) receptor antagonist **aprepitant.** This combination is highly effective.
- Cisplatin is nephrotoxic and this may be dose-limiting. Intensive intravenous hydration reduces the risk. This risk is greatly reduced with carboplatin and oxaliplatin.
- All these drugs are neurotoxic and visual and hearing disturbances are not unusual. Other neuropathies can also occur. Cisplatin is also directly ototoxic, and the hearing loss may be permanent.
- Electrolyte disturbances occur.
- Myelosuppression is common and is particularly troublesome with carboplatin. Opportunistic infections are relatively common.
- Hypersensitivity reactions occur and can be severe. Anaphylaxis has occurred, as has autoimmune haemolytic anaemia.

Another problem is that many cancers become resistant to the effects of these drugs with repeated use. The problematic adverse effects and the issue of resistance have spurred the development of new platins. An example is **nedaplatin**, which is available in some countries.

Other Cytotoxic Drugs

There are a number of cytotoxic drugs that are in current use that have mechanisms of action that do not fall into the groups already discussed. Some examples follow:

Procarbazine is used in the treatment of lymphomas. Nausea is less likely if the drug is given after meals and it may have to be combined with an antiemetic. If alcohol is taken at the same time as the drug, it may produce a reddish flush.

Dacarbazine is largely used in treating Hodgkin's lymphoma and melanomas. It has to be given intravenously and is highly irritant, so it must be injected very slowly into a fast-running infusion. It also causes considerable vomiting and severe myelosuppression.

Bleomycin has relatively weak anticancer effects and is used in combination to treat lymphomas and testicular cancers. However, unlike all the drugs already discussed, it does not depress the bone marrow. It is usually injected at weekly intervals, and a spike of fever may follow injection. Prolonged use, however, leads to lung fibrosis.

Dactinomycin is used to treat childhood cancers, including soft tissue sarcomas and Wilms' tumour of the kidney.

Mitomycin is used to treat anal and bladder cancer.

Ixabepilone is a new cytotoxic that interferes with microtubule function in a manner similar to the taxanes. It can be used for breast cancers that have become resistant to the taxanes.

TARGETED THERAPIES

In the past 20 years, there has been an explosive growth in new anti-cancer therapies that are referred to as 'targeted therapies'. In many cases, they have offered new therapeutic opportunities to treat cancers that were either difficult to treat with cytotoxics or where such treatment had failed. The implication of the name is that these therapies are specifically targeted at cancer cells and kill them without causing harm to other normal cells. This is unfortunately untrue, and the search for a true 'magic bullet' with these properties continues. However, some of these drugs do *come closer* to the magic bullet ideal. One of the best examples is **imatinib**, which inhibits a mutated protein kinase enzyme that is only found in tumour cells in chronic myelogenous leukaemias that are positive for an abnormality called the 'Philadelphia chromosome'. Normal cells do not express this enzyme and so imatinib is able to target cancer cells with a high degree of accuracy. However, for most of this group of drugs, targeted is a relative term.

The distinguishing feature of these drugs is that they target specific metabolic pathways in cells, and unlike cytotoxics, these are not directly related to DNA transcription or replication. They thus kill or suppress malignant cells in a more subtle manner than cytotoxics. If a particular metabolic pathway is greatly over expressed in a cancer cell compared to a normal cell, then a therapy that targets that pathway will kill many more of those cells than normal cells and so adverse effects should be reduced. Many targeted therapies are immunomodulators, enabling the immune system's normal mechanisms for removing abnormal cells to 'see' cancer cells that otherwise 'hide' from immune surveillance. There is therefore an overlap with other immunotherapies for cancer, considered later. These 'non-targeted' immunotherapies, such as interferons or corticosteroids, are conceptually perhaps more like the cytotoxics in that, to use an analogy, they stick a very large 'spanner' in the immune system's works and the 'spanner' is much smaller and more carefully aimed in the targeted immunotherapies.

It is usually necessary to biopsy the cancer in order to identify specific cell biomarkers that indicate whether a specific targeted therapy is likely to work.

Although many targeted therapies are better tolerated than cytotoxics, they have specific adverse effects related to their many modes of action, and these can sometimes be severe or even catastrophic. Hypersensitivity reactions can occur, particularly to therapies that involve monoclonal antibodies, and immunomodulators can sometimes lead to profound and lasting immune system dysfunction.

There are targeted therapies for lung cancer, colorectal cancer, head and neck cancer, breast cancer, multiple myeloma, lymphoma, prostate cancer, melanoma and other cancers. This is a rapidly expanding field that has had some major successes and a number of relative failures. It is a characteristic of most of these therapies that they are extremely expensive, when compared with older treatments.

Classifying targeted therapies in a useful way is difficult, as each drug is developed to target a very specific pathway or receptor. However, there are some large groupings that are useful, and a few examples of the many possibilities are outlined below. Further reading about specific drugs is essential. The broadest grouping is between:

- Monoclonal antibodies (names mostly end in '*mab*')
- Small molecules (names often end in '*nib*')
  - Tyrosine kinase inhibitors
  - mTOR inhibitors

- PARP inhibitors
- Retinoids
- Histone deacetylase inhibitors
- Other mechanisms.

Monoclonal Antibody Targeted Therapies

These are yet another example of Biologic therapy (see Appendix), derived from and manufactured using recombinant DNA technology and biological systems. They are antibodies that have been engineered so that, instead of binding to foreign antigens, they bind to specific surface receptors on cells, and trigger changes that either stimulate or inhibit metabolic pathways that eventually lead to cell death. They are all given intravenously or subcutaneously. As they are proteins, they may themselves trigger immune responses and hypersensitivity, as well as the adverse effects that are a consequence of their specific effects on cell metabolism. An accepted abbreviation for monoclonal antibody is **MAb**.

A few examples of many anti-cancer MAbs available and under development:

- trastuzumab
- bevacizumab
- rituximab
- pembrolizumab
- antibody-drug conjugates.

Trastuzumab for the treatment of HER2-positive breast cancer was mentioned in the introduction. HER2 stands for Human Epidermal Growth Factor Receptor 2 and is a cell membrane protein that, when activated, sends signals that control cell growth. It is one of many examples of the *tyrosine kinase* family of protein kinases, which have a key role in cancer formation, when they are abnormal in some way. Protein kinases will be discussed further later, as many small molecule anti-cancer drugs are tyrosine kinase inhibitors. Many cancers, but particularly breast cancers, greatly over express HER2. Around 30% of breast cancers are HER2-positive and they tend to be aggressive and difficult to treat. Trastuzumab binds to HER2 and prevents it from functioning, thus preventing abnormal cell growth.

It is given by intravenous infusion or subcutaneous injection and may be given as monotherapy, combination therapy or adjuvant therapy after surgery. In this case, it is given at 3-week intervals for a year, although there is some evidence that shorter courses may be as effective.

Trastuzumab treatment has made a significant improvement in survival for patients with HER2-positive breast cancers. It offers no benefits in HER2-negative cancers and its adverse effects may decrease survival in these patients. Apart from hypersensitivity reactions and acute allergic reactions, the biggest problem with trastuzumab is cardiotoxicity, as it may lead to cardiomyopathies. Patients need to be carefully assessed for cardiac problems before and during treatment. It may also trigger respiratory disorders. Trastuzumab has also been used to treat some stomach cancers and offers possibilities in other cancers that overexpress HER2.

Bevacizumab is a MAb used to treat metastatic colorectal, breast and renal cancers and as first-line treatment for some non-small cell lung cancers, and certain ovarian, cervical and fallopian cancers. It is no longer licensed for breast cancer treatment in the USA. It is licensed for palliative treatment of glioblastomas in some countries. It is used in combination with cytotoxic drugs and is given by intravenous infusion. It is an *angiogenesis inhibitor* that interferes with the growth of blood vessels. Many cancers have abnormal blood supplies that support their growth and interfering with this can cause cancer regression. It works by binding to a protein called 'Vascular Endothelial Growth Factor-A' (VEGF-A). This protein is released by tissues in areas of low oxygenation due to poor perfusion and stimulates new blood vessel formation. Bevacizumab inactivates VEGF-A and so reduces new blood vessel formation. On its own, it only shrinks tumours and slows their growth, which is why it is always combined with cytotoxic therapies.

Apart from hypersensitivity and allergic reactions, the major adverse effects stem from its inhibitory effect on blood vessel formation, which may seriously delay wound healing, promote skin ulcers, abscesses, fistulae and perforations and also may trigger osteonecrosis of the jaw, a problem also seen with bisphosphonate treatment for osteoporosis (see Chapter 15). Previous or concurrent bisphosphonate treatment may increase this risk. The weakening effect on blood vessels may also lead to an increased risk of bleeding.

Bevacizumab is also used to treat wet age-related macular degeneration, an eye disorder characterized by new blood vessel formation on the retina. It is given by direct injection into the eye.

Rituximab was one of the earliest MAb therapies to be widely used and remains an important treatment for non-Hodgkin's lymphoma and chronic lymphocytic leukaemia, used in conjunction with other drugs. It is also an important treatment for rheumatoid arthritis and other conditions in which abnormal lymphocytes feature. It has been used outside of its licence to treat a range of other autoimmune conditions. It is given by intravenous infusion or subcutaneous injection and it binds to a protein called 'CD20', which is present mainly on B lymphocytes. When it binds to the protein, it triggers lysis and cell death in the lymphocytes. It has this effect on both normal and cancerous lymphocytes, so while it is more selective than cytotoxics, it is still something of a 'blunt instrument'. Hypersensitivity reactions are common and anaphylactic reactions have occurred. Increased susceptibility to infections occurs and myocardial infarction is a recognized adverse reaction. It may lead to reactivation of hepatitis virus infections and has been associated with a progressive fatal neurological condition, progressive multifocal leukoencephalopathy (PML). This is thought to be due to reactivation of human polyoma-2-virus (otherwise known as the 'JC virus'). Despite these alarming sounding adverse effects, rituximab has been widely used and is generally well-tolerated in clinical practice.

CLINICAL NOTE

There is a high risk of anaphylaxis during administration of rituximab and to reduce this, administering paracetamol and a corticosteroid prior to treatment may be necessary. Emergency treatment such as adrenaline, antihistamines and corticosteroids should be available during treatment.

Pembrolizumab is an example of an immunomodulator, of a specific type known as a *checkpoint inhibitor* that disrupts an immune regulation mechanism ('checkpoint'), which normally controls the activity of the body's own anti-cancer cells ('killer T cells'). Some cancers are able to use this mechanism to hide from the killer T cells, and pembrolizumab removes this hiding place. It is used to treat many difficult to treat cancers, such as melanoma and stomach cancer.

Antibody-drug conjugates represent an attempt to design the fabled 'magic bullet' in cancer treatment. A MAb is chemically linked to a cytotoxic agent. This uses the greater specificity of the MAb for cancerous cells combined with the toxicity of the cytotoxic to deliver cytotoxics more accurately to where they are needed. The history of this type of drug has been disappointing to date, but some are available, and many are in development. An example is **gemtuzumab ozogamicin**. The double name indicates a conjugate of a MAb – here targeted to a cell surface protein found on myeloid cells – with another agent – here an extremely potent cytotoxic agent, too toxic to be used alone. It can be used in acute myeloid leukaemia, where it rapidly depletes abnormal (and normal) myeloid cells. It has had a chequered history, having been withdrawn from sale, and then reintroduced, and this perhaps typifies the hopes and disappointments associated with this class of drugs.

Small Molecule Targeted Therapies

These are referred to as 'small molecule' because, by comparison to the large protein chains that make up MAbs (5000–50,000 atoms), they are indeed relatively small (20–100 atoms) and behave like typical drugs in their pharmacology. Many are, for instance, active orally. They are synthesized chemically rather than grown using recombinant DNA technology, so for all of the these reasons they are not Biologics (although they are sometimes confused with them). They sometimes target the same cell surface molecules that the MAbs target and sometimes are active intracellularly. There are a great many drugs in this class, but they fall into a number of major groups, as follows:

Tyrosine Kinase Inhibitors

These form a large class of new medications. Tyrosine kinase and the protein kinases in general are part of a family of proteins found on cell membranes that, when activated, act as on or off switches for protein synthesis within cells. Protein synthesis is a key factor in cell growth, including the abnormal cell growth found in cancers. There are many different tyrosine kinases that are activated by various different signalling proteins and which activate different cellular protein synthesis pathways. Many drugs have been developed which inhibit specific tyrosine kinases and which have proved useful cancer therapies.

A problem with the tyrosine kinase inhibitors is the development of resistance to their effects, often after a year or so of treatment.

Examples include:

- imatinib
- erlotinib.

Imatinib, mentioned earlier, is mainly used to treat Philadelphia chromosome-positive acute lymphoblastic leukaemia and chronic myeloid leukaemia, as well as some other cancers. It is particularly active in inhibiting an abnormal tyrosine kinase enzyme found on the cell surface of these types of cancers. While it does inhibit other tyrosine kinases to some extent, it is relatively specific for the abnormal tyrosine kinase and so particularly targets these types of leukaemia. It is orally active. It can cause myelosuppression leading to an increased risk of infection and anaemias and low platelet counts can also occur. Gastrointestinal upsets are fairly common. Oedema is relatively common. Other specific serious side-effects are rare, but pericardial effusions and high uric acid levels have been reported.

Erlotinib is a specific tyrosine kinase inhibitor that blocks the cell surface epidermal growth factor receptor (EGFR). EGFR is particularly expressed in certain cancers and in some cancers is present in a mutated form. Erlotinib is particularly active against this mutated form. EGFR inhibition prevents some important pathways in cell growth. Erlotinib is used, with cytotoxic drugs, to treat non-small cell lung cancers and metastatic pancreatic carcinoma, and as maintenance therapy in non-small cell lung cancers in remission. As it affects epidermal cells, it is unsurprising that its major adverse effects involve the skin. Rashes are usual and resemble acne. They normally resolve, but severe and dangerous skin reactions have occurred. Pulmonary toxicity is a rare and sometimes fatal sequel to treatment, and intestinal perforations have also occurred. Resistance to erlotinib can develop between 8 and 12 months after treatment commences.

mTOR Inhibitors

This class of drugs are also inhibitors of a particular group of protein kinases, otherwise known as PI3K or AKT, that are signalling proteins that control several major metabolic pathways involved in cell growth. These pathways are dysregulated in some cancers and there is considerable interest in drugs that target them. The mTOR inhibitors also have an important role in immunosuppressive treatment and in topical form are used in dermatology. There are two current anticancer drugs in this class:

- everolimus
- temsirolimus.

Both of these drugs are derivatives of the immunosuppressive drug sirolimus. **Everolimus** is orally active and is used to treat renal cell cancer, neuroendocrine tumours and breast cancer. **Temsirolimus** is given intravenously to treat renal cell tumour and mantle cell lymphoma. For both drugs, metabolic disturbances of lipids, electrolytes and glucose are common as is bone marrow depression. More severe side-effects are uncommon but have included cardiac failure and thrombosis.

Poly(ADP-ribose) Polymerase Inhibitors (PARP inhibitors)

PARP is an enzyme that is involved in the repair of DNA. If it is inhibited in cancers where the BRCA protein (also involved in DNA repair) is defective, then cell death is triggered. There are several drugs in this class, of which **olaparib**, licensed in 2014, was the first and is used to treat advanced ovarian cancer if proven to be BRCA deficient. Others in this class are being developed and licensed to treat epithelial derived cancers and breast cancers, if BRCA deficient. Fast growing cancers seem to be particularly sensitive to PARP inhibitors.

Retinoids

Retinoids are most commonly used to treat skin conditions including severe acne. They also have a role in treating several skin cancers, but some are also used to treat promyelocytic leukaemia and neuroblastoma. They are agonists for the retinoic acid receptor (RAR) and/or the retinoid X receptor (RXR). They are used orally or topically. Examples include:

- isotretinoin
- bexarotene.

All retinoids can cause skin reaction, sometimes severe and also can cause marked hypercholesterolaemia and other metabolic disturbances. While many anti-cancer drugs are teratogenic, the retinoids are unusually so, and highly effective contraception is essential when they are used.

Histone Deacetylase Inhibitors

Histone deacetylase is an enzyme that helps control the packing of DNA in cell nuclei. If it is inhibited, then cell death can be triggered through multiple mechanisms. Some tumours are particularly sensitive to its effects. The earliest drug known to have this effect is the antiepileptic drug valproate, which has been used (out of licence) to treat a variety of tumours. In the UK, the only currently licensed drug is **panobinostat**, although a few others have been developed. It is used, in combination with other agents, to treat refractory multiple myeloma. Gastrointestinal disorders, including diarrhoea, are common. Anaemia, metabolic disorders and ECG abnormalities are also common.

Other Small Molecule Targeted Therapies

There are many other small molecule therapies available or under development, targeting different pathways involved in cell growth and replication. Examples include **asparaginase**, used to treat acute lymphoblastic leukaemia and **vemurafenib**, which inhibits the enzyme BRAF kinase and kills melanoma cells if they have a particular common mutation in the BRAF gene. It improves survival and disease-free progression in people with advanced melanoma.

IMMUNOTHERAPY

Several approaches to cancer chemotherapy involve drugs that affect the immune response. As noted earlier, there is a considerable overlap here with the MAbs in particular. The immune checkpoint inhibitor pembrolizumab has been considered earlier, and several other MAb checkpoint inhibitors exist. Other approaches to cancer immunotherapy include:

- corticosteroids and other immunosuppressants
- cytokines
- adjuvants.

Corticosteroids and Other Immunosuppressants

Prednisolone is a synthetic corticosteroid (a glucocorticoid), the properties and adverse effects of which have already been discussed elsewhere in this book (see Chapter 17). This steroid is used to suppress the immune response in several autoimmune diseases and to suppress organ transplant rejection. It can cause tumour regression in some cancers, including hormone-responsive breast cancer, Hodgkin's disease, non-Hodgkin's lymphomas and lymphoblastic leukaemia. Prednisolone is also useful as part of palliative care in end-stage malignant disease, as it lifts the patient's mood and to some extent restores appetite.

The **mTOR inhibitors** have already been discussed and are related to immunosuppressants such as tacrolimus and sirolimus.

Cytokines

Cytokines are chemical signals produced by body cells to modulate other cell growth and activity. **Interferons** are substances produced by cells that are infected by viruses and that stimulate antiviral activity. There are three types of human interferon: alpha (from white blood cells), beta (from fibroblasts) and gamma (from lymphocytes). Interferon alpha (IFN-α) has a number of forms that have been of some value in the treatment of some leukaemias, melanoma and sarcomas. They are used more frequently in the treatment of chronic viral infections.

Interleukins (IL) are a family of proteins that are part of the control mechanisms of the immune response; an example is IL-2, which is used clinically as **aldesleukin**. It is used to treat metastatic renal cell carcinoma and promotes tumour shrinkage but has not been shown to increase survival. It is extremely toxic to several organs, including the thyroid, bone marrow, liver, kidney and brain.

Adjuvants

These agents activate pathways involved in the innate immune system that can stimulate general immune responses and ultimately promote adaptive immune responses. **Imiquimod** is an agent that is applied to skin and can promote resolution of actinic keratoses, which are precancerous. They also may promote resolution of the superficial form of basal cell carcinoma.

Imiquimod can promote healing of warts and this is particularly useful in the anogenital region. **Poly ICLC** is an agent that is licensed in some countries to treat some types of squamous cell skin cancer. Both of these agents bind to the TLR3 receptor, which is involved in pattern recognition in the innate immune system.

SEX HORMONES AND HORMONE ANTAGONISTS

The growth of some cancers can be affected by the presence or absence of sex hormones. Breast cancers and prostate cancers are often hormone-dependent, and castration was often performed to slow the growth of prostate cancer before less drastic therapies became available. Several drugs have been developed to block the effects of oestrogens and androgens and these have made a major difference to the outlook in several common cancers.

Oestrogens were used to treat breast cancers, as in some cases the high doses of potent synthetic oestrogens caused regression of these normally oestrogen-dependent tumours. Oestrogens were also used to treat prostate cancer but are little used for either indication today. **Progestogens (progestins)** are used to treat endometrial cancers where the hormones have a strongly suppressive effect on endometrial growth. They are rarely used to treat other cancers today. **Androgens** have been used in the treatment of breast cancer, but very rarely today.

Hormone Antagonists

The introduction of drugs that block the action of the sex hormones or which block their production has been a major step forward in the treatment and palliation of common cancers.

Sex Hormone Receptor Antagonists

Tamoxifen and toremifene are oestrogen receptor antagonists, whereas cyproterone acetate, flutamide and bicalutamide are androgen receptor antagonists.

Tamoxifen

Has been used for over 30 years to treat women with breast cancer. It is also used to prevent recurrences among women with early breast cancer. The drug works by competing with the body's oestrogen for its receptor sites, thus blocking the accelerating effects of oestrogens on the disease. It is usually used in addition to treatment with surgery and/or other chemotherapy. Clinical trial evidence shows that most of the benefit occurs in the first 5 years of use and lasts for at least 15 years after diagnosis.

There is good evidence that it can prevent breast cancer among healthy women who are considered at high risk for breast cancer.

Tamoxifen is associated with a two- to three-fold increase in the risk of endometrial cancer and a two- to three-fold increase in the risk of thromboembolism. Nevertheless, tamoxifen remains probably the most widely used drug for breast cancer.

Therapeutic Use. Tamoxifen is prescribed for women whose breast cancer shows positive for the presence of oestrogen receptors. Some tumours are oestrogen receptor-negative, and tamoxifen is not effective in these cases. About 60%–65% of women with oestrogen receptor-positive tumours respond to initial tamoxifen treatment, while less than 10% of patients with oestrogen receptor-negative tumours will respond. Tamoxifen is supplied in tablet form for oral administration to be taken daily for breast cancer.

Tamoxifen is also prescribed for anovulatory infertility, when the drug is taken on days 2, 3, 4 and 5 of the menstrual cycle.

Adverse Effects and Contraindications. Adverse effects are mild and include occasional nausea, oedema, flushing and bone pain and a slightly increased risk of endometrial cancer. The drug is contraindicated in breastfeeding and should be stopped before planned pregnancy.

Toremifene

Is another oestrogen receptor antagonist. It is chemically similar to tamoxifen (it is a chlorinated analogue). It is used to treat hormone-dependent metastatic breast cancer in postmenopausal women. It is, like tamoxifen, taken orally.

Cyproterone acetate, **flutamide**, **bicalutamide**, **apalutamide** and **enzalutamide** block the actions of the male sex hormones (androgens) at their receptor sites. They are licensed to be used alone or with other treatments for the treatment of prostate cancer. They should be prescribed before treating patients with GnRH agonists (see later), since GnRH agonists cause an initial large release of testosterone from the testes before shutting them down, and this burst of testosterone can exacerbate the cancer, and even prove fatal. **Abiraterone** works by a different mechanism and is used in metastatic prostate cancer resistant to GnRH agonists or castration. It is used in conjunction with a corticosteroid and castration or a GnRH analogue.

Adverse Effects. Androgen receptor antagonists can cause gynaecomastia and other problems associated with androgen lack, such as decreased libido and weight changes. Cyproterone acetate has been reported to cause direct hepatic failure in some patients after prolonged use, and patients should have blood counts and tests of hepatic function before and during treatment with these drugs. Other unwanted effects include hirsutism due to partial agonist activity, and nausea, vomiting and changes in appetite. With apalutamide, enzalutamide and abiraterone, a condom and another highly effective form of contraception must be used if a man's partner is of childbearing age.

Contraindications. Cyproterone acetate is less favoured in the UK. With the other drugs, hepatic and adrenal impairment might pose problems and the patient should be tested for adrenal and hepatic function before and during treatment.

Aromatase Inhibitors

Aromatase inhibitors block the ***production*** of oestrogens and are used in the treatment of breast cancer.

Anastrozole and **letrozole** are non-steroidal aromatase inhibitors and they prevent the production of oestrogens in peripheral tissues. In postmenopausal women, no oestrogen is produced in the ovaries and so these drugs can reduce residual oestrogen production by 98%. They are used in the treatment of oestrogen receptor positive breast cancer in postmenopausal women. There is trial evidence to support switching to them after 5 years' treatment with tamoxifen.

Adverse Effects. These are generally restricted to mild menopausal symptoms, but serious skin and allergic reactions have occurred with anastrozole and embolism, thrombosis and myocardial infarction with letrozole. All the aromatase inhibitors provoke loss of bone density and can lead to osteoporosis.

Exemestane is a steroidal aromatase inhibitor. It may be used as an adjuvant treatment in early breast cancer but is more commonly used for advanced breast cancer in postmenopausal women in whom tamoxifen has failed.

GnRH Analogues

These are synthetic analogues of the hypothalamic hormone GnRH (gonadorelin), which is physiologically released in *pulses* and which stimulates luteinizing hormone (LH) release from the anterior pituitary. However, if GnRH is given as a *continuous* treatment, it shuts down the production of LH and therefore stops gonadal sex hormone production.

They are prescribed not only for prostate cancer but also for early oestrogen receptor-positive breast cancer and advanced breast cancer. Some also have a role in women with severe endometriosis, particularly before surgery. Here it is oestrogen production which is being suppressed. They are also used in many other conditions where suppression of sex hormones is useful, including delaying puberty, as part of assisted conception treatment and for the treatment of hypersexuality.

There are many agents marketed, generally as controlled release preparations given 1- or 3-monthly. Implants lasting a year are also available. Examples include:

- buserelin
- goserelin
- histrelin
- leuprorelin
- nafarelin
- triptorelin.

Gonadorelin is also a GnRH analogue, with a very short duration of action. It is used in diagnostic testing to assess pituitary function, but has also been used to treat hypogonadism caused by pituitary dysfunction, as its short duration of action mimics natural GnRH release and, rather than suppressing LH production, it stimulates it – unlike all of the long-acting GnRH analogues.

CLINICAL NOTE

As mentioned earlier, before these substances are administered to men with prostate cancer, the patient should first be given an androgen receptor antagonist such as flutamide or cyproterone acetate, for at least 3 days before the GnRH analogue. Similar to many drugs described in this chapter, there is a risk of liver toxicity and the patient should be monitored for signs of this during treatment.

Adverse Effects. The GnRH analogues all produce the typical effects of gonadectomy. In women, these effects include the symptoms of menopause – hot flushes, sweating, vaginal dryness, changes in breast size and anorexia – and in men there may be gynaecomastia. In both sexes, there may be sleep disorders and mood swings.

COMBINATION THERAPY

In most forms of malignant disease that can be treated successfully by drugs, better results with less toxicity are achieved if several cytotoxic agents are combined in the course of treatment. Most regimens consist of repeated courses given at intervals of 1–2 weeks and extending over 6–12 months or even longer. This enables the malignant cells to be attacked at different stages in their cell cycle; also, careful timing enables the normal cells of the body to recover while the malignant cells remain suppressed. Treatment is usually carried out in day units. As an example of a treatment that has been used for widespread lymphomas, the **CHOP** regimen, is shown below:

- Cyclophosphamide: days 1 and 8
- Hydroxydaunorubicin (**doxorubicin**): day 1
- Oncovin (**vincristine**): days 1 and 8
- Prednisolone daily for 5 days.

Rituximab is now often added to this, to create the **R-CHOP** regimen.

The course is given in cycles of 3–4 weeks and repeated about six times.

Many combination regimens are being used in the treatment of various types of cancer. Among the malignant diseases that can often be improved or cured by chemotherapy are:

- various leukaemias, particularly acute lymphoblastic in children
- Hodgkin's disease
- non-Hodgkin's lymphomas (some types)
- testicular cancer
- ovarian cancer
- retinoblastoma
- choriocarcinoma.

Other types of cancer can often be improved but may not be cured so frequently; these include carcinoma of the breast and prostate, and myeloma. Some cancers are very difficult to improve and are rarely cured. Many sarcomas and advanced melanoma fall into this category. The targeted therapies have opened new avenues of treatment for some of these cancers, offering new hope for some patients.

Although much cancer is still treated in general hospitals, it is preferable for this to be carried out in special units experienced in this type of work and such units are being widely established. In terms of nursing organization, it requires frequent short-term admissions or special outpatient facilities and careful checks on the general health of the patient and the blood count. Oncology nurses are very highly trained to play an important role in specialist and non-specialist units.

ADJUVANT TREATMENT

It is common experience that, although a malignant growth appears to have been totally removed, a recurrence may occur somewhere else in the body at a later date. This must mean that at the time of operation there was already a seedling deposit. The object of adjuvant treatment is to give cytotoxic drugs after surgery, even if there is no evidence of spread, to eradicate hidden small deposits which are particularly susceptible to drug treatment. For example, over half the women who have only had surgery for carcinoma of the breast will ultimately develop metastases, although these were not apparent at the time of the initial operation. Results of trials in this condition have made it clear that adjuvant treatment improves the long-term prognosis in all age groups. The type of chemotherapy is determined by the age of the patient, the nature of the cancer cells and whether the axillary nodes are involved. It varies from tamoxifen given alone to postmenopausal low-risk patients, to polychemotherapy, perhaps combined with ovarian ablation, for high-risk younger patients. A related strategy is to give chemotherapy before operation (primary treatment).

PALLIATIVE CHEMOTHERAPY

In some types of advanced cancer, chemotherapy can relieve symptoms and prolong life, but is not curative. Most regimens have some side-effects, and before embarking on palliative chemotherapy it is very important to weigh possible benefits against disadvantages. This will require a compassionate discussion with the patient and ascertaining the views of relatives, doctors and nursing staff, and others who are involved. As with all chronic diseases, much supportive care will be necessary, and, generally, such treatment should be given in specialist oncology units.

PRACTICAL POINTS

Storage of Drugs and Preparation of Solutions

Oncology units should have a pharmacist with special experience and expertise in handling cytotoxic drugs to advise and supervise others. Solutions for injection should be prepared in a designated area by:

- nurses who have received special training
- pharmacists
- medical staff.

Some of these substances are irritants, and, in addition, can be highly dangerous if absorbed.

CLINICAL NOTE

Although some cytotoxic drugs can be used for some time after the solutions have been prepared, it is usually best to discard all unused remnants at the end of the treatment session.

The following precautions should be observed:

- Wear plastic gloves and a plastic apron when making up solutions. If any of the drug splashes onto the skin, it should be washed off immediately. Some of the drugs are irritants and there is always the risk of an allergic reaction.
- Wear protective spectacles to protect the eyes. If the drug comes into contact with the eyes, they should be washed out with water and further advice should be sought.
- Care should be taken to avoid absorbing the drug either systemically or by inhalation. Hands should be washed after preparing a drug (even when gloves are worn). Although at present there is no evidence that those who handle cytotoxic drugs are more liable to suffer long-term ill-effects, there are certainly no grounds for complacency and every care must be taken.
- Pregnant staff should not prepare cytotoxic solutions.
- If spillage occurs, it should be mopped up with absorbent paper, which must be disposed of properly, and the whole area washed down thoroughly.
- Waste material should be disposed of safely.

CLINICAL NOTE

Areas that are administering cytotoxic drugs should have the following available and in easy reach:

- Cytotoxic spillage kits – to assist in cleaning up any accidental spillages safely and ensuring safe disposal of the medication.
- Cytotoxic splash kits – which should include eye wash and burn wash.
- Cytotoxic extravasation kits – if an intravenous cannula is dislodged.

Administration of Cytotoxic Drugs

Cytotoxic drugs are, by their nature, dangerous drugs. In the UK NHS, cancer networks have been established to develop safe systems for their delivery.

Safe systems require that (BNF, 2020):

- cytotoxic drugs for the treatment of cancer should be given as part of a wider pathway of care coordinated by a multidisciplinary team
- cytotoxic drugs should be prescribed, dispensed, and administered only in the context of a written protocol or treatment plan
- injectable cytotoxic drugs should only be dispensed if they are prepared for administration
- oral cytotoxic medicines should be dispensed with clear directions for use.

Dose calculations for parenteral drugs is complex and may be based on weight or on body surface area. Clear written protocols are essential and doses need careful checking and challenging if there is any doubt. Oral anti-cancer drugs need to be prescribed with similar care and patients must be provided with clear written information.

CLINICAL NOTE

Inadequate health literacy or knowledge of why chemotherapy is prescribed, how it should be taken and the importance of adherence to guidance may impede cancer survival. Service user–clinician trust, exploration of health beliefs and a person-centred approach to drug counselling are recommended as strategies to optimize medicines in people with cancer (Costa and McGraw, 2020).

Extravasation of Cytotoxic Drugs on Injection

Even if great care is taken, some leaking of the injected drug may occur around the vein and this can cause problems. **Vesicant drugs** carry a high risk of severe tissue necrosis if they extravasate. They are:

- chlormethine
- dactinomycin
- daunorubicin
- doxorubicin
- epirubicin
- melphalan
- mitomycin
- vinblastine
- vincristine
- vindesine.

Bleomycin and ifosfamide are irritant drugs which cause pain, but do not lead to tissue damage. For vesicants, a **practical summary** of the full extravasation procedure is given below:

1. The needle should be left in situ, the infusion stopped and as much as possible of the extravasated fluid removed.
2. The needle can now be removed.
3. Ice packs should be applied to the area.
4. The area should be kept cool for the next 24 h and 1% hydrocortisone cream applied twice daily.
5. The episode and subsequent progress should be recorded in the patient's notes.
6. An expert should be consulted.
7. The area should be inspected after 24 h and as often as necessary thereafter.

TABLE 29.1
Vomiting with Cytotoxic Drugs

Severe	Moderate	Mild
Chlormethine	Cytarabine	Bleomycin
Cisplatin	Etoposide	Busulfan
Cyclophosphamide (high dose)	Procarbazine	Chlorambucil
Dacarbazine	Vinblastine	Fluorouracil
Daunorubicin		Melphalan
Doxorubicin		Mercaptopurine
Lomustine		Methotrexate
		Vincristine

Policies may vary in different units, and local policies and procedures should be available and strictly followed. Occasionally, necrosis occurs despite all the measures, and skin grafting may be required.

Vomiting with Cytotoxic Drugs

Many cytotoxic drugs cause the patient to vomit a few hours after administration (Table 29.1).

There is as yet, no complete remedy for this troublesome adverse effect. A variety of regimens may be tried in an attempt to mitigate the symptoms, and patients vary in their preference. It is usual to give cytotoxic drugs in the late evening, so that the patient may sleep as much as possible through the period of nausea. For mildly or moderately emetic cytotoxic drugs, dexamethasone, prochlorperazine, domperidone or low-dose metoclopramide can be used. Combinations are often more effective and intravenous dexamethasone and metoclopramide initially, followed by both orally, is useful.

It is believed that the most severely emetic drugs such as the platins stimulate the 5-HT$_3$ receptors in the gastrointestinal tract and brainstem. Ondansetron, a 5-HT$_3$ antagonist, combined with dexamethasone given intravenously and aprepitant given orally immediately before treatment and followed by further doses of ondansetron, either orally or intravenously is the most effective antiemetic regime for this type of cytotoxic drug.

Some patients, particularly towards the end of their course of treatment, become anxious and tense before treatment and may indeed vomit before receiving their drugs. This is a difficult problem. Lorazepam an hour before coming to hospital may be tried and sometimes psychiatric support with a desensitization programme helps.

Care of the Mouth

Mouth ulceration may occur with many cytotoxic regimens. This is partially due to the direct effect of the drugs on the mucous membrane of the mouth. Also, the general suppression of immunity, particularly of the leucocytes, encourages infection. This unpleasant complication can be minimized and a practical summary is given below:

1. Before starting treatment, the patient should be seen by a dentist or dental hygienist and have any infections treated.
2. If the white blood cell count drops or the mouth becomes sore, the patient should have nystatin pastilles (for candida) every 6 h and Corsodyl mouthwashes twice daily. Some units use fluconazole systemically.
3. If ulceration develops, the pain can be relieved by Difflam Oral Rinse, which contains benzydamine, a local anaesthetic. The mouth is rinsed out every 3 h with the undiluted solution. Lidocaine gel can also be applied to the painful area.

CLINICAL NOTE

Oral hygiene is essential for patients who are receiving chemotherapy. The patient should be encouraged to attend to this regularly if they are able to or if not, a nurse should assist them with regular (maximum 4-hourly) with this care. It should include not only teeth cleaning and mouthwash but oral artificial saliva, lip care and if ulcers or pain in the mouth is present, medication to relieve this.

Alopecia

Hair loss may occur with many cytotoxic drugs (particularly doxorubicin, etoposide and ifosfamide). It will recover, but causes embarrassment to patients. With doxorubicin, ice-cold water caps applied to the scalp during treatment may decrease the loss, otherwise wigs may help, although some patients will tolerate the hair loss. However, it is important to warn the patient of this problem before treatment is started.

CLINICAL NOTE

Many units offer specialist advice on hair loss, obtaining wigs, head coverage and coping with the psychosocial aspects of hair loss. Patients should be referred to these services early and have the side-effects explained to them.

Bone Marrow Suppression and Infection

Cytotoxic drugs (except bleomycin and vincristine) depress bone marrow function. This leads to a low white blood cell count and, sometimes, to low platelet and red blood cell counts, usually after 7–10 days. As a result, immunity is suppressed and the patient is liable to develop an infection or to bleed. In addition to those caused by the usual bacteria, infections may be due to fungi, viruses and even organisms which do not normally cause disease in healthy people. Attempts have been made to diminish the risk of infection by isolating the patients, but this is difficult and, if strictly implemented, very expensive. In most cases it appears to be sufficient to avoid obvious sources of infection. Those caring for these people should always watch for signs of infection and the patients should be told to report any suspicious symptoms. Immunosuppressed patients often respond poorly to antibacterial treatment and the infecting organism may be obscure, so a combination of antibiotics is often used.

The extent and duration of the low blood count can be minimized by giving haemopoietic growth factor and this has proved a useful adjunct to the more intense courses of chemotherapy.

Sometimes, very large doses of cytotoxic drugs are given in an attempt to eradicate a tumour that is poorly sensitive to chemotherapy and this will destroy the blood-forming cells in the bone marrow. In these circumstances, bone marrow is removed from the patient before starting treatment, or stem cells, which can form bone marrow, are harvested from the patient's peripheral blood and stored. After the chemotherapy is finished, the stored cells are injected back into the patient to multiply and restock the bone marrow. This is a high-risk procedure with an appreciable morbidity and mortality, but can lead to cures which were previously not possible.

LONG-TERM RISKS OF THE USE OF CYTOTOXIC DRUGS

Most cytotoxic drugs interfere in some way or other with the structure of the cell nucleus and this can have serious long-term implications.

Second Malignancy

These drugs may induce changes in normal cells so that they ultimately become malignant. This means that although the original cancer is eradicated, a different malignancy may develop at a later date. Second malignancies are more common after certain cytotoxic drugs and if drugs are combined with radiotherapy. The risk is greater with drugs which inhibit topoisomerase II than with most other cytotoxics. It is necessary to put this risk in perspective, as the chance of dying from the initial cancer, if untreated, is much greater than that of developing a further cancer. This risk will be one factor to be considered when choosing a suitable regimen.

Gonadal Damage

Many cytotoxic drugs damage the gonads. In men, permanent sterility may result; in women, amenorrhoea is common, but periods usually return after stopping treatment. It is sensible to store a man's sperm before treatment in case gonadal function is permanently suppressed by treatment with cytotoxic drugs.

Teratogens

Most cytotoxic drugs are potentially teratogenic, especially in early pregnancy. However, if pregnancy is avoided during and for 6 months from the end of treatment, there does not seem to be an increased risk of an abnormal infant being born.

THE ROLE OF THE NURSE IN CANCER CHEMOTHERAPY

The establishment of units specializing in oncology has enabled nurses to receive advanced training which is of direct benefit to patients and their families. A multidisciplinary approach is important in the treatment of cancer and the team will consist of nurses, doctors, pharmacists and social workers. In most centres, part of the work will be concerned with therapeutic trials and this will require ancillary staff.

The management of malignant disease may be by chemotherapy alone or may involve surgery or radiotherapy. In this book, only the problems of chemotherapy are considered. In addition to technical knowledge, the nurse will have a most important role in patient support. The distress and fear of having cancer is enough to shake even the strongest personality and chemotherapy is usually prolonged and often unpleasant.

In the initial assessment, nurses should try to establish what patients know about malignant disease and their beliefs, if any, about treatment. They will appeal to the nurses for information and this provides an opportunity to dispel myths and at the same time, explain what treatment will entail. Patient education is multifaceted and can take the form of booklets, videos, question-and-answer sessions and group discussions, so that sufferers can gain support from others in similar circumstances. Patients usually attend oncology units at regular intervals for treatment and follow-up, so it is possible for the nursing staff to build up a supportive relationship with those who know and trust them.

Chemotherapy is now delivered in many different clinical settings as well as the home setting. Patients have the opportunity to develop a strong understanding of their care and the providers of this care.

REFERENCES AND FURTHER READING

Affronti, M.L., Schneider, S.M., Herndon 2nd, J.E., et al., 2014. Adherence to antiemetic guidelines in patients with malignant glioma: a quality improvement project to translate evidence into practice. Support Care Cancer 22 (7), 1897–1905.

Birand, N., Boşnak, A.S., Diker, Ö., et al., 2019. The role of the pharmacist in improving medication beliefs and adherence in cancer patients. J. Oncol. Pharm. Pract. 25 (8), 1916–1926.

BNF, 2020. Cytotoxic drugs. https://bnf.nice.org.uk/treatment-summary/cytotoxic-drugs.html.

Costa, A., McGraw, C., 2020. Exploring perceptions and experiences of oral chemotherapy in people with cancer. Cancer Nurs. Pract. 19 (1), 35–41.

Dougherty, L., Lister, S., West-Oram, A., 2015. Royal Marsden manual of clinical nursing. Student Edition, ninth ed. Wiley, London.

Farrell, C., McCulloch, E., Bellhouse, S., et al., 2017. Peripheral cannulae in oncology: nurses' confidence and patients' experiences. Cancer Nurs. Pract. 16 (3), 32–38.

Henke Yarbro, C., Wujcik, D., Holmes Gobel, B., 2011. Cancer nursing: principles and practice. Jones and Bartlett, London.

Nagaya, N., Horie, S., 2018. [Endocrine therapy for prostate cancer.]. Clin. Calcium. 28 (11), 1527–1533.

NICE, 2020. Browse Guidance by Topic: Cancer. https://www.nice.org.uk/guidance/conditions-and-diseases/cancer.

Prezioso, D., Iacono, F., Romeo, G., et al., 2014. Early versus delayed hormonal treatment in locally advanced or asymptomatic metastatic prostatic cancer patient dilemma. World J. Urol. 32 (3), 661–667.

Priestman, T., 2012. Cancer chemotherapy in clinical practice. Springer Verlag, London.

Ream, E., 2007. Fatigue in patients receiving palliative care. Nurs. Stand. 21 (28), 49–56.

Treister, N.S., Sankar, V., 2017. Chemotherapy-induced oral mucositis treatment and management. https://emedicine.medscape.com/article/1079570-treatment.

Vickers, V., Uzzell, M., Burnet, K., 2012. Understanding how targeted therapies work. Cancer Nurs. Pract. 11 (7), 14–22.

USEFUL WEBSITES

American Cancer Society. https://www.cancer.org/docroot/ETO/content/ETO_1_4X_Monoclonal_Antibody_Therapy_Passive_Immunotherapy.asp.

Lymphoma Info. https://www.lymphomainfo.net/therapy/immunotherapy/mab.html.

30 DRUGS USED IN THE TREATMENT OF TROPICAL DISEASES

CHAPTER OUTLINE

LEARNING OBJECTIVES

At the end of this chapter, the reader should be able to:

- discuss the impact of modern air travel on the spread of diseases
- describe the symptoms and treatment of tropical diseases that affect the gastrointestinal tract
- give an account of the cause and treatment of leprosy
- give an account of the cause, symptoms and use of drugs to suppress and treat malaria, and the limitations of treatment
- give an account of the protozoan infections such as leishmaniasis
- describe the treatments for the various worm infestations
- describe the precautions to take in order to reduce the chances of being bitten by flying insects, and provide sensible bite avoidance strategies

INTRODUCTION

Most tropical diseases are caused by infectious agents or by dietary deficiency. In former times, epidemics caused widespread disease and death rates were high. 'New' infectious diseases have been widely reported in the scientific literature and the media, e.g. the Coronavirus (COVID-19), sudden acute respiratory syndrome (SARS), Middle East Respiratory Syndrome (MERS) and the Zika virus. COVID-19 is a novel coronavirus, which forms part of a large family of coronaviruses including the common cold and more severe diseases such as SARS and MERS. The outbreak was reported from Wuhan, China in December 2019. COVID-19 is transmitted easily between people and causes respiratory symptoms, including cough, fever, shortness of breath and death. Current figures suggest the fatality rate to be much higher than influenza (Gates, 2020) and the genome of the virus has been sequenced and vaccines have been developed (see Chapter 28). More studies are presently underway. Health authorities have recommended hygiene recommendations to prevent infection such as self-isolation if travelled from high-risk areas, wearing of face-coverings, undergoing testing if symptomatic, social distancing and regular handwashing.

Previously known tropical infections have also been reported: in 2015, the largest ever outbreak of Ebola virus disease was reported in West Africa. Although the death rate was high, survival was improved compared with former outbreaks, mainly through better supportive nursing and medical care. An Ebola vaccine, *Ervebo*, was approved in the USA in December 2019, for the prevention of Ebola virus. Other diseases such as the Zika virus as yet do not have any approved therapy and members of the public visiting affected countries should be concerned about the risks they pose. The public are also increasingly aware that air travel has brought tropical infections nearer to home, although the risk of catching Ebola or Zika is low. However, it is possible to be infected with malaria when travelling to a country known to be a high-risk area, and not become ill until after returning to the UK. Some knowledge of these disorders are therefore necessary for all health practitioners. NHS Choices and Public Health England offer up-to-date information about tropical infections. The World Health Organization (WHO) is another useful resource providing useful information on international travel, health and disease.

In this chapter, the consideration of tropical disease will be carried out under headings of the disease, rather than any drugs used to treat these conditions.

PREPARATIONS AND BITE AVOIDANCE

Sensible precautions can be taken to minimize contraction of disease transmitted through drinking-water, food and insect bites, especially if one knows some of the habits of the insects whose bite one wishes to avoid. General advice is as follows:

- Prepare for the trip by getting all necessary vaccinations, and if a trip to a malaria-infested area is planned, take the necessary drugs. Take medical advice well before the trip.
- Maintain good handwashing hygiene.
- Take water-purifying tablets to countries where water is likely to be contaminated, and drink only bottled water if available.
- Ascertain whether rivers, dams and pools have bilharzias before swimming, especially in Africa.
- Reduce exposure to insects through knowledge of their behaviour and what attracts a bite.
- Use insect repellents on the skin, including soap and hair wash.
- Use insecticides impregnated into materials – clothing, tents and nets.
- Use contact insecticides, i.e. knock-down sprays or burners/mats.

Mosquitoes

- Do not wear dark clothing, which attracts mosquitoes.
- Powerful perfumes and other strong smells attract mosquitoes.
- *Anopheles* mosquitoes carry malaria, and are most active in the early evening and at night.
- Wear long-sleeved, loose-fitting clothing, especially at and after sunset.
- Apply insect repellents to the skin.
- Ensure that mosquito nets are not torn and are sprayed with an insect repellent.

Sandflies

- Sandflies can pass through mosquito nets, so the nets should be treated with an insecticide.
- Sandflies fly low, so it is best to sleep high up, e.g. on the upper floors.

DISEASES AND INFESTATIONS

Travellers' Diarrhoea

A holiday in tropical or subtropical countries can often be interrupted by an attack of diarrhoea, colic and vomiting. It is believed that there is usually an infective cause and the organism most often implicated is an unusual variant of *Escherichia coli*.

Prevention should include care over drinking water and washing uncooked foods such as fruit and vegetables in chlorinated water. The prophylactic use of antibiotics is not recommended except for those at special risk (e.g. patients with bowel disease or those with immunosuppressant drugs). Due to the complexity of geographical variation of pathogens causing disease and thus the choice of appropriate antibacterial prophylaxis, it is recommended that specialist advice is sought. For the affected patients who are otherwise fit, **fluid replacement** with added **glucose** and **electrolytes** (e.g. *Dioralyte* or a similar preparation) is important. Mild to moderate symptoms can be improved with **loperamide**, which should not be given to children under 4 years and should be avoided in patients with a fever.

Amoebiasis (Amoebic Dysentery)

Amoebiasis is an infection of the lower bowel by an organism called *Entamoeba histolytica* and is characterized by chronic diarrhoea, abdominal pain and can be accompanied with per-rectal bleeding. Sometimes the infection spreads outside the bowel, particularly to the liver, where it causes an abscess. It occurs through ingestion of food and water contaminated with human faeces containing amoebic cysts.

The most important drug used for the treatment is **metronidazole**, which is now the first choice in treating amoebic infection of the bowel and abscess of the liver. A 5–10-day course is recommended, but vomiting can be troublesome at the dose levels used to treat amoebic dysentery. Metronidazole is followed by **diloxanide furoate**, which is active against organisms in the bowel lumen, but not in the tissues. The combination appears to be even more efficient at eradicating the infection. An alternative to metronidazole is **tinidazole**.

Giardiasis

Giardiasis is due to the organism *Giardia lamblia*, which affects the intestine and causes distension, flatulence and frothy very offensive stools. Infection can occur in many parts of the world, and symptoms often develop on return from a holiday abroad. Varying dosage of **metronidazole** is an effective treatment.

Shigellosis (Bacillary Dysentery)

This may be caused by a variety of organisms of the *Shigella* group. In mild cases, symptomatic treatment only is required and there is no evidence that antibiotics produce a more rapid cure. In severe cases, the organism should be cultured and its sensitivity to antibiotics defined. **Ciprofloxacin** or **azithromycin** are the treatments of choice. However, **trimethoprim** or **amoxicillin** can also be used if the culture shows the pathogen is sensitive. **Fluid** and **electrolyte** replacement are important.

Cholera

Cholera is due to the organism *Vibrio cholerae*, which invades the intestine, producing severe and copious diarrhoea and vomiting. This leads to intense dehydration along with sodium and potassium deficiency and is often fatal. The most important part of treatment is to replace the lost water and salts orally or by intravenous infusion.

Although the mainstay of treatment is rehydration, for severe cases, antibiotics are recommended. It is prudent that local antibiotic guidelines are adhered to. The cholera *Vibrio* organism is sensitive to treatment with **tetracycline** and **ciprofloxacin**, which can be used to eradicate the infection and shorten the course of the illness.

In developing countries, where this disease reaches epidemic proportions, large-scale intravenous infusion may be difficult. An important advance has been the discovery that if glucose is added to the electrolyte replacement solution and given orally, water and electrolytes are well-absorbed and intravenous infusion is less often required. As per WHO, 80% of the cases can be successfully treated with oral rehydration salts (ORS). Improvements in water and sanitation is crucial to help improve outbreaks in high-risk areas. ORS (WHO/UNICEF 2006) contains:

- Sodium chloride 2.6 g
- Glucose, anhydrous 13.5 g
- Potassium chloride 1.5 g
- Trisodium citrate, dihydrate 2.9 g
- made up to 1 litre.

The volume given is titrated against the loss in the stools and by vomiting.

Oral cholera vaccines are available, but are of little use as they do not provide complete protection and hygiene measures should still be strictly followed. However, it should be considered for individuals travelling to endemic/epidemic areas who are at increased risk, e.g. occupational risk relief aid workers, cleaners, who may also have limited access to medical care.

Leprosy

Leprosy is a disease of great antiquity and is referred to in the *Bible*. It is caused by the bacterium *Mycobacterium leprae*; these bacteria cause chronic infection of the skin, visceral nerves and other parts of the body. Leprosy has long resisted treatment, but in recent years the introduction of new drugs has made the outlook more hopeful. It is common in areas of poverty due to increased susceptibility to infection due to overcrowding. The incubation of *Mycobacterium leprae* is about 5 years and symptoms can take as long as 20 years to appear. The WHO confirms that the highest cases of new diagnosis are found in India.

Mycobacterium leprae can become resistant to the drugs used in treatment. To prevent the emerging resistance, the WHO recommends a three-drug regimen for *multibacillary leprosy* and a two-drug regimen for *paucibacillary leprosy*. Three drugs are used in leprosy at present: dapsone, clofazimine and rifampicin.

- **Dapsone** is widely used. It is given orally, usually over long periods.
  - *Adverse effects* are uncommon, but include headaches, cyanosis, anaemia and blood dyscrasias.
- **Clofazimine** is useful in treating leprosy and is combined with other agents. It is given orally over long periods.
  - *Adverse effects* are rare, but it may cause pigmentation of the skin.
- **Rifampicin** is also effective against *Mycobacterium leprae*, although resistance may develop.

Malaria

Malaria has been known for thousands of years and is one of the most widespread diseases which afflicts humans. Although it is largely confined to tropical and subtropical zones, air travel has led to its increased frequency in the UK. Malaria is most active in the broad band between the tropics. Increasing tourism to such areas has resulted in malaria presenting as a significant risk. Every year, about 2000 travellers from the UK contract malaria and up to a half dozen deaths occur as a result of infection. Over one-third of such cases occur in those from ethnic groups resident in Britain who have visited their country of origin.

Malaria is caused by a small organism called 'a plasmodium' (Goodyer, 2000). There are four main varieties of plasmodia, which cause malaria in humans. They are:

- *Plasmodium vivax*
- *Plasmodium malariae*
- *Plasmodium ovale*
- *Plasmodium falciparum*.

P. vivax is the commonest cause of the disease. Most forms of malaria cause the less severe and 'benign' disease except *P. falciparum*, which causes the most severe and fatal disease. Rarely, *P. knowlesi* which normally infects animals can occasionally infect humans.

These plasmodia are injected into the bloodstream of humans by the mosquito. They are carried to the liver, where they go through a stage of division known as the exo-erythrocyte stage. After a short period, some plasmodia enter the red cells of the bloodstream. Here they divide in a simple asexual fashion to form more plasmodia, which rupture the red cells and then re-enter further red cells; the breaking up of the red cells corresponds with the rise of temperature with rigor and later sweating, which is so characteristic of the disease.

Other plasmodia that have entered the red cells form male and female gametes. These may be sucked out by the mosquito when it bites, and they then continue the cycle in the infected mosquito. The cycle is shown graphically in Fig. 30.1.

The Treatment of Malaria

It is impossible to give precise instruction as to the best drug or drugs in the treatment of malaria, as this is always changing and may also vary with different forms of malarial infection.

It must be realized that there are two possible ways in which malaria may be attacked by drugs:

- suppressive
- treatment of established disease.

Suppressive treatment means the regular administration of a drug to prevent the clinical manifestation of the disease. Full details are given in the *British National Formulary* (BNF).

The best drug for this purpose varies in different parts of the world. This is because the widespread use of antimalarial drugs has led to the development of

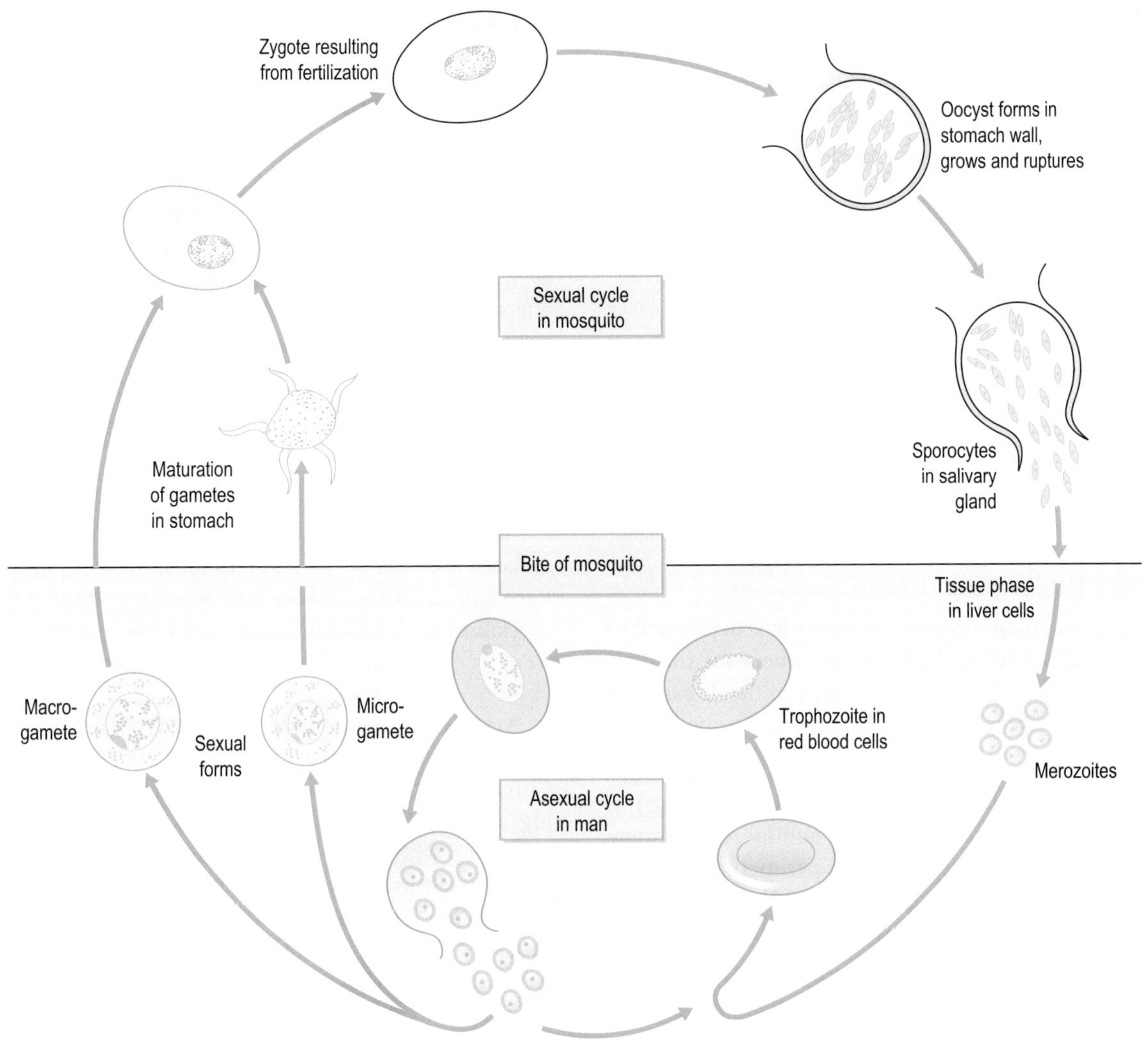

Fig. 30.1 ■ The malarial cycle.

resistant strains of *P. falciparum*, particularly in South-East Asia, but also in South America and parts of Africa. It is wise to obtain up-to-date advice before travelling.

CLINICAL NOTE

Any unexplained fever occurring within 1 year (and especially the first 3 months) of returning from a risk area could be due to malaria.

The chosen drug must be started before entering the malarial area and continued after leaving it, according to specific instructions. In addition, precautions should be taken against mosquito bites, including the use of nets at night, as drug prophylaxis is not totally effective (see also later). Travellers in highly malarious areas who are likely to be remote from medical care should take an emergency treatment kit.

Treatment of Established Disease. The really dangerous type of malaria is caused by *P. falciparum*, which may prove fatal unless treated rapidly. Strains from many parts of the world are resistant to one or more antimalarial drugs and it is safest to regard all *P. falciparum* infections as chloroquine-resistant.

CLINICAL NOTE

Quinine is the preferred drug for treating *P. falciparum* malaria during pregnancy. Recommendations for prevention and treatment are always changing and clinicians are advised to seek up-to-date advice from the Travel Clinic of the Hospital for Tropical Diseases.

Patient information and education surrounding malaria is important and should include advice on new treatments, clothing, nets and hats impregnated with mosquito repellent, as well as advice on new soaps and shampoos that are also effective in reducing mosquito bites.

Drugs Used to Treat Malaria

The appropriate treatment for malaria is dependent on the species causing the infection, where the infection was acquired, as well as the severity of the disease. The drugs effective in treating malaria may be divided into two groups:

- Drugs which act on the **asexual stage** of the malarial parasite in the blood: quinine, chloroquine, proguanil, mefloquine and pyrimethamine
- Drugs which act on the **exo-erythrocyte stage** in the liver and the gametocytes: primaquine.

Quinine is described first, because it was the first effective remedy. It is one of the alkaloids obtained from the bark of the cinchona tree and has been known to be effective against 'fever' for several hundred years.

For some years it was largely replaced by newer antimalarial drugs, but is now proving very useful in the treatment of *P. falciparum* infection when it is resistant to other drugs.

Quinine is given either orally or intravenously. It is well absorbed from the intestine. It suppresses the multiplication of the plasmodia in the bloodstream. It does not, however, have any effect on the gametes or exo-erythrocyte stages of the malarial life cycle; thus, symptoms may recur when quinine is stopped.

Quinine has a number of other actions. It has a depressing action to the heart similar to that of quinidine and can be teratogenic in the first trimester; therefore, it should be avoided in pregnancy unless the benefits are outweighed by the risks. It is sometimes used in the treatment of muscle cramps but this is now rare as it is associated with prolonged QT-interval.

Adverse effects. Adverse effects are common with quinine; the syndrome produced is known as cinchonism. This may occur with large doses. Some people, however, are hypersensitive to the drug and develop toxic effects after small amounts; the chief symptoms are vertigo, tinnitus, deafness and visual disturbances. In addition, it can cause delirium, haemolytic anaemia, thrombocytopenia and renal failure.

CLINICAL NOTE

If quinine is given intravenously, which is required in the treatment of fulminating malignant tertiary malaria, it should be given as quinine dihydrochloride. Receiving the correct advice and instruction from specialist travel nurses or travel clinics will help the traveller decide on the treatment that is right for them.

Artemisinin and its derivatives are obtained from a plant called sweet wormwood, which originated in China. They appear to be rapidly effective in treating severe *P. falciparum* infections, either alone or combined with other antimalarials, and are given by injection, although oral and rectal routes are possible. Artemisinin derivatives include artemether and artesunate. Artemisinin combination therapy is the preferred therapy for mixed malaria infection. **Artesunate** is given for treatment of severe or complicated malaria and is the **first-line treatment**; it is not used for prophylaxis. The medication is generally well-tolerated and its mechanism of action is unclear.

Chloroquine is a useful drug to treat malaria, but resistant strains of *P. falciparum* are common and therefore it is used to treat the other varieties of plasmodium. It can be given orally, intramuscularly or intravenously. It is rapidly absorbed and is stored in various organs of the body, part being destroyed and part excreted in urine. It is effective against the asexual forms of the plasmodia in the bloodstream, but has no effect on the gametes or on the exo-erythrocyte stages. Strains of malaria resistant to chloroquine have appeared in South-East Asia, South America and Central and East Africa.

Adverse effects. These are rare, but include nausea and headaches and, as chloroquine may cause fetal damage, it should not be used during pregnancy.

Mefloquine is effective against chloroquine-resistant *P. falciparum* and is used in parts of the world where this is common. It is excreted very slowly, so single or divided doses once weekly, but not for more than 1 year, are used.

Adverse effects. Nausea and giddiness are fairly common. Psychotic disturbances, including hallucinations, panic attacks and depression can occur and the patient should be warned of this possibility. Mefloquine should not be used during pregnancy or in people with epilepsy.

Atovaquone acts against the different types of malaria, but, if used alone, relapses are common. However, when combined with proguanil, it is effective both in treating *P. falciparum* malaria and also as a prophylactic.

Proguanil is given by mouth. It is rapidly absorbed but disappears rapidly from the bloodstream. It is effective against the bloodstream asexual phase of the plasmodia and also has some action against the gametocytes, and against the exo-erythrocyte stage of *P. falciparum*. It is, however, slower at relieving an acute attack of malaria than is chloroquine and, furthermore, resistant strains of plasmodia have been encountered. Toxicity is very low.

Proguanil is very slow in its antimalarial action and it is therefore largely used as a suppressant.

Doxycycline is effective against resistant *P. falciparum* and has been used with success in the Far East. It should be taken after meals with copious fluids. It is usually combined with quinine when used.

Pyrimethamine is effective against the asexual bloodstream phase of the malarial parasite but is too slow to be used in treating an acute attack. Owing to the emergence of resistant strains, it is now only used in combination, e.g. pyrimethamine/sulfadoxine (*Fansidar*). It is associated with significant adverse effects and must be discontinued at appearance of rash (as associated with Stevens–Johnson syndrome), as well as toxic epidermal necrolysis and development of active infection. It should also not be used in patients with megaloblastic anaemia caused by folate deficiency. Pyrimethamine/sulfadoxine remains on the WHO essential list of medication for malaria treatment but has been discontinued in the UK.

It can be seen that all the drugs so far described, with the possible partial exception of proguanil, while effectively suppressing the asexual bloodstream phase of the malaria organism and relieving acute symptoms, are ineffective against the exo-erythrocyte stage in the liver and against the gametocytes. This is particularly important when the malaria is caused by *P. vivax* or *P. malariae*, as a relapse may occur on stopping treatment. In these types of malaria, the initial treatment should be followed by a drug which acts against the parasites in the exo-erythrocyte stage.

Primaquine is effective against the exo-erythrocyte stage and against the gametocytes. It is not free from toxic effects and may produce nausea and vomiting. It is not used alone in the treatment of the acute malarial attack, but may follow treatment of *P. vivax* with chloroquine, when it is particularly valuable in eradicating benign tertian malaria. Relapses will not occur unless there is reinfection.

Before starting treatment, it is important to test the patient for G6PD deficiency, an inherited disorder of the red blood cells, which results in severe haemolysis with primaquine and some other drugs, which can be fatal.

Leishmaniasis (Kala-Azar)

There are several varieties of kala-azar caused by closely related organisms. These organisms may invade the spleen, liver, lymph glands and bone marrow, producing a generalized disease with constitutional symptoms or a local ulcerative lesion. This disease may also complicate HIV infection.

Leishmaniasis is caused by a small protozoan organism transmitted by the bite of a sandfly. It is found in Africa, South America and the Mediterranean. It is often missed by physicians who are not familiar with this condition, as relatively few cases are reported annually in travellers from the UK.

The most useful drug for treating leishmaniasis are those which contain antimony. They are believed to interfere with enzymes within the parasite.

Sodium stibogluconate is given intravenously or by intramuscular injection. Early non-inflamed lesions can be treated with intralesional injections. The patient usually responds within 2 weeks and should be restored to full health within 2 months.

Adverse effects. Effects include irritation at the site of injection, muscle aches and cardiotoxicity with arrhythmias.

Paromomycin (unlicensed), an aminoglycoside antibiotic, is also effective, either alone or combined with sodium stibogluconate.

Adverse effects. Adverse effects are uncommon but include ototoxicity.

Amphotericin given intravenously, can be used for visceral leishmaniasis in patients who are unresponsive to antimonial.

Schistosomiasis (Bilharzia)

This disease is caused by a parasitic flatworm, which inhabits the veins of the bladder and the lower bowel, leading to haematuria and rectal bleeding.

Praziquantel has now emerged as the most useful drug. It is effective against all types of the disease and, unlike formerly used drugs, it appears free from serious adverse effects.

ANTHELMINTICS

Anthelmintics are drugs used to treat worm infestations. Although such infestations, with the possible exception of threadworms, are not common in the UK, they may occur in immigrants, being endemic in some regions of the world, and are of great medical and economic importance. The anthelmintics are a diverse group of substances with widely differing properties and they will be described under the headings of the type of infestation they are used to treat.

Threadworms

Threadworms (*Enterobius vermicularis*) appear like short lengths of thread. They live in the caecal region of the gut and the females migrate to the anus, where they lay eggs and provoke intense itching. The resulting scratching leads to the hands becoming contaminated with eggs, which may then be transferred to food, and thus further infestation occurs.

General cleanliness and scrubbing of the nails before meals is important in treating this disorder.

It must be remembered that the whole family of an infected patient must be examined for infestation, as it is common to find several members of a family harbouring worms, and reinfection will occur unless the worms are eradicated from the whole family.

Mebendazole as a single dose is effective. It is unlicensed in children under 2 years (but can be given to children over 6 months old) or during pregnancy and, rarely, can cause nausea and diarrhoea. A second dose can be given after 3 weeks, as reinfection is common. It is available without prescription.

Strongyloides Stercoralis

This worm, which is common in the tropics, lives in the intestines. The larvae of *Strongyloides stercoralis* can penetrate the anal skin and thus reinfect the host, so infection can last for a long time. Usually they only cause mild intestinal symptoms, but if the patient is immunosuppressed (i.e. as a result of treatment with large doses of steroids or has HIV), widespread penetration of the bowel occurs, which may be fatal.

Ivermectin (unlicensed use) daily for 2 days is effective and is better-tolerated with fewer adverse events but with similar cure rates in comparison to **thiabendazole** (Henriquez-Camacho et al., 2016).

Tapeworms

There are two common types of tapeworm, *Taenia solium* and *Taenia saginata*. Both these worms inhabit the small intestine of humans, where they may reach several feet in length. They consist of a head, which is embedded in the wall of the intestine and a body consisting of a large number of segments. These segments, which contain eggs, are shed and pass out in the faeces.

The eggs may then infect an animal host, which is the pig in the case of *Taenia solium* and the bullock in the case of *Taenia saginata*. In the animal's gastrointestinal tract the larval form is released and migrates, via the bloodstream, throughout the body, where it remains until the animal is killed; the meat is eaten by humans and reinfection occurs.

There are several drugs which can be used to treat tapeworms, the most effective being **niclosamide** (unlicensed). No preparation is required. In the morning, the drug is chewed and swallowed on an empty stomach. After 1 h, the dose is repeated. This is followed 3 h later by a saline purge. In *Taenia solium* infestation, a more powerful laxative should be used as it is important to clear all the ova from the gut. Treatment may be preceded by **metoclopramide** to minimize the risk of vomiting.

The drug appears to have minimal side-effects and acts by actually killing the worm.

Alternatively, a single dose of **praziquantel** (unlicensed) is effective.

Roundworms

The roundworm (*Ascaris lumbricoides*) is similar to a pale-coloured earthworm. It lives in the small intestine and its eggs are passed out in the faeces. If reinfection occurs, the larval forms are liberated in the gastrointestinal tract and pass via the bloodstream to the lungs. They then migrate up the trachea to the pharynx and are swallowed, thus completing the cycle.

Piperazine is useful for treating roundworms. It paralyses the muscle of the worm, which is passed through the faeces alive via the rectum. A single dose of the elixir for an adult is effective and should be repeated after 14 days. Alternatively, one *Pripsen* sachet (containing piperazine + sennosides) may be used, the purgative helping to clear the bowel of worms.

Mebendazole twice-daily for 3 days is an alternative.

Hookworms

The hookworm, although not seen in the UK, is extremely common in tropical and subtropical countries in both the Old and New World.

This worm lives in the small intestine of humans; the fertilized eggs are passed out in the faeces and develop into larvae in the soil. The larvae penetrate the skin and pass via the bloodstream to the lung. Here they enter the bronchial tree and migrate to the intestinal tract via the trachea. Severe infestation can cause iron deficiency anaemia.

Mebendazole twice daily for 3 days is effective. It should not be used during pregnancy and is unlicensed for children under 2 years old. In addition to anthelminthic medication, iron supplements may also need to be prescribed for the anaemia.

Filariasis

The parasitic worms *Loa loa*, which causes subcutaneous swellings, and *Wuchereria bancrofti*, another filarial parasite, which causes elephantiasis, may be eradicated by **diethylcarbamazine** (unlicensed).

Onchocerciasis (River Blindness)

Onchocerciasis (river blindness) is caused by *Onchocerca volvulus*, a parasitic worm that can live for up to 14 years in the human body. It is mainly prevalent in Africa, although it does occur in Canada and the USA during wet seasons, and in Latin America and the Yemen. It is the leading cause of infection-mediated blindness. The host is infected through the bite of the black fly (family *Simuliidae*), whose saliva contains the larvae of the parasite. The larvae migrate to the subcutaneous tissues, including those of the eye, and there mature into adult worms. The host's immune system attacks the parasite, causing tissue damage. Symptoms include skin itchiness and skin rashes. Cattle are also infected through fly bites and may die from the disease. If left untreated, blindness can result.

Treatment is with **ivermectin** (unlicensed), which is very effective, although there are some reports of resistance development in flies. A single dose is given followed by follow-up doses at 6–12-month intervals until the infestation is eliminated.

REFERENCES AND FURTHER READING

Boyne, L., 2005. Providing a travel health service in primary care. Pract. Nurse 30 (8), 25–28.

Bradwisch, S.A., 2013. Malaria: has your patient travelled recently? Nurs. Made Incred. Easy 11 (4), 1–3.

Davies, H.G., Bowman, C., Luby, S.P., 2017. Cholera management and prevention. J. Infect. 74 (Suppl. 1), S66–S73.

Gates, B., 2020. Responding to Covid-19 – a once in a century pandemic? N. Engl. J. Med. 382 (18), 1677–1679.

Gray, D.J., Ross, A.G., Li, Y.S., McManus, D.P., 2011. Diagnosis and management of schistosomiasis. BMJ 342, d2651.

Goodyer, L., 2000. Malaria. Pharmaceut. J. 264, 405.

Henriquez-Camacho, C., Gotuzzo, E., Echevarria, J., et al., 2016. Ivermectin versus albendazole or thiabendazole for Strongyloides stercoralis infection. Cochrane Database Syst. Rev. (1), CD007745.

Lalloo, D.G., Shingadia, D., Bell, D.J., et al., 2016. UK malaria treatment guidelines 2016. J. Infect. 72 (6), 635–649.

PHE, 2013. The Green Book: Immunisation against Infectious Disease. Public Health England. https://www.gov.uk/government/collections/immunisation-against-infectious-disease-the-green-book.

RCN, 2014. Delivering Travel Health Services: RCN Guidance for Nursing Staff. Royal College of Nursing. https://www.trectravel-health.co.uk/wp-content/uploads/2014/03/RCN-Travel-Health-Guidelines.pdf.

Ryan, E.T., Wilson, M.E., Kain, K.C., 2002. Illness after international travel. N. Engl. J. Med. 347 (7), 505–516.

Scaggs Huang, F.A., Schlaudecker, E., 2018. Fever in the returning traveler. Infect. Dis. Clin. North Am. 32 (1), 163–188.

Turner, H.C., Walker, M., Lustigman, S., et al., 2015. Human onchocerciasis: modelling the potential long-term consequences of a vaccination programme. PLoS Negl. Trop. Dis. 9 (7), e0003938.

Wasihun, A.G., Wlekidan, L.N., Gebremariam, S.A., et al., 2015. Diagnosis and treatment of typhoid fever and associated prevailing drug resistance in northern Ethiopia. Int. J. Infect. Dis. 35, 96–102.

Wendt, S., Trawinski, H., Schubert, S., et al., 2019. The diagnosis and treatment of pinworm infection. Dtsch. Arztebl. Int. 116 (13), 213–219.

Winner, D., 2017. Ending Malaria: How Nursing Research and Training Is Playing a Part. Seed Global Health. https://seedglobalhealth.org/ending-malaria-nursing-research-training-playing-part.

WHO/U.N.I.C.E.F., 2006. Oral Rehydration Salts: Production of the New ORS. https://apps.who.int/iris/bitstream/handle/10665/69227/WHO_FCH_CAH_06.1.pdf.

WHO, 2012. International Travel and Health. World Health Organization, Geneva. https://www.who.int/publications/i/item/9789241580472.

Xavier, G., 2006. Management of typhoid and paratyphoid fevers. Nursing Times 102 (17), 49–52.

USEFUL WEBSITES

Medscape. https://reference.medscape.com/slideshow/travel-diseases-6006331.

NICE. Clinical knowledge summaries: Malaria. https://cks.nice.org.uk/topics/malaria.

Public Health Scotland. Fit For Travel. https://www.fitfortravel.nhs.uk.

WHO. International Travel and Health. https://www.who.int.

31 DRUGS USED IN THE TREATMENT OF OPHTHALMOLOGICAL DISEASES

CHAPTER OUTLINE

LEARNING OBJECTIVES

At the end of this chapter, the reader should be able to:

- list the different types of local preparations used in the eye
- state which antibiotics and antivirals are used to treat conditions affecting the eyes and list some of the more common infections treated
- explain what is meant by protozoan infections and how they are treated
- list steroids used topically to treat eye conditions
- explain what is meant by mydriasis and miosis; give examples of drugs that produce these effects and their uses for patients with eye conditions
- describe the different types of glaucoma and how they are treated
- list the local anaesthetics that can be topically applied to the eyes
- list that stains are used when the eyes are examined and explain their purposes

STRUCTURE OF THE EYE

The structure of the eye and orbit are shown in Fig. 31.1.

Conditions Affecting the Eye

Eyecare includes eye disorders and their prevention, treatment and patient education. This is an important area of practice. Eye problems and traumatic disorders of the eye account for over 6% of all attendances at Accident and Emergency Departments in the UK, while worldwide, approximately 5,000,000 blinding injuries occur annually. Eye disorders are particularly common in older people and as the population ages, the number of people affected is increasing rapidly. Examples are cataracts, glaucoma and macular degeneration. Glaucoma and macular degeneration are both chronic conditions and it is very important that patients should be able to apply their own medication if possible, in order to maintain independence. Cataract removal is a common operation, now usually undertaken as a day-case procedure. The nurse plays an important role preparing patients undergoing cataract extraction preoperatively and teaching them how to use local medication during the postoperative period at home.

CLINICAL NOTE

Drugs used in the treatment of osteoporosis may cause adverse events affecting the eye. A retrospective review carried out in Canada cited a higher incidence of both uveitis and scleritis in people who were prescribed bisphosphonates (Etminan et al., 2012). Patients on this medication should be regularly screened for symptoms of intraocular inflammation, including redness, blurred vision and pain.

Local Use of Drugs on the Eye: Types of Applications

The following preparations are used in the local treatment of eye diseases:

- eye lotions
- eye drops
- eye ointments
- subconjunctival injections
- injections into the anterior chamber at operation.

Whenever administering local preparations to the eye, it is of paramount importance to ensure that the eye to receive treatment is clearly designated. Patients going to theatre for eye operations will usually have an arrow marked on the forehead pointing to the eye to be treated to avoid any confusion. Often only one eye is to be treated or the two eyes are to be treated differently. For example, after an operation for angle closure glaucoma in one eye, it may be necessary to dilate the pupil with mydriatic drugs. Instilling mydriatic eye drops into the incorrect eye could impair vision in the normal eye and be very disabling for the patient.

Eye Lotions

Occasionally referred to as *collyrium*, these are used to wash foreign material and irritants from the eye, and some have a mild antiseptic action. They are applied using a giving set, eye bath or a soft plastic irrigation bottle. In an emergency, the priority is to administer treatment quickly to the contaminated eye before damage is done to the conjunctiva and cornea.

The patient should lie back or sit in a chair with the head extended back. The lotion should preferably be warmed to body temperature and before washing the eye, the lotion should be run into the medial

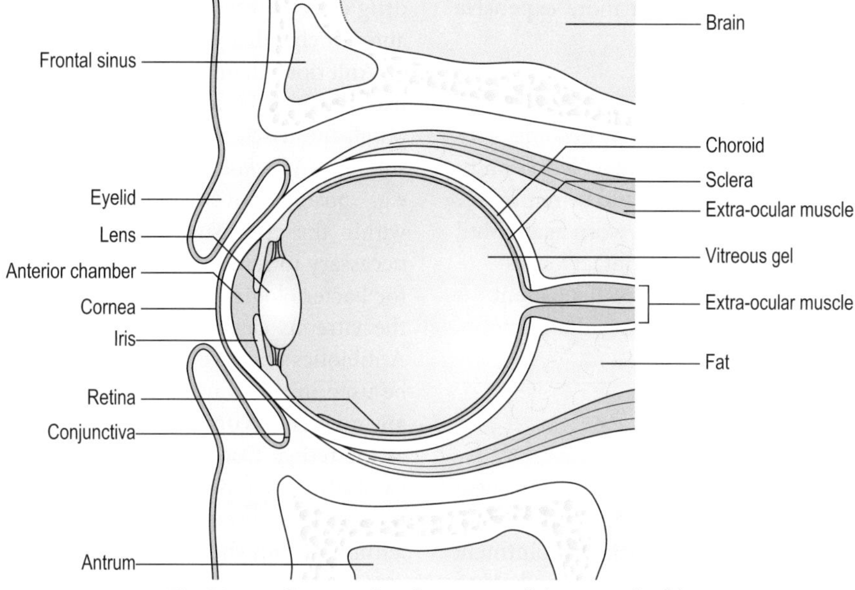

Fig. 31.1 ■ Cross-sectional anatomy of the eye and orbit.

canthus, the lids being firmly separated by the fingers. A towel held by the patient close to the face will absorb the runoff. This is less unpleasant than pouring the lotion directly onto the cornea. The lotion should be irrigated slowly but steadily from the irrigation receptacle, the patient being instructed to move the eyes in all directions.

In emergency cases, as in chemical contamination, it is better to use plenty of running cold tap water at once rather than to lose time in starting the treatment. The irrigating fluid most commonly used in the clinical situation is normal saline. Alkaline chemical contamination can penetrate the eye by saponifying cell membranes, causing local production of soap and causing erosion to the cornea, tissue destruction and secondary vascular thrombosis; therefore, immediate treatment should be sought. At least 1 litre of normal saline solution should be used. Afterward, use litmus paper to check the pH of the eye. If it is over pH 7, repeat with another irrigation of 1 litre of normal saline solution until the pH is 7 or below.

In cases of corneal damage, topical **citrate** and **potassium ascorbate** eye drops can improve the prognosis, though patients should be warned they do produce stinging. They can be used for acid or alkali burns to the cornea and are often supplemented with oral **ascorbic acid** (vitamin C) at high doses of 1.5 g/day to promote healing.

Eye Drops

Occasionally referred to as *guttae*, some drugs can be applied to the eyes by means of drops, which should be instilled into the lower conjunctival sac. The patient should look upwards and the lower lid is held down with the finger. A drop is instilled into the 'gutter' that is thus formed, and the patient is then told to close the eye for a short while and the excess is wiped away Without these instructions, patients often tilt their heads back and try to aim drops at the open eye. They generally miss! When two or more eye-drop preparations are used at the same time of day, an interval of 3–5 min should be left between instilling two preparations, in order to avoid dilution and the overflow effect.

All drops and ointment should be sterile when supplied, and once opened, can no longer be considered so.

Single dose unit packs are particularly useful for patients who require medication over long periods and who may develop sensitivity to benzalkonium chloride, the preservative present in most eye drops.

However, unit doses packs are a lot more expensive and are wasteful of packaging.

CLINICAL NOTE

Drugs or preservatives in eye drops may become absorbed into or onto hydrophilic contact lenses and cause irritation. Therefore, lenses should be removed before eye drops are instilled and not worn again until the treatment is finished. Similarly, contact lenses should not be used with eye ointments. If a patient develops an eye infection, contact lenses should not be worn until it has resolved.

Eye Ointments

Occasionally referred to as *oculentum*, these are usually supplied in 4 or 5 g tubes with a long plastic nozzle. To apply, the lower lid is pulled down and the ointment is placed in the lower fornix of the eye. About half an inch or 1 cm of ointment is squeezed from the tube at each application. It is important to twist the tube upward so that the strip of ointment remains in the fornix as the tube is moved away from the eye.

Subconjunctival Injections

This method of application is used to immediately obtain a high concentration of drugs such as anti-infective agents, corticosteroids or mydriatics in the anterior chamber. This would be appropriate in the treatment of an acute intraocular infection. This treatment is painful, and the eye must first be thoroughly anaesthetized by the instillation of several drops of local anaesthetic. The injection is given with a hypodermic syringe and a fine needle. Some drugs are manufactured in a depot form and are bound to a base substance from which they are released slowly. For example, *Depo-Medrone* (methylprednisolone acetate) can be used as a steroid preparation for the local treatment of iridocyclitis (inflammation of the iris and ciliary body). It is given as a subconjunctival injection and its action is continuous over a period of 3–4 days.

Intracameral Injections

For some conditions, it may be desirable to achieve high therapeutic concentrations of antibiotic drugs with a minimum of delay. This calls for delivery of the drug directly into the globe of the eye, either into the anterior chamber or the vitreous cavity.

Anterior chamber administration is frequently used during cataract operations, when, to constrict the pupil, the iris is irrigated directly with acetylcholine solution (*Miochol-E*). In severe intraocular infections, e.g. postoperative endophthalmitis (inflammation within the eye, usually due to infection), it may be necessary to remove a sample of the vitreous humour for bacteriological examination. It is timely to inject the vitreous cavity with broad-spectrum antibiotics. Antibiotics effective against a range of organisms can be used in this way, although care is needed to avoid any toxic effects on delicate intraocular structures such as the retina. Consequently, the injections need to be carefully prepared and used only in the recommended dosage, in volumes not exceeding 0.05–0.1 mL, and administration should generally be under sterile theatre conditions.

TYPES OF DRUGS USED

The following types of drug are in frequent use in the treatment of eye disorders:

- anti-infectives:
  - antibiotics
  - antifungals
  - antivirals
- steroids and other antiinflammatory drugs
- those which affect pupil size
- those used in the treatment of glaucoma
- local anaesthetics
- stains
- miscellaneous preparations.

Drugs can be administered to the eye by either local or systemic routes.

ANTIBACTERIAL AGENTS

The three main classes of anti-infectives used in the eye are: antibacterials (also known as antibiotics), antivirals and antifungals. There are also antiamoebics and other antiprotozoals. While many of the dose forms are available from proprietary manufacturers as standard drugs, some must be ordered from special manufacturers who manufacture limited quantities in batches.

TABLE 31.1

Antibacterial Agents Used in the Eye[a]

Drug(s)	Spectrum
Amikacin	Gram-negative, *Mycobacteria* (Specialist use)
Bacitracin zinc + polymyxin B sulphate	Broad, Gram-negative, coliforms, *Pseudomonas*
Ceftazidime	Broad, *Pseudomonas*
Cefuroxime	Broad, *Staphylococcus*
Chloramphenicol	Broad
Ciprofloxacin, levofloxacin, moxifloxacin, **ofloxacin**	Broad, Gram-negative, *Pseudomonas* (not moxifloxacin)
Azithromycin	Broad, *Streptococcus, Chlamydia*
Framycetin sulphate	Broad, Gram-negative
Fusidic acid	Staphylococcus
Gentamicin, tobramycin	Broad, Gram-negative, *Pseudomonas*
Neomycin sulphate + gramicidin + polymixin B sulphate	Broad
Trimethoprim + polymixin B sulphate	Broad, Gram-negative, coliforms
Vancomycin	*Staphylococcus, Clostridium*

[a]More commonly used agents are in bold.

The antibacterial agents are summarized in Table 31.1.

Antibiotics are used to treat a wide range of eye infections and they may be administered in three ways:

- Drops are satisfactory for superficial inflammation such as conjunctivitis, but rapid dilution occurs because of the tears. The drops should be instilled at 2 hourly intervals at least, if a reasonable concentration of antibiotic is to be maintained. Frequency of application may be reduced when improvement is noted.
- Ointments release the antibiotic more slowly and their action is helped by the eye being covered; they are especially useful for overnight use.
- Subconjunctival injection is the best way of ensuring a rapid and high concentration of anti biotic within the anterior ocular segment. The maximum volume that can be injected at one time is 1.0 mL.

Although, owing to the accessibility of the eye, diseases of the anterior segment can usually be effectively treated by means of the local administration of drugs, for those diseases which affect the posterior part, or the deeper intraocular structures, systemic administration is generally necessary.

Eye infections may be due to a variety of agents, both bacterial and viral. The correct antibiotic in the case of bacterial infections can be selected as a result of clinical observation and should be validated by bacterial or viral diagnostic tests.

Chloramphenicol and the quinolones are widely used in the treatment of superficial eye infections. They are active against a broad spectrum of bacteria and are particularly suitable for local administration as this avoids systemic toxicity. They include:

- **chloramphenicol 0.5% drops or 1.0% ointment**
- **ciprofloxacin 0.3% drops and ointment**
- **levofloxacin 0.5% drops**
- **ofloxacin 0.3% drops.**

These drugs are active against both Gram-positive and Gram-negative organisms.

Chloramphenicol is widely used as first-line empirical therapy in most eye infections. It functions by inhibiting peptidyl transferase, thus preventing peptide bond formation causing misreading of messenger RNA, which leaves the bacteria unable to synthesize proteins vital to their growth.

Ofloxacin, **levofloxacin** and **ciprofloxacin**, members of the quinolone group, have a broad spectrum of antibacterial action, including activity against *Pseudomonas aeruginosa*. The fluoroquinolones work by inhibiting DNA gyrase, an enzyme necessary to separate replicated DNA, thereby inhibiting cell division. They have a broader spectrum of activity than chloramphenicol and fewer local side-effects than gentamicin, while maintaining a similar spectrum of activity to those agents. Ofloxacin rivals chloramphenicol as a general prophylactic antibiotic.

Antibiotics of the **penicillin** group are rarely, if ever, used as local eye applications as they have a marked tendency to cause allergic reactions. However, they have an important place in the treatment of spreading infections of the eyelids, which are commonly of staphylococcal origin (provided the infection has not developed resistance). In such cases, the infection is deep in the tissues, requiring systemic rather than local administration. In general, a broad-spectrum penicillin is best, but if the infection is acquired in hospital, one of the penicillinase-resistant types is preferable. β-Lactam antibiotics work by inhibiting the formation of peptidoglycan cross-links in the bacterial cell wall. The β-lactam part of the molecule of penicillin binds to the enzyme (DD-transpeptidase) that links the peptidoglycan molecules in bacteria, and this weakens the cell wall of the bacterium, leading to cell death.

Azithromycin eye drops (and orally, or in combination with oral doxycycline) is used to treat chlamydial conjunctivitis and trachoma, but has a broad spectrum of activity.

Sodium fusidate is particularly active against penicillin-resistant staphylococci. It has the property of being concentrated in bone and other connective tissues, including the sclera of the eye and the vitreous, and is therefore useful in treating intraocular infections, especially those acquired in the operating theatre, which can often be due to resistant organisms. **Fusidic acid** is also used as eye drops in gel, which liquefies on contact with the conjunctiva, for a variety of superficial infections. It has been shown to be as effective as other commonly used antibiotics for first-line use in community-acquired bacterial conjunctivitis, and the twice daily dosage is an advantage when treating children (Doughty and Dutton, 2006). Fusidic acid works by interfering with bacterial protein synthesis, preventing the translocation of the elongation factor G (EF-G) from the ribosome, thus inhibiting bacterial replication.

Prophylaxis against postoperative infection is a routine part of eye surgery. Common procedures such as removal of cataracts are now performed as day-cases. It is important to ensure that the eye is protected from infection; therefore, broad-spectrum agents are preferred, such as **gentamicin**, which interrupts protein synthesis in Gram-negative bacteria, and **cefuroxime**, a cephalosporin with effectiveness against both Gram-positive and Gram-negative organisms.

Bacterial Conjunctivitis

Conjunctivitis is a common complaint with various causes. The bacterial infection is usually caused by *Streptococcus pneumoniae* or staphylococci; therefore a topical antibiotic effective against Gram-positive bacteria is indicated.

Empirical treatment is with **chloramphenicol** eye drops, every 4 h, but more florid infections may require more frequent application. Chloramphenicol ointment may be used at night. The alternative is **fusidic acid** eye drops twice daily.

Acute Intraocular Infections

In acute bacterial infection of the eye, much of the damage occurs as a result of the inflammatory response rather than the direct activity of the bacteria. Consequently, it is important to use steroids at the same time as effective antibiotics.

A particular problem exists in severe intraocular infections such as those following eye surgery. In post-surgical infection, it is essential that vigorous antibiotic and antiinflammatory treatment is started without delay to prevent damage to delicate eye structures and consequent loss of vision. As time cannot be allowed to obtain the results of bacterial investigations before commencing treatment, a combination of broad-spectrum antibiotics and steroids can be used by both subconjunctival and systemic routes and even by direct intravitreal injection, together with a mydriatic (a drug that causes the pupil to dilate). The ophthalmologist should be consulted for the combinations and doses to be used.

Systemic administration of antibiotics can be either orally or by injection. Their use may be indicated in spreading infections involving the eye, the eyelids and ocular adnexa (adnexa means adjoining parts) such as the lacrimal sac. Sepsis around the eye, in particular in the vicinity of the internal angular vein, is of particular clinical importance, as it may lead to a septic cavernous sinus thrombosis in the brain. Cellulitis around the eye therefore normally requires intravenous antibiotics.

Other Antibiotics

In certain severe cases of intraocular infection, the following antibiotics have been used successfully when injected directly into the vitreous. Some of these antibiotic preparations are only available in specialist units and hospitals. Preparations of a suitable strength for intraocular injection are not generally available and the following must be diluted following local guidelines devised by specialist practitioners and pharmacists.

Vancomycin is effective against Gram-positive bacteria. Vancomycin prevents incorporation of N-acetylmuramic acid (NAM)- and N-acetylglucosamine

(NAG)-peptide subunits into the peptidoglycan matrix, which forms the major structural component of Gram-positive cell walls but is ineffective against most Gram-negative bacteria.

Ceftazidime is active against Gram-negative organisms and can be used simultaneously with vancomycin. Like other cephalosporins, it disrupts the synthesis of the peptidoglycan layer of bacterial cell walls, which is needed for cell wall structural integrity.

Amikacin is mainly used to treat infections due to *Mycobacteria* organisms; its toxicity to the intraocular tissues precludes wider use against Gram-negative infections. It works by binding to the bacterial ribosomal subunit, causing misreading of mRNA and leaving the bacteria unable to synthesize proteins vital to their growth.

ANTIFUNGAL DRUGS

None of the antifungal preparations described here are currently licensed for or commercially available as eye medications in the UK. Fungal infections are relatively rare compared with bacterial and viral eye infections. Symptoms are likely to present as keratitis or endophthalmitis in patients who are immunocompromised. Keratitis is usually susceptible to the imidazole class of antifungal. The drops should be applied topically every hour initially and under specialist supervision.

Imidazoles such as **clotrimazole**, **econazole** and **miconazole** inhibit the enzyme cytochrome P450 14α-demethylase, which converts lanosterol to ergosterol required for fungal cell wall synthesis. Fungal endophthalmitis is more resistant to topical application and **amphotericin** is used via intravitreal injection as well as topically; systemic therapy may also be required. It is effective against organisms such as *Aspergillus*, *Fusarium* and *Candida* species. **Voriconazole, fluconazole and flucytosine** have been used by intravitreal injection for severe fungal infections; they may also be used systemically.

ANTIVIRAL AGENTS

The antivirals used are listed in Table 31.2.

Viral eye infections can be caused by herpes simplex and herpes zoster (shingles).

TABLE 31.2
Antiviral Agents Used in the Eye

Drug	Spectrum
Aciclovir	Herpes simplex, varicella zoster
Ganciclovir	Herpes simplex. (Retinal inserts can be used to treat CMV retinitis)
Trifluridine (Trifluorothymidine, F3T)	Herpes simplex. (Not routinely available in UK)

As a treatment for ocular herpes simplex infections, **aciclovir** has become the drug of choice. It is highly effective when applied in the form of a 3% ointment 5 times daily and has minimal, if any, toxic effects. Its action can be supplemented by oral administration and this may well be helpful in cases of herpes simplex keratitis which have been previously treated in error with preparations containing steroids, which greatly reduce the rate of healing. Aciclovir is also commonly available as a 5% topical cream for the treatment of cutaneous cold sores and this preparation should not be confused with the ophthalmic ointment, as it is not suitable for use in the eye.

Aciclovir is a prodrug converted into acycloguanosine monophosphate (acyclo-GMP) by viral thymidine kinase. Subsequently, it is converted into an active form, acycloguanosine triphosphate (acyclo-GTP), by cellular kinases. Acyclo-GTP is a potent inhibitor of viral DNA polymerase and is incorporated into viral DNA, resulting in chain termination.

Herpes zoster virus may affect the eye, especially when it involves the nasociliary branch of the ophthalmic division of the trigeminal nerve. Provided that treatment is commenced at the first appearance of the vesicular rash, aciclovir can significantly reduce the severity of this painful disorder. For this indication, higher oral doses are required, and if started promptly, shorten the time before cutaneous healing occurs and materially reduce the pain in the acute stage and possibly also the post-herpetic pain, which often lasts for many years after healing has taken place.

Trifluridine (trifluorothymidine, F3T) has good activity against herpes simplex; consequently it may be used for herpes simplex keratitis and stromal herpes simplex keratitis. As it is not available as a proprietary drug, its use is mainly limited to specialist eye units, but it can be obtained from the pharmacy manufacturing department of specialist eye hospitals. It is not a particularly stable preparation and must be freshly prepared and kept refrigerated.

Ganciclovir (0.15% eye gel) is an alternative herpes simplex keratitis. It can also be given by local intravitreal injection or as an intraocular, slow-release implant (available as an imported preparation) for cytomegalovirus retinitis. It is teratogenic and effective contraception should be used during and after use in women and men.

ANTIPROTOZOAN DRUGS

Onchocerciasis

Onchocerciasis is a protozoan infection of the eye, which is common in some tropical countries in Africa and South America. The disease is spread by flies which transfer the microfilariae from one human host, who harbours the adult worms in cutaneous nodules, to another individual, in whom they spread throughout the body. In the eye, they set up inflammation in both the superficial and deeper tissues. Typically, they can be seen with a microscope, swimming in the aqueous humour. The drug of choice for treating this disorder is **ivermectin**, which is a semi-synthetic macrocyclic lactone. It binds and activates glutamate-gated chloride channels (GluCls) present in neurones and myocytes, resulting in parasite neuromuscular paralysis and death. It is readily available in many tropical countries; it is unlicensed for oral use in the UK and may need to be specially ordered.

Acanthamoeba Keratitis

With the increased popularity of hydrophilic (soft) contact lenses, infections of the cornea with *Acanthamoeba* keratitis, a sight-threatening condition, have increased in frequency. The risk is increased if daily care instructions are not followed scrupulously, and particularly if hands are not washed before handling, and if storage solutions are reused. Overnight wear (even of lenses designed for this) is associated with increased risk. Daily disposable lenses have the lowest risk. The amoeba occurs in soil and water. Diagnosis is made by microscopic examination of deep corneal scrapings and treatment is with the drug **polyhexanide**, also known as **polyhexamethylene biguanide (PHMB)**. This drug is an antiseptic agent. It is chemically related to **chlorhexidine** and **hexamide**, which have also been used to treat acanthamoeba. These drugs are made up in 0.02% strength and are applied as eye drops. Treatment is lengthy and recurrence is not unusual.

Propamidine is also sometimes used. It is available over-the-counter as *Brolene* eye drops and ointment. Treatment should be under specialist supervision and be prolonged to ensure that the amoebic cysts are eradicated. Frequent use over long periods can produce epithelial toxicity.

Steroids and Non-steroidal Antiinflammatory Drugs (NSAIDs)

One of the many commonly used steroids for local ophthalmic application is **betamethasone disodium phosphate** (*Betnesol*). This can be used in 0.1% drops or ointment. In some preparations the steroid is combined with an antibiotic, e.g. *Betnesol-N* contains neomycin. Application can be as frequent as hourly, and drugs of this type are used to suppress a wide variety of inflammatory processes within the eye. Steroids should not be used indiscriminately as their improper use may be followed by serious complications. This is particularly so for infective processes, which may spread rapidly if steroids are given without a suitable antibacterial agent. For similar reasons, they are rarely applied to virus infections of the eye and never in the presence of active herpes simplex (dendritic ulcer).

Administration of dilute steroid eye drops is often beneficial in the treatment of herpetic corneal infection, when corneal stromal opacification threatens and ***when the viral activity has already been contained***. For this purpose, **prednisolone** eye drops of 0.1% administered 2 or 3 times daily can, by suppressing the antibody–antigen reaction in the deeper layers of the cornea, prevent serious loss of vision. For local administration in the form of eye drops, **dexamethasone** (*Maxidex*) is often used. This drug has good penetration into the eye and is useful in the routine treatment of inflammatory disorders such as iritis. It is available in 1% suspension and may be combined with neomycin and polymyxin B sulphate, available as *Maxitrol*. In severe ocular inflammation, a subconjunctival injection of **methylprednisolone acetate** (*Depo-Medrone*) produces a continuous level of steroids in the anterior chamber for several days.

In inflammation of the posterior uvea (choroiditis), it is necessary to administer steroids systemically, as local applications do not readily reach the site of the disease. In this case, **prednisolone** may be used and is generally given in a very high dosage for a short period, followed by a rapid reduction at first, which is tailed off more slowly.

All steroid drugs, whether administered locally or systemically, can result in a rise in intraocular pressure. **Fluorometholone** and the more recently developed steroid **rimexolone** have lower penetration than some of the older steroids; they are therefore less likely to produce side-effects.

One of the challenges in the use of steroid eye drops is using topical steroids for superficial conditions and deeply penetrating steroids for posterior conditions. **Hydrocortisone** has superior penetration into the aqueous humour following topical application than **hydrocortisone acetate**. However, **prednisolone acetate** has superior penetration into the aqueous humour following topical application than **prednisolone**. Penetration of all steroids is increased if the cornea is abraded. Side-effects include corneal oedema, raised intraocular pressure, delayed healing and corneal ulceration.

For superficial inflammation of allergic origin such as vernal conjunctivitis, mast-cell stabilizing drugs such as **sodium cromoglicate** and **nedocromil sodium** are often useful. To be effective, the concentration in the conjunctival sac must be maintained at a high level, necessitating frequent or continuous administration. This must be done over the entire period of exposure to the antigen, i.e. throughout the pollen season or on exposure to grass seeds. Histamine (H1) receptor antagonists available as eye drops, such as **antazoline** 0.5% (commercially available in combination with a vasoconstrictor xylometazoline 0.05%), **azelastine** 0.05%, **emedastine** 0.05%, **epinastine** 0.05%, **lodoxamide** 0.1%, **olopatadine** 0.1% and **ketotifen** 0.025%, are used in allergic conjunctivitis.

The value of NSAIDs for ocular use lies in their ability to reduce the synthesis of proinflammatory prostaglandins. In cataract surgery, prostaglandins are liberated as a response to tissue trauma. These mediators of inflammation can cause constriction of the pupil with consequent surgical difficulties. **Diclofenac sodium**, as a preservative-free 0.1% solution marketed as *Voltarol Ophtha*, seems to protect against this effect. There is also evidence that patients who receive NSAIDs preoperatively show a lower incidence of macular oedema following cataract removal. **Flurbiprofen sodium** (*Ocufen*) and **ketorolac trometamol** (*Acular*) are newer NSAIDs used perioperatively; their use is also increasing for seasonal allergic conjunctivitis and episcleritis, and conditions where steroids are contraindicated such as following trabeculoplasty. Oral **flurbiprofen** may be indicated in more severe cases of episcleritis and scleritis.

CLINICAL NOTE

People with HIV infection may be particularly susceptible to opportunistic intraocular inflammation. To avoid long-term damage to sight in this group, long-term monitoring and antimicrobials are recommended (Testi et al., 2020).

DRUGS AFFECTING PUPIL SIZE

These can be divided into:

- those which enlarge the pupil (mydriatics)
- those which constrict it (miotics).

Mydriatics

Mydriatics are of two sorts:

- *antimuscarinic drugs:* these cause paralysis of the muscular sphincter of the iris; the sphincter muscle is innervated by the parasympathetic nervous system (see Chapter 4)
- *sympathomimetic drugs:* these stimulate contraction of the radial dilator pupillae muscle, which is sympathetically innervated.

Antimuscarinics

These are also known as anticholinergics as they block the actions of the parasympathetic nervous system by antagonizing the effects of ACh acting on muscarinic receptors.

Atropine. One of the earliest known drugs of this type, **atropine** is the active principle in the poisonous berry of the Deadly Nightshade plant. Its mydriatic properties have been known for centuries and in the

Middle Ages, it was used as a cosmetic, hence its scientific name *atropa belladonna* (Italian for 'beautiful woman'). Today one of its main uses is to dilate the pupil in patients with iritis, where the inflamed iris goes into spasm and adheres to the lens of the eyes. Because the ciliary muscle has the same nerve supply as the sphincter muscle of the iris, atropine can be used to paralyse the focusing of the eye (cycloplegia) for sight-testing young children.

Therapeutic use. It is used as eye drops of 1% or 0.5% strength and in the form of ointment. The action of this drug lasts for about 2 weeks and it is not reversible by means of miotics. It is, therefore, unsuitable for dilating the pupil for fundal examination.

Adverse effects. Atropine can be dangerous as it can cause acute angle closure glaucoma in patients with narrow anterior chamber angles. This will not respond to miotic treatment and will almost certainly require an emergency operation.

Homatropine. For most purposes, a mydriatic with a shorter duration of action is appropriate. **Homatropine**, which is a homologue of **atropine**, can be used in 1% or 2% strengths. This has a rapid action, producing pupillary enlargement in 5–10 min, and its effect rarely lasts for more than 24 h and can be reversed with miotics.

Cyclopentolate. A synthetic drug, **cyclopentolate** is now commonly used as a mydriatic and as a cycloplegic for sight tests in young children, in whom it is necessary to abolish their accommodation reflex. It has a rapid onset and short duration of action. Its action is reversed by **physostigmine** eye drops.

Tropicamide. This is another short-acting mydriatic which, although it is a rapid pupillary dilator, is a weak cycloplegic and causes less blurring of vision. It is therefore useful for clinical fundal examination, as it has only a slight effect on the patient's ability to read afterwards.

Both **tropicamide** and **cyclopentolate** are synthetic compounds less likely to cause contact sensitization produced by the other alkaloid compounds; they are commonly used in outpatient clinics for eye examinations. Reversal with miotics is not usually required but patients should be warned of blurred vision and advised not to drive until the effect wears off. Patients with darker eyes may require higher doses, as they dilate less readily than those with a lighter pigmented iris.

Sympathomimetics

Also known as adrenergic drugs, they mimic the actions of **adrenaline** and **noradrenaline** in the sympathetic nervous system. In addition to their mydriatic effect they increase outflow of aqueous humour. Traditionally, **phenylephrine** was used as eye drops in 10% strength. Increasingly, **Dipivefrine**, a prodrug of adrenaline, is now used under the brand name *Propine*; it is more lipid-soluble, enabling lower doses with fewer systemic sympathomimetic side-effects (see section later on the treatment of glaucoma).

Sympathomimetic drugs can be used synergistically with muscarinic receptor antagonists in cases where dilatation is difficult.

Miotics

Miotic drugs act on the sphincter muscle of the iris, either directly or indirectly constricting the pupil. They are also known as cholinergics as they mimic the actions of ACh in the parasympathetic nervous system. Their main action is to reduce intraocular pressure by increasing outflow of aqueous humour.

Pilocarpine is used to treat angle closure glaucoma and some chronic glaucomas. It is available in strengths of 1%–4% in the form of eye drops and has been in use successfully for many years (see section later on the treatment of glaucoma).

Acetylcholine is used during intraocular surgery such as cataract extraction, where a rapid miosis may be required. This can be achieved by the injection of **acetylcholine** directly into the anterior chamber. It is marketed as ***Miochol-E***, a dry powder in a sterile ampoule containing its own diluent fluid. Mixing is done by breaking an inner seal but, as the preparation has limited stability, it should be made up just before use. Its effect is dramatic but short-lived. After the insertion of an iris-supported acrylic lens replacement, a longer-acting miotic is often advisable.

THE TREATMENT OF GLAUCOMA

Glaucoma is a group of diseases of the optic nerve involving loss of retinal ganglion cells in a characteristic pattern of optic neuropathy. Raised intraocular pressure is a significant risk factor for developing glaucoma. There may also be a relationship between fluctuating intraocular blood flow caused by hypertension and glaucoma. Optic nerve damage may occur at relatively low pressure, while prolonged elevated eye pressure may never develop into glaucoma. There are two common types of primary glaucoma:

- acute angle closure: this can occur suddenly and may be acutely sight-threatening
- chronic open angle: this is long term and causes gradual loss of peripheral vision.

These are two entirely different diseases, but the one common factor is that the eye pressure is raised above normal by the failure of the aqueous humour to pass through the outflow channels. The continuous secretion of aqueous by the ciliary body causes a build-up of pressure within the eye.

In acute angle closure glaucoma, the draining of aqueous into the canal of Schlemm through the trabecular meshwork is obstructed by the root of the iris. The eye becomes acutely painful, red and sensitive. Vision becomes cloudy and may rapidly be lost. The pupil becomes paralysed and the cornea rapidly becomes cloudy. To treat this disorder, **miotics** are used to constrict the iris sphincter muscle and pull the root of the iris centrally, thus relieving the obstruction. In patients with shallow anterior chambers and therefore narrow angles, both mydriatics and strong miotics can precipitate acute angle closure glaucoma. This is termed either 'mydriatic glaucoma' or, in the case of miotics, 'paradoxical glaucoma'. In such subjects both groups of drugs should be used with extreme caution.

Chronic open angle glaucoma develops slowly, and the patient may notice nothing until peripheral vision is largely lost. It is usually diagnosed by routine screening at an optician. A loss of peripheral vision with raised intraocular pressure may be noted.

Drugs used in the treatment of glaucoma work by increasing the outflow of the aqueous humour or by reducing its production by the ciliary body. Some drugs seem to work in both ways. There are several broad categories of drugs, described as follows:

Drugs Acting on the Autonomic Nervous System

In acute angle closure glaucoma, intensive administration of 4% **pilocarpine** eye drops is often the first part of the treatment. This means giving 1 drop/min for 5 min; 1 drop every 5 min for half an hour; and quarter-hourly thereafter. If this is successful in reopening the angle, the pupil will become small and the corneal oedema will clear in an hour or so.

It is easy to see why miotics are effective in angle closure glaucoma, as they help outflow by relieving the obstruction of the drainage angle. It is more difficult to understand why they should work in glaucoma of the open angle type. It has, however, been shown that they act by speeding up the passage of aqueous humour through the trabecular meshwork, which is the band of specialized tissue, which separates the anterior chamber from the canal of Schlemm, thus increasing the facility of outflow. In chronic open angle glaucoma, **pilocarpine** was used previously in strengths of between 1% and 4%, applied 4 times a day, as it is only effective for 6 h. For this reason, its use as a drug for chronic treatment has declined and longer-acting once-a-day therapies have gained popularity.

β-Blockers

Timolol is one of the most commonly used β-blockers, causing a reduction in aqueous secretion. A once daily long-acting preparation is available. It reduces the amount of aqueous humour that is formed and thereby lowers intraocular pressure. It has the advantage that it does not cause unwanted changes in pupillary size and is therefore a very useful drug in the treatment of open angle glaucoma. For this reason, however, it is not suitable for glaucoma of the closed angle type unless a miotic is used simultaneously. Another advantage of **timolol** is that it is well-tolerated by the eye with prolonged use in strengths of 0.5% or less. **Timolol** can, however, be absorbed systemically to an extent that it may produce an unwanted fall in blood pressure in some subjects due to its action on β_1 receptors producing vasodilation, resulting in dizziness or even collapse. It is also contraindicated in patients with asthma and care is needed in those with chronic obstructive airways disease, due to the systemic absorption and the subsequent action on β_2 receptors in the lung producing bronchospasm and bronchoconstriction.

Betaxolol, another β-blocker, is similar but less likely to produce systemic effects as it acts more selectively on β receptors but is less effective than timolol in lowering the intraocular pressure. There is, however, some evidence that its absorption via the conjunctiva results in a systemic effect, which may increase the blood supply to the optic nerve. It is available as a 0.5% solution or preferably as a 0.25% suspension, which produces fewer systemic side-effects being weaker but produces a more prolonged effect due to its suspension formulation.

Levobunolol, carteolol and **metipranolol** are other β-blockers, which can all be administered twice a day, although the latter two are no longer available in the UK and some other markets. **Carteolol** has intrinsic sympathomimetic activity which may additionally be of therapeutic value.

Sympathomimetics

Brimonidine tartrate is available as 0.2% eye drops. It is an α_2-stimulant and can be used when β-blockers are contraindicated, e.g. in patients with asthma, which is mediated by β receptors. **Lofexidine** is a similar drug. **Apraclonidine**, another α_2-stimulant, has a short duration of action and is used commonly to prevent postoperative elevation of intraocular pressure after laser eye surgery; its effectiveness decreases over time. In some markets, the prodrug **dipivefrine hydrochloride** remains available. This is converted by intraocular enzymes to **adrenaline**.

Prostaglandin Analogues

The use of prostaglandin analogues in the treatment of glaucoma has risen rapidly in 20 years. All four agents **latanoprost**, **bimatoprost, travoprost** and **tafluprost** increase the aqueous outflow and are analogues of prostaglandin $F2_{\alpha}$. Latanoprost, travoprost and tafluprost are further examples of prodrugs. The main side-effect is redness of the conjunctiva in about 10% of patients. They may cause permanent darkening of the iris to brown with prolonged use. Care is required in patients with light-coloured eyes, mixed-coloured eyes and in those having only one eye treated. The prostaglandins are generally well-tolerated, and have gradually replaced other agents as the first-line treatment for chronic open angle glaucoma. All drugs in this class are available as single preparations and in a combination with **timolol** for patients who fail to be controlled with either drug alone. Bimatoprost is also available as a cosmetic preparation to encourage growth and thickness of eyelashes.

Carbonic Anhydrase Inhibitors

Acetazolamide has the action of inhibiting the enzyme carbonic anhydrase, which is necessary for the secretion of aqueous humour. In acute glaucoma, the drug is very useful, as, by reducing the aqueous production, the intraocular pressure can be at least temporarily lowered, and this may have the effect of allowing better penetration of locally applied anti-glaucoma treatment.

Acetazolamide may also be used to avoid having to operate on a hard and inflamed eye; it does unfortunately have some unwanted side-effects. It is an effective diuretic, which may be inconvenient with chronic use, and it almost always causes paraesthesia of the extremities, though neither of these effects is permanent. Gastric irritation, nausea and depression are, however, more serious and if they occur, the drug should be discontinued.

Acetazolamide is available in tablets and also as a sustained-release capsule. The sustained-release capsule produces a more even and prolonged action, and, as it is absorbed in the intestine, avoids the gastric side-effects.

Dorzolamide and **brinzolamide** are carbonic anhydrase inhibitors, which can be administered locally in the form of eye drops. This is of value in view of the great reduction in systemic side-effects. They can also be given in combination with other anti-glaucoma drugs with a different mechanism of action.

Dehydrating Agents

Another method of reducing the pressure in acute glaucoma before surgery involves the intravenous infusion of certain hypertonic solutions such as **mannitol**. This has the effect of producing a vigorous diuresis and causes dehydration of the body tissues, including the eye, and at the same time, produces an inhibition in the secretion of aqueous humour. **Glycerol** 50% is the drug of choice if oral administration is possible. It produces a quick but short-lived reduction of intraocular pressure.

Cytotoxics

Fluorouracil is a cytotoxic drug more commonly used in cancer therapy; however, it has found a place in eye surgery as it exerts a delaying effect on the healing of scleral wounds. This is useful after drainage operations for glaucoma, such as trabeculectomy. The drug is given as a subconjunctival injection into the lower fornix, taking care that the bleb does not abut on the cornea. **Mitomycin-C**, another cytotoxic drug, is used when indicated to minimize postoperative scar formation and for conjunctival or corneal squamous cell carcinoma.

THE TREATMENT OF AGE-RELATED MACULAR DEGENERATION

AMD is the progressive destruction and dysfunction of the central retina, leading to blindness. In its more common form, dry AMD, the onset is very gradual and there are as yet no treatments available. The use of nutritional supplements has not been shown to prevent the onset of dry AMD; however, for established intermediate severity dry AMD, the use of antioxidant **vitamins C** and **E with lutein, zeaxanthin, copper and zinc salts** (known as the **ARED2 combination**) has been shown to reduce the risk of progression by up to 25%. The use of beta-carotene supplements is no longer recommended.

Wet AMD is characterized by blood vessel formation around the macula with more rapid onset. Older treatments such as laser coagulation have been superseded by the introduction of drugs that block the action of vascular endothelial growth factor (VEGF), which is implicated in the choroidal neovascularization (CNV) that produces wet AMD. The anti-VEGF drugs include **pegaptanib**, **ranibizumab, bevacizumab** and **aflibercept.** They are administered by intravitreal injection, usually initially every month. Around one-third of patients gain improvement in their vision and most of the rest maintain their level of vision. The drugs are expensive and the route of administration is unpleasant.

LOCAL ANAESTHETICS

Ophthalmic anaesthetics comprise:

- **tetracaine**
- **oxybuprocaine (benoxinate)**
- **proxymetacaine**
- **lidocaine**
- **bupivacaine.**

As the eye is a surface organ and covered with mucous membrane, it is particularly responsive to topically applied anaesthetics, which produce good operative conditions by stabilizing the cell membranes.

Cocaine has been in use for over a century, its application to ophthalmic surgery being first described in 1884. Although still one of the most effective longer-acting anaesthetics, it is no longer widely used owing to the advent of highly successful synthetic homologues. As an unfortunate result of its frequent abuse, the Controlled Drug Regulations, which apply to all its legitimate clinical applications, have reduced its popularity. In addition, it causes clouding of the corneal epithelium. Nevertheless, the impact it had on ophthalmic surgery when first introduced will be appreciated if a moment's thought is given to the experience of an eye operation without anaesthesia of any kind!

For surface anaesthesia of the cornea and the conjunctival sac, topical **tetracaine** 1% solution produces rapid anaesthesia which lasts for up to 20 min. The anaesthesia is profound and suitable for the removal of corneal sutures. It does cause stinging when first instilled and for this reason, either **oxybuprocaine** or **proxymetacaine** may be preferred, especially in children. The action is rapid but less well-sustained, which makes it very useful for accident and emergency work, as corneal sensitivity is regained relatively soon. **Lidocaine** is used as an injection both into the eyelids and as retrobulbar and peribulbar injections for globe surgery.

Injection of Local Anaesthetics

Retrobulbar Injection

For the performance of eye operations under local anaesthesia, an injection is often given behind the eyeball and within the cone of muscles that surround the optic nerve. This is known as 'retrobulbar injection' and may only be given by someone who is specially trained to do so. For this purpose, **lidocaine** 1% can be used, up to a total volume of 2–4 mL. When a prolonged period of analgesia is required, a mixture of **lidocaine** and **bupivacaine** is effective. All of these anaesthetic agents can be combined with **adrenaline** (epinephrine), but these combinations are usually avoided by ophthalmic surgeons, in view of the danger of injecting directly into an orbital vein.

Peribulbar Anaesthesia

A more recent technique involves the injection of local anaesthetic into the tissue space surrounding the globe and extra-ocular muscles of the eye, rather than directly into the muscle cone. This is known as 'peribulbar anaesthesia' and is less likely to cause the embarrassing and highly inconvenient, if rarely dangerous, complication of a retrobulbar haemorrhage.

For this procedure, a larger-volume injection is given, amounting to 8 or 10 mL. As a preliminary, the conjunctiva is anaesthetized using a few drops of tetracaine. A mixture of **lidocaine** and **bupivacaine** is used, and a diluted fraction is injected into the medial and lateral angles and, after a minute or so, the remainder of the main injection is given into the peribulbar space, half-medially and half-laterally. Such a volume does cause an excessive pressure on the outside of the eye for intraocular surgery to be safely performed. A balloon is therefore secured onto the front of the closed eyelids with a *Velcro* strap and is inflated to a pressure of 40 mmHg.

After 5 min, all the excess fluid will have been dispersed from the orbit and the effect of the anaesthesia and akinesia (absence of movement) will be complete. To ensure rapid spread of the local anaesthetic agent, a proteolytic enzyme, **hyaluronidase** (*Hyalase*), is often included in the injection.

OCULAR LUBRICANTS

Tear Supplements

Acetylcysteine is a mucolytic, which breaks up surface mucin; it is commonly used in combination with ophthalmic lubricants in the treatment of tear deficiency. Conversely, **polyvinyl alcohol** increases the tear film in the absence of mucin.

Carbomers are high molecular weight polymers, which are formulated in thick, viscous solutions that stick to the surface of the eye, trapping moisture to prevent dryness. A number of cellulose products are commonly used to replace tears, such as **hypromellose**, **carmellose** and **hydroxyethyl cellulose**. These all act like sponges, trapping moisture onto the surface of the eye. Oily preparations such as **liquid paraffin** and **yellow soft paraffin** are messy to use and will smear into the surrounding skin; however, they are useful lubricants in cases of corneal erosion and for prolonged therapy overnight.

STAINS USED IN OPHTHALMOLOGY

Fluorescein

Fluorescein is applied locally to the eye to stain ulcers and abrasions of the cornea and thus allow them to be easily seen. It is usually dispensed as 1% minims, which should be discarded immediately after use to prevent microbial contamination.

It can also be used in photographic investigations of patients with retinal diseases. Here it is injected rapidly into the antecubital vein using 5 mL of a 5% or 10% solution. As it passes through the retinal blood vessels, it causes them to fluoresce and any leakage through blood vessel walls as may occur in diabetic retinopathy, can be vividly demonstrated using a fundus camera. As anaphylactic reactions can occur, it is recommended to give a small test dose in patients with a history of allergy or adverse drug reactions.

Rose Bengal

This is a stain of carmine hue, which is taken up actively by injured or infected cells. It is thus very useful for detecting an active virus infection of the corneal epithelium, e.g. in herpes simplex. It is more effective than fluorescein in the diagnosis of conjunctival epithelial damage, but, as it stings sharply, a short-acting topical anaesthetic is instilled beforehand.

Lissamine Green

Lissamine green is a newer agent for conjunctival staining, with a similar activity to that of rose bengal. However, patient tolerance to **lissamine green** is reported to be better, thanks to a reduced stinging sensation. **Lissamine green** is available in impregnated paper strips. It is currently unlicensed in the UK.

DRUGS WITH ADVERSE EFFECTS ON THE EYE

Many drugs in general use have an unwanted, sometimes disastrous effect on the eye. Nurses in charge of patients receiving these drugs should be aware of the likely problems, as their early recognition may help to avoid permanent ocular damage and possibly total blindness. It should be remembered that where a drug is being administered systemically, both eyes may be at risk. Only a few examples are described here.

Chloroquine

Chloroquine was first used as an antimalarial drug and now plays a part in the management of rheumatoid disorders and tropical diseases. It can cause opacities in the cornea and has a toxic effect in the retina. The corneal disorder is reversible when the treatment is stopped, but that in the retina is permanent and visual loss can be severe. All patients receiving this drug should be under regular ophthalmic supervision.

The Autonomic Nervous System

A variety of drugs have a sympathomimetic or anticholinergic action as their primary or secondary effects, including antidepressants of the tricyclic group, and drugs used for the treatment of parkinsonism such as **trihexyphenidyl** and **levodopa**.

All these drugs have dangers when used in patients with glaucoma, but here a distinction must be made between the open and the closed angle types of disease. A patient with open angle glaucoma may merely show a relative increase in the resistance to aqueous outflow, with the result that the ocular pressure becomes more difficult to control. One with narrow filtration angles may suffer an acute attack which can be bilateral, resulting in rapid and perhaps complete blindness. In the open angle type the use of such drugs may be justified provided the risk is recognized and the glaucoma treatment suitably adjusted. In patients with narrow angle filtration these drugs should be avoided unless they are essential. When in doubt, an ophthalmic opinion should be sought.

Corticosteroids

Corticosteroids which are widely used to suppress the inflammatory response can have serious side-effects on the eye. They are also used as immunosuppressants in the longer-term following organ transplantation. Such patients are subject to three major side-effects on the eye:

- **corneal infection**
- **open angle glaucoma**
- **cataracts.**

Steroids can precipitate a corneal infection with herpes simplex but with prolonged administration they can induce glaucoma of the open angle variety and can cause cataracts. The two latter effects can be produced by either local or systemic administration.

Phosphodiesterase Inhibitors

PDE5 inhibitors are widely used as treatments for erectile dysfunction, including **sildenafil**, **vardenafil** and **tadalafil.** Drugs in this class can cause ocular side-effects including changes in light and colour perception, as well as blurred vision. Ocular adverse effects are dose-dependent and reversible.

Ethambutol

This antituberculous agent can cause inflammation of the optic nerve with some visual disturbance. Fortunately, these effects regress spontaneously when treatment is discontinued.

Isotretinoin

Isotretinoin, a synthetic retinoid derivative, has shown multiple, mainly dose-related ocular effects, including dry eye complaints, blepharoconjunctivitis, transient blurring of vision and acute transient refractive changes.

Voriconazole

Visual disturbances, including altered/enhanced visual perception, blurred vision and photophobia, occur in nearly 30% of patients treated with intravenous therapy and to a lesser extent with oral **voriconazole**. These effects, although distressing for patients, are reversible and transient.

Antiepileptic Drugs

Vigabatrin may induce visual field abnormalities. These may commence after several years of treatment and are sometimes irreversible. Baseline evaluation of visual field and 6-monthly tests are advisable to detect early changes.

Topiramate has been associated with acute bilateral angle closure glaucoma with an array of associated presenting symptoms. The glaucoma usually, but not always, develops within the first month of starting treatment. In cases of symptoms developing, specialist ophthalmological advice must be sought.

Amiodarone

Amiodarone is used to treat some types of cardiac arrhythmias. It does, however, produce corneal deposits similar in appearance to those caused by chloroquine. Fortunately, retinal side-effects are absent, and the corneal changes do not affect vision.

Tamoxifen

This drug, used in carcinoma of the breast, has been reported to cause blurring of vision as the result of changes in the cornea, lens and retina. This occurs mainly after high doses.

Chemical Toxicity

Ocular irritation may result from substances contained in ophthalmic preparations; either the active principle, the preservative or the greasy base of ointments. Prolonged use can cause chronic and sometimes permanent pathological changes in the conjunctiva. This effect can also be seen with the proprietary cleaning and sterilizing fluids used in the care of hydrophilic contact lenses. Systemic drugs can also adversely affect wearers of contact lenses:

- Sedatives can reduce blinking, leading to dry eyes.
- Antimuscarinics cause decreased production of tear fluid, leading to dry eyes.
- Aspirin, rifampicin and sulfasalazine taken systemically may affect contact lenses adversely.

SUMMARY

- Ensure that the eye to be treated is clearly delineated.
- Warm lotions to 35°C (95°F) before applying them to the eye.
- In cases of corneal damage, topical **citrate** and **potassium ascorbate** eye drops can improve the prognosis.
- Antibiotics used as drops are rapidly diluted by tears, and ointments release antibiotics more slowly.
- Any intraocular infections following eye surgery must be tackled promptly and aggressively.
- Be aware of the dangers of infection with *Acanthamoeba* associated with soft contact lenses.
- Infective processes can spread rapidly if topical steroids are used alone without the inclusion of an antibacterial agent.
- Steroids are never applied to the eye in the presence of active herpes simplex.

REFERENCES AND FURTHER READING

Doughty, M.J., Dutton, G.N., 2006. Fusidic acid viscous eyedrops – an evaluation of pharmacodynamics, pharmacokinetics and clinical use for UK optometrists. Ophthal. Physiol. Opt. 26 (4), 343–361.

Etminan, M., Forooghian, F., Maberley, D., 2012. Inflammatory ocular adverse events with the use of oral bisphosphonates: a retrospective cohort study. CMAJ (Can. Med. Assoc. J.) 184 (8), E431–E434.

Feldman, R.M., Cioffi, G.A., Liebmann, J.M., Weinreb, R.N., 2020. Current knowledge and attitudes concerning cost-effectiveness in glaucoma pharmacotherapy: a glaucoma specialists focus group study. Clin. Ophthalmol. 14, 729–739.

Hadavand, M.B., 2013. Role of ophthalmic nurses in prevention of ophthalmic diseases. NCBI Winter 2 (4), 92–95.

Sadda, S.R., Guymer, R., Monés, J.M., et al., 2020. Anti-vascular endothelial growth factor use and atrophy in neovascular age-related macular degeneration: systematic literature review and expert opinion. Ophthalmology 127 (5), 648–659.

Santaekka, R.M., Fraunfelder, F.W., 2007. Ocular adverse effects associated with systemic medication. Drugs 67 (1), 75–93.

Shaw, M., 2016. How to administer eye drops and eye ointment. Nurs. Stand. 30 (39), 34–36.

Testi, I., Ahmed, S., Shah, C., Agrawal, R., 2020. Challenges in treating intraocular inflammation in HIV patients. Ocul. Immunol. Inflamm. 28 (7), 1094–1098.

USEFUL WEBSITES

NICE. Age related macular degeneration [NG82]. https://www.nice.org.uk/guidance/ng82.

NICE. Glaucoma: diagnosis and management [NG81]. https://www.nice.org.uk/guidance/ng81.

32 SPECIAL CONSIDERATIONS IN DRUG USE
Pregnancy, Paediatrics and the Older Patient

CHAPTER OUTLINE

LEARNING OBJECTIVES

At the end of this chapter, the reader should be able to:

- list the four stages of pregnancy when drugs may damage the fetus
- provide examples of drugs known to or be suspected of causing fetal abnormalities
- enumerate the general rules to be observed when thinking of treating pregnant women with drugs
- explain why dosages need to be altered in pregnancy and in babies, children and older people
- list the problems experienced by the newborn infant when dealing with drugs given to the mother during labour and breastfeeding
- explain why drug administration to children and older people sometimes needs consideration of problems such as swallowing tablets
- recognize that older people have impaired abilities to metabolize and excrete drugs, and this can cause toxicity
- explain how adverse reactions to drugs are more likely in older patients
- understand the risks of polypharmacy
- list the main drugs used in palliative care, and their uses

INTRODUCTION

Most facts about drugs are obtained from observations on young and middle-aged adults. Age, however, may modify the way drugs are handled by the body and also the way the body reacts to the actions of drugs. It is important to understand the effects of drugs given at the extremes of age and in pregnancy.

DRUGS IN PREGNANCY

Drugs can affect the fetus either by interfering with some important function in the mother, which indirectly damages the fetus or by passing across the placenta and acting directly on the fetus. Many drugs cross the placenta and thus caution must be exercised when treating pregnant women.

Stages of Pregnancy

In obstetric practice, pregnancy is divided into periods known as **trimesters**: the first trimester is from week 1 to the end of week 12. The second trimester is from week 13 to the end of week 26. The third trimester is from week 27 to the end of the pregnancy. However, from the perspective of toxicology, four stages are generally recognized:

- **Implantation** (5–15 days). Drug toxicity at this stage usually results in abortion.
- **Embryo** stage (15–55 days). During this period, the embryo is changing from a group of cells into a recognizable human being. The embryo is particularly susceptible to drug toxicity at this time, which leads to fetal malformation (teratogenesis) such as occurs with thalidomide.
- **Fetogenic** stage (55 days to birth). As the fetus continues to grow and develop, drug damage becomes less likely, but it is still possible.
- **Delivery.** Drugs at this stage may interfere with labour and modify the behaviour of the neonate immediately after birth.

While drugs can cause harm at any stage, it will be seen that the first two stages, corresponding to the first part of the first trimester, are the most dangerous to the fetus.

In the UK, about 30% of women take some drugs during pregnancy, although only 10% take one in the first trimester when the fetus is most vulnerable to damage. Those most commonly taken are mild analgesics and antibiotics.

It is important to discover which drugs can produce fetal damage and which are safe to use. This is difficult for two reasons:

- Fetal abnormalities can occur for various reasons, even when no drugs are taken. About 2% of babies have some abnormality at birth, but only about 5% of these are believed to be drug-related.
- If the drug only rarely causes an abnormality, thousands of pregnant women need to be studied before a connection between a certain drug and fetal damage can be confirmed.

Experiments with pregnant animals are necessary but are not able to predict all possible types of toxicity.

Drugs and Fetal Abnormality

Online and printed resources such as Appendices 4 and 5 of the *British National Formulary* contain detailed information on the safety of specific drugs in pregnancy and breastfeeding (https://bnf.nice.org.uk/guidance).

Drugs can be divided into three groups:

1. Some drugs known to produce fetal abnormalities (this is not a comprehensive list; always check when in doubt before prescribing or administration of any drugs):
   - Thalidomide
   - Folic acid antagonists
   - Tetracyclines
   - Androgens
   - Danazol
   - Warfarin (during the first 4 months of pregnancy)
   - Diethylstilbestrol
   - Etretinate
   - Lithium
   - Some anticonvulsants, especially sodium valproate and valproic acid
   - Retinoic acid and derivatives
2. Drugs suspected of producing fetal abnormalities:
   - Oral hypoglycaemic agents as they can cause neonatal hypoglycaemia
   - Various cytotoxic drugs

- Amphetamines (used to treat ADHD, also a drug of abuse)
- Angiotensin-converting enzyme (ACE) inhibitors and thiazides

There are a number of other drugs which are under suspicion or for which information is not available.

3. Drugs which *probably* do not harm the fetus:

Simple analgesics	Paracetamol for minor pain. NSAIDs can be used if really necessary; ibuprofen being amongst the safest
Cough	Codeine
Powerful analgesics	Opioids can be used (but see later)
Diabetes	Insulin
Drugs for dyspepsia	Antacids – advice on diet advisable
Drugs for constipation	Bulk purges, lactulose
Drugs for nausea	Avoid if possible and treat by modifying diet
Antibacterial drugs	Penicillins, cephalosporins, erythromycin; avoid trimethoprim in the first 3 months of pregnancy if possible
Hypotensive agents	Methyldopa; hydralazine for rapid lowering of blood pressure; β-blockers may be used but may retard fetal growth. Labetalol is preferred. Long-acting nifedipine
Antimalarial drugs	Chloroquine (low dose); proguanil
Anti-asthmatic drugs	β2 agonists; inhaled steroids; a short course of systemic steroids if absolutely necessary
Centrally-acting drugs	Benzodiazepines (but see later); neuroleptics and tricyclic antidepressants are probably safe; antiepileptics
Hay fever (allergic rhinitis)	Topical preparations; H1 receptor antagonists (antihistamines, such as chlorphenamine and loratadine)

SAFETY POINT

The golden rule is: pregnant or breastfeeding women should seek the advice of their doctor, pharmacist or midwife before taking any medicine, whether over-the-counter (OTC) or otherwise.

When treating pregnant women, some **general rules** should be observed:

- Avoid giving drugs if possible, especially in the first 3 months of pregnancy.
- Give drugs at the lowest effective dose for as short a time as possible.
- Avoid newly marketed drugs if possible.
- Drugs on lists 1 and 2 (see earlier) should be avoided if possible. The problem arises when there is no satisfactory substitute and treatment is vital. This is a matter of risk to the fetus against risk to the mother (and often, therefore, the fetus as well).
- Alcohol and street drugs: alcohol taken by the mother during pregnancy can damage the fetus, resulting in an infant with a small head, facial abnormalities and of low intelligence. Current advice is to avoid alcohol altogether in pregnancy, although it is very unlikely that a small amount taken very infrequently will cause harm. If the mother is dependent on opioids, the newborn infant may suffer acute withdrawal symptoms. Regular use of cocaine is associated with an increased risk of fetal abnormality.

CLINICAL NOTE

Pregnant women in the third trimester of pregnancy are often advised to avoid NSAIDs as they may delay the onset of labour.

Pregnancy and Dosage

Pregnancy causes a number of changes in the way a drug is handled by the body:

- The volume of water in the body is increased, so the concentration of a given dose will be decreased, although this may be offset by a fall in protein binding, which leaves more unbound active drug in the blood.
- Liver enzymes increase, so some drugs are broken down more rapidly and renal excretion may also be enhanced. Where dosage is not critical,

this does not matter, but for a few drugs (e.g. anticonvulsants and theophylline) adjustment of the dose may be necessary during pregnancy.

DRUGS IN NEWBORN INFANTS

During the hours of labour, drugs may be given to the mother and some of these can pass via the placenta to the neonate. Among those which are important are the following:

Analgesics and Hypnotics.

- Morphine and similar drugs affect the fetus and may lead to difficulties in establishing respiration immediately after birth.

Barbiturates and Benzodiazepines.

- Excessive dosing of the mother with barbiturates and benzodiazepines leads to accumulation of these drugs in the fetus and after birth, the infant will be floppy with depressed breathing and will show a failure to suck.

β-Blockers.

- These drugs pass into the fetus and produce a slow pulse rate.

Chloramphenicol.

- Newborn infants are not able to break down drugs as effectively as older children or adults; thus, accumulation may occur after repeated dosing. With chloramphenicol this can be dangerous, as accumulation of the drug produces the 'grey baby syndrome', which is due to collapse of the circulation.

Oxygen.

- Treating a newborn, usually preterm, infant with a high concentration of oxygen is known to cause blindness due to retrolental fibroplasia (abnormal proliferation of fibrous tissue behind the lens of the eye, causing blindness).

Drugs Triggering Kernicterus

- Certain drugs given to the mother late in pregnancy or to the infant in the first few days of life bind onto the plasma protein and displace bilirubin from the binding sites. This can be dangerous because too much unbound bilirubin in the blood causes brain damage. Drugs that have been implicated are:
  - sulphonamides
  - tolbutamide
  - aspirin.

Kernicterus is the staining of, and subsequent damage to, the newborn infant's brain by the bile pigment bilirubin, which may occur due to a haemolytic disease of the infant or through drugs displacing bilirubin from its binding sites on plasma proteins. Neurones in the basal ganglia are especially affected, and at about 6 months, a form of cerebral palsy emerges, with feeding difficulties, disturbed vision, deafness and uncoordinated movements. Speech, when it develops, is impaired.

BREASTFEEDING AND DRUGS

Most drugs will pass into the breast milk, but usually at very low and innocuous concentrations. However, this is not always the case, and a few drugs being taken by the mother can be a hazard to the baby. As a general principle, the lowest effective dose should be used, and drugs with a short half-life, such as sertraline are preferred over drugs with a long half-life such as fluoxetine. Ideally, drugs should be avoided by nursing mothers, but if a drug is essential, the baby should feed just before the mother takes her dose, when blood levels will be low.

CLINICAL NOTE

It is important to check the manufacturer's recommendations regarding breastfeeding before prescribing any drug. In some cases, there will be insufficient information available to be certain of safety, in which case the decision whether to prescribe must be made on the basis of the balance of possible risks and benefits. National drug formularies, e.g. the *British National Formulary*, are a good resource to consult when caring for women who are breastfeeding.

Certain drugs should not be used by nursing mothers, but if their use is unavoidable, then it will require transfer of the baby to bottle-feeding.

Commonly used drugs include:

- codeine
- nasal decongestants in tablet form
- aspirin
- herbal remedies – there is insufficient information on safety for most herbal remedies.

Less commonly used drugs include:

- anticancer drugs
- lithium
- oral retinoids
- amiodarone
- iodine
- gold salts.

DOSAGE OF MEDCINES IN CHILDREN

Children should *not* be regarded as small adults when prescribing for them, particularly in the first few months of life. Drugs dosage should be always based on weight and it is important to weigh the child to ensure a correct dosage.

They differ from adults in:

- body composition
- elimination of drugs.

In the first few weeks of life, the breakdown of drugs by the liver is reduced, but thereafter, because of the relatively large size of a child's liver, the rate of breakdown is greater, weight for weight, than in adults. This discrepancy progressively disappears until adulthood.

Renal excretion is similarly reduced in the first few weeks of life but reaches normal levels by about 6 weeks. It follows therefore that except for the first few weeks of life, weight-related doses of most drugs are higher in children than in adults. This means that dosage has to be carefully considered for each individual drug. Young children find it difficult to swallow tablets, so liquid preparations are preferable. However, they should not be mixed in the feeding bottle, as milk may interfere with drug absorption. Older children respond to drugs more like adults but, even here, there may be differences.

There is no completely satisfactory way of calculating the correct dose of a medicine for children.

In practice, three Formulas may be used:

1. $\text{Dose} = \text{Adult dose} \times \dfrac{\text{Patient's weight in kg}}{70}$
2. $\text{Dose} = \text{Adult dose} \times \dfrac{\text{Patient's body surface area (meters}^2\text{)}}{1.8}$
3. Dose as follows:

Age	Weight (kg)	% of adult dose[a]
Newborn	3.5	12.5
4 months	6.5	20
1 year	10	25
3 years	15	33
7 years	23	50

[a]This assumes that the child is 'average'.

Formula 1 is most satisfactory in deciding the initial loading dose, but Formula 2, which takes into account the rate of breakdown of the drug, is to be preferred for maintenance dosage. These methods are only approximate and with certain drugs, the dose in adults and children differs considerably.

Administration of drugs to children may present difficulties (see Chapter 2). Children under 5 years of age cannot usually swallow tablets and will require liquid preparations. Volumes of less than 5.0 mL should be given via an oral syringe. These should be free of sucrose, which causes dental damage. For certain drugs (e.g. diazepam) the rectal route is useful.

Further information can be found in the *British National Formulary for Children* or in various other paediatric formularies.

USE OF DRUGS IN THE OLDER PATIENT

In the UK, older people are responsible for about one-third of the expenditure on drugs by the NHS, and a high proportion of them receive regular medicine treatment. It is therefore important to know whether the action of drugs is modified by old age and how advancing years may alter the handling of drugs by the body.

Absorption, Distribution, Metabolism and Excretion

Drug Absorption

At present, there is little evidence that the absorption of drugs after oral administration changes with age, provided there is no disease of the gastrointestinal tract.

Drug Distribution

After absorption, drugs are carried round the body in the blood. They are to a greater or lesser extent bound to the plasma proteins, particularly albumin. Older people have less albumin in the blood; therefore, with certain drugs, less is protein-bound, and more is free in the blood and tissue fluids and can therefore produce a greater pharmacological effect.

Drug Metabolism (Breakdown)

Many drugs are broken down by enzymes in the liver, but with advancing age, these enzymes become less active and, in addition, the blood supply to the liver decreases. Some drugs may therefore be more slowly broken down and their blood concentrations may rise to toxic levels. Those implicated include:

- lidocaine
- tricyclic antidepressants
- propranolol
- caffeine
- benzodiazepines.

Drug Excretion

Drugs are also excreted via the kidney. Old age, sometimes associated with kidney disease, leads to a decline in renal function, so that by the age of 80 years, renal function is only half that at age 40. This again may cause drug accumulation. Among the most important drugs in this case are:

- digoxin
- aminoglycosides
- propranolol.

Organ Sensitivity

This is more difficult to assess, but there is evidence that certain systems become more sensitive to drug action with advancing years. Brain function is easily disturbed in older people, so hypnotic and other centrally-acting drugs can easily produce confusion and excessive drowsiness. The control of blood pressure is more easily disturbed, causing fainting, not only with hypotensive drugs, but also with tricyclic antidepressants and levodopa.

Adherence

Complicated medicine regimens (see Polypharmacy, later) may be impossible for older people to follow, so they either give up taking their drugs or take the wrong doses at the wrong times, sometimes with disastrous results. Dispensing of drugs for older and confused people is made easier through the supply of colour-coded, compartmentalized and labelled calendar packs in which the different drugs can be placed.

NURSING NOTE

Always assess the patient's ability to open medicine packets, bottles or boxes. If necessary, a single dispensing device should be offered, as being unable to use the drugs is obviously a barrier to compliance.

Adverse Reactions

Adverse reactions to a drug are two or three times more common in the older people than in younger adults and there are several reasons for this:

- Older patients often need several drugs at the same time and there is a close relationship between the number of drugs taken and the incidence of adverse reactions.
- For the reasons given earlier, the elimination of drugs may be impaired in older patients, so that they are exposed to higher concentrations unless the dose is suitably adjusted.
- Older patients are often severely ill, and this may interfere with elimination.
- Drugs associated with adverse reactions, such as digoxin, diuretics, NSAIDs, anti-hypertensives and various centrally acting agents, are often prescribed for older patients.

All this does not mean that diseases should not be treated in older people, but drugs must be prescribed with care.

Some General Principles

All these considerations have made it necessary to observe certain general principles when using drugs for older/elderly patients, and a **practical summary** is given below:

- **A full drug history** is important, as the patient may have experienced an adverse effect from a drug in the past. Medication already being taken (including OTC preparations) may raise the possibility of an interaction. It will also enable the prescriber to assess the patient's ability to manage the regimen alone or whether help may be needed.
- **Keep the regimen simple** and use as few drugs as possible.
- Prescribe the **smallest effective dose** and, if possible, use drugs which are short-acting.
- Do not continue to use a drug for longer than necessary.
- If an older person's condition deteriorates, remember that a drug may be responsible.
- **Ease of administration**: certain formulations such as elixirs may be easier than tablets for an older person to take, particularly if the tablets are very large or very small.
- **Clear and simple instructions** should be given to the patient and the container must be clearly labelled. Various types of calendar packs are available, but it is important to ensure that the patient can use them.

CLINICAL NOTE

Most countries have an adverse drug reaction reporting mechanism and in many countries, patients, relatives and carers can report known or suspected adverse drug reactions. These groups should be encouraged to report adverse reactions.

Polypharmacy

Polypharmacy (from the Greek *polus*, meaning 'many' and *pharmakeia*, meaning 'the use of drugs') refers to an increasing problem in medical practice, particularly in high-income countries. Polypharmacy is the prescription of many drugs to one individual. The rapid increase in the use of drugs (such as statins) for the primary and secondary prevention of cardiovascular disease, combined with a huge increase in the prevalence of type two diabetes in high- and middle-income countries has driven polypharmacy. It is often defined as the concurrent prescription of five or more different medications to a patient (but definitions vary). Polypharmacy has increased in high-income countries. In a recent Dutch study, polypharmacy prevalence increased from 3% to 8% over the 15 years to 2014, and the evidence suggests this trend continues. The highest rates of polypharmacy are seen in the over 65s.

Polypharmacy can be appropriate if all the drugs prescribed have a clear purpose, are working and are not causing significant adverse effects. Polypharmacy is inappropriate when they have no clear purpose or are no longer needed, are not working, are prescribed at too high a dose, are having adverse interactions with other drugs or are causing unacceptable adverse effects.

It has been estimated that in the UK 11% of unplanned hospital admissions are related to harm from medicines, and over 70% of these are over the age of 65 on multiple drugs. Older people are both more likely to be on many medications and are more likely to have adverse reactions to them.

While the problem of polypharmacy is increasingly recognized, the best approach to managing it is not yet agreed. It is clearly important for the prescriber to review all a patient's medication when considering a new prescription. The review needs to consider the indications, dose, monitoring requirements, effectiveness, adverse reactions and drug interactions for that individual patient. Inappropriate drugs should be stopped. Clinical pharmacists and general physicians are best placed to make such evaluations, but they can be lengthy, and sometimes difficult. Some patients can be surprisingly attached to their drugs (while others refuse to take drugs of clear benefit)! Deprescribing of drugs in polypharmacy is likely to be an area of clinical practice that develops considerably in the next few decades. Elderly care physicians have often noted that apparently moribund patients admitted to hospital make remarkable recoveries when all of their routine drugs are stopped. It is, of course, better to avoid inappropriate polypharmacy in the first place.

CLINICAL NOTE

Polypharmacy is a key consideration in the World Health Organization's Medication Without Harm document (WHO, 2016). When assessing a patient, always consider adverse drug reactions and interactions and ask yourself whether the drug you propose to prescribe is really needed, **and** whether any of the patient's other drugs could be stopped. A systematic approach, e.g. the 7-steps approach recommended in the UK, may be helpful. This approach encourages the clinician to consider the necessity of the drug from both a patient and evidence-based perspective and the likelihood that the patient will take the medication as prescribed (NHS Scotland, 2018). The SIMPATHY project is a European-wide initiative designed to reduce inappropriate use of medicines over the next decade (European Union, 2020).

Specific Therapeutic Problems

Sleep. Older people generally require less sleep than younger adults, and broken sleep during the night is common. They do not usually require medication but should avoid sleeping during the day and take more exercise. Alcohol, taken in the evening, may induce sleep, but often leads to waking in the night because its hypnotic effect wears off rapidly. If, however, the patient is used to a little alcohol before sleep, it is usually best not to interfere. Various disorders can cause sleeplessness and they should be sought and treated if possible:

- pain
- depression
- urinary frequency
- heart failure
- constipation
- dementia
- caffeine taken in the evening.

Hypnotic drugs (sleeping tablets; 'hypnotic', from Greek *hypnos* = sleep) are not prescribed as often as they used to be, but still are prescribed and can cause problems. For older people who are on hypnotic drugs, these are:

- **confusion** – drugs may cause mental confusion during the night
- **hangovers** – they may have hangover effects into the next day
- **falls** – older people on hypnotic drugs may fall more easily and can sustain serious injuries.

Those most commonly used for insomnia are the benzodiazepines and the 'Z-drugs' (cyclopyrrolones). Temazepam is a short-acting benzodiazepine and is preferred over longer acting drugs in this class. Zopiclone (eszopiclone in the USA) or zolpidem are commonly prescribed Z-drugs. All of these drugs have potential for abuse and dependence and are legally restricted in some countries (named 'controlled drugs' in the UK). Although relatively safe in short courses, these drugs can produce excessive drowsiness, confusion and ataxia, and the smallest possible dose must be used. They should only be given for short periods and a careful watch kept for adverse effects and falls.

Agitation. Agitation with restlessness is common in older people living with dementia. Drug treatment has often been used, but dementia sufferers are extremely sensitive to sedatives and antipsychotic drugs and are often over-sedated with a consequent loss of quality of life and dignity. Behavioural approaches and environmental changes are often helpful and should be tried before medication. Ensuring the person is comfortable, has diversions and adequate exercise in an environment that is calm and familiar, are part of these measures. Training of carers is very important to enable this. Drugs are sometimes required if these measures are inadequate, but doses should be low and the patient's condition frequently reassessed. Advice from an elderly care psychiatrist should be sought if drugs are considered. **Risperidone** has the best evidence for effectiveness and safety and is the first-choice medication. However, there is an increased risk of stroke associated with the use of antipsychotics in people with dementia. Other drugs have less evidence for effectiveness and safety but are sometimes used when agitation is severe. Older phenothiazine-like antipsychotic drugs should not be used unless there is no alternative, as side-effects (particularly over-sedation and falls) are common.

Depression. Of the selective serotonin reuptake inhibitor (SSRI) antidepressants, sertraline has the fewest anticholinergic side-effects and is the antidepressant of choice in older people. Anticholinergic side-effects such as postural hypotension, urinary retention, dry mouth, exacerbation of glaucoma and falls can occur with many antidepressants but are most marked with the older tricyclic-type drugs, such as amitriptyline. Amitriptyline is useful when used cautiously in low doses for neuropathic pain, but this class of antidepressants should not usually be used for other indications.

Hypertension. Older people benefit from control of hypertension, particularly in reducing the risk of stroke. However, the cardiovascular systems of older people do not adapt to change as well as in younger patients; therefore, a gentle approach is needed. Calcium channel blockers such as amlodipine are the first-line of treatment. Lymphatic mediated swelling of the ankles, especially in hot weather, is a common, dose-related adverse effect. Constipation may also occur in the elderly. If calcium channel blockers are not tolerated, a thiazide-like diuretic, such as indapamide, is a good alternative. ACE inhibitors are also effective and well-tolerated, but renal function must be monitored. Postural hypotension is common, and symptoms of this should be enquired for. Sitting and standing blood pressure should be checked for a large postural blood pressure drop. Blood pressure treatment targets should be considerably less aggressive than in younger people. The 2019 NICE target suggests <150/90 in people aged 80 or over.

Chronic Heart Failure. This condition is increasingly common and is usually, but not always, due to coronary artery disease. Treatment is along the same lines as in younger patients (see Chapter 5), but certain problems are more liable to arise in older people:

- **Diuretics:** sodium deficiency may develop with diuretics, causing postural hypotension and fainting on standing. With loop diuretics, the rapid diuresis can cause acute retention in men with enlarged prostates. With large doses, potassium deficiency occasionally occurs, requiring potassium supplements or the addition of a potassium sparing diuretic.
- **ACE inhibitors** can cause hypotension, particularly with the first dose and in those already receiving diuretics. Renal failure can develop, and renal function should be monitored.
- **Digoxin toxicity** may be a problem due to reduced renal elimination. If used, doses are lower than in younger people.

CLINICAL NOTE

Ankle oedema can occur during long periods of sitting and is not always associated with heart failure. If there is a suspicion that ankle oedema is associated with heart failure and is in the presence of decreased exercise tolerance and fatigue, the patient may require referral to cardiology.

Antibiotics. There is no particular contraindication to antibiotics in older patients as long as care is taken with aminoglycosides, as reduced renal function can lead to high blood levels and toxic effects.

Analgesics. Older patients are more sensitive to opioids and particular care is necessary if the patient has chronic obstructive airways disease. Co-codamol (codeine and paracetamol) can be used, but the resulting constipation may require a laxative. Paracetamol is preferred for minor pains because NSAIDs are especially liable to cause gastric bleeding in older people.

PALLIATIVE CARE

Palliative care is medical and nursing care at the final extremes of life – often, but not always – in old age. It does not aim to cure, but to control distressing symptoms in people with terminal illness, while maximizing their quality of life and addressing their psychosocial and spiritual needs and supporting their families. Quantity of life is regarded as being less important than quality, and if a treatment, such as morphine, controls distressing symptoms, then it is used, even if it also will hasten death. This approach is known by ethicists as the principle of **Double Effect** and refers to situations where it is morally permissible to perform an action in pursuit of a good end (control of severe pain) in full knowledge that the action will also bring about bad results (hastened death).

Palliative care is not the same as euthanasia, which is currently legal in only a few countries and states. Palliative care as a discipline arose from the hospice movement in the UK, and over the last 70 years has gradually spread around the world, making a huge difference to quality of life for people in their final months, weeks and days. Even so, the principle of Double Effect took a time to be accepted widely, and in some countries until recently, the use of morphine and similar drugs was restricted in terminal care on the absurd grounds that they might cause the patient to become addicted! Some cultures still have a tendency to prioritize quantity of life even in the face of suffering, and here, it is important to understand the patient's preferences and recognize that they are more important than the wishes of family members. Most patients understand that they are dying and have no wish to endure intolerable suffering.

Palliative Care Drugs

Drugs have an important role in palliative care but are only part of a holistic and patient-focussed package. They aim to deal with distressing symptoms that may be associated with terminal illness.

Routes of administration: All the usual routes of administration may be used, but as patients become more unwell, they will often be unable to manage oral drugs. Transdermal patches may be useful for analgesics and for reducing secretions. Often drugs need to be given intramuscularly or subcutaneously. The most effective way of doing this is with a syringe driver or infusion pump, providing a constant low dose infusion of analgesics and other agents. Syringe drivers are relatively inexpensive but may be unaffordable in some health systems. Here, intermittent injections should be given. If no other means of administration is possible, many palliative care drugs can be given rectally.

Drugs for Specific Symptoms

Pain: Bone pain from metastatic cancer often responds well to oral NSAIDs (some **bisphosphonates** are also used to treat bone pain), but for other pain, when simple analgesics are insufficient, opiates are generally used (see Chapter 20). These may be given orally, transdermally or parenterally. **Morphine** is often used, and intermittent dosing with morphine solution orally may be the first step in treatment. If regular dosing with oral morphine is required, then a modified release preparation should be prescribed, with once or twice daily dosing, depending on the preparation. If breakthrough pain occurs, oral morphine can be taken 2–4-hourly if necessary, and the additional amount required can be used to guide a dose increase in the modified release preparation. **The dose of modified release morphine should be increased, not the frequency of dosing.** Practitioners often fear overdosing their patients and are hesitant about increasing morphine doses. In reality, serious sedation or respiratory depression is unlikely to occur when patients are in pain, and it is generally safe to increment morphine doses by one-third to one-half of the previous total daily dose if the patient remains in pain.

If a patient taking oral morphine becomes unable to swallow, then the parenteral dose is approximately half the daily oral dose.

Other opiates, such as **codeine**, **tramadol**, **buprenorphine**, **hydromorphone**, **diamorphine**, **oxycodone** or **methadone** are also used. Oxycodone is a useful alternative to morphine if the latter is not tolerated.

- **Constipation:** When taking opiates, particularly more potent ones, constipation is almost inevitable and can be very distressing; it is important to prescribe an appropriate laxative such as **co-danthramer** or **lactulose** with **senna** at the same time as the opiate is started. The possibility of constipation should always be considered in terminally ill patients.
- **Nausea and vomiting:** Nausea and vomiting are frequent symptoms in terminal illness but are also a common adverse effect of treatment with opiates. Opiate-related nausea normally settles after the first few days of treatment. It is wise to prescribe an antiemetic such as **metoclopramide** or **haloperidol** when starting opiates, but the antiemetic can often be discontinued after a few days. If the cause of the nausea can be determined, this can guide prescription of an appropriate antiemetic. Metoclopramide increases gastric emptying and can help in vomiting from gastric stasis. Haloperidol is useful for vomiting due to metabolic causes such as uraemia and hypercalcaemia. **Cyclizine** is helpful for nausea from bowel obstruction and raised intracranial pressure. **Dexamethasone** may also be used for nausea and headache associated with raised intracranial pressure. **Levomepromazine** is also used as an antiemetic.
- **Convulsions** may be treated with phenytoin, carbamazepine, diazepam, phenobarbital or midazolam.
- **Excess respiratory secretions:** The sound of rattling secretions may be more distressing to relatives than to the terminally ill patient, but they may be reduced by a subcutaneous injection of hyoscine hydrobromide, hyoscine butylbromide, or glycopyrronium. These drugs may also be helpful in reducing painful intestinal colic.
- **Dyspnoea:** Dyspnoea may be very distressing. Paradoxically, given its respiratory depressant effect, small doses of oral morphine can be benefi-

cial. Diazepam can help with associated feeling of panic or anxiety.

- **Hiccup:** is relatively common. Metoclopramide or haloperidol can help.
- **Cough:** Morphine is the most effective treatment for severe cough associated with terminal illness.
- **Itch:** Pruritus is common in cholestatic jaundice but occurs with severe uraemia as well. If emollients and antipruritics such as topical **crotamiton** are ineffective, oral **cholestyramine** can help reduce the itch associated with cholestasis.
- **Agitation and confusion:** If this cannot be controlled after ensuring that pain, constipation and other symptoms are adequately managed, then **haloperidol** or **levomepromazine** may be used, orally or parenterally.

CLINICAL NOTE

Specialist teams exist in many countries to provide support for patients and relatives and their medical attendants. They are often associated with hospices and can also provide inpatient and home-delivered palliative care. In particular, they are able to provide clinicians with advice about symptoms control and drug choice and dose. Many of these teams are nurse-led. In the UK, the Marie Curie Cancer Care and Macmillan Cancer Support provide these and other services for terminally ill people – not only those suffering with cancer.

Further information about issues raised in this chapter can be obtained from:

- The *British National Formulary* – individual drug monographs
- NHS Regional Drug & Therapeutics Centre (RDTC) website: http://rdtc.nhs.uk/
- Hospital drug information units.

REFERENCES AND FURTHER READING

Arfman, I.J., Wammes-van der Heijden, E.A., Ter Horst, P.G.J., et al., 2020. Therapeutic drug monitoring of antiepileptic drugs in women with epilepsy before, during, and after pregnancy. Clin. Pharmacokinet. 59 (4), 427–445.

Assiri, G., Shebl, N., Mahmoud, M., et al., 2018. What is the epidemiology of medication errors, error-related adverse events and risk factors for errors in adults managed in community care contexts? A systematic review of the international literature. BMJ Open 8 (5), E019101.

Bennett, S., 2014. Pharmacology in neonatal care: prescribing considerations. Nurse Prescribing 12, 87–91.

Bennett, S., 2015. Prescribing in pregnancy: effects on the fetus. Nurse Prescribing 13, 24–29.

Cavallari, J., Bridgeman, P.J., Awad, N.I., et al., 2017. 114 A survey of emergency medicine resident education in prescribing medications for pregnant and breastfeeding women in the emergency department. Ann. Emerg. Med. 70 (4), S46–S47.

Chappell, F., 2015. Medication adherence in children remains a challenge. Prescriber 26 (12), 31–34.

European Union, 2020. Stimulating Innovation and Management of Polypharmacy and Adherence in the Elderly (SIMPATHY). http://www.simpathy.eu.

Hales, C.M., Kit, B.K., Gu, Q., Ogden, C.L., 2018. Trends in prescription medication use among children and adolescents—United States, 1999–2014. J. Am. Med. Assoc. 319 (19), 2009–2020.

Kaufman, G., 2013. Prescribing and drugs management in older people. Nurs. Older People 25 (7), 33–41.

Naughton, C., Hayes, N., 2017. Deprescribing in older adults: a new concept for nurses in administering medicines and as prescribers of medicine. Eur. J. Hosp. Pharm. 24 (1), 47–50.

NHS Scotland, 2018. Polypharmacy Guidance and Medicines Review. http://www.polypharmacy.scot.nhs.uk/polypharmacy-guidance-medicines-review.

NICE, 2020. Prescribing in Pregnancy. https://bnf.nice.org.uk/guidance/prescribing-in-pregnancy.html.

Tomlin, S., 2015. Medicine doses in children. Nurse Prescribing 13, 352–356.

Walson, P.D., 2020. Drug exposure and effects in pregnancy and lactation. Ther. Drug Monit. 42 (2), 169–171.

WHO, 2016. The Third WHO Global Patient Safety Challenge: Medication without Harm. https://www.who.int/patientsafety/medication-safety/en.

USEFUL WEBSITES

BMJ. http://www.bmj.com.
BBNF. https://bnf.nice.org.uk/guidance.
Nurse Prescriber. https://www.nurseprescriberforum.co.uk.
RCN. http://www.rcn.org.uk.

33 TOXICITY OF DRUGS AND TREATMENT

CHAPTER OUTLINE

LEARNING OBJECTIVES

At the end of this chapter, the reader should be able to:

- list and discuss circumstances that can result in accidental poisoning in adults and children
- name the three criteria on which the severity of poisoning is based
- describe the non-specific measures for treatment of poisoning
- describe the strategies for treating poisoning for the medicine examples given in this chapter

INTRODUCTION

The treatment of acute poisoning has of recent years become increasingly important. About 10% of acute medical admissions to hospital are due to an overdose of a medicine or ingestion of a poison. However, 80% of these patients require only observation until the effects of the poison wear off. Most of this chapter applies to the more severely-poisoned patient. This may be due to attempted suicide, less often to accidental poisoning and very rarely to homicide. Perhaps the commonest cause of overdosage is an attempt by the patient to draw attention to, or modify, some intolerable situation. In these circumstances, he or she is not seeking death, but merely trying to shock relatives or friends into the realization of their problems.

In children, poisoning occurs most commonly in the 1–5-year age group, as the child becomes mobile and is inclined to put everything in their mouth. Medicines and other harmful substances must be kept not only out of reach, but also out of sight, as children are adept at reaching 'impossible' places. Occasionally, poisoning may be due to accidental overdose of a medicine.

The most frequently used agents to attempt suicide are centrally-acting medicines such as sedatives, hypnotics and antidepressants, analgesics such as aspirin, paracetamol and opioids, and a mixed bag, which includes some cardiovascular drugs. In addition, poisoning can occur, particularly in children, from various chemicals used domestically or in the garden, from a number of berries. Carbon monoxide poisoning is also a concern in people living in poorly-ventilated accommodation.

This chapter briefly summarizes the approach to the treatment of relatively common poisons. It is not a substitute for expert advice from specialist poisons units.

GENERAL MANAGEMENT

The main principles when managing a patient with poisoning is life-support, ongoing assessment and drug decontamination or detoxification. When a patient is admitted to hospital suffering from poisoning, the first step is to decide if life is at immediate risk from airway obstruction or respiratory arrest (Resuscitation Council UK, 2015). If so, the appropriate measures should be taken immediately for life-support. The next steps are to assess the severity of the poisoning, the nature of the poison used (overdose by more than one drug is common) and to institute appropriate treatment.

Severity of Poisoning

The severity of the poisoning will be assessed largely on three criteria:

- level of consciousness
- respiration
- circulation.

CLINICAL NOTE

An illness severity track and trigger system, e.g. the National Early Warning Score (NEWS)2 will assist in risk stratification of the person who has been exposed to poisoning (Royal College of Physicians, 2017). A systematic approach to management and treating the reversible cause will improve the outcome for the patient.

This is usually classified by the Glasgow Coma Scale or in the case of NEWS2, the AVPU score. This categorizes conscious level into four grades:

A – Alert: awake and alert and responding appropriately to verbal questions
V – Verbal: responsive to verbal stimulus but may be confused
P – Pain: responsive to painful stimulus, such as nailbed stimulus or periorbital stimulus, but is not to voice: unconscious, but responds to severe stimulation
U – Unresponsive: with no response to verbal or painful stimulus.

Level of Consciousness

A person responsive to only pain correlates with a Glasgow Coma Scale of 8 or less and is at risk of airway compromise; at this stage, the patient requires immediate and urgent review by critical care or if at home, emergency services.

Respiration

Depression of respiration so that less oxygen reaches the lungs is a common cause of death following overdosage. Respiratory rate should be charted at regular intervals. Blood oxygen saturation measurement is very useful and monitors are now inexpensive and readily available. If oxygen saturations are less than 94% and in a previously fit and healthy individual, the airway should be maintained and oxygen commenced (BTS, 2017).

Circulation

Many medicines in overdose cause circulatory failure. The nurse is frequently asked to measure the blood pressure at intervals and a low blood pressure is indicative of a failing circulation. However, it must be realized that what really matters is the perfusion of vital organs such as the brain and kidney. It is possible to have a reasonable blood pressure maintained by intense constriction of blood vessels, but organ perfusion will then be poor. In such a situation the hands and feet will be cold and blue, and this may be a useful sign. In addition, certain drugs (particularly antidepressants) can cause cardiac arrhythmias, so ECG monitoring is necessary.

Nature of Poison Used

The identification of the poison used will depend on history and circumstantial evidence on clinical signs, and on analysis of gastric aspirate, blood and urine. Samples should be collected, carefully labelled and analysed as soon as possible. The results may not only be useful in the management of the patient as they may help in identifying the intoxicant, but the results may also have medico-legal implications.

TREATMENT

The treatment of poisoning can be divided into:

- non-specific measures
- specific measures, which are considered by individual poisons (discussed later).

Non-specific Measures

Non-specific measures comprise five procedures, described as follows:

Maintenance of Ventilation

In the unconscious patient, the reflexes which protect the airways may be lost, so there is a danger of respiratory obstruction by the tongue and the aspiration of vomit. These patients should be nursed in the coma position with an airway in place until it is possible to insert a cuffed endotracheal tube, which can be kept in place for up to 72 h. Secretions should be aspirated regularly.

With severe respiratory depression, oxygen and/or assisted ventilation will be required.

Reducing Absorption of Poisons

It is desirable to minimize the absorption of poison from the gastrointestinal tract. While in the past it was normal practice to empty the stomach of the conscious patient by induction of vomiting, there is now evidence that this practice has little effect on absorption of poisons and carries a risk of aspiration. Therefore, this is no longer a recommended treatment. In the unconscious patient, gastric lavage was often performed, but again has fallen out of favour. For most substances, activated charcoal and similar treatments are more effective and much safer. Gastric lavage should only be performed if a life-threatening amount of a substance has been taken in the previous hour that cannot be removed by other means. Iron or lithium salts are examples of such substances. The airway must be protected before lavage is attempted. Induction of vomiting or gastric lavage must not be attempted for poisoning with petroleum distillates, or corrosive substances such as bleach.

Activated Charcoal. Activated charcoal reduces the absorption of many poisons. Treatment should be started as soon as possible but may be of value even an hour after poisoning for modified release drugs and anticholinergic drugs and antidepressants. Repeated doses are needed for poisoning with carbamazepine, dapsone, phenobarbital, quinine and theophylline.

Activated charcoal should not be used for poisoning with petroleum distillates, corrosive substances, alcohols, malathion, cyanides and metal salts, including iron and lithium salts.

Maintenance of Blood Pressure

Some patients will have a low blood pressure and failing circulation. Adequate ventilation will often improve matters. Raising the foot of the bed is simple and is usually successful in mild poisoning. With severe hypotension, intravenous fluids or vasopressors may be required.

Increasing Elimination of Poisons

This can be achieved by increasing elimination via the kidneys or by hemoperfusion. *Renal elimination* of some medicines can be increased by altering the pH of the urine and an example is in the treatment of salicylate poisoning. **Haemodialysis** may be used to directly remove poisons from the blood in the case of poisoning with ethylene glycol, lithium, methanol, phenobarbital, salicylates and sodium valproate.

Nutrition, Hydration and Electrolyte Disturbances

In comatose patients, the problems of nutrition, hydration and electrolyte disturbances will require consideration, although intravenous infusion will not usually be necessary unless the coma is prolonged.

Follow-up

When the patient has recovered, it is important that the social and mental health background to a suicide attempt is investigated and most of these patients will require continued supportive treatment.

INDIVIDUAL POISONS

See Table 33.1 for individual poisons and plasma concentration levels for therapeutic use and severe overdose.

Benzodiazepines

These medicines are widely used, so it is not surprising that overdose is common. They produce coma without any specific features, and cardiorespiratory depression is usually minimal. However, death can occur from respiratory depression and/or the aspiration of stomach contents, particularly if they have been combined with other more sinister agents. There is some evidence that death from temazepam overdose is more frequent. Some of this group of medicines have long half-lives and/or active metabolites, and full recovery may take several days.

Treatment

It is usually sufficient to maintain a clear airway and give general nursing care. **Flumazenil** is a specific antidote, which reverses the actions of this group of medicines, but it is only rarely required in severe overdose.

CLINICAL NOTE

Flumazenil is usually used as a reversal agent when a benzodiazepine has been used as a sedative during a procedure, e.g. endoscopy. It allows the patient to recover more quickly and be discharged sooner. Although flumazenil is normally well-tolerated, side-effects include agitation, shivering, nausea and vomiting. A review by Penninga et al. (2016) noted that in the emergency situation, when compared with placebo, it was associated with worse outcomes.

Salicylates (Aspirin)

Aspirin has long been a common cause of poisoning, although in recent years, its place has been partially taken by paracetamol. In addition to suicide attempts, it is particularly dangerous as a cause of accidental overdosage in children, who are more sensitive to its toxic effects than adults.

Symptoms

Symptoms of aspirin poisoning include nausea, vomiting, tinnitus, increased respiration and, with severe overdose, confusion, convulsions and coma.

Aspirin also produces complicated changes in the acid–base state of the body. Early on, it causes increased respiration and thus washes carbon dioxide out through the lungs and causes an alkalosis. However, aspirin is an acid and therefore tends to produce an acidosis after some hours.

Treatment

- Activated charcoal can be given in the first hour after ingesting salicylates.

TABLE 33.1

Individual Poisons and Plasma Concentration Levels

	Plasma Concentration Producing Severe Overdose	Upper Limit of Therapeutic Plasma Level
Hypnotics		
Barbiturates	50 mg/L	5 mg/L
Diazepam	5 mg/L	1 mg/L
Anticonvulsants		
Phenobarbital	100 mg/L	30 mg/L
Phenytoin	35 mg/L	20 mg/L
Analgesics		
Salicylates	600 mg/L	250 mg/L
Paracetamol	200 mg/L (4 h after ingestion)	20 mg/L
	30 mg/L (15 h after ingestion)	
Miscellaneous		
Amitriptyline	1 mg/L	0.2 mg/L
Ethanol	3 g/L	0.8 g/L is the legal limit for driving

- Plasma salicylate levels may rise slowly and require repeated measurements.
- In severely ill and unconscious patients (serum salicylate ≥500 mg/L for adults and ≥300 mg/L for children) intravenous fluid and electrolyte (particularly potassium) replacement is essential. Elimination of salicylate by the kidneys can be enhanced by infusing sodium hydrogen carbonate solution to make the urine alkaline (forced alkaline diuresis), but if available, haemodialysis is the treatment of choice.

Paracetamol

Overdosage with paracetamol produces liver necrosis, which has often been fatal. This is due to abnormal breakdown products that do not occur with normal dosage, but only when excess has been taken. As little as 7.5 g (15 of the usual tablets) can be fatal. Early symptoms, usually nausea and vomiting, are minimal and it is only after 2 or 3 days that jaundice with hepatic failure and/or, more rarely, renal failure develop. The risk of serious liver damage can be predicted by the plasma paracetamol concentration plotted against the time since ingestion. Such graph plots are readily available, and treatment should be given if the plasma–paracetamol concentration falls above the *treatment line* on the graph (Fig. 33.1). Fatalities from paracetamol have fallen in countries where restrictions have been placed on the number of tablets that can be purchased without a prescription. Similarly, foil packs of individual tablets rather than sale in bottles has reduced the risk of overdose.

Treatment

Activated charcoal should be given if a large dose of paracetamol has been taken in the previous hour. Acetylcysteine is effective in protecting the liver from damage from paracetamol overdose, provided it is given promptly.

Acetylcysteine should be given if the plasma paracetamol concentration is above the treatment line (see Fig. 33.1) or if more than 150 mg/kg paracetamol has been ingested in the previous 8–24 h, even if the plasma paracetamol level is not known. Three infusions of acetylcysteine are given over 20 hours. The amount given depends on body weight.

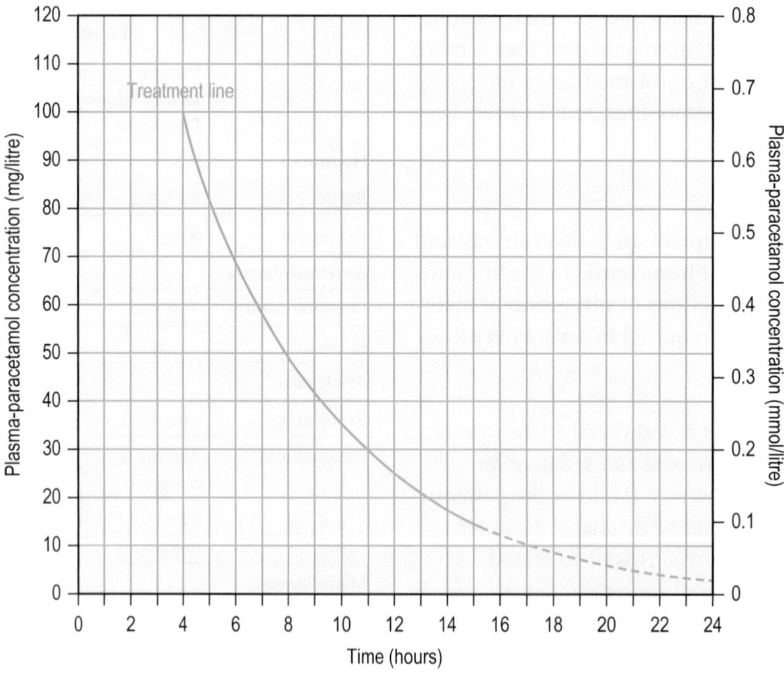

Fig. 33.1 ■ Plasma-paracetamol concentration.

Methionine given 4-hourly for four doses is an option if intravenous access is not possible. Acetylcysteine may also be given by mouth; however, the intravenous route is much preferred.

Need for Rapid Treatment. These treatments are very effective if given within 8–10 h of ingestion of paracetamol; after this, their efficacy declines, although there may be benefit in treatment up to 24 h after ingestion. They should therefore be given immediately to all patients in whom there is good evidence of overdose, even if a plasma level estimation is not immediately available. When this information becomes available, treatment can be modified if necessary.

CLINICAL NOTE

Refer to local paracetamol overdose guidelines to ensure treatment and monitoring is consistent. During administration, patients may experience mild reactions, which may improve when the infusion is stopped or slowed down and an antihistamine given. More severe anaphylactoid reactions may occur such as rash bronchospasm and hypotension. In these cases, anaphylaxis protocols should be followed (Resuscitation Council UK, 2015). People with asthma may be hypersensitive to the drug and additional bronchodilators may be required during administration.

Opioids

Opioids include:

- **morphine**
- **heroin**
- **dihydrocodeine**
- **oxycodone.**

Morphine and related substances are common causes of poisoning. This may occur as a suicide attempt or because an addict has misjudged his or her 'fix'. Although morphine and heroin are the best known of this group, serious overdosage can occur with so-called weak narcotics such as codeine and dihydrocodeine, provided a large enough dose is taken. Overdose of **dextropropoxyphene** was a substantial problem and has resulted in restrictions on prescribing this drug in many countries. Deaths from overdose have fallen substantially in those countries where prescribing has now been restricted.

Symptoms

The classic symptoms are coma, depressed respiration and pinpoint pupils. The patient sweats and is liable to develop hypothermia. The pulse is slow. Pulmonary oedema may develop rapidly and is often fatal.

Treatment

Respiratory depression is reversed by **naloxone** given intravenously. It is, however, short-acting and repeated doses may be required. Respiratory arrest will require full resuscitation with assisted ventilation. Hypothermia should be treated in the usual way.

CLINICAL NOTE

Constant monitoring of patients who are having naloxone is essential due to the short action of this medicine. If naloxone is given to reverse the effect of accidental overdose, e.g. in the case of postoperative pain control, the analgesic effect of morphine will also be reversed and a replacement analgesic may be required. Following evidence-based guidance on postoperative pain management will reduce the risk of adverse events (Aubrun et al., 2012).

The central effects of all opioids are increased by concurrent consumption of alcohol.

Tricyclic Antidepressants

Amitriptyline is the only commonly prescribed tricyclic antidepressant in most countries today. It is often prescribed for chronic pain, rather than depression. Both chronic pain and depression increase the risk of suicide attempts and tricyclic antidepressants are very dangerous in overdose, largely because of their effects on the heart.

Symptoms

With small overdosage, the patient is flushed, agitated with some blunting of consciousness and has a rapid pulse. The pupils are dilated, and accommodation paralysed. The QRS interval on the ECG becomes progressively longer, with increasing severity of poisoning. Larger doses cause fits, coma, depression of respiration and blood pressure, and various cardiac arrhythmias.

Treatment

There is no specific treatment for overdose with these drugs, and diuresis and dialysis are no help. Activated charcoal is beneficial. Cardiac arrhythmias are treated along the usual lines (see Chapter 5). Hypotension can be reversed by raising the cardiac output with dopamine, and fits controlled by diazepam. Systemic acidosis may require correction by infusion of sodium hydrogen carbonate.

The newer SSRI antidepressants are much less dangerous in overdose. Treatment of overdose involves the use of activated charcoal and supportive measures.

Alcohol

The patient may be conscious, but mentally disorientated or may be unconscious. There is a smell of alcohol on the breath. Acidosis may occur, and hypoglycaemia, particularly in children. Aspiration of vomit is the greatest risk.

Treatment

Most patients will recover if kept warm and allowed to sleep it off. Care of the airway is essential. It is very important to remember that patients who are intoxicated from alcohol may have received injuries of which they are not aware. It should also be remembered that patients may have taken other drugs in addition to alcohol.

NURSING NOTE

The risk of head injury during alcohol intoxication is reportedly as high as 65% (Shahin and Robertson, 2012). Patients who are intoxicated must be monitored to ensure no other injury (such as a head injury) has been sustained. If presenting to the emergency department, assessment of conscious levels should be monitored using standardized scoring systems such as the Glasgow Coma Scale or AVPU Scores (Hoban, 2017).

Barbiturates

Symptoms

The patient is confused or in a coma. Respiration is depressed and the blood pressure is low. Skin blistering is a fairly common feature of barbiturate overdose.

Treatment

In barbiturate poisoning, death is usually due to respiratory depression, circulatory failure or pneumonia at a later date. Care of the airway is essential and mechanical ventilation may be required.

Carbon Monoxide

Carbon monoxide is a common cause of fatal poisoning. It may be accidental or a suicide attempt. It may be due to the escape of gas from faulty heating or lighting installations, to car exhaust fumes or to combustion stoves in poorly-ventilated rooms.

Symptoms

These comprise confusion or coma, usually combined with cyanosis or pallor. The classic bright red colour of the skin and mucous membranes due to carboxyhaemoglobin is rare. After recovery, a few subjects may develop symptoms similar to Parkinson's disease.

Treatment

Give 100% oxygen through a **tight-fitting** mask. Mechanical ventilation may be required, and occasionally hyperbaric oxygen is necessary. If cerebral oedema occurs, intravenous **mannitol** infusion may be needed.

Phenothiazines

Symptoms

Phenothiazines such as chlorpromazine produce coma, with hypotension and sometimes hypothermia. Chronic intoxication causes a parkinson-like state.

Treatment

Treatment is largely symptomatic along with activated charcoal to reduce absorption. Parkinson-like states and other forms of dystonia respond to orphenadrine or similar drugs.

Iron Compounds

These substances, particularly ferrous sulphate, are sometimes taken by children because of their colour and sugar coating.

Symptoms

These include vomiting with haematemesis, pallor, collapse and tachycardia. Fatal collapse sometimes occurs after apparent recovery. **Iron overdose in children must always be taken very seriously.**

Treatment

- Gastric lavage may be required to prevent absorption.
- The iron chelating agent **desferrioxamine**, which combines with iron and prevents absorption, should be used in severe cases. Desferrioxamine can be given intravenously to a maximum dose of 80 mg/kg of body weight in 24 hours.

Organophosphorous Insecticides

Organophosphorus insecticides are widely used and inhibit the action of cholinesterase, thus prolonging the activity of acetylcholine in the central and peripheral nervous systems. They can be absorbed through gut, skin and bronchi and cause many symptoms. Severe poisoning leads to convulsions and paralysis of skeletal muscle, including respiratory muscles. Practitioners attending such patients need to protect themselves from exposure to the poison. The airway must be protected, and artificial ventilation may be needed. Gastric lavage may be used. **Atropine sulfate**, given intravenously, reverses some of the effects of these poisons. **Pralidoxime chloride** reactivates cholinesterase and may be used in moderate to severe poisoning. It is only available from specialist poisons centres.

Nerve agents such as **Sarin** and **VX** are highly active organophosphorus compounds, occasionally encountered in acts of war or terrorism. Treatment is similar to that of the insecticides, but personal protection is essential, as even tiny quantities can be fatal.

CHELATING AGENTS

Chelating agents combine with metals and thus render them inactive. They are used for the treatment of heavy metal poisoning.

Dimercaprol (British Anti-Lewisite; BAL)

Some heavy metals produce their toxic effects by combining with a chemical grouping found in living tissues called 'sulfhydryl (-SH) groups'. Their toxic effects can be prevented by giving **dimercaprol**, which also contains SH groups and thus combines with and inactivates heavy metals.

Therapeutic Use. Dimercaprol is useful in poisoning by arsenic, mercury, lead and gold. It is given by intramuscular injection.

Penicillamine

Copper poisoning can be treated with **Penicillamine**, a drug used to treat Wilson's disease, which is due to the excessive deposition of copper in the brain and liver, and rheumatoid arthritis. Penicillamine chelates the copper, which is then excreted. It can be given orally, daily. Penicillamine chelates various other metals and can be used to treat copper, iron, lead, mercury and zinc poisoning, although it is more commonly used in veterinary practice than in human medicine.

The chelation agent **DMSA** is also used to treat lead poisoning with good evidence for effectiveness. This agent is also used by practitioners of complementary and alternative medicine to 'treat' spurious 'heavy metal toxicity'.

GENERAL INFORMATION

Many countries have national resources to support the identification and treatment of poisoning. In the UK and the Republic of Ireland, these are Poisons Information Centres. They can be contacted day or night by telephone and will give information about poisoning and its treatment. Telephone numbers of these centres can be found in the *British National Formulary*. The BNF also contains useful current treatment summaries for common poisons, but expert advice should always be sought. The UK National Poisons Information Service (NPIS) is available to healthcare professionals 24 hours a day. The NPIS provides a detailed online resource called *TOXBASE*. This is available for any UK NHS practitioner: http://toxbase.org.

REFERENCES AND FURTHER READING

Aubrun, F., Mazoit, J.X., Riou, B., 2012. Postoperative intravenous morphine titration. Br. J. Anaesth. 108 (2), 193–201.

Avau, B., Borra, V., Vanhove, A.C., et al., 2018. First aid interventions by laypeople for acute oral poisoning. Cochrane Database Syst. Rev. 12 (12), CD013230.

Bonilla-Velez, J., Marin-Cuero, D.J., 2017. The use of activated charcoal for acute poisonings. Int. J. Med. Students 5 (1), 45–52.

BTS, 2017. BTS Guideline for Oxygen Use in Healthcare and Emergency Settings. British Thoracic Society. https://www.brit-thoracic.org.uk/quality-improvement/guidelines/emergency-oxygen.

Chiew, A.L., Gluud, C., Brok, J., Buckley, N.A., 2018. Interventions for paracetamol (acetaminophen) overdose. Cochrane Database Syst. Rev. 2 (2), CD003328.

Hoban, C., 2017. Assessing for head injury in alcohol-intoxicated patients. Emerg. Nurse 25 (5), 30–33.

Juurlink, D.N., 2016. Activated charcoal for acute overdose: A reappraisal. Br. J. Clin. Pharmacol. 81 (3), 482–487.

Penninga, E.I., Graudal, N., Ladekarl, M.B., Jürgens, G., 2016. Adverse events associated with flumazenil treatment for the management of suspected benzodiazepine intoxication – a systematic review with meta–analyses of randomised trials. Basic Clin. Pharmacol. Toxicol. 118 (1), 37–44.

Resuscitation Council UK, 2015. 2015 Resuscitation Guidelines. https://www.resus.org.uk/resuscitation-guidelines.

Royal College of Physicians, 2017. National Early Warning Scoring (NEWS)2. https://www.rcplondon.ac.uk/projects/outputs/national-early-warning-score-news-2.

Shahin, H., Robertson, C., 2012. Alcohol and the head-injured patient. Trauma 14 (3), 233–242.

USEFUL WEBSITES

BMJ. Best practice: Paracetamol overdose in adults. https://bestpractice.bmj.com/topics/en-gb/3000110.

NICE. Clinical Knowledge Summary: Poisoning or overdose. https://cks.nice.org.uk/poisoning-or-overdose.

34 HERBAL MEDICINES AND HOMEOPATHY

CHAPTER OUTLINE

LEARNING OBJECTIVES

At the end of this chapter, the reader should be able to:

- be aware of the increase in self-medication with herbal and other alternative treatments, and appreciate the need to find out from the patient whether they are self-medicating
- recognize that many herbal remedies are in fact potent drugs that can poison and interact with other drugs, and be able to give examples
- describe how some herbal remedies may actually exacerbate problems rather than cure them
- be familiar with the names of commonly used herbal remedies and what they are used for
- respect the decision of the patient to seek alternative therapies, but be prepared to research and advise
- understand the principles of homeopathy and its associated problems

HERBAL MEDICINES

Introduction

The use of herbal remedies worldwide is growing at an immense rate. Alternative therapies include licensed and unlicensed herbal medicines, homeopathic remedies and essential oils used for aromatherapy. The growing trend for alternative therapies globally reflects a degree of disaffection with conventional medicine, which may be perceived as harsh or 'unnatural' or simply ineffective for some conditions.

Most of this alternative treatment is virtually unregulated, although efforts are being made to ensure that standards of quality and integrity among suppliers can be put in place, as well as efforts to educate the public and health professionals about the uses, effects, limitations, adverse effects and potential drug interactions of this bewildering array of 'therapies'.

Many medical schools, particularly in the USA, are now instituting training courses in alternative forms of therapy, at both the undergraduate and postgraduate level, such as the Program of Integrative Medicine at the College of Medicine at the University of Arizona.

Healthcare practitioners, particularly if working in the community, will quickly realize that many people use various types of alternative or complementary medicines. This chapter provides an overview from the perspective of UK practice. Other countries will differ. Some knowledge of herbal medicines is important for several reasons:

- Herbal medicines may have pharmacological actions which affect the patient.
- Not all herbal medicines are free from adverse effects.
- Herbal medicines may interact with orthodox medicines if they are taken concurrently.

History of Herbal Medicine

Medicines derived from plants have been used for centuries. The pragmatic and most definitive classics on Oriental medicine are *Shang Han Lung* (*Treatise on Febrile Disease*) and *Chin Kuei Yao Lueh* (*Summaries of Household Treatments*) described in southern China by Chang Chung Ching in the eastern Han dynasty (CE 25–220). This empirical system has been followed for the past 2000 years and many of the formulae in these two books are still used today.

Many herbs have found their way into the pharmacopoeias of orthodox medicine, sometimes as the isolated and chemically standardized active ingredient. Drugs such as cocaine, coumarin, curare, digoxin, ephedrine, morphine, quinine and quinidine, reserpine, senna and the ergot and vinca alkaloids entered orthodox medicinal use by this route.

Many other herbal substances are freely available to the public, and in the UK, only a small proportion comes under the direct control of current regulation. Individual unprocessed traditional herbs are not considered as medicines and, therefore, do not require product licences in the UK. In Britain alone, it has been estimated that 6000–7000 tons of herbs are extracted annually for use as ingredients of herbal remedies.

Categories of Traditional Herbs

Traditional herbs (including Chinese herbs) can be divided into three categories:

- licensed herbal products
- dried herbs, which are exempt from licensing requirements
- herbal products sold as food supplements with no medical claims.

Licensed Herbal Products

Licensed herbal products are those which are sold or supplied with claims for use as medicines (currently over 500 products are licensed). Almost all the licensed herbal medicines on the UK market have been available for some time and most are licensed on the basis of long historical use. Since 1995, new regulations have been applied such that prior to marketing, all new licensed herbal products are assessed for quality, safety and efficacy.

Dried Herbs Exempt from Licensing Requirements

Dried herbs are currently exempt from regulatory requirements, as long as they are not sold or supplied with medicinal claims on the labelling. These products, often sold as 'teas', are prepared from dried, crushed or comminuted (reduced to small fragments) plants, and sold under their botanical names. These exemptions provide herbal practitioners with the flexibility to prepare their own remedies for individual patients, with no need to prove quality, safety and efficacy.

Herbal Products Sold as Food Supplements

This category includes herbal products sold as food supplements with no medical claims, although some therapeutic value may be implied.

The Practice of Herbal Medicine

Medical practitioners rarely prescribe herbal remedies, and medical herbalists, who constitute only a small professional body, are not consulted by most people who purchase herbal products. Consequently, the principal outlets are health food stores or mail order firms advertising in health magazines and the internet. Herbal products are also increasingly available at community pharmacies and are stocked by some supermarkets.

Groups of people who have moved from other countries will often bring their own medical traditions. Oriental medicine in particular has remained the most widely used traditional medicine. Oriental drugs are alleged to have specific characters such as the 'four properties' ('chill' and 'cool' of yin and 'lukewarm' and 'heat' of yang with 'intermediate') and the 'five flavours' ('acrid', 'sour', 'sweet', 'bitter' and 'salty'). Drugs are dispensed according to their character (e.g. diseases with fever are treated with chill and cool drugs). Over 500 herbal remedies are used in Chinese medicine and there are about 600 or more varieties of crude drugs.

Asian medicine is also relatively popular, following the traditional practices of Unani and Ayurvedic medicine. The traditional healer is termed *hakim* if they practise the Unani system or *vaidya* if they practise the Ayurvedic. Unlike Oriental medicine, which follows traditional formulae, the philosophy behind the Asian system is that preparations are not uniform from country to country, i.e. a preparation sold in India under a certain name will differ from the nominally identical product prepared for sale in Britain. The addition or omission of certain herbs is usually explained by reference to different climates or temperaments of the person being treated.

In general, herbal medicines claim to use the patient's natural resistance and to restore the balance of health. They are commonly used in treating chronic disorders, which often respond poorly to orthodox remedies, such as the common cold, arthritis, back pain, mental and stress problems and, sometimes, malignant disease.

Safety and Efficacy

Many of the plants used in herbal medicine contain principles whose effects can be demonstrated pharmacologically, and the action of the whole plant extract can usually be related to that of the isolated constituents. However, for some herbal remedies, it is not possible to demonstrate or evaluate their pharmacological activity and the situation is further complicated by the fact that the supposed active ingredients have not been identified.

It should be appreciated that even if a herbal medicine can be shown to work, this does not imply that the underlying diagnostic and treatment system (such as Ayurveda) is itself scientifically validated. Many effective herbal treatments have been identified through trial and error over centuries of use, but frameworks such as Ayurveda or traditional Chinese medicine do not themselves conform to any recognizable chemical or physical scientific understanding of the world. They may, however, still be of pragmatic use.

It is a common belief that herbal remedies, being natural products, are inherently safer than the potent synthetic drugs used in orthodox medicine. However, toxicity from herbal medicines does occur, although it is rarely an acute episode due to accidental consumption or an overdose. Herbal remedies are often taken over long periods and the appearance of toxicity may be considerably delayed and may even appear after the remedy has been discontinued. The quality of the product can be affected by environmental factors, such as climate and growing conditions before harvesting, and toxicity may vary with the part of the plant used, time of harvesting, post-harvest factors and method of preparation. Concern over the uncontrolled supply and administration of these products has led the UK regulatory authorities to remind practitioners that the 'yellow card' scheme for reporting adverse events applies as much to these natural products as it does to conventional medicines. However, the regulatory authorities can take little action, as these medicines do not have a product licence.

CLINICAL NOTE

When taking a drug history from a patient, it is important to include a specific question on herbal, complimentary or alternative medicines. Many side-effects are mild but some are severe and most commonly involve liver or renal impairment (Posadzki et al., 2013).

Herbal Extracts of Proven or Suspected Toxicity

Herbal Teas

Traditionally, **comfrey** has been used as a demulcent in the treatment of chronic catarrh, as a treatment for gastrointestinal disorders and less specifically as a tonic. In the UK, it is used by herbalists as a demulcent, an antihaemorrhagic and antirheumatic agent, and as an antiinflammatory agent. Safety concerns over comfrey centre on its content of pyrrolizidine alkaloids; their toxic effects are due to activation in the liver, leading to liver cell necrosis. Human hepatotoxicity of comfrey has been illustrated by characteristic veno-occlusive lesions with hepatomegaly and inhibition of mitosis. Hepatotoxicity has also occurred with other herbal teas containing pyrrolizidine.

A 'Babchi' herbal tea has been associated with photosensitivity. The seeds of this plant contain psoralen, isopsoralen and psoralidin, known to cause photosensitivity reactions.

Contamination of Natural Remedies

Herbal medicines may be contaminated with microorganisms, pesticides, mycotoxins (fungi) or substituted herbs, e.g. herbs containing podophyllum or substances with anticholinergic effects. On occasion, an orthodox drug, such as aspirin, steroids or paracetamol, has been found in supposedly herbal remedies. This adulteration is both dishonest and potentially dangerous. Patients using herbal medicines should be encouraged to use reputable suppliers and to be sure they know what they are taking.

Metals in Herbal Mixtures

Metals may be added to Asian and Oriental medicines in varying amounts, sometimes in sufficient quantities to cause toxicity. Some Asian and East African preparations called 'Kushta', also used in the Unani tradition, contain oxidized heavy metals such as arsenic, mercury, tin, zinc and lead. A Kushta may contain 10%–12% of each of several of these metals. Chronic arsenic toxicity has been documented in clinical studies of the uses of some of these preparations. Skin-lightening preparations containing mercury salts are popular in some parts of Africa and find their way to other parts of the world. Mercury toxicity has been demonstrated with long-term use of these products.

Other Herbal Preparations

Table 34.1 summarizes some reported adverse effects of herbal medicines. There are also problems with the apparently widespread use of khat and betel nut. Concern has been expressed about the incidence of carcinoma of the oral cavity when these are chewed for their stimulant properties.

Aconitine, the poisonous alkaloid in the plant aconite, is cardiotoxic and can induce life-threatening arrhythmia. *Aconitum* is used predominantly in Chinese medicine.

TABLE 34.1

Possible Adverse Reactions when Using Herbal Remedies (Short List of Examples)

Preparation	Indication for Use	Adverse Effects
Alfalfa seeds	Urinary, bowel problems; cholesterol lowering	May activate SLE (lupus)
Comfrey	Bruising, cuts, indigestion	Cancer, cirrhosis, some fatalities
Echinacea	Immune stimulant	Aggravation of SLE
Ephedra (Ma huang)	Decongestant	Cardiac stimulant; toxic in overdose; fatalities reported
Gingko biloba	Antioxidant	Bleeding
Ginseng	Fatigue, stress	Hypertension, oestrogenic
Kava	Narcotic, sedative	Possible liver toxicity; aggravation of Parkinson's disease
Margosa (neem tree)	Skin problems, stimulant, insecticide	Some reports of hepatotoxicity
European mistletoe	Headaches, seizures, antispasmodic	Diarrhoea, hepatitis; US mistletoe is toxic
Pennyroyal	Indigestion	Dangerous to liver – do not use
St. John's wort	Depression	Allergic reactions, dizziness, fatigue, confusion
Willow bark	Pain, inflammation	Gastric irritation

Source: D'Arcy, P.F., 1991. Adverse reactions and interactions with herbal medicines. Part 1. Adverse reactions. Adverse Drug React. Toxicol. Rev. 10(4):189–208.

CLINICAL NOTE

Since 2002, kava-containing medicinal products have been banned in the UK, and not permitted for use in the USA. Kava root has been used by some herbal practitioners for many years as a treatment for anxiety, insomnia and mental tension. It also acts as a diuretic and a genitourinary antiseptic. The substance can be toxic to liver tissue; the incidence is relatively rare but appears to be idiosyncratic, meaning that it is impossible to predict under which circumstances and in which patients this is more likely to happen.

TABLE 34.2
Some Reported Interactions between Herbal and Orthodox Medicines

Herbal Preparation	Conventional Medicine	Effect
Capsicum	ACE inhibitors	Cough
Ephedra (Ma huang)	Conventional ephedrine preparations	Overdose, cardiovascular events, e.g. arrhythmias
Garlic	Anticoagulants	Bleeding
Gingko biloba	Thiazide diuretics	Hypertension
Ginseng	Warfarin, paracetamol	Bleeding
Hypericum (St. John's wort)	Serotonin reuptake inhibitors	Gastrointestinal upsets, tremor, headache
Kava	CNS depressants	Additive effects
Licorice	Antihypertensives	Hypokalaemia, hypernatraemia

ACE, Angiotensin-converting enzyme; *CNS*, central nervous system.
Sources: Cupp, M.J., 1999. Herbal remedies: adverse effects and drug interactions. Am. Fam. Physician 59(5):1239 -1245; D'Arcy, P.F., 1993. Adverse reactions and interactions with herbal medicines. Part 2. Drug interactions. Adverse Drug React. Toxicol. Rev. 12(3):147–162; Editorial, 2000. Herbal medicines interactions. Pharmaceutical J. 264(7081):173.

Interactions Between Herbal Medicines and Drugs Used in Orthodox Treatment

In view of the large quantities of drugs consumed, both prescribed and over-the-counter, it is not surprising that interactions (some dangerous) are possible. As well as interactions between orthodox drugs, interactions may also occur with herbal remedies, some of which are shown in Table 34.2.

Use of Some Common Herbal Remedies

There are numerous herbal drugs and just a few of those most commonly used, together with their suggested therapeutic effects, are described here. There is no doubt that many people obtain benefits from herbal remedies and they should not be disregarded. However, if they can be shown to work, then it is because they contain active substances (even if these are not yet identified) and their use should be attended with the same caution as orthodox medicine. Medications of any sort should be tested for safety and efficacy. This approach is established in orthodox medical practice and is gradually being extended to herbal medicines.

- **Valerian** contains volatile oils and alkaloids. Its main use is as a tranquillizer, but it is also recommended for a variety of other disorders.
- **Ginseng** (Asiatic) contains saponins, glycosides and sterols. It is claimed to have a wide variety of actions, including improvement in adrenal, muscular and cerebral function. It is used for debility and as an antidote to stress. Long-term use may result in increased tension and sleeplessness. Although widely used, it has not been demonstrated to have a clear benefit for any one condition.
- **Echinacea** root contains a mixture of high molecular weight branched polysaccharide and caffeic acid derivatives. It produces a non-specific stimulation to the immune system and may be useful both as a prophylactic and a treatment in common infectious diseases. It is available as an alcoholic extract in a liquid form or in the dry state as capsules or tablets. The tincture is now licensed for the relief of colds, influenza and other respiratory infections. However, clinical trials of echinacea for prevention or treatment of colds have been generally disappointing.

CLINICAL NOTE

Some rheumatologists are concerned about the use of echinacea in patients with autoimmune diseases such as rheumatoid arthritis, lupus and psoriatic arthritis. Echinacea, being an immune stimulant, may cause flares, and this highlights the need for the doctor to know what the patient is taking. Unfortunately, from experiences of doctors both in the UK and elsewhere, patients are often unwilling to admit to doctors that they are seeking medical help on their own. They may perhaps be more willing to talk to a nurse or pharmacist.

Agnus castus contains volatile oils, castine and alkaloids. It is used to treat the symptoms of hormonal imbalance associated with menstruation and the menopause and is said to improve the function of the corpus luteum. The powdered fruit can be incorporated into tablets or used as a liquid extract or tincture.

Feverfew has active ingredients called *sesquiterpene lactones* from the aerial parts of the plant and is recommended for the prophylaxis of migraine. The sesquiterpene lactones are spasmolytic and render smooth muscle less responsive to noradrenaline, acetylcholine, bradykinin, histamine, prostaglandins and serotonin (5-hydroxytryptamine). Feverfew's activity in migraine is thought to be due to its inhibition of: (a) the production of the inflammatory, platelet-aggregating prostaglandins and (b) serotonin release from the platelets.

Chamomiles contain aliphatic esters of angelic and tiglic acids, and other oils extracted from the flowers. Roman chamomile promotes digestion, increases appetite and is antiemetic, antispasmodic and mildly sedative when taken orally. German chamomile or *matricaria* is used most extensively as a panacea. Preparations of warm and cold infusions of both chamomile and matricaria serve as medicinal agents and as health-related drinks. Teas, made by steeping loose fresh or dried flowers in water or teabags, are used both orally and externally.

Herbal diuretics include bearberry, celery and dandelion. These herbal diuretics are used traditionally by herbalists in the treatment of microbial infections and chronic inflammatory disorders. In more recent years, they have been incorporated in over-the-counter products used for other applications, such as the symptomatic relief of premenstrual syndrome, and as slimming aids. Dandelion is probably the preferred diuretic, as it is unlikely to result in toxicity and the roots and leaves contain high quantities of potassium, which reduces the likelihood of hypokalaemia. Bearberry is primarily of use as a urinary antiseptic and is effective only if the urine is alkaline. Celery may cause allergic reactions or photodermatitis in some subjects.

Garlic contains various volatile oils including allicin, which is believed to form other sulphur-containing compounds responsible for its cholesterol-lowering effects. Studies have used doses of 600–900 mg of garlic powder a day or one-half to one garlic clove a day to produce reductions in cholesterol of 9%–12% compared with placebo in patients with hyperlipidaemia. Interest has been shown in using garlic as an antihypertensive, but clinical trials have not shown significant results. Garlic has also been proposed to have antithrombotic activity. Traditionally, garlic has been used to treat a wide range of conditions, including chronic bronchitis, coughs, colds and influenza, and is also believed to have expectorant, antiviral, bacteriostatic and anthelmintic properties.

St. John's wort (*Hypericum perforatum*) is used extensively in both homeopathic and herbal preparations traditionally as a sedative and for wound healing. However, clinical trials have demonstrated that St. John's wort at doses of 350–900 mg daily have a similar effectiveness to amitriptyline in the treatment of mild or moderately severe depressive disorders (Apaydin et al., 2016).

CLINICAL NOTE

St. John's wort is generally well-tolerated, but photosensitivity is a recognized adverse effect and so patients should be advised of this when taking it. **It interacts with a number of important drugs, including a number of antiretroviral HIV drugs, warfarin, digoxin and theophylline** (Henderson et al., 2002). Most extracts of hypericum are standardized on their hypericin content, although it is considered that the effects of hypericum may be due to a variety of constituents.

Ginkgo biloba (maidenhair tree) has been used medicinally for thousands of years. Traditionally, it has been used as a tea for the treatment of asthma and bronchitis. It is widely used in France and Germany in licensed herbal remedies for the treatment of circulatory insufficiencies (peripheral and cerebral) (Mei et al., 2017). Many clinical studies of varying quality have examined its use in cerebral insufficiency, employing doses of 120 mg daily for 4–6 weeks or 50 mg three times a day for up to 52 weeks. Further study is required but clinically significant effects have been found for improving cognitive impairment and daily living/social behaviour. Naturally occurring receptor antagonists for the inflammatory mediator *platelet activating factor* have been identified from extracts of ginkgo biloba, some of which have shown promise in the treatment of inflammatory conditions.

Coltsfoot (*Tussilago farfara*): the leaves and flowers from this common wild plant have long been used in the form of tea as a popular remedy for coughs and bronchial congestion. The mucilage produced from the leaves is thought to produce a throat-soothing effect. The preparations available often contain complex mixtures of different medicinal plants. However, safety concerns have been expressed about its long-term use and use in pregnancy due to its content of pyrrolizidine alkaloids, which could be potentially tumour-inducing.

Essential Oils

Essential oil constituents are found in conventional medicinal products, e.g. peppermint oil for the relief of abdominal colic and distension. However, the practice of aromatherapy for the palliative care of patients with cancer and for hospice patients has brought the use of essential oils into a different area for the nurse. Some midwives are using aromatherapy for pregnancy and childbirth and for both the mother and infant after birth.

Essential oils are obtained from plant material, e.g. root, leaves, flowers, seeds, usually by distillation, although physical expression is used to obtain some essential oils, mainly those from citrus fruit. It should be noted that there are no controls on the quality of the products sold to the consumer. The concentration of constituents can vary between plant sources and adulteration and contamination is known to occur with pesticides, synthetic oils and other oils. The chemistry of essential oils is complex. A typical essential oil will contain about 100 or more chemical constituents, but most will be present in concentrations below 1%. In aromatherapy, it is the constituents of the oils that are thought to provide the 'relaxant' or 'stimulant' effect. Examples of constituents found in some essential oils are given in Table 34.3.

TABLE 34.3
Constituents Found in Essential Oils

Constituent	Source
Limonene	Citrus oils, e.g. bergamot
Thymol	Thyme oil
Cineole	Eucalyptus oil
Citral	Lemongrass
Linalyl acetate	Lavender oil

Essential oils are believed to act in two ways:

- By exerting pharmacological effects following absorption into the circulation. It is not clear what these effects are, or if they occur at all
- Via the effects of their odour on the olfactory system
- It may be that it is the act of massage using a pleasant-smelling substance that brings the most benefit, particularly in helping relaxation.

Topical application (i.e. massage) and inhalation have been shown to result in constituents being absorbed into the circulation. However, some oils can cause skin irritation or contact dermatitis, even when highly diluted in a bath, and some, particularly citrus fruit (with the exception of mandarin), have resulted in photosensitivity. Tea tree oil has been used for the treatment of certain skin infections and clinical trials have shown its potential for use in treating acne.

Patients wishing to consult an aromatherapist should be advised to choose one who has undertaken relevant training, is registered with an appropriate professional body and who has adequate professional indemnity.

HOMEOPATHY

Homeopathy is a controversial alternative therapy. It is very popular, particularly in France and Germany. The maxim that '*there is no such thing as alternative therapy, there are only therapies that can be shown to work, and therapies that can be shown not to work*' certainly can be applied to homeopathy. It is an eminently testable therapy. When it is tested, the results are almost always negative, and even the few positive clinical studies can be shown to be of poor quality and their results cannot be replicated in higher quality trials. There is no substantial evidence that homeopathy is clearly efficacious for any single clinical condition. When the same standards of testing are applied to homeopathy as are applied to conventional drugs, homeopathy is shown to be no better than a placebo. Fascinatingly, none of this evidence is enough to convince enthusiasts that homeopathy is ineffective.

History and Philosophy of Homeopathy

In the 18th century, Dr. Samuel Hahnemann (1755–1843), a German-born physician, appalled by the medical practices of the day, sought a method of healing, which would be safe, gentle and effective. He believed that human beings have a capacity for healing themselves and that the symptoms of disease reflect the struggle of individuals to overcome their illness. He reasoned that instead of suppressing symptoms, he could seek to stimulate them and so encourage and assist the body's natural healing process.

Hahnemann discovered that when he self-administered an infusion of cinchona bark (quinine) it produced the symptoms of malaria. When given to a patient suffering from the disease it alleviated the symptoms. He used this procedure with numerous active substances from animal, vegetable and mineral sources in healthy volunteers to determine the 'symptom picture' of each substance. This approach came to be known as 'proving'. He then went on to establish the smallest effective dose to reduce the toxicity of the substance. He diluted his medicines and subjected them to vigorous shaking ('succussion') at each dilution step. He claimed that the more dilute the remedies were, the more potent they became; this process of serial dilution and succussion became known as 'potentization'.

Homeopathy became extremely popular in Europe, especially in France, and all but dominated medicine in the USA, not least because it offered another, gentler route than the drastic and damaging treatments such as bleeding, purging and violent emesis that were all that conventional medicine had to offer for many of the diseases that contemporary doctors did not understand at the time.

Homeopathy's run of popularity ended abruptly with the discovery of antibiotics, whose dramatic, fast and life-saving actions swept it away for much of the 20th century. Homeopathy was still taught and practised and retained much respectability. Now, however, there is a great resurgence in the use of homeopathy, due perhaps to a combination of an accumulation of knowledge of the adverse effects of many of our modern drugs.

Features of Homeopathy

Classical homeopathy has the following characteristics:

- Medicines are chosen on the basis of the similarity between the symptoms they produce in healthy people and the symptoms from which the patient is suffering.
- The medicines are given singly.
- The medicines are given in very minute doses.
- Medicines are not repeated routinely, but only when the patient's symptoms demand it.

In practice, there are wide variations in how these principles are applied; a good deal depends on the orientation of the particular homeopath, with respect to the symptoms he or she considers important (physical and psychological), the type of illness and whether the illness is acute or chronic. Many homeopaths ignore the 'single remedy' rule, preferring to adopt a multiple prescribing approach, such as in remedies for hay fever.

Diagnosis and Treatment

In addition to the basic principles of classical homeopathy, there are other basic tenets of homeopathy. Homeopaths believe that illness results from the body's inability to cope with challenging factors, such as poor diet and environmental conditions, and that the signs and symptoms of disease represent the body's attempt to restore order. Homeopathic remedies are believed not to act directly on the disease process but to stimulate the body's own healing activity known as the 'vital force'. As homeopaths believe that the 'vital force' is expressed differently in each individual, their choice of treatment is based on each individual's unique set of symptoms. It is usual for a homeopath during a first consultation to take a very detailed history to determine the patient's physical, mental and emotional symptoms. A homeopath may then use a 'homeopathic repertory' to choose a remedy that most closely fits a patient's symptom picture. Computerized repertories are now available, which greatly facilitate this process.

Having chosen the remedy, the homeopath must select the potency and the form, e.g. tablets, pills or powders. The method of preparing a homeopathic medicine usually commences with the 'mother tincture', which is usually a concentrated alcoholic extract. One drop of this is mixed with 99 (or sometimes 9) drops of water and shaken hard to give the first potency, i.e. 1c the first centesimal dilution. One drop of this preparation is then mixed with 99 drops of water and shaken to give the second potency (2c), and this process is repeated for as many times as required. Insoluble substances, such as metals, are ground up in a mortar and mixed with lactose. Some commonly used potencies are the 6c, 12c and 30c.

Modern molecular theory suggests that the 12th centesimal potency is the limit beyond which no molecules of the original substance would be present. This is therefore taken as the boundary between 'low' and 'high' potencies. In practice, the high potencies are considered more powerful than the low ones, despite the near absence of any of the original substance. This claim is justified by suggesting that the medicine has been 'dynamized' to a greater extent. The 'seriousness' of the symptoms determines how frequently the remedy is administered and the number of total doses.

Mechanism of Action

The lack of an even slightly plausible mechanism of action continues to be one of the strongest arguments against homeopathy, when combined with a lack of evidence of efficacy in well-controlled clinical trials. Numerous hypotheses of the supposed mechanism of action of homeopathic potencies exist. How the solution 'remembers' information from the original substance (without 'remembering' information from any of the contaminants that will also have been in it) is speculation that bears no relation to our current understanding of physics and chemistry.

The Placebo Response

The placebo response is a beneficial effect of a preparation that has no medicine in it and contains only vehicle (e.g. lactose in pills). No health professional these days dismisses the placebo response out of hand; too many have seen dramatic cures and improvements in symptoms from patients who have taken treatments such as homeopathy, faith healing or who take placebos in clinical trials. It is a matter of debate whether a practitioner should knowingly prescribe a placebo to a patient without informing them. To inform the patient they were being given a placebo would undermine the basis of the placebo effect, but many medical ethicists and medical regulatory authorities consider it to be unethical to knowingly prescribe a placebo to a patient without their knowledge.

Safety

Homeopathic remedies are often claimed to be entirely free from adverse effects. However, there are isolated reports in the literature of suspected adverse effects, usually allergic reactions, following the use of homeopathic remedies. It is difficult to assess these claims without a detailed chemical analysis of the preparation used, which might have contained impurities. Also, it is often stated that a patient may experience an 'aggravation' (a temporary worsening of symptoms) within a few days of starting treatment. Homeopaths claim that this is a sign that the correct remedy has been chosen and that it is working. It is also possible for a patient to suffer harm from the use of an ineffective treatment, instead of using a potentially effective orthodox treatment.

Certain homeopaths (usually lay practitioners) have been criticized in the past for advocating the use of homeopathic remedies as an alternative for immunization in childhood. Patients seeking a consultation should be advised to check that the homeopath has recognized qualifications, is registered with a relevant professional body, e.g. the British Homeopathic Association, the Society of Homeopaths, the UK Homeopathic Medical Association, and has adequate professional indemnity. There is also a plethora of remedies available for self-administration.

It is often claimed that the use of caffeine, aromatic substances (e.g. peppermint, essential oils) or certain orthodox drugs (e.g. corticosteroids) can inactivate homeopathic remedies if used concurrently. However, there does not appear to be any reliable evidence to support this and there is no evidence that homeopathic remedies interact with conventional medicines, although homeopaths may claim that a patient's symptoms may be 'masked' by conventional medicines, therefore making an accurate choice of homeopathic remedy more difficult.

REFERENCES AND FURTHER READING

Apaydin, E.A., Maher, A.R., Shanman, R., et al., 2016. A systematic review of St. John's wort for major depressive disorder. Syst. Rev. 5 (1), 148.

Ekor, M., 2014. The growing use of herbal medicines: issues relating to adverse reactions and challenges in monitoring safety. Front. Pharmacol. 4, 177.

Henderson, L., Yue, Q.Y., Bergquist, C., et al., 2002. St John's wort (Hypericum perforatum): drug interactions and clinical outcomes. Br. J. Clin. Pharmacol. 54 (4), 349–356.

Johnson, T., Boon, H., 2007. Where does homeopathy fit in pharmacy practice? Am. J. Pharm. Educ. 71 (1), 7.

Mantle, F., 2008. Homeopathy: History, Treatment Options and Evidence Base for Homeopathic Remedies. Nursing Times. article https://www.nursingtimes.net/archive/homeopathy-21-07-2008/.

Mathie, R.T., Ramparsad, N., Legg, L.A., et al., 2017. Randomised, double-blind, placebo-controlled trials of non-individualised homeopathic treatment: systematic review and meta-analysis. Syst. Rev. 6 (1), 63.

Mei, N., Guo, X., Ren, Z., et al., 2017. Review of Ginkgo biloba-induced toxicity, from experimental studies to human case reports. J. Environ. Sci. Health C Environ. Carcinog. Ecotoxicol. Rev. 35 (1), 1–28.

Nelson, D.H., Perchaluk, J.M., Logan, A.C., Katzman, M.A., 2019. The bell tolls for homeopathy: time for change in the training and practice of north American naturopathic physicians. J. Evid. Based Integr. Med. 24, 2515690X18823696.

Posadzki, P., Watson, L.K., Ernst, E., 2013. Adverse effects of herbal medicines: an overview of systematic reviews. Clin. Med. 13 (1), 7–12.

Salamonsen, A., Wiesener, S., 2019. 'Then I went to a hospital abroad': acknowledging implications of stakeholders' differing risk understandings related to use of complementary and alternative medicine in European health care contexts. BMC Complement. Altern. Med. 19 (1), 93.

Stub, T., Quandt, S.A., Arcury, T.A., et al., 2016. Perception of risk and communication among conventional and complementary health care providers involving cancer patients' use of complementary therapies: a literature review. BMC Complement. Altern. Med. 16 (1), 353.

Zamanzadeh, V., Jasemi, M., Valizadeh, L., et al., 2015. Effective factors in providing holistic care: a qualitative study. Indian J. Palliat. Care 21 (2), 214–224.

USEFUL WEBSITES

Homeopathic Nurses Association (HNA). http://www.nursehomeopaths.org.

Patient. http://www.patient.co.uk/patientplus.asp.

APPENDIX

BIOLOGIC AGENTS

INTRODUCTION

While biopharmaceutical drugs and therapies have been used for a long time, it is only in the last 20 years or so that the agents most commonly referred to as 'Biologics' – monoclonal antibody (MAb)-based therapies – have appeared and come into use. Since the introduction of the first TNF-α blocking biologics for the treatment of rheumatoid arthritis, in the mid-1990s, there has been a huge growth in the field of 'MAb-based biologics', with new agents being introduced all the time, and for an increasing range of conditions. By 2017, there were MAbs targeted at 37 diseases or more, and more are being developed (Shepard et al. 2017).

It is not an exaggeration to say that biologics have led to a revolution in therapeutics that has enabled more precise targeting of disease processes than was often possible with traditional small molecule drugs. Almost every area of clinical practice has benefitted but in particular, rheumatology, oncology, gastroenterology and dermatology have seen the introduction of new treatments for diseases that were previously difficult or impossible to treat. This Appendix is intended to provide an overview of these agents, but can only skim the surface of a complex and fascinating new area of therapeutics.

All treatment revolutions have downsides, and for the biologics, there are several. Perhaps most striking is the fact that these agents are complex and difficult to develop and test and then manufacture. This is reflected in their prices, which are generally orders of magnitude greater than most small molecule drugs. For instance, in 2020, one pre-filled syringe of golimumab 100 mg had a UK NHS indicative price of £1525 and a US retail price of around $5700. As this dose is given monthly, the costs are considerable and may be beyond the reach of healthcare systems in middle- and lower-income countries. The introduction of 'Biosimilars' (see later) is leading to some reduction in the cost of some treatments.

Another issue with these agents is that they are large molecules, based on antibodies that are meant to interact with the immune system. The earliest of them were modified mouse antibodies and all of these factors mean that allergic reactions to them are relatively common. Newer agents have been altered to resemble human antibodies or are constructed to be identical to human antibodies, and this reduces their immunogenicity.

These agents affect cellular function at a profound level and can have adverse effects related to their mechanisms of action. Many affect immune functioning, and increased susceptibility to infection is a common and sometimes serious, unwanted effect. Some have idiosyncratic adverse effects: the TNF-α inhibitors may increase the risk of worsening or even inducing multiple sclerosis (MS), although this seems rare and the mechanism by which this might occur remains obscure. Several biologics were withdrawn from use when it became clear that their risks outweighed their benefits.

All Mab-related agents need to be given by infusion or injection, which may limit their availability and acceptability, although self-administered injections are possible with some of these agents.

Types of Biological Therapy

Any medicinal product that is extracted from or manufactured by biological sources can be referred to as a biopharmaceutical or a biologic, although, as noted, in common usage a 'biologic' is generally taken to refer to MAb-based agents.

Before MAbs, there were many biopharmaceuticals in clinical use, and many continue to be developed and used today. Important examples are:

- blood and blood products
- immunoglobulins, containing antibodies from hyperimmune individuals (to treat or prevent some viral infections by passive immunization)
- tissue and organ transplants
- stem cells
- erythropoietin
- insulins.

Insulins are an important example because of their widespread use over the past century, and the fact that they were originally extracted from animal tissue, but are now made using the recombinant DNA technology that is used to make many other biologics. Recombinant human identical insulin (*Humulin*) was the first biopharmaceutical to be made using this technology.

MONOCLONAL ANTIBODY-BASED BIOLOGICS

This section provides an overview of the production, nomenclature, mechanisms of action and therapeutic use of MAb biologics and agents based on similar technologies.

Antibodies

All MAbs are, or are based upon, ***antibodies***. These are complex protein molecules, otherwise known as ***immunoglobulins***, and in mammals are produced by specialized B lymphocytes as an immune response to the presence of 'foreign' proteins – proteins not found within the host organism – such as bacteria and viruses. They have a distinctive Y-shaped structure (Fig. A1) made of gamma globulin proteins of two sorts, known as *heavy chains* and *light chains*. The stem of the 'Y' is relatively unchanging and is known as the *constant region* and at its base is a protein structure that enables it to interact with other cells of the immune system, such as the neutrophil white blood cells, triggering them to kill the bacterium or other organism that the antibody has bound to. Antibodies bind to specific structures on bacteria and other organisms (and also non-living allergens). These are known as *antigens* and it is the ends of the two limbs of the 'Y' that bind to them. These two limbs are known as the *variable region* of the antibody. The ends of these limbs can take very many forms, corresponding to a huge range of possible antigens, and act as 3-dimensional 'locks' into which specific 'keys' – the antigens – bind. Any one antibody will normally only bind to one antigen and it does so with extreme precision. It is this specificity that makes antibodies of such value, if they can be designed to target antigens they would not normally target, such as particular cellular signalling molecules involved in inflammatory or neoplastic diseases. When an antibody binds to an antigen on a cell, it may block the function that the antigen has in that cell, or it may trigger the other cells of the immune system to destroy the antigen-bound cell. Both of these mechanisms may be used by MAb-based biologic therapies.

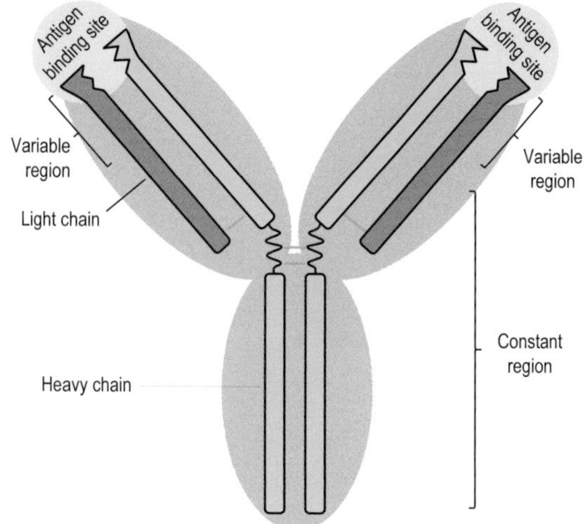

Fig. A1 ■ Antibody structure.

How MAb Biologics are Made

Monoclonal means '*one* (*mono*) and *copy* (*clone*)'. A monoclonal antibody is a single antibody, directed against a single antigen, grown in cell culture bioreactors. The earliest MAbs were produced by inoculating a mouse with the specific human antigen of interest so that the mouse produced antibodies against that antigen. The mouse B lymphocytes producing that one particular antibody were then extracted and fused with human myeloma cells. These abnormal blood cancer cells constantly produce abnormal antibody fragments, but when fused with the mouse cells they produce a constant large supply of the one specific mouse antibody. The fused myeloma cells can be grown at scale and the monoclonal antibodies they produce can be extracted, purified and used therapeutically.

As noted earlier, mouse antibodies are immunogenic and provoke allergic reactions when used in humans. Various approaches have been developed to reduce this problem. Initially, recombinant DNA technology was used to alter the mouse antibodies by replacing large segments of the mouse antibody with segments of human antibody. This produces ***chimeric*** antibodies that are structurally about 65% human and are less likely to provoke allergic reactions. More recently, ***humanized*** antibodies have been produced using transgenic mice and other technologies. These are structurally about 95% human and are much less likely to provoke allergic reactions. Only the very end of the variable region – the 'lock' – remains from the original mouse antibody. The most recent technologies enable the production of ***fully human*** antibodies (Fig. A2).

More recently, agents have been introduced that are fragments of antibodies, comprising only the ends of the variable regions that contain the 'locks' for the antigen 'keys'. These can be produced by recombinant technology directly from bacterial cultures, in a manner similar to human insulins. This technology reduces costs somewhat. Examples include **abciximab** and **certolizumab pegol**.

The technology of MAb production is extremely sophisticated and difficult and accounts for the high cost of these agents.

MAb Biologic Names

MAb biologics have difficult to pronounce non-proprietary (generic) names and are generally known by their manufacturers' trade names. There is, however, a rationale behind the generic names, which is the *WHO nomenclature of monoclonal antibodies*. Key parts of this nomenclature are:

- Most importantly, MAb names always end in '*-mab*'.

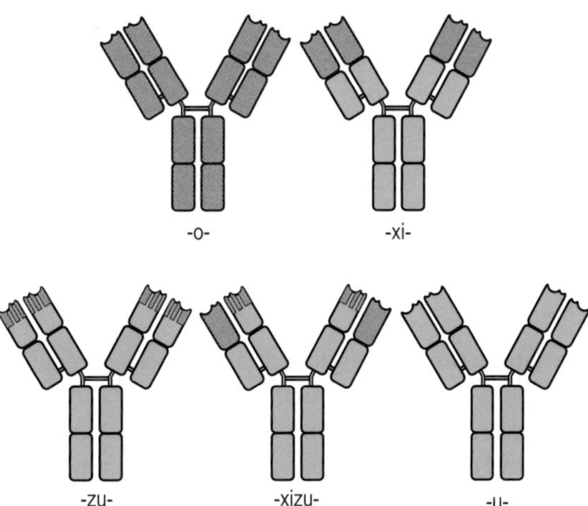

Fig. A2 ■ Mouse, chimeric, humanized, chimeric humanized and fully human antibodies. The grey areas indicate mouse protein and the blue areas human protein. The letters in the generic names associated with these types of antibodies are shown below each one.

- The first part of the name is a combination of unique identifier and a letter combination that indicates the main target of the agent. So, '*t(u)*' indicates it is targeted at a tumour. '*l(i)*' indicates an immunomodulating function. Other targets exist and are indicated by other letter combinations.
- The last part, before the '*-mab*', indicates the origin of the antibody. Fully murine antibodies have the letter '*-o*' in the name. Chimeric antibodies contain '*xi*'; humanized antibodies contain '*zu*'; mixed chimeric/humanized antibodies contain '*xizu*'; and fully human antibodies contain '*(m)u*'. Fig. A2 demonstrates this aspect further.

Thus, for example, for **rituximab** the suffix *-mab* indicates that it is a monoclonal antibody, the *-xi-* denotes that it is of chimeric origin, the *-tu-* shows that it targets a tumour, and the prefix *ri-* is its individualized prefix.

For **golimumab**, the suffix *-mab* indicates that it is a monoclonal antibody, the *-u* indicates that it is a fully human antibody, the *-li* indicates that it modulates immune responses and the prefix *go-* is its individualized prefix.

The fusion protein biologics (see later), although often based on an immunoglobulin structure, are not MAbs and do not share these naming conventions.

Several of the agents currently in use share the suffix '...*cept*'. **Etanercept** is an example of this.

Monoclonal Antibody Biologics

MAb biologics are used for many different therapeutic purposes, and examples of these are to be found throughout this book.

Most MAb biologics work in one of three ways (Fig. A3):

- Some work by binding to and effectively neutralizing circulating signalling substances that may be present in excessive amounts. MAbs exist that bind to many different substances, but among the most important are those that bind to circulating TNF-α. This substance is an important promoter of inflammatory responses in many conditions, but particularly rheumatological conditions, psoriasis and Crohn's disease. By binding to the excessive circulating TNF-α and rendering it biologically inactive, MAbs such as **adalimumab** and **certolizumab pegol** dramatically reduce inflammation. Other circulating MAb targets include various interleukins and other substances, including drugs.
- Many MAbs work by binding to cell surface proteins and either render them inaccessible to circulating signalling substances or alter their function (stimulate or block) and so change intracellular activities, such as growth or protein synthesis. Important examples of this are the anti-cancer agents **trastuzumab** and **pertuzumab** that bind to the abnormal HER2 receptor that is present in some breast cancers. In different ways, they affect the functioning of the receptor and have a marked effect in reducing the growth of the cancer cells. MAbs have been developed that bind to many other types of cell surface receptor.
- A subset of the type of MAb described previously act like natural antibodies and trigger the destruction of cells that they bind to. Several MAbs used in haematological cancers utilize this mechanism. An example is **rituximab**, which binds to CD20 proteins on circulating B lymphocytes and causes them to die. It destroys both normal and malignant B cells but is very useful in B cell malignancies. More sophisticated MAbs of this type have a different binding site 'lock' on each arm of the variable region and so can bind two different antigens simultaneously. These *bispecific* MAbs are used in cancer immunotherapy where they bind an antigen on a tumour cell and an antigen on an immune system cytotoxic T cell, bringing them into close proximity and activating the T cell to destroy the tumour cell. An example is **blinatumomab**, used to treat some lymphoblastic leukaemias.

1. Bind and neutralize ligand.
e.g. Adalimumab + TNFα

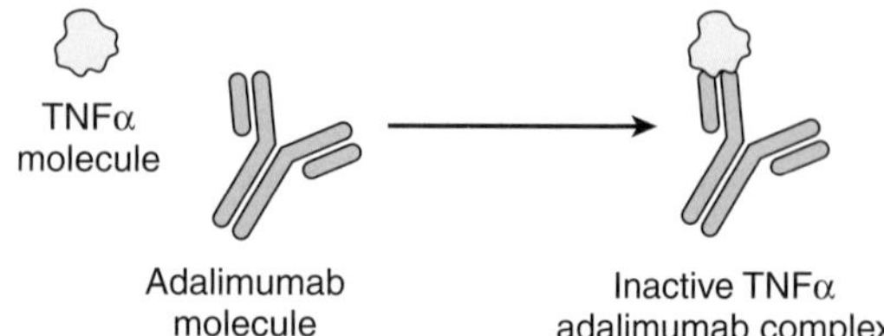
TNFα
molecule
Adalimumab
molecule
Inactive TNFα
adalimumab complex

2. Bind and inactivate cell membrane receptor.
e.g. Trastuzumab + breast cancer HER2 receptor
[Some MAbs *activate* cell membrane receptors]

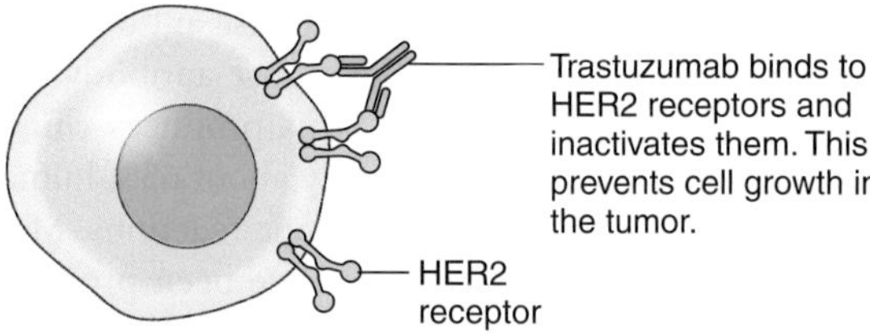
Trastuzumab binds to
HER2 receptors and
inactivates them. This
prevents cell growth in
the tumor.
HER2
receptor
Breast tumor cell

3. Bind to cell surface antigen and trigger cell death.
e.g. Rituxumab and B cell lysis

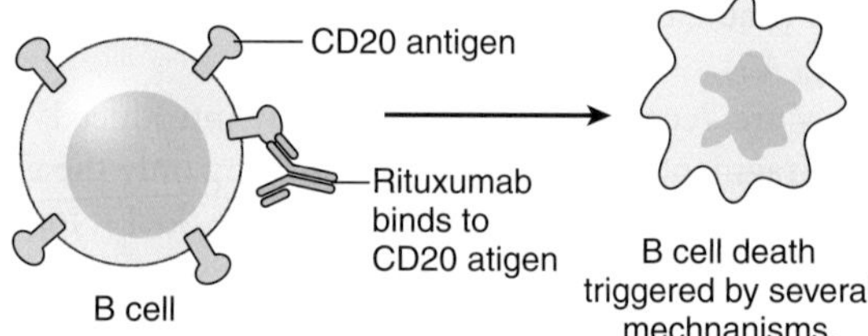
CD20 antigen
Rituxumab
binds to
CD20 atigen
B cell
B cell death
triggered by several
mechnanisms.

Fig. A3 ■ Main mechanisms of MAb biologic action.
1. Bind and neutralize ligand, e.g. adalimumab and TNF-α.
2. Bind and inactivate cell membrane receptor, e.g. trastuzumab and breast cancer HER2 receptor (some MAbs activate cell membrane receptors).
3. Bind to cell surface antigen and trigger cell death, e.g. rituximab and B cell lysis.

There are many MAbs with many different targets. It is important to become familiar with those most used in your own speciality of practice. MAb development proceeds apace and dynamically updated lists of the agents offer the only possibility of keeping up-to-date with developments. One such list contains over 500 MAbs, including those that are under development and those which have been withdrawn. (A website for access to this list is given in the Useful Websites section at the end of this Appendix.)

FUSION PROTEIN BIOLOGICS

These drugs are conceptually closely related to MAbs, and they are often based upon part of the antibody molecule framework. Commonly, they retain the constant region of the antibody but do not have the arms of the variable region. Instead of the 'lock' formed by the variable region, they instead have a different type of protein 'lock' fused to the constant region. Often, this will be a fragment of a cell surface receptor, and these ***fusion protein*** constructs can be used to bind circulating signalling substances in a similar manner to the first MAb mechanism described earlier. **Etanercept** was an early example. Here, the 'lock' is a fragment of the natural tumour necrosis factor receptor, and it binds circulating TNF-α in a similar manner to adalimumab. Other fusion protein biologics bind to cell surface receptors and alter their activity. **Abatacept** binds to receptors on T lymphocytes and prevents them from becoming activated. It is of value in autoimmune conditions, such as rheumatoid arthritis.

Other types of 'biologic drug' exist or are being developed. There is continued interest in combining the target sensitivity of MAbs with cytotoxic or other drugs, to provide targeted 'magic bullets' in cancer and other therapies. To date, progress in this area has been slow and somewhat disappointing.

USES OF BIOLOGICS

Disordered cell growth and disorders of immune system regulation feature in many diseases, but particularly in cancers and rheumatological diseases. Biologics have had a major impact in both of these groups of diseases, but also in other conditions associated with inflammation, abnormal blood vessel development and many others. In principle, any condition that depends in some way on cell-to-cell communication by signalling molecules can be targeted by MAb or fusion proteins. In clinical practice, they have transformed the treatment of inflammatory arthritis and have improved the chances of remission or cure in some difficult to treat cancers. They have offered improvements in therapy for inflammatory bowel disease, psoriasis and some types of macular degeneration. However, against these positives, it should be noted that for some cancers, biologics do not offer the possibility of cure or prolonged remission and in some cases, offer only a brief extension to life at sometimes dramatically high cost. It is possible that the use of biologics earlier on in the course of cancers, rather than after other treatments have failed, may improve these outcomes, and research is ongoing. More than most therapies, the introduction of biologics in cancer care have forced clinicians and healthcare providers to face difficult questions about costs versus benefits of treatment in healthcare systems with finite resources. These drugs are also relatively new and their long-term effects are not yet fully understood. However, the increased risk of infections with many of these agents, and other risks, such as increased cancer risk, MS or cardiomyopathy risk among others; need to be carefully considered before these treatments are used.

Biologic MAb-based drugs have been used to treat these (and more) conditions:

- Cancers: leukaemias, lymphomas, breast, colon, stomach, brain, melanoma and childhood solid tumours and others
- Rheumatoid arthritis
- Ankylosing spondylitis
- Crohn's disease
- Ulcerative colitis
- Psoriasis and psoriatic arthritis
- Multiple sclerosis
- Acute coronary syndrome
- Systemic lupus erythematous
- Wet macular degeneration
- Diabetic retinopathy
- Anaemias
- Migraine
- Osteoporosis
- Asthma
- Urticaria
- Paroxysmal nocturnal haemoglobinuria.

ADMINISTRATION OF BIOLOGICS

MAb-based biologics are not absorbed by mouth and are usually given by intravenous infusion or subcutaneous injection. Injection technique can be taught and automated delivery devices can enable patients to self-administer these agents. They have a long half-life in the circulation and typically last 2–4 weeks after administration, so dosing can be infrequent. MAbs do not pass through an intact blood–brain barrier.

Unlike other drugs, it is important that biologic drugs (and biosimilars – see later) are prescribed by brand name, in order to avoid drug errors.

Patients should be carefully assessed prior to commencement of biologic treatment. In particular, the risk of current infection or reactivation of latent infections, such as TB, HIV or hepatitis needs careful assessment. For most agents, liver function and blood counts need to be assessed and then monitored and for some agents, other parameters, such as urinary protein and total immunoglobulin levels, need assessment and monitoring. Patients should normally be up-to-date with all routine vaccinations, particularly pneumococcal, influenza, hepatitis, measles, mumps and rubella. Live vaccinations may be contraindicated if the patient is already using immunosuppressive therapy, and should not be given while patients are using biologic treatments. If a vaccine is required before treatment starts, it should be given at least a month before treatment start, or vaccine response may be poor. Risk of malignancy can be assessed based on family history and lifestyle factors, and any suspicion of malignancy must be excluded before biologic treatments for inflammatory conditions are started.

It is important to be able to recognize and manage allergic reactions to these agents.

During treatment, patients and their carers should be advised of the signs of infection and of blood dyscrasias (such as bleeding or easy bruising) and these should be enquired about before each treatment. Individual agents will have particular high-risk side-effects that should also be enquired about. Monitoring investigations vary between agents, but are often less intensive than with older treatments. The practitioner should assess the response to treatment and enquire about concerns and adverse effects.

Adequate monitoring of biologic agents requires a good knowledge of the agents used, and the conditions they are being used to treat. Although there are a bewildering number of these agents, those in use in any one therapeutic field are relatively limited and it is important to have a good understanding of the agents you are using.

BIOSIMILARS

Similar biologics or ***Biosimilars*** are analogous to generic small molecule drugs, in that they are versions of biologics introduced after the original's patent has expired. In principle, they should be cheaper than the original, as their development costs are somewhat less. However, there are important differences between biosimilars and generic small molecule drugs. The most important is that biosimilars are not structurally identical to the original agent. Unlike generic drugs, in which the active agent is identical to the original (although some of the inactive ingredients may differ), a biosimilar is *similar* in structure, and for all clinical purposes, *identical* in activity, to the original biologic. MAbs are huge molecules, relative to small molecule drugs, and the process of creating and then manufacturing them from living organisms means that they can never be identical to the original agent, even though they are directed against the same antigen. In view of this, the process of creating and gaining approval for a biosimilar is much more complex than that for a generic drug. Some of the safety and efficacy testing needed for the original agent can be reduced for its biosimilar, but cannot be removed altogether. All of these factors mean that, while biosimilars will generally cost less than the original agent, they are still expensive drugs. However, they do offer the potential for wider use within healthcare systems because of their reduced cost. It should always be remembered that they are not identical to the original agent and this may occasionally show itself in different efficacy or adverse effects in some patients. Unlike generic drugs, where generic dispensing of a branded prescription may be acceptable (if legally permitted), a biosimilar must never be substituted for an original biologic, without careful assessment and discussion.

Biosimilar Names

As with all biologics, biosimilars must be prescribed by brand name. Different approaches exist in different countries to biosimilar nomenclature. In the UK and EU, biosimilars and their original biologic share the same generic (non-proprietary) name, and the only way of distinguishing them is by the brand name. Canada takes the same approach but requires both brand and generic names to be shown on all prescriptions. The USA requires that all biosimilars' generic names contain a four-character suffix that is unique to that particular brand of biosimilar.

Thus, in the UK **adalimumab** may be prescribed as the original biologic brand name, *Humira*, or as the biosimilars, *Amgevita*, *Hulio*, *Hyrimoz* or *Imraldi*. In the USA, the biosimilar would be additionally identified by a four-character suffix. So, the FDA approved biosimilar of adalimumab is *Hadlima*, and its generic name is **adalimumab-bwwd**.

It is important to become familiar with the approved nomenclature in your country of practice.

REFERENCES AND FURTHER READING

Shepard, H.M., Phillips, G.L., Thanos, C.D., Feldmann, M., 2017. Developments in therapy with monoclonal antibodies and related proteins. Clin. Med. (Lond.) 17 (3), 220–232.

USEFUL WEBSITES

Wikipedia. List of therapeutic monoclonal antibodies. https://en.wikipedia.org/wiki/list_of_therapeutic_monoclonal_antibodies.

A list of 500 MAbs – an up-to-date online list of (almost) all MAbs in use, in development and withdrawn from use.

GLOSSARY

ACE inhibitors: Drugs that inhibit angiotensin converting enzyme (see also **ARB**)

Acetylsalicylic acid: Aspirin

ACh: Acetylcholine

Acidosis: Abnormal acidity of body fluids and tissues

Acid reflux: Backflow of acid from the stomach into the oesophagus

Acquired specific immune responses: The responses of the immune system which are able to recognize as foreign specific proteins of invading organisms or of neoplastic cells and make antibodies against them

Acromegaly: Excessive production of growth hormone by a tumour of the pituitary gland in adults leading to abnormal bone overgrowth, especially in the face

Active immunization: Promotion of the production by the patient, of antibodies or sensitized lymphocytes to certain bacteria or toxins produced by bacteria before infection occurs (see also **passive immunization**)

Acute: Sudden, recent onset of a disease process. Does *not* mean severe (see also **chronic**)

Acute confusional states (called delirium by some practitioners): States of impaired cognition, mood and self-awareness or attention that are often superimposed on an underlying disease such as dementia or schizophrenia

Acute coronary syndrome: Any acute reduction or interruption of coronary artery blood flow; may lead to myocardial infarction (see also **myocardial infarction**, **STEMI**, **NSTEMI**)

Acute inflammatory reaction: Part of the body's defence mechanism against invading pathogens. Redness, swelling and pain are typical

Addison's disease: Disease caused by deficiency of corticosteroid production and release from the adrenal cortex. The main symptoms are loss of energy, muscle weakness and hypotension. Low corticosteroids lower the body's defences against stress and infectious diseases

Adherence: The degree to which a patient follows medical advice. Related to the idea of **compliance**, but felt to be less paternalistic (see also **concordance**)

Adjuvant therapy: In cancer treatment, refers to the use of cytotoxic drugs to kill remaining cancer cells after surgery or radiotherapy, particularly if there is a high risk of recurrence of the tumour

Adrenaline (epinephrine): Hormone released from the adrenal medulla; one of the **catecholamines**

Adrenergic: Describes nerves of the sympathetic nervous system that release noradrenaline, or receptors that respond to noradrenaline (norepinephrine) and sympathomimetic drugs (see also **noradrenergic**)

Adverse effects: Unwanted effects; also called side-effects

Aerobes: Bacteria that require oxygen to grow

Afterload: The arterial resistance against which the heart must pump

Affinity: Describes the tightness of the binding reaction between drug and receptor

Agonist: Drug that reacts with a cell receptor, activating a cellular response similar to the physiological response of the cell

AIDS: Acquired immune deficiency syndrome

Akathisia: Feeling of restlessness with an inability to stand still

Alzheimer's disease: A progressive dementia characterized by short-term memory loss and progressive loss of cognitive ability

Anabolic: Promoting tissue growth; forming complex substances such as proteins and laying down glucose as glycogen

Anaemia: Clinically significant reduction in haemoglobin in blood

Analogue: Drug that is chemically related to a parent substance, e.g. ethinyloestradiol is an analogue of the hormone oestradiol, and has similar oestrogenic properties but, unlike oestradiol, can be taken by mouth

Anaerobes: Bacteria that can live and multiply in the absence of oxygen

Androgen: One of a group of compounds, including testosterone, which develops and maintains male sexual function and secondary male characteristics, e.g. hirsutism (hair growth)

Analgesic: Drug that relieves pain

Anaphylactic shock: Widespread release of histamine as part of an allergic response; can be fatal unless dealt with immediately

Angina: Crushing chest pain, often on exertion, generally due to ischaemic heart disease (see also **Chronic coronary syndrome**)

Antagonist: Drug that reacts with a cell receptor, blocking the cell activity that normally occurs when that receptor is stimulated

Anthelmintic: Chemical used to destroy parasitic worms

Anti-arrhythmic: Any drug used to treat heartbeat irregularities

Antibiotic: Any drug used to treat bacterial infections

Antibody: An immune system protein produced by **B lymphocytes** that binds to specific **antigens** and blocks their action, or triggers immune responses to them

Anticholinesterase: A drug that blocks the enzyme acetylcholinesterase, which breaks down the neurotransmitter acetylcholine

Anticoagulant: Agent that prevents or slows down the clotting of blood

Anticonvulsant: Drug that prevents or reduces the severity of epileptic seizures

Antidepressant: Drug that alleviates the symptoms of depression

Antiemetic: Agent that inhibits or reduces vomiting

Antigen: Any substance seen by the body as foreign, and against which the body may make a specific **antibody**

Antihistamine: Agent that blocks the action of histamine, usually by blocking histamine receptors

Antiinflammatory: Reducing or blocking inflammation reactions

Antimetabolite: Drug that blocks a metabolic pathway; commonly used in cancer treatment

Antimuscarinic: Drug that blocks **muscarinic** receptors

Antioxidant: Any substance that neutralizes oxygen free radicals

Antipsychotic (neuroleptic): Drug used to treat **psychosis**

Antipyretic: Lowering of body temperature (e.g. aspirin is antipyretic)

Antiserum: Serum containing antibodies directed against specific antigens; used clinically for **passive immunization**

Antitussive: Agent to treat coughs

Antithrombin III: A protein that is part of the system that regulates clotting. It binds to certain clotting factors and renders them inactive

Anxiety: A term used to describe a condition of generalized, all-pervasive fear

Anxiolytic: Drug that reduces anxiety

Aqueous humour: Fluid that fills the chamber of the eye behind the cornea and in front of the lens (see also **vitreous humour**)

ARB: Angiotensin receptor blocker (see also **ACE inhibitor**)

Ariboflavinosis: Deficiency of riboflavin (vitamin B_2) in humans causes several symptoms, including cracking and fissures at the corner of the mouth and a sore tongue and skin lesions

Arrhythmia: Deviation from the normal sinus rhythm of the heart

Aromatase inhibitor: Drug that blocks the biosynthesis of oestrogens by inhibiting the aromatase enzyme

Arteriole: Small branch of artery, important in the control of blood flow and blood pressure, since it is innervated by nerves and responds to drugs that may either dilate or constrict it

Arthritis: Inflammation of joints (see also **osteoarthritis** and **rheumatoid arthritis**)

Ascites: Accumulation of fluid in the peritoneal cavity, which causes the abdomen to swell

Atheroma: Degeneration of the inner arterial wall (intima) due to the deposition of fatty plaques and scarring; also called atherosclerosis

Athlete's foot: Fungal infection of the skin between the toes (tinea pedis)

Atrial fibrillation: Atrial arrhythmia marked by rapid, randomized contraction of small areas of the atrial myocardium, causing an irregular and often rapid ventricular rate

Atrial flutter: An arrythmia in which the atria contract at very high speed, usually about 240–300/minute

Atrioventricular (AV) node: A part of the heart in the lower part of the right ventricle that receives contractile impulses from the atria and transmits these to the ventricles through the **bundle of His**

Atrium: Either of the two upper chambers of the heart

Atrophy: Wasting away of tissues or organs due to cellular degeneration

Atypical antipsychotic agent: Second generation antipsychotic drugs with fewer side-effects than first generation (typical) antipsychotics

Aura: Distinctive sensory phenomena that may be the prelude to a migraine attack or to an epileptic seizure

Auscultation: Listening to sounds made by fluids or gas in the body, usually with a stethoscope

Autocrine: Hormones that act on the cell that produced them

Autonomic nervous system: Part of the nervous system that controls functions over which there is little or no conscious control; consists of sympathetic and parasympathetic divisions

Bactericidal: Able to kill bacteria, usually rapidly

Bacteriostatic: Able to stop bacteria from replicating, but not killing them

Basal ganglia: Areas of brain grey matter embedded within the white matter of the cerebral hemispheres; they are concerned mainly with control of voluntary movements at a subconscious level

B cell: see **B lymphocyte**

Beriberi: Disease caused by thiamine (vitamin B_1) deficiency caused by eating a diet rich in polished rice; leads to nervous degeneration and often death from heart failure unless treated with vitamin B_1

Bile acid-binding resins: These drugs combine with bile acids and cholesterol in the gut, thus preventing their absorption and increasing faecal excretion

Bioavailability: The proportion of a dose of a drug that reaches the circulation and is therefore available to have an action on body tissues

Biologics: Any drug made using biological methods such as recombinant DNA technology. Commonly used to describe monoclonal antibody-based drugs (see also **Biosimilars**)

Biosimilar: 'Similar biologic'; a biologic drug with similar structure and identical action to an earlier, established and more expensive biologic. Conceptually like a **generic drug**

Blood–brain barrier: A physiological barrier that selectively restricts the passage of many drugs and chemicals from the blood to the brain

B lymphocyte: White blood cell made in the bone marrow, which matures in the lymph nodes and spleen before entering the blood. B lymphocytes make antibodies

Bronchiole: A small subdivision of the bronchial tree

Bradycardia: Slowing of the heart rate; pulse rate falls below 60

Bronchiectasis: Chronic bronchial inflammation with pus formation

Bronchospasm: Narrowing of the bronchial tubes through contraction of bronchial smooth muscle

Bullous rash: Rash with blisters

Bundle of His (also called atrioventricular bundle): Bundle of modified heart muscle fibres called Purkinje fibres that conduct waves of electrical stimulation from the atria to the ventricles

Calcium antagonist: Drug that blocks calcium channels; used in hypertension and cardiac arrhythmias

Carcinogen: Anything that may cause cancer

Cardiac: Pertaining to the heart; also used to describe the upper end of the stomach

Cardioversion: The application of a controlled direct current shock to the heart of an anaesthetized patient using electrodes placed on the chest wall to restore the normal rhythm of the heart (see also **defibrillator**)

Catabolic: Breakdown of complex substances such as proteins and glycogen to glucose to release energy

Cataract: Development of an opaque lens; generally caused by ageing, but can be caused by occupational injuries or diseases such as diabetes

Catecholamine: An amine that contains the catechol ring, e.g. **noradrenaline** (norepinephrine) and **adrenaline** (epinephrine)

CD4: A protein on the surface of **helper T cells** that is important in the development of immunity to viral infections

Cerebral palsy: Disorder of movement, caused by brain damage before, during or soon after birth; brain damage is permanent, but the disorder is non-progressive

Chelating agents: Chemicals that form complexes with some metal ions, thus rendering them harmless; the complex is safely excreted. Chelating agents are useful in cases of, e.g. copper poisoning

Chemoreceptor trigger zone: Nerve centre in the medulla of the brain that, when stimulated by drugs such as apomorphine, triggers the **vomiting centre**

Chemotherapy: Treatment or prevention of disease with chemicals; commonly refers to treatment of cancer with **cytotoxic** drugs

Chimeric: A **biologic MAb** produced using proteins or genes from two or more different species

Cholecalciferol: Vitamin D

Cholinergic: Usually refers to any function or nerve where acetylcholine is the mediator

Chronic: A disease process that is long established and ongoing

Chronic coronary syndrome: Chronic **ischaemic heart disease**, mainly manifested as **angina**

Cirrhosis: Formation of a damaging network of fibrous tissue and regenerating cells in the liver in response to, e.g. alcohol, hepatitis or chronic heart failure

Claudication: Muscle pain due to impaired blood supply. Commonly in the calf muscles on exertion

Clotting factors (coagulation factors): Components of blood that are part of a cascade of reactions that result in coagulation

Clotting time (coagulation time): The time taken for blood or plasma to coagulate under controlled laboratory conditions

CNS: Central nervous system

Coagulation: In the case of blood, the conversion of liquid blood to a solid clot

Coeliac disease: Disease where the small intestine is unable to digest and absorb food; successfully treated by adopting a strictly gluten-free diet

Co-enzyme: Non-protein chemical essential for the function of some proteins; several co-enzymes contain B vitamins as part of their molecular structure

Colic: Severe abdominal pain caused by blockage of a tube such as the ureter

Collyrium: Medicated sterile **lotion** for bathing the eye

Compliance: The degree to which a patient takes a prescribed drug, as it has been prescribed (see also **Adherence** and **Concordance**)

COMT: Catechol-O-methyltransferase; an enzyme that breaks down **catecholamines**

Concordance: An agreement between clinician and patient on a course of treatment, after a shared decision-making process. Concordance should lead to greater **compliance/adherence**

Congenital: Any disorder recognized at birth, whether caused genetically or by environmental factors

Conjunctiva: Delicate membrane covering the front of the eye and lining the inner surface of the eyelids

Conjunctivitis (pink eye): Inflammation of the conjunctiva causing discomfort and discharge; caused by viral or bacterial infection

Constipation: Difficult, painful or infrequent evacuation of bowel contents

Contractility: Degree of power of the muscle to contract

Contraindications: Conditions that mean a drug should not be used

Coronary: Relating to the heart

Coronary angioplasty: Opening a narrowed part of a coronary artery using a balloon catheter in the artery (see also **stent**)

Coronary thrombosis: Thrombus (blood clot) formation in the coronary artery, leading to **STEMI** or **NSTEMI**

Corpus striatum: Part of the **basal ganglia** in the cerebral hemispheres of the brain

Corticosteroid (corticoid): Any steroid hormone synthesized in the adrenal cortex: the two main types are glucocorticoids, e.g. cortisol and mineralocorticoids, principally aldosterone

COX: Cyclooxygenase; an enzyme involved in inflammation

Cranial nerves: 12 pairs of nerves arising directly from the brain, e.g. vagus (X)

Creatinine: A chemical derived from creatine in muscle; excreted in the urine

Crohn's disease (regional enteritis, regional ileitis): Inflammation of segments of the alimentary tract, which become ulcerated, thickened and inflamed. The cause is unknown

Cushing's disease: Disease caused by excessive production and release of corticosteroid hormones due to an ACTH-secreting tumour in the pituitary or elsewhere in the body. *Cushing's syndrome* is a condition where the patient has the symptoms of Cushing's disease, but is caused, e.g. by large amounts of steroid medication

Cyanocobalamin: Vitamin B_{12}

Cyanosis: Skin and mucous membranes turn blue due to inadequate oxygen supply to the tissues

Cycloplegic: Drug that paralyzes the ability of the eye to focus

Cytokine: Proteins released by cells to signal to other cells. Important regulators of cell differentiation and inflammation

Cytomegalovirus (CMV): One of the herpes group of viruses

Cytopenia: Depression of the blood count

Cytotoxic: A type of cancer **chemotherapy** that destroys cells by blocking cell division

Decompensated liver disease: Cirrhosis of the liver with a build-up of **ascites**

Defibrillator: Device that delivers a controlled electric shock to restore normal heart rhythm in cardiac arrest due to ventricular fibrillation

Dementia: Chronic mental disorder of intellectual function and behaviour due to brain degenerative disease or destruction of brain tissue through physical trauma such as stroke

Dependent oedema: Oedema of ankles caused by sitting, mainly in elderly people

Depolarization: Transient change in the voltage potential across a cell membrane, caused by rapid influx of sodium ions. In nerve cells, this may spread as an action potential down the nerve

Depolarizing blocking drugs: Neuromuscular blocking drugs that depolarize muscle cell membranes and then block any further membrane depolarization by acetylcholine released from nerve endings at the neuromuscular junction (e.g. suxamethonium)

Diabetes: A term to describe a metabolic disorder characterized by production of abnormally large volumes of dilute urine. When used alone, it usually refers to **diabetes mellitus**

Diabetes insipidus: This is a rare disease when the patient produces large amounts of dilute urine due to a deficiency of vasopressin

Diabetes mellitus: Raised blood sugar due to a deficiency of insulin; there are two types. Type I (juvenile onset; insulin-dependent) diabetes mellitus is an autoimmune disease that destroys the body's ability to make insulin. Type II (non-insulin-dependent) diabetes mellitus is a consequence of **insulin resistance** rather than reduced ability to make insulin

Diarrhoea: Abnormally high frequency of bowel evacuation, often with soft or liquid stools; it can cause serious loss of water, salts and nutrients

Diastole: Period between two contractions of the heart

Diastolic blood pressure: The pressure recorded at diastole when the heart is filling; the value obtained reflects predominantly the total peripheral resistance in the vascular beds

Differentiation: The process by which immature or embryonic cells mature and become specialized into tissues

Diuretic: Drug that increases urine flow

DMARD: Disease-modifying antirheumatic drug

DNA: Deoxyribonucleic acid

DOAC: Direct acting oral anticoagulant drug

Dopaminergic: Refers to nerve cells that use dopamine as neurotransmitter

Drug absorption: Movement of the drug into the internal environment

Drug dependence: Patient either craves a drug (psychological dependence) or suffers physical symptoms of withdrawal without the drug (physical dependence)

Drug distribution: The tissues to which a drug gains access

Drug elimination: Movement of the drug out of the body into the external environment (see also **excretion**)

Drug metabolism: How the body chemically alters a drug. This may activate the drug or may allow it to be excreted

Drug tolerance: More of a dose of a drug is required in order to achieve the same effect

Dysmenorrhoea: Painful menstruation

Dyspepsia (indigestion): Disorder of digestion during which there may be pain and discomfort in the abdomen or lower chest, and perhaps nausea and vomiting

Dyspnoea: Shortness of breath

Dystonia: Uncontrolled movements

Eclampsia: Convulsions not caused by epilepsy in a pregnant woman after a sudden rise in blood pressure (**pre-eclampsia**) that may be accompanied by **oedema** and **proteinuria**

Ectopic beat: see **extrasystole**

Eczema: Dry, flaky, itchy skin disorder; there are several types

Efficacy: How effective the drug is (see also **potency**)

Embolism: Condition when an **embolus** becomes lodged in an artery and blocks blood flow

Embolus: Anything such as air, fat, blood clot, amniotic fluid or a foreign body carried in the blood to lodge elsewhere, e.g. a lung (pulmonary) embolism

Embryo: In humans, the product of conception up to the 8th week of pregnancy

EMEA: The European Agency for the Evaluation of Medicinal Products

Emetic: Substance that causes vomiting

Emphysema (pulmonary emphysema): Difficulty with breathing caused by damaged alveoli of the lungs. Smoking is the most important cause

Emulsion: A mixture of two immiscible liquids (e.g. oil and water) in which one is dispersed through the other in a finely divided state, e.g. Milk of Magnesia

Endocarditis: Inflammation and/or infection of the lining of the heart cavity (the endocardium)

Endocrine gland: Hormone producing gland, making hormones have their effect elsewhere in the body (see also **paracrine**)

Endometriosis: Abnormal presence of endometrial tissue in other parts of the pelvis

Enema: Fluid infused into the rectum through a tube that has been passed through the anus

Enzyme: Protein that catalyses biochemical reactions

Epidural injection: The injection of a local anaesthetic into the epidural space in the lumbar region of the spinal cord

Epinephrine: see **adrenaline**

Erythema: Skin redness due to capillary dilatation in the dermis

Erythematous: Appearing red (see also **erythema**)

Erythropoietin: Hormone secreted by some kidney cells in response to reduced oxygen tension in the blood; erythropoietin increases the rate of red blood cell production

Essential hypertension: Clinically high blood pressure with no clear single cause

Euphoria: Elation and optimism for no apparent reason; in extreme form it is called **mania**

Excretion: Ejection of anything from the body

Exfoliation: Flaking off of the upper layers of the skin; separation of the surface epithelium from underlying tissue

Expectorants: Drugs that supposedly loosen the sputum and thus aid its ejection from the bronchial tree. Most do no such thing

Extrasystole: Also called an **ectopic beat**, it is a heartbeat that originates in the heart away from the sinoatrial node; may be ventricular or supraventricular

FDA: The Food and Drugs Administration of the United States.

Febrile: Relating to fever

Ferritin: A complex of iron and a protein that is one of the ways in which iron is stored in the tissues

Fetus: Unborn child from the 8th week of development

Fibrates: Fibrates alter the metabolism of lipoproteins, and so lower blood cholesterol and triglycerides

Fibrillation: Rapid, chaotic beating of individual cardiac muscle fibres

Fibrin: Fibrous insoluble protein in blood clots

Fibrinogen: Soluble protein converted to insoluble fibrin by **thrombin**

First pass metabolism: Metabolism of a drug in the liver after its absorption from the gastrointestinal tract (**GIT**)

Flukes: Parasitic flatworms; they cause, e.g. bilharziasis

Focal epilepsy: A seizure that arises from a focal electrical discharge in the brain. Awareness may be normal or impaired. Focal epilepsy may be motor (abnormal movements) or non-motor (sensory abnormalities)

Focal to bilateral epilepsy: A focal seizure that spreads to the whole brain. Consciousness is impaired as the abnormal electrical activity spreads

GAD (general anxiety disorder): The patient feels apprehensive and tense for no particular reason, or as a result of some minor problem

Gallstone (cholelithiasis): A hard body made of cholesterol, bile pigments and calcium that forms in the gallbladder

GAS: General adaptation syndrome; a three-stage physiological and psychological response to stress

Gastric: Relating to or affecting the stomach

Generalized epilepsy: Epilepsy with impaired consciousness from the outset and abnormal electrical activity affecting all or most of the brain. May be motor (tonic-clonic fits; grand mal) or non-motor (absence attacks; petit mal)

Generic drug: A chemically identical copy of a branded drug manufactured after the patent on the original drug has expired. Generally much less expensive than branded drugs

GIT: Gastrointestinal tract

Glaucoma: Loss of vision partly caused by abnormally raised intraocular pressure

Glomerulus: Usually refers to the network of blood capillaries in the Bowman's capsule of the kidney; an important function is to filter substances out of the blood into the urine

Glycogen: Principal storage form of glucose in the body, consisting of branched chains of glucose

Gonadotrophins: FSH (follicle stimulating hormone) and LH (luteinizing hormone) are hormones released from the anterior pituitary gland and from the placenta; they are mainly concerned with the synthesis and release of the sex hormones and control of the menstrual cycle

Gonads: Male or female reproductive organs (testis and ovary, respectively)

Gout: Disease in which uric acid metabolism and excretion are impaired, leading to very painful acute arthritis

Guttae: Latin term sometimes used in prescriptions meaning 'drops'

Haemoglobin: Iron containing protein in the red blood cell that carries oxygen

Haemolytic anaemia: Anaemia due to destruction of red blood cells (see also **anaemia**)

Haemorrhage: Serious escape of blood from blood vessels

Haptens: Small molecules that combine with larger molecules such as proteins and turn them 'foreign', e.g. aspirin

Heart attack: Colloquial term for **acute coronary syndrome**

Heart block: Complete or partial failure of the **bundle of His** to transmit electrical impulses from the atria to the ventricles. Can lead to a dangerously slow heart rate

Heart failure: Inadequate pumping power of the ventricles of the heart leading to symptoms that may include oedema and shortness of breath

Helper T cells: Type of white cell called a lymphocyte that stimulates the production of **killer T cells**, which attack and destroy target cells

Hepatic: Relating to the liver

Heroin: Diacetylmorphine; diamorphine. A powerful analgesic opioid. Often abused by addicts

Herpes: Infection of mucous membranes or skin caused by the herpes virus. Herpes simplex virus type I causes the cold sore and type II causes genital herpes; herpes zoster causes shingles

Hirsutism: Inappropriate and unwanted growth of body hair

HIV: Human immunodeficiency virus: **retrovirus** responsible for **AIDS**

HRT: Hormone replacement therapy

Hypercalcaemia: High blood calcium

Hypercalciuria: Raised calcium level in the urine

Hyperglycaemia: High blood glucose

Hyperkalaemia: High blood potassium

Hyperlipidaemia (hyperlipaemia): Abnormally high concentration of fats in the bloodstream. Commonly used to imply high blood cholesterol levels

Hypernatraemia: Abnormally high blood sodium

Hyperparathyroidism: Overactivity of the parathyroid glands, leads to **hypercalcaemia**

Hyperplasia: The increased production and growth of normal cells in any organ or tissue, e.g. benign prostatic hyperplasia (BPH) in older men

Hypertension: Abnormally raised blood pressure that could damage perfused tissues

Hyperthyroidism: Over-secretion of thyroid hormone

Hypertrophy: The enlargement of the cells themselves without necessarily an increase in cell number; the increase in muscle size following exercise or 'pumping iron' is an example of hypertrophy

Hypervolaemia: Overfilling of the vascular system

Hypnotic: Drug that induces sleep

Hypoglycaemia: Clinically low blood glucose

Hypokinesia: Inhibition of voluntary movements

Hypotension: Clinically low blood pressure

Hypothyroidism: Under-secretion of thyroid hormone

Idiopathic: A condition, the cause of which is unknown and which appears to arise spontaneously

IM: Intramuscular
Incontinence: Involuntary passage of urine
Inert: Describes a drug ingredient that has no medicinal properties, e.g. lactose in a tablet
Inflammation: Redness, swelling and associated pain that are signs of the **innate immune response** in action
Inflammatory bowel disease: Any of a group of inflammatory conditions of the intestine, including Crohn's disease and ulcerative colitis
Infusion: Slow injection of a volume into the body, usually into a vein
Innate immune response: The immediate protective reaction to local damage or the presence of pathogens. Leads to **inflammation**
Insomnia: Inability to fall asleep or remain asleep for an adequate time
Insulinoma: Insulin-producing tumour
Insulin resistance: A metabolic abnormality where body tissues are resistant to the effects of insulin. Typically seen in Type 2 **diabetes**
Intercurrent illness: The occurrence of an illness that may modify the course and treatment of another illness that is present at the same time
Interferons: Peptides that are produced by cells to fight viral infections. May be used therapeutically
Interleukins: Peptides produced by leukocytes that regulate the immune response
Intraosseous injection: Injection into the bone marrow
Intrathecal injection: The administration of the drug directly into the central nervous system (**CNS**), thus bypassing the blood–brain barrier
Ionization: Conversion of an electrically neutral chemical into a charged one either by gaining or losing electrons
Ischaemia: Inadequate blood flow to a part of the body
IV: Intravenous

JAK inhibitors (Janus kinase inhibitors; jakinibs): A class of **protein kinase inhibitors** that inhibit **cytokines** involved in cell differentiation and inflammation. Used to treat inflammatory and neoplastic diseases

Kaolin cephalin time: A method of measuring the clotting time
Kernicterus: Staining of the newborn brain by the bile pigment bilirubin, which is displaced from its blood-binding proteins by drugs such as sulphonamides, tolbutamide or aspirin taken by the mother in late pregnancy. It causes brain damage, with subsequent development of symptoms of cerebral palsy about 6 months after birth
Killer T cells: Lymphocytes that target and destroy other cells
Korsakov's psychosis: Memory defect with failure to learn new information, although already learned information is retained. The usual cause is alcoholism, leading to vitamin B_1 deficiency, and it is treated with high doses of vitamin B_1

Laxative: A drug used to treat constipation
LDL: Low-density lipoprotein that carries cholesterol in the bloodstream
Leukaemia: Overproduction of leukocytes by the bone marrow and other blood-forming organs due to malignant disease, and suppression of production of platelets, other white cells and of red cells, resulting in immunodeficiency and bleeding; may be acute or chronic
Lewy body dementia: Dementia with symptoms overlapping those of Alzheimer's, with loss of cognition, hallucinations and symptoms of Parkinson's disease. Lewy bodies are abnormal lumps seen in degenerating cells of the cortex and substantia nigra
Libido: Sexual drive
Ligand: Any chemical that binds to another (in pharmacology, usually refers to drugs that bind to receptors)
Linctus: A liquid that contains some sweet syrupy substance, which is used for its soothing effect on coughs. It may also contain a cough suppressant such as dextromethorphan
Lipid: Fat
Lipoproteins: Molecules in the blood and lymph consisting of protein and lipids; important in the transport of cholesterol and the uptake of cholesterol into cells
Loop diuretics: Diuretics such as furosemide that act in the ascending limb of the loop of Henle

Malignant tumour: A tumour that invades and destroys a tissue or organ in which it occurs, and which may then spread to other tissues and may prove fatal

Malnutrition: Condition arising from improper balance between an individual's diet and what is required in diet for maintenance of health

Mania: Wild, extravagant and incoherent speech and behaviour

MAOI: Monoamine oxidase inhibitor

Meniere's disease: A disease of the inner ear with episodes of tinnitus, deafness and vertigo. The medical name is endolymphatic hydrops

Meningitis: Inflammation of the meninges, the three membranes that enclose the brain and spinal cord. Symptoms include severe headache, photosensitivity, fever, loss of appetite, muscle rigidity, especially in the neck and, in severe cases, delirium, convulsions and death

Menopause: When cessation of ovulation and menstruation start to occur

Menorrhagia: Abnormally heavy bleeding during menstruation

MHRA: In the UK, The Medicines and Healthcare products Regulatory Agency regulates medicines, medical devices and blood components for transfusion

Miotics: Drugs that cause contraction of the pupil

Mixtures: Liquids that contain several ingredients dissolved or diffused in water or some other solvent, e.g. kaolin mixture for diarrhoea

MMR vaccine: Combined vaccine against measles, mumps and German measles (rubella)

Monoamine oxidase inhibitor (MAOI): Drug that inhibits the enzyme monoamine oxidase, that breaks down catecholamines such as noradrenaline and adrenaline; used chiefly to treat depressive illness

Monoclonal antibody (MAb): Antibody produced from an artificial cell. Used to make **Biologic** and **Biosimilar** drugs

Monocyte: Type of white blood cell with kidney shaped nucleus, whose function is to take in foreign particles such as bacteria and debris

Morbidity: Condition or state of being diseased

Mortality: Death, i.e. mortality rate; death rate

MRSA: Methicillin-resistant *Staphylococcus aureus*

Mucolytic: Agent that liquefies phlegm

Muscarinic: Describes drugs that bind to and activate muscarinic acetylcholine receptors of the parasympathetic division of the autonomic nervous system or drugs that mimic the effects produced by stimulation of muscarinic receptors

Mydriasis: Dilation of the pupil

Mydriatic: Drug used to dilate the pupil, e.g. atropine, tropicamide

Myocardial infarction (MI): Damage or death of part of the heart muscle, usually in the left ventricle, following interruption of the blood supply (see also **STEMI** and **NSTEMI**)

Myoclonic jerks: Sudden jerking of the limbs that occurs in some patients with epilepsy and in those with degenerative neurological disease

Myopathy: Any disease of muscle (e.g. cardiomyopathy)

Necrosis: Death of cells within a tissue or organ

Negative feedback: A regulatory system whereby the end-product controls its own synthesis and/or release by inhibiting the system that stimulates its production

Negative inotropic: Drug that decreases heart contractility

Neoplastic growth: Any new and abnormal growth, which may be either benign or malignant

Nephrotic syndrome: Heavy protein loss in urine as a consequence of one of several disease processes. Severe oedema is a consequence

Nephrotoxic: Toxic to the kidneys

Neuroleptic: Antipsychotic drug

Neutropenia: Clinically significant reduction in the numbers of neutrophils in the blood

NICE: National Institute for Health and Care Excellence: reviews the cost-effectiveness of drugs and treatments and clinical guidelines

Non-depolarizing blocking drugs: Drugs that block muscle contraction without themselves causing any depolarization of the muscle fibre membrane (e.g. **tubocurarine**)

Noradrenaline (norepinephrine): A **catecholamine** neurotransmitter released from noradrenergic nerve terminals; small amounts are also released from the adrenal medulla

Noradrenergic: Describes nerves that release noradrenaline as neurotransmitter or receptors that respond to noradrenaline (norepinephrine)

Norepinephrine: see **Noradrenaline**

NSAID: Non-steroidal antiinflammatory drug

NSTEMI: Non-ST elevation myocardial infarction. A type of **acute coronary syndrome**

Nucleoside: A chemical consisting of a pyrimidine or purine base attached to a sugar, e.g. adenosine

Nucleotide: A pyrimidine or purine base attached to a sugar, to which is attached a phosphate group; the building blocks of **RNA** and **DNA**

Obsessive compulsive disorder (OCD): Characterized by repetitive, anxiety-driven behaviour such as the repeated washing of hands or obsessive thoughts and doubts

Oedema: Accumulation of excess fluid in body tissues leading to swelling

Oesophageal varices: Veins that have dilated in the lower oesophagus because of portal hypertension (high blood pressure in the hepatic portal vein). They can rupture and cause dangerous bleeding

Oestrogen: One of a group of chemicals, including oestradiol, which develops and maintains female sexual function and secondary female characteristics such as breast development

Oliguria: Abnormally low urine production

Oncogene: A gene that is known to have a number of possible mutations associated with increased risk of malignancy

Opioid: Natural substances (e.g. morphine, codeine, endorphins) or synthetic derivatives (e.g. diacetylmorphine) that produce morphine-like effects such as analgesia or sedation

Oral: By mouth

Oral anticoagulants: Anticoagulants that can be taken by mouth, e.g. warfarin (see also **DOAC**)

Oral contraceptive: Tablet taken orally that blocks conception

Osmosis: Flow of water through a semi-permeable membrane (e.g. the proximal tubule of the kidney) from a region of lower salt concentration to a region of higher salt concentration

Osteoarthritis (osteoarthrosis): Degenerative joint disease, involving wear of articular cartilage, which may cause secondary changes in underlying bone. It can be primary, or secondary to abnormal loads to joints or damage to cartilage due to trauma or inflammation

Osteoporosis: Loss of bone mineral density, resulting in fracture-prone brittle bones

Ototoxic: Toxic to the organs of hearing or balance in the inner ear or to the vestibulocochlear nerve

PABA: Para-aminobenzoic acid, a precursor of folic acid, which is essential in cell division

Palliative therapy: Drug treatment to relieve symptoms, without actually curing a disease; commonly used in cancer

Pallidotomy (pallidectomy): Introduction of electrodes into the brain to destroy a particular part of the brain in an area called the globus pallidus

Panic attacks: Unexpected attacks of anxiety, often with marked physical symptoms such as tremor, palpitation and dry mouth due to overactivity of the sympathetic nervous system

Paracrine: Hormone that acts on cells in the region of those that produced it, rather than on tissues to which it has to be carried in the bloodstream

Parasympathomimetic: Drug that mimics the stimulation of the parasympathetic division of the autonomic nervous system

Parenteral: Administration of a drug by any route other than orally, e.g. by injection

Parkinsonism: A term used to describe the symptoms of **Parkinson's disease**, which may result not only from the degeneration of the nigrostriatal pathway but also from drugs or infections

Parkinson's disease: Degenerative brain disorder in the basal ganglia with the loss of dopaminergic neurones, resulting in rigidity, tremor and progressive difficulty in initiating and stopping movement

PARP inhibitor: A class of **targeted therapy** drugs, mainly for cancers, but other indications are emerging. Inhibits the enzyme poly ADP ribose polymerase (PARP), that is involved in DNA repair

Partial agonist: A drug that is both an agonist and antagonist under different conditions (usually dose)

Parturition: Childbirth

Passive immunization: A pre-formed antibody against the invading organism or toxin is injected (see also **active immunization**)

Patch: Adhesive impregnated with medicine and applied to the skin for slow, continuous release of active agent

Pathogen (pathogenic): Any substance (generally an organism) that causes disease

Pediculosis: Infestation of the skin with lice

Pegylated interferons: Interferons to which are attached molecules of polyethylene glycol, prolonging its duration of action

Pepsin: Stomach enzyme that breaks down proteins

Peptic: Relating to pepsin or to digestion

Peptide: Molecule consisting of two or more amino acids, e.g. oxytocin

Pernicious anaemia (Addison's anaemia): Anaemia caused by deficiency of vitamin B_{12} (cyanocobalamin)

Pessary: Device for insertion into the vagina (also called a vaginal suppository). May contain drugs or provide support for vaginal prolapse

Petit mal (absence) seizure: Older term for generalized non-motor seizure

pH: Measure of acidity or alkalinity in units from 1 to 14: the pH is the negative logarithm of the hydrogen ion concentration

Pheochromocytoma: A catecholamine-secreting tumour of the adrenal gland

Pharmacodynamics: Study of how drugs exert their effects at a cellular level

Pharmacokinetics: Study of how the body processes drugs: absorption, metabolism and excretion

Pharynx: Muscular tube lined with mucous membranes that extends from the base of the skull down to the beginning of the oesophagus; its functions are to carry air from the nose and mouth to the larynx, to act as a resonating chamber for the larynx, and to carry food from the mouth to the oesophagus

Phlebothrombosis: Obstruction of a vein by a blood clot

Phobic states: A condition of fear and panic associated with situations or objects. The commonest is agoraphobia, in which the subject is frightened to go outside

Phosphodiesterase: Enzyme that breaks down cyclic AMP

Phytomenadione: Vitamin K

Plasma: Straw-coloured fluid in which the blood cells are suspended

Plasma half-life: The time taken for the plasma concentration of the drug to decline to one-half of its value

Plasmodium: Genus of **protozoans** that live in human red blood and liver cells; they cause, e.g. malaria

Platelet (thrombocyte): Disc-shaped body in blood, 1–2 μm in diameter, with functions related to stopping bleeding

Platelet aggregation: Sticking together of platelets in the blood

PMS: see **premenstrual syndrome**

Pneumocystis pneumonia: Pneumonia that is caused, usually in immunosuppressed patients, by a protozoan called *Pneumocystis*

Polyarteritis nodosa (periarteritis nodosa): Potentially dangerous inflammation of the walls of the arteries, producing symptoms of, e.g. arthritis, asthma, fever and hypertension, kidney failure and neuritis. It is treated with prednisolone or other corticosteroids

Positive inotropic: Drug that increases heart contractility (see also **negative inotropic**)

Post-traumatic stress disorder: The anxiety that follows traumatic experiences such as rape or warfare

Potency: How strong/powerful the drug is

Pre-eclampsia: Sudden rise in blood pressure (over 140/90) in a pregnant woman, in whom blood pressure was previously normal

Preload: The pressure in the venous system filling the heart and stretching the heart muscle

Premenstrual syndrome (premenstrual tension): Irritability, nervousness and depression before menstruation, associated with accumulation of water and salts in the tissues. The condition usually disappears when menstruation begins

Prodrug: A drug that is metabolized to a therapeutically active metabolite

Prosthesis: Any artificial aid attached to the body, e.g. prosthetic heart valve

Protease: Enzyme that catalyses the splitting of proteins

Protein kinase inhibitors: Any of a large class of **targeted therapy** drugs that inhibit protein kinase enzymes, involved in cell growth and differentiation. Important cancer therapies, also used for other indications

Proteinuria: Protein in the urine

Prothrombin: Protein that is converted to thrombin by thromboplastin. Part of the blood clotting cascade

Prothrombin time (PT): The time taken for clotting to occur in a sample of blood to which **thromboplastin** and calcium have been added

Protozoa: Group of microscopic, single-celled organisms, e.g. *Trypanosoma* (malaria)

Psoriasis: Common chronic skin disease, in which scaly, pink patches occur on scalp, elbows, knees and other parts of the body

Psoriatic arthritis: Inflammatory arthritis that is often associated with psoriasis

Psychomotor seizure: Type of focal motor seizure. Involuntary movements, without loss of consciousness

Psychosis: A term used to describe any of a group of psychiatric disorders where thought and perceptions are disturbed

Purgatives: Drugs that cause fluid **diarrhoea** – a strong **laxative**

Pyridoxine: Vitamin B_6

RA: Rheumatoid arthritis

Receptor: Cell surface protein that binds another chemical (including drugs), usually affecting the function of the cell in some manner

Refractory period: Period between muscle contraction or nerve impulse generation when the muscle or nerve recovers and is unable to respond to an incoming impulse

Renin: Enzyme protein released into the circulation by the kidney in response to stresses such as haemorrhage or other causes of low blood pressure

Retinoids: Group of drugs derived from vitamin A and used to treat skin disorders such as acne

Reverse transcriptase: An enzyme, usually viral, which converts single-stranded RNA into single stranded DNA

Retrovirus: RNA-containing virus that converts its **RNA** into **DNA** using an enzyme called **reverse transcriptase**

Reye's syndrome: Childhood symptoms of encephalitis with symptoms of liver failure; aspirin is implicated and contraindicated in children

Rheumatic fever: Mainly affecting children and young adults as a delayed complication of haemolytic streptococcal infection of the upper respiratory tract. It may progress to chronic rheumatic heart disease

Rheumatoid arthritis: An autoimmune disease, rheumatoid arthritis is a common form of inflammatory arthritis

Riboflavin: Vitamin B_2

Rickets: Disease caused by vitamin D deficiency in children, whose bones do not develop properly and may be deformed

RNA: Ribonucleic acid

SC: Subcutaneous

Scabies: Skin infestation caused by the mite *Sarcoptes scabiei*

Schizophrenia: Change of personality with disordered thought processes, which may be associated with hallucinations, delusions and withdrawal

Scurvy: Disease caused by vitamin C deficiency

Second messenger: Chemical within the cell that carries the message that a hormone, neurotransmitter, etc. has bound to its receptor on the cell membrane; cyclic AMP and inositol triphosphate are examples of second messengers

Seizure: Convulsion, fit

Serum: Fluid that separates from clotted blood. It is essentially plasma without fibrinogen and other factors involved in **coagulation**

Serum sickness: A delayed hypersensitivity reaction to injection of foreign proteins; symptoms include fever, rashes, lymph node enlargement and joint pain

Sinoatrial (SA) node: Tiny, modified area of heart muscle in the upper right ventricle near the entry point of the vena cava; called the pacemaker because it has an independent rhythmic beat of about 70/minute

Sinus rhythm: The normal heart rhythm that originates in the **sinoatrial node**

Skeletal (striated) muscle: Muscles attached to the skeletal frame, which are under voluntary control

Small molecule drugs: Essentially, any drug that is not a large protein molecule such as a **MAb**. Often used to distinguish non-MAb **targeted therapies**

Smooth muscle: Muscle of the **autonomic nervous system** that mediates involuntary contractions, e.g. of arterioles and bronchi

Specificity: Describes the selectivity of a receptor for drugs

Splanchnic: Refers to the **viscera**, which in turn means the organs within the body cavities, especially those in the abdominal cavities

Statins (HMG-CoA reductase inhibitors): Drugs that block the synthesis of cholesterol in the liver

Steatorrhoea: Fatty stools

STEMI ST-segment elevation myocardial infarction

Stent: A device introduced into a tubular organ to hold it open. Typically used to hold coronary arteries open

Stethoscope: Instrument used to listen to body sounds

Stomatitis: Inflammation of the mucous lining of the mouth

Stroke: Weakness or paralysis on one side of the body caused by interruption of blood flow to the brain; in bygone days was called apoplexy

Sublingual: Under the tongue

Suppository: Formulation for administration of medicine into the rectum

Supraventricular: Above the ventricles

Supraventricular rhythm: Any cardiac rhythm originating above the ventricles

Sustained release: Refers to a medicinal formulation that continuously releases the active agent, e.g. from the **GIT**. Also called 'retard' preparations

Sympathomimetic: Drug that mimics the stimulation of the sympathetic division of the autonomic nervous system

Systole: Period of the cardiac cycle when the heart is contracting

Systolic blood pressure: The blood pressure at **systole**, when the ventricles contract and pump blood into the arterial circulation

Tachycardia: Very rapid heart rate

Tachyphylaxis: The action of a given dose of a drug becomes successively less effective

Tardive dyskinesia: Abnormal movements of the mouth and tongue and sometimes the upper limbs

Targeted therapy: A general name for drugs that target a specific metabolic pathway aiming to minimize unwanted effects. Mainly cancer treatments

Teratogenic: May cause birth defects

Therapeutic index: Ratio of a therapeutic dose to one that is actually toxic. The higher the therapeutic index, the safer the drug

Thiamine: Vitamin B_1

Thrombin: Enzyme that converts soluble **fibrinogen** to insoluble **fibrin** in the clotting process

Thrombocytopenia: Reduction in the number of platelets in the blood. It results in bruising of the skin and prolonged bleeding of wounds

Thrombolytic: A drug that dissolves a thrombus

Thromboplastin (thrombokinase): Enzyme that converts **prothrombin** to **thrombin**

Thrombosis: Solidification of blood in a blood vessel through clot formation

Thrombus: Blood clot

Tincture: Alcoholic extract from natural tissues such as plants, e.g. tincture of belladonna

Tinnitus: Sensation of sounds without any external stimulus

T lymphocytes: White blood cells that mature in the thymus gland before they enter the circulation

Tocolytic agents: Drugs that inhibit uterine contractions

Tocopherol: Vitamin E

Tonic-clonic (grand mal) seizure: Older names describing **generalized** seizures or the latter stages of **focal to bilateral** seizures. Awareness is always impaired in generalized seizures

Total peripheral resistance (TPR): Resistance to blood flow caused by resistance only in the peripheral vascular beds, i.e. when the heart is in diastole

Toxic: Poisonous to the tissues

Transient insomnia: This occurs in people who usually have no sleep problem and is due to altered circumstances, i.e. admission to hospital or travel

Trophic: Causing growth

Tubocurarine: A non-depolarizing neuromuscular blocker extracted from curare

Ulcer: Break in skin through all its layers or break in any mucous membrane

Ulcerative colitis: Inflammatory and ulcerative disease of the colon and rectum

Uric acid: Chemical excreted in the urine; an end-product of nucleic acid metabolism, which causes gout if deposited in joints

Uricosuric drugs: Drugs that increase uric acid excretion in the urine

Urinary retention: Difficulty with micturition, e.g. in benign prostatic **hyperplasia** (BPH)

Vaccine: A drug prepared from components of pathogenic organisms or killed pathogens or weakened (attenuated) living pathogens. When introduced into the body, often by injection, a vaccine induces an immune response that protects against infection by that pathogen

Vagolytic: An effect that lessens the influence of the vagus nerve. The vagus slows the heart, so a vagolytic effect is one that speeds up the heart

Vasoconstriction: Decrease in diameter of blood vessels, especially arterioles

Ventricle: Either of the two lower chambers of the heart: also refers to fluid-filled chambers of the brain

Ventricular fibrillation: Cardiac arrhythmia marked by fine, irregular contractions of the ventricular muscle due to rapid, repetitive excitation of myocardial fibres without coordinated ventricular contraction. It is usually fatal unless treated immediately with a **defibrillator**

Virus: Particle visible only with an electron microscope that multiplies within living cells. It can infect other microorganisms such as bacteria, plants and animals

Viscera: The organs within the body cavities, especially those in the abdominal cavities (see also **splanchnic**)

Vitamin: One of a group of chemicals not synthesized in the body but taken in the diet. Vitamins are required in tiny amounts for normal development and cellular function

Vitreous humour: Jelly-like transparent substance that fills the chamber of the eye behind the lens

Vomiting centre: Nerve centre in the medulla of the brain that when stimulated electrically causes vomiting (see also **chemoreceptor trigger zone**)

Wernicke's encephalopathy: Brain disorder with delirium or mental confusion caused by vitamin B_1 deficiency, usually associated with alcoholism. It is treated with vitamin B_1

White coat hypertension: Measurement of raised blood pressure only when the patients' pressure is measured in a clinical environment or in unfamiliar environments

INDEX

Page numbers followed by "*f*" indicate figures, "*t*" indicate tables, and "*b*" indicate boxes.